REHABILITATION NURSING

PROCESS AND APPLICATION

REHABILITATION NURSING

PROCESS AND APPLICATION

Sharon S. Dittmar, RN, PhD

Associate Professor,
School of Nursing;
Assistant Clinical Professor,
Department of Rehabilitation Medicine,
State University of New York,
Buffalo, New York

with 175 illustrations

Medical illustrations by
John A. Nyquist, MS, Medical Illustrator

THE C. V. MOSBY COMPANY

ST. LOUIS • BALTIMORE • TORONTO   1989

Mosby

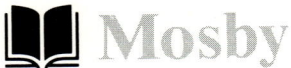

Editor: William Grayson Brottmiller
Senior developmental editor: Sally Adkisson
Project manager: Carol Sullivan Wiseman
Book designer: Susan E. Lane
Editing and Production: Top Graphics

The authors and publisher have made every effort to make sure
drug selections and dosages are in agreement with the
recommendations and practice at the time of publication of this text.
However, in view of ongoing research, changes in governmental
regulations, and increasing publication of drug information, the reader is
advised to check the package insert of each drug for any change in
indications for use, dosage, side effects, and warnings.

Printed in the United States of America

The C.V. Mosby Company
11830 Westline Industrial Drive, St. Louis, Missouri 63146

Library of Congress Cataloging in Publication Data

Dittmar, Sharon S.
    Rehabilitation nursing: process and application/Sharon S.
Dittmar; medical illustrations by John A. Nyquist.
        p.   cm.
    Includes index.
    ISBN 0-8016-1319-1
    1. Rehabilitation nursing. I. Title.
    [DNLM: 1. Nursing Care. 2. Rehabilitation. WY 150 D617r]
RT120.R4D58   1989
610.73′6—dc19
DNLM/DLC
for Library of Congress   88-38164
                                                         CIP

GW/D/D 9 8 7 6 5 4 3 2 1

Contributors

Mila A. Aroskar, RN, EdD
Associate Professor,
School of Public Health,
University of Minnesota,
Minneapolis, Minnesota

Rita J. Boucher, RN, EdD
Former Chairman (retired),
Department of Nursing,
Emmanuel College,
Boston, Massachusetts

Dorothy P. Byers, RN, MS
Clinical Specialist,
Rehabilitation Nursing,
Veteran's Administration Medical Center,
Buffalo, New York

Sandra Chenelly, RN, MS
Clinical Specialist,
Gerontological Nursing,
Veterans Administration Medical Center,
Batavia, New York

Sharon S. Dittmar, RN, PhD
Associate Professor,
School of Nursing;
Assistant Clinical Professor,
Department of Rehabilitation Medicine,
State University of New York,
Buffalo, New York

Theresa P. Dulski, RN, C, MS
Lecturer,
College of Nursing,
University of North Carolina,
Charlotte, North Carolina

Susan M. Evans, RN, MS
Patient Care Coordinator,
Millard Fillmore Hospital,
Buffalo, New York

Kathy M. Graham, RN, MS
Head Nurse—Oncology,
Veterans Administration Medical Center,
Buffalo, New York

Denise Hanlon, RN, MS
Clinical Instructor,
School of Nursing,
State University of New York,
Buffalo, New York

Brenda P. Haughey, RN, PhD
Associate Professor,
School of Nursing;
Assistant Professor,
Social and Preventive Medicine,
State University of New York,
Buffalo, New York

Margaret M. Hens, RN, MS
Buffalo General Hospital;
Clinical Instructor,
School of Nursing,
State University of New York,
Buffalo, New York

Linda M. Janelli, RN, C, MS, EdD
Assistant Professor,
School of Nursing,
State University of New York,
Buffalo, New York

Judith A. Laughlin, RN, PhD
Vice-President,
Computer Professionals Unlimited, Inc.,
South Wales, New York

Martha F. Markarian, RN, MS
Clinical Instructor,
School of Nursing,
State University of New York,
Buffalo, New York

Elizabeth A. Moody-Szymanski, RN, MS
Former Clinical Instructor,
School of Nursing,
State University of New York,
Buffalo, New York

Mary Sue Niederpruem, RN, MS
Coordinator,
Home Infusion Therapy Team,
Episcopal-General Home Care,
Buffalo, New York

Elizabeth C. Phelps, RN, MS
Executive Director,
Gerontological Professional Consulting
    Services,
Vestal, New York;
formerly Chief of Clinical Practice,
Robert Wood Johnson Teaching Nursing
    Program, in conjunction with SUNY
    Binghamton School of Nursing and Willow
    Point Nursing Home,
Binghamton, New York

Joyce Santora, RN, MS
Coordinator, Spinal Cord Unit,
Erie County Medical Center;
Clinical Assistant Professor,
School of Nursing;
Clinical Instructor,
Department of Rehabilitation Medicine,
State University of New York,
Buffalo, New York

Yvonne Krall Scherer, RN, EdD
Clinical Assistant Professor,
School of Nursing,
State University of New York,
Buffalo, New York

Jill A. Scott, RN, MS
Consultant, Rehabilitation Nursing,
Mayville, New York;
Clinical Instructor,
State University of New York,
Buffalo, New York;
Satellite Program,
Fredonia, New York

Margie L. Scott, RN, EdD
Associate Professor,
State University of New York,
Brockport, New York

Elizabeth L. Sharkey, RN, MS
Instructor in Nursing,
Jamestown Community College,
Jamestown, New York

Margaret A. Umhauer, RN, MS
Clinical Instructor,
Millard Fillmore Hospital,
School of Professional Nursing,
Buffalo, New York

Barbara G. White, RN, EdD
Nurse Public Health Coordinator,
Veterans Administration Medical Center,
Salisbury, North Carolina

Barbara Wisnom, RN, MS
Consultant, Loss Control,
Hospital Underwriters Mutual Insurance Co.,
Tarrytown, New York

In memory of
Halys McEachron

A special friend and
an exemplary role model
for rehabilitation nurses.
We were fortunate to have known her.

Preface

Advances in science, medicine, technology, and information systems have contributed to the long-term survival of persons with physical disabilities and chronic illnesses. Often, however, the years added to life are accompanied by dependence in performing activities of daily living and in fulfilling social roles. Functional dependence may affect individual quality of life, family dynamics, and ultimately, society. As rehabilitation nurses, we can significantly influence the level of function and quality of life achieved by disabled individuals.

The goals of rehabilitation are to prevent further disability, maintain existing ability, and restore maximum levels of function within the limits of the client's impairment. The contributors to this text believe each individual is unique and has a right to participate in and contribute to society. During the rehabilitation process, the rehabilitation nurse and client form a partnership in which their interactions are characterized by mutual decision making and goal setting. Although these interactions may take place in a variety of rehabilitation settings, the nurse uses the nursing process consistently to assist the client and family. In this textbook, the nursing process is described as it applies to the client with functional limitations resulting from impairment.

Few books have addressed rehabilitation nursing. With some exceptions, existing books focus on diseases and disorders or are written by a number of rehabilitation team members. Although we recognize the important contributions of the interdisciplinary rehabilitation team, the contributors and I have searched without success for a textbook that addresses the unique contribution of nurses to rehabilitation and that uses a nursing process approach. An increasing number of undergraduate nursing education programs are offering courses in rehabilitation nursing, and more graduate programs each year are developing rehabilitation clinical nurse specialist options, yet few books are available to support these educational offerings. Thus this book is written for both undergraduate and graduate students in nursing. It also should be a helpful reference for new graduates practicing in rehabilitation settings. Publication by rehabilitation nurses for rehabilitation nurses is critical to advancing knowledge and improving practice in the field.

Functional ability in performing activities of daily living and fulfilling social roles is emphasized throughout this book. The book contains five sections. Part I presents a foundation for rehabilitation nursing practice and includes chapters addressing the scope of rehabilitation, theoretical bases for rehabilitation nursing, the rehabilitation team, the nursing process, the teaching-learning process, and the professional practice of rehabilitation nursing.

Part II focuses on function in activities of daily living necessary to sustain life, and part III addresses function in activities of daily living necessary to participate in life. Each chapter in part II discusses an essential life function: breathing, controlling body temperature, eating and swallowing, bladder elimination, bowel elimination, sleep and rest, and maintaining skin integrity. Each chapter in part III presents a function that either promotes or requires interaction with another person. Functions discussed are personal hygiene and grooming; communication, including speech and language, vision and hearing, and sensation and perception; movement; sexuality and sexual function; work and recreation; accessing home and community, and coping with disability.

To determine the effectiveness of any venture, evaluation is necessary. Thus part IV presents different aspects of evaluation in rehabilitation nursing. Functional evaluation, a method whereby client outcome is quantified; quality assurance, a method of evaluating structure, process, and outcome; and cost-effectiveness, one method of evaluating nursing process and client outcome from a societal perspective are included. The final section addresses further dimensions in rehabilitation nursing. Chapters include planned change, consultation, research, ethical issues, and future directions. Parts IV and V may be of particular interest to the graduate student preparing as a clinical specialist in rehabilitation nursing.

A textbook in a field as broad as rehabilitation nursing must have limitations. Therefore topics such as pediatric and geriatric rehabilitation are beyond the scope of this book. Similarly, rehabilitation of clients with specific diseases such as cardiac disease or cancer are not included as separate chapters. Examples of specific conditions, however, are given when appropriate to illustrate the functions affected.

Each chapter begins with objectives for the reader and ends with recommendations for additional readings. Test questions and learning activities follow the chapters in parts II and III. The appendixes include information and resources to assist the disabled client and the professional nurse.

We, the contributors, would like to communicate to others what we have learned from clients, families, colleagues, and students. After many combined years of experience in practice, education, and research, we would like to share with others the challenges and rewards of working with disabled clients and their families. We hope the material contained in this book will touch the professional lives of students and young nurses and encourage them to consider a career in rehabilitation nursing. We hope that the content will promote dialogue, offer guidance to students and rehabilitation nurses, and inspire further publication.

Encouragement, support, and the hard work of many people made this book possible. Special thanks to Kenneth Stengel and Fred Kwiecien for photography; to Drs. Brenda P. Haughey and Carol Maull for editing; to Sandra Bennett Illig, Doris Farzan, and Sheila Marks for invaluable assistance; to Patricia Brock-Eisenstein for typing; and to staff members at Erie County Medical Center and the university for posing for pictures. Friends, nursing staff members at Erie County Medical Center, professional colleagues, and graduate students in rehabilitation nursing provided the moral support to continue and complete this project.

Sharon S. Dittmar, RN, PhD

Contents

REHABILITATION NURSING

PROCESS AND APPLICATION

PART I

Foundations of
Rehabilitation Nursing

CHAPTER 1

Scope of Rehabilitation

Sharon S. Dittmar

OBJECTIVES

After completing Chapter 1, the reader will be able to:

1. Describe the historical events contributing to the development of rehabilitation.
2. Articulate a philosophy of rehabilitation.
3. Define chronic illness, impairment, functional limitation, handicap, rehabilitation, and health.
4. Identify the numbers and nature of recipients of rehabilitation services.

Disability and chronic illness are conditions that affect the physical, social, emotional, economic, and vocational status of individuals and their families. As a result, functional losses and limitations occur, and changes in life-style often become necessary. Many individuals and families affected by disability receive rehabilitation services.

Rehabilitation is an approach, a philosophy, an attitude, and a process involving the specialized techniques and interactions of members of the rehabilitation team. The individualized rehabilitation plan is developed by all rehabilitation team members, including the client and the family. This chapter introduces the reader to the historical evolution of rehabilitation, a rehabilitation philosophy, terms commonly used in rehabilitation, and clients served by rehabilitation providers.

HISTORICAL PERSPECTIVE

Disabled individuals have been subjected to different kinds of treatment during history. They have been killed, ridiculed, given asylum, offered physical and custodial care, or taught to care for themselves.

Before the nineteenth and twentieth centuries, attitudes toward an individual with a disability varied according to the culture and the time. The ancient Greeks disposed of crippled children, whereas in the Middle Ages the French gave blind persons a place of privilege. Even the precision by which disabilities were defined varied among cultures. For example, the Eskimo language included only a few general terms for disability, whereas other languages used many differentiating terms, such as epileptic, handicapped, mental retardate, emotionally disturbed, and more.[8]

Religious organizations were among the first groups to show concern for the disabled. From primitive times throughout the Middle Ages, monasteries and temples were noted for providing tender loving care.[11]

Society slowly began to recognize a responsibility to assist disabled citizens and their families. During the sixteenth and seventeenth centuries in England, hospitals were established, and laws passed to assist the poor and disabled. Marine hospitals cared for disabled individuals as early as 1588, at a time when other persons were punishing disabled individuals. Shortly afterward, in 1601, the Poor Relief Act was passed to outlaw begging, classify dependent people, and assist both the poor and disabled. These events helped the poor and disabled become more self-sufficient by improving their health and decreasing their dependence on public welfare.[18]

The practice of housing together the aged, insane, blind, deaf, drunks, prostitutes, and other citizens without resources also began in England. Although the care was poor, the establishment of almshouses, formerly viewed as the responsibility of religious institutions, marked the beginning of social responsibility for the poor, sick, and aged. Pilgrims brought this philosophy to the New World and established almshouses in Boston in the 1660s. The limits of these facilities soon became apparent.[11]

In the eighteenth century, British physician John Hunter described the basis of muscle reeducation and focused on the relationship between patient will and range of motion. The liberation of the insane at the Asylum De Bicêtre by Philippe Pinel occurred at the end of the century, signifying the beginning of physical *and* psychological care. Occupational and recreational treatment methods were used for the first time during this century.[18]

A series of advances in medicine around the turn of the nineteenth century generated an interest in rehabilitation. The first evidence of this interest was in the training of crippled children. Physical restoration was incorporated to help continue the gains made through medical care. Occupational therapy, at that time, was referred to as putting idle time to use. A shift from a totally medical approach to the inclusion of the work goal in rehabilitation occurred. During this period, the first medical social service department was established at Bellevue Hospital in New York, the first visiting nursing service was begun by Lillian Wald in New York City, and the first visiting professorship of physical therapy was established at the University of Pennsylvania.[18]

War and the introduction of sophisticated weaponry have greatly influenced the development of rehabilitation. With the advances in warfare, injuries and resulting disability were occurring for reasons other than accidents of birth. To return injured soldiers to the front lines or to productive lives in the community, approaches beyond pain relief and comfort giving became necessary. In 1918 the United States government initiated a national rehabilitation program for disabled World War I veterans. Although the goal was to help disabled veterans secure jobs, the program continued to stress the physical rather than the psychological aspects of disability. The more comprehensive World War II program reached a larger number of veterans. It included work and community reintegration, thus combining a physical and psychosocial approach to rehabilitation.

Other contributions to the development of rehabilitation as a concept occurred during the twentieth century. Evolution from an agrarian to an industrial society and then to an information society took place. Industrial accidents, motor vehicular injuries, trauma from leisure and sports activities, and injuries from gunshot wounds have increased the number of disabled people in this country. Simultaneous advances in science, medicine, technology, and information systems have made it possible for increasing numbers of persons with disabilities and chronic illnesses to live normal life spans. The life span of individuals in Western society also has increased, and consequently the probability of contracting one or more chronic diseases has increased. In contemporary society, disability is perceived now as something that will probably happen to everyone rather than as something that happens to others.

Medicare legislation of the 1960s further stimulated the demand for rehabilitation. Impending legislation for catastrophic health insurance may increase the need for rehabilitation services even more. Diseases such as cancer, formerly seen as terminal in all cases, and new diseases of the twentieth century, such as acquired immune deficiency syndrome (AIDS), may place demands on the health care system for more rehabilitation professionals and more rehabilitation services.

Professional organizations for physicians specializing in rehabilitation (physiatrists) and nurses now exist. Rehabilitation became a board-certified specialty in 1947 with the establishment of the American Board of Physical Medicine and Rehabilitation. In 1974 the Association of Rehabilitation Nurses was formed, followed closely thereafter with recognition of rehabilitation nursing as a specialty of nursing by the American Nurses' Association.

With the discovery of antibiotics, the leadership of outstanding rehabilitation professionals, philanthropic efforts of private individuals, legislative changes, and economic support of the government, rehabilitation became a viable societal solution for returning disabled individuals to productive roles and/or improving their quality of life.

PHILOSOPHICAL APPROACH

A philosophy is a composite of personal feelings and beliefs about individuals, their interactions with social groups, effects of environmental influences, and professional beliefs. A philosophy emerges from life experiences and evolves over the course of time. The personal feelings and beliefs underlying the information in this text are presented here.

Beliefs About Individuals

Each individual is unique and complex. Despite the severity of an injury or illness, every person has the potential to maintain or regain self-esteem and dignity and to transcend disability. Physical, emotional, social, economic, and spiritual attributes act synergistically to give identity to the total being. Although an individual is more than the sum of parts, alteration in any part or area affects total function. Separating the physical effects of disability and chronic illness from the behavioral manifestations is difficult. When a person is affected by a disability, observable behaviors often indicate the individual's attempt to gain control over the environment or frustration at the inability to do so. For example, a woman who has lost sensation in her hands may no longer feel the warmth of her child; may no longer be able to type, an activity that brought in money for the household; and may no longer feel comfortable outside her home because of fear of injury from heat, cold, or mechanical irritation. These losses affect her responses to social situations and to the environment and alter their effects upon her.

Each individual must satisfy many needs to enjoy and experience life. Physical needs necessary to maintain life include obtaining oxygen through breathing, controlling body temperature, eating and swallowing food and liquids, eliminating wastes from the body, obtaining adequate sleep and comfort, and maintaining skin integrity. Psychosocial needs necessary to participate in life include keeping the body clean and well-groomed; communicating with others through speaking, understanding, seeing, hearing, sensing, and perceiving; expressing self as a sexual being; working and playing; accessing the environment; and coping with life events. Physical disability and chronic illness may alter an individual's ability to satisfy these needs.

Individuals have in common the uniquely human need to hope. Stotland[17] defines hope as an expectation greater than zero. Everything a person does in life is done with some expectation that what is wanted will happen. Hope is at its most intense level when one is suffering or experiencing a personal trial. The intensity and character of hope change over time, and one hopes for different things. Hope is necessary for individuals, families, and other rehabilitation team members to continue with the rehabilitation process.

Individuals have a constant and reciprocal interaction with the environment. A feeling of control over one's environment helps to maintain dignity and encourages participation in life. I once worked with a gentleman dying of cancer who said the worse part of his physically and mentally incapacitating illness was the loss of a feeling of control. When he wanted to eat or drink, he had to rely on others to bring nourishment; when he wanted to go to bed, he had to wait for someone to assist him; and when he wished to know the time, he had to ask someone, because he was unable to interpret the time shown on his watch. He depended on others to accomplish physical and mental functions "healthy" persons control and take for granted in daily life.

Individuals can achieve optimum independence within the limits of impairment, provided they are included in decisions about the rehabilitation plan. Full participation in such decisions is just one of the many rights to which the disabled person is entitled throughout the rehabilitation process. More important, however, is that failure to participate in decision making may seriously hinder a person's motivation to maintain or regain function. The following are rights of individuals during the rehabilitation process[3]:

- Accurate and adequate knowledge

- An equal voice in plans and decisions surrounding own care
- Reassurance and hope
- Self-determination
- Equal status as a participating member of the rehabilitation team, family, and society
- Opportunities for increasing independence in performing self-care or managing self-care
- Opportunities to resume social roles

Individuals can be taught to perform self-care. When this is physically impossible, the person can take responsibility for supervising personal care when the opportunities are provided. Learning self-care requires intact mental abilities and a belief that the information or skill to be learned has immediate applicability. Persons are ready to learn when they are faced with a problem to be solved and are participants in the problem-solving process.

Beliefs About Social Groups

Beliefs about social groups include beliefs about family and society.

Family

Persons regarded as "the family" are affected by disablement of a family member, and they have been identified as one of the most important variables in determining outcomes of care.[21] Wright[23] perceives the individual who is disabled and the family as co-managers of care.

The degree to which time, energy, feelings, and resources must be accommodated to assist an individual who is disabled dictates, to some extent, the requirements for changes in family methods of handling interpersonal conflict, making decisions, allocating tasks, performing specific roles, and communicating. Often, roles of family members shift, and it becomes necessary for individual family members to alter their lifestyles. For example, the wife of a man with arthritis may become the major economic support of the household, and the husband and children may take responsibility for household chores. Thus the reaction of the individual and other family members to the disability and the interaction of these responses influence the health of each family member and the family as a whole. The time required for family members to reallocate roles, change functions, and renegotiate relationships to reestablish equilibrium depends upon the type and degree of disability, the meaning of disability to each member, previous methods of coping, and the family's resources.

The family should be included as an integral part of the rehabilitation team from the outset of the rehabilitation process. Working with family members and using family resources as desired by the client and family can facilitate community reintegration for the client and preserve the health of the family unit. The rights of the family during the rehabilitation process are as follows[3]:

- Sound medical knowledge regarding the chronic illness, injury, and disability
- Continual reevaluation of the disabled family member
- Helpful, relevant, and specific information about their role in the rehabilitation process
- Reassurance, human consideration, and hope
- Help in seeing the disabled member's potential
- Knowledge of educational opportunities, community resources, and rehabilitation services
- Demonstrations of caretaking procedures and printed instructions regarding care
- Interaction with other families of disabled individuals
- Assertions of their rights as individuals

Society

Members of society determine group attitudes toward particular segments of the group, establish laws to govern the society, allocate monies for services to maintain and perpetuate the society, and set up norms based on values of the group. Although individuals and families have a role in determining societal directions, groups within society often compete for the same resources. These subgroups have their own ideas, skills, arts, and other unique features. As their numbers increase, disabled individuals as one subgroup are becoming more visible and more forceful in expressing their needs and feelings. They are emerging as social and political forces in this nation, while at the same time contributing to the nation's economy either by offering their skills or by using the skills of others.

Members of society have certain expectations of individuals. These expectations have shaped the development of rehabilitation in Western culture. According to Granger,[9] our society believes the individual should:

1. Receive signals from surroundings (such as seeing, listening, smelling, or touching), assimilate these signals, and express a response to what is assimilated.
2. Maintain a customarily effective independent existence with regard to the more immediate physical needs of the body, including feeding, personal hygiene, and other activities of daily living.
3. Move about effectively in the environment.
4. Occupy time in a manner customary to age, sex, and culture, including performance within a work or home environment and participation in recreational activities.
5. Participate in and maintain social relationships with others.
6. Sustain socioeconomic independence by virtue of some form of work carried out in the home or community and support family members and societal members who are physically and/or mentally unable to carry out such activities.

Beliefs About the Environment

Although the concept of environment has often been viewed by nursing theorists as synonymous with society, it also can be conceived as a separate entity, controlled and manipulated to some extent by individuals and groups comprising society. Environment has many dimensions, including temperature, barometric pressure, wind, rain, sun, and other atmospheric conditions. These atmospheric conditions can influence the signs and symptoms of such diseases as multiple sclerosis and arthritis. Furthermore, physical aspects of the environment—such as stairs, curbs, and placement of telephones, electrical outlets, mirrors, appliance controls, and sinks—can inhibit or facilitate independence and can make the difference between complete independence and total dependence in daily activities.

In addition to having physical characteristics, the environment also has psychosocial components. People, objects, animals, technology, and information within the environment can create an emotional tone that stimulates an individual to strive for optimum functional independence or discourages such efforts. More specifically, the attitudes of personnel providing rehabilitation services have an impact on the outcome of rehabilitative efforts.

The technology and information systems for controlling and manipulating the environment to meet the needs of disabled persons exist. The expense of these systems currently prohibits maximum use. As computer technology becomes more available and economically feasible, however, the potential for controlling the environment will have fewer limits. The opportunities for exerting control over activities of daily living and making life more meaningful for those with disabilities increases each day.

Beliefs About Rehabilitation Nursing

Rehabilitation is an important component of nursing practice overall, but it also is an area of specialized practice implemented within rehabilitation settings. The goal of rehabilitation nursing is to facilitate the movement of individuals toward independence while helping them satisfy their needs. Therefore the approach to rehabilitation is holistic, creative, caring, and optimistic. Focusing on one need to the exclusion of others negates the interaction of these needs and denies the totality of the individual.

The rehabilitation nurse works with the client, the family, and other members of the rehabilitation team to satisfy current needs and anticipate potential and future needs as well. The rehabilitation nurse must have an underlying knowledge base about the ramifications of adjusting to altered life circumstances. This knowledge base includes an understanding of normal anatomy and physiology, especially of the circulatory, respiratory, musculoskeletal, neurological, genitourinary, and gastrointestinal systems; kinesiology; psychological responses to disability; and personal and community resources. Furthermore, the rehabilitation nurse must understand group dynamics in order to work effectively with professional and lay members of the interdisciplinary rehabilitation team, paraprofessionals, and members of volunteer, community, and governmental agencies. Additionally, knowledge of educational principles and strategies is necessary for implementation of client and family education. The philosophy, knowledge, and skills of the rehabilitation nurse are implemented through use of the nursing process.[18]

Rehabilitation nurses should include the family in the rehabilitation process from the outset. Understanding ways in which disability affects the total family unit is necessary. Through direct, daily, and consistent interaction with clients and families, the nurse occupies a pivotal position for assisting clients with reintegration into their own environment. Helping clients move toward optimum function in self-care tasks and in social roles presents a challenge to the rehabilitation nurse to act as an expert practitioner, coordinator, educator, counselor, change agent, client advocate, and researcher. Working with other members of the rehabilitation team is the most effective way to plan, implement, and evaluate the rehabilitation process. The professional practice of rehabilitation nursing is further described in Chapter 6.

DEFINITIONS

Many terms are used to describe the situation of an individual with a disability. To establish a common frame of reference, chronic illness, impairment, functional limitation, disability, handicap, rehabilitation, and health are defined. Confusion results when these terms are used without clear differentiation.

Chronic Illness

Historically, chronic illness was defined by the Commission on Chronic Illness[13] as:

> All impairments or deviations from normal which have one or more of the following characteristics: are permanent, leave residual disability, are caused by a nonreversible pathological condition, require special training of the patient for rehabilitation, may be expected to require a long period of supervision, observation, or care.

More recently, a number of definitions of chronic illness have been proposed. After examining these definitions, Lubkin[12] points out the problems in definition. Many chronic conditions have multiple contributing factors; origin is sometimes difficult to determine but can influence prevention and amelioration of disease, many conditions can accumulate over a number of years and are difficult to pinpoint as to time of onset, chronic illnesses have different implications for different people, and chronic illnesses are never

completely cured or prevented. She gives this definition of chronic illness[12]:

> Chronic illness is the irreversible presence, accumulation, or latency of disease states or impairments that involve the total human environment for supportive care and self-care, maintenance of function, and prevention of further disability.

Although Lubkin states that chronic illness is mentioned only in passing in rehabilitation literature and individuals with mobility problems seem to receive priority for rehabilitation, the ideas of impairment and disability are implicit in the definition of chronic illness.

Impairment, Functional Limitation or Disability, Handicap

Impairment refers to the residual limitation resulting from disease, injury, or a congenital defect.[10] Functional limitation results from an impairment and refers to the loss of ability to perform self-care tasks and fulfill usual social roles and normal activities.[14] Disability is defined as the inability to perform some key life functions and is often used interchangeably with functional limitation. Handicap refers to the interaction of a person with a disability with the environment.[10] The same types and degrees of limitation can lead to varying degrees of social disability. For example, the concert pianist with amputation of the right hand would be more disabled than the teacher with the same amputation. The pianist would be unable to fulfill a social role in relation to work, whereas the teacher could continue to carry out teaching functions.

In previous years, an individual whose situation departed from the social norm was referred to as "handicapped." Although this term is still used by government agencies, it is now rarely seen in rehabilitation literature and is rarely used by individuals with disabilities. Some persons may be disabled but not handicapped, whereas others are both disabled and handicapped by their disability. For example, the person who is paraplegic may be handicapped by not being able to climb stairs, but if elevators are installed in the home and work place, the person can access the home and fulfill the preinjury role as breadwinner.

Health

To assist individuals with disabilities to move toward health, rehabilitation nurses should have a common reference for the concept "health." The World Health Organization[22] defines health as "a state of complete physical, mental, and social well-being and not merely the absence of disease or infirmity." This definition has been criticized because of its utopian character and because it provides little direction for measurement. It also refers to health as a state rather than a process. According to this definition, very few persons would qualify as healthy.

Twaddle and Hessler[20] view health as three dimensional and as "an ideal toward which people are oriented but not one they expect to attain." According to their model (Figure 1-1), health has three components: (1) biological health—a state in which all the cells of the body are functioning at optimum capacity and in perfect harmony with one another, (2) psychological health—a state in which the individual is in perfect harmony with the environment and capable of meeting any obligations, and (3) social health—a state in which an individual's capacity for role performance is optimized. Nonhealth is defined on a biological level by signs and symptoms of illness, on a psychological level by depression, and on a social level by a reduced capacity for role performance.

Rogers[16] proposes a health status scale that includes optimum health, suboptimum health, overt illness or disability, approaching death, and death (Figure 1-2). He recognizes that it is sometimes difficult to identify overt illness or disability because the onset may be insidious, such as in multiple sclerosis. In contemporary society, approaching death does not necessarily mean that death will occur because available treatments may reverse the health status on this scale.

Dimond and Jones[6] conclude that "evaluations of health and nonhealth depend implicitly on the value orientations and life situations of the people involved. Illness to one person is not necessarily illness to another." Clearly, health is a difficult concept to define. It is rarely achieved, although most individuals attempt to move toward health. Health is determined by the physical state, the psychological state, and the ability to function within society. Furthermore, it is defined by our culture, society, and environmental conditions. Ideal health is achieved when a balance is present between and within these forces, and when individual and societal views of health are consonant.

Rehabilitation

Rehabilitation is the process by which we facilitate an individual's movement toward health. Rehabilitation has been defined by many rehabilitation team members.[2,7,10,18,19] However, a previously unpublished definition by McEachron, a rehabilitation nurse, captures the essence and philosophical approach taken in this text:

Rehabilitation is a dynamic process of planned adaptive change in life-style in response to unplanned change imposed on the individual by disease or traumatic incident. The focus is not on cure, but on living with as much freedom and autonomy as possible at every stage and in whichever direction the disability progresses.

Rehabilitation is founded upon the uniqueness of the individual and the commonality of man. It recognizes the right to separateness as an individual and to togetherness with other human beings. It revolves around and evolves from the disabled person's goals, choices, and decisions, shared and shaped in an integrative way by all who have impact upon the individual. It means operating with the knowledge that the nurse is only one of many important influences upon the

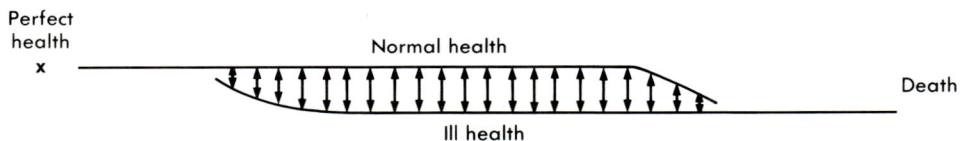

Figure 1-1
Relationships among perfect health, normal health, ill health, and death. *(From Twaddle AC and Hessler RM: A sociology of health, St Louis, 1977, The CV Mosby Co.)*

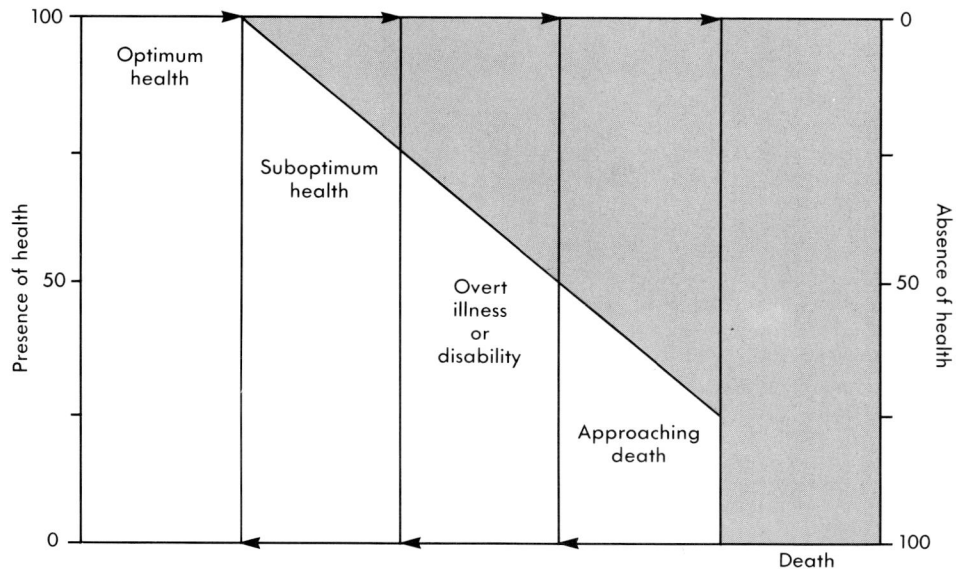

Figure 1-2
Health status scale indicating declining health and improving health *(bottom arrows)*. *(From Itoh M and Lee MHM: The epidemiology of disability as related to rehabilitation medicine. In Kottke FJ, Stillwell GK, and Lehmann JF, editors: Krusen's handbook of physical medicine and rehabilitation, Philadelphia, 1982, WB Saunders Co; modified from Rogers ES: Human ecology and health: introduction for administrators, New York, 1960, Macmillan Publishing Co, Inc.)*

client's life. It can mean having compassion and understanding for those who feel uncomfortable about their disabilities, knowing that ignorance and lack of understanding are rehabable *[sic]* disabilities. It is not confined to a hospital but should take place wherever individuals attempt to reclaim as much of their former territory as possible or to stake out a claim on new territory—unfamiliar terrain.

Rehabilitation is communication—to listen and *hear*, to observe and *see*, to speak and *be understood*. It is interpretation of the unspoken word, of "noes" which mean "yes," of vague and spastic gestures, and of body language. It is relaying of messages from those who can't be articulate about their needs. It is to touch a body and a life with acceptance, guidance, and support.

Rehabilitation is an endless search for possibilities, yet learning to accept that limitations of body, mind, money, time, architecture, and society are real. It means the recognition and acknowledgment of one's own limitations without shame. It is aiming toward independence, but identifying areas where dependence is appro-

priate and necessary. It is fostering an atmosphere of trust and understanding between the dependent and the depended upon.

Rehabilitation is directed toward strength, but realistic about weakness; it strives for strength in the midst of weakness. It is measuring strength, endurance, progress in millimeters instead of feet, yards instead of miles, seconds instead of minutes, weeks instead of days.

Rehabilitation is flexibility and improvisation. It is continuous validation of the accuracy and depth of our assessments of needs, our communication, our effectiveness as helpers. It is willingness to change our ideas, our direction, our approach. It is testing inner strength hour by hour, day by day, year by year. It is seeking self as a facilitator, not omnipotent or omniscient.

Rehabilitation is harsh realities. It is being burned up and burned out because of the inadequacies of the system, of self. It can be awesome, overwhelming in the immensity of scope, touching all aspects of life with its demanding goals of maximum, optimum. It can be ugly, smelly, noisy, painful, exhausting, embarrassing—but hopefully not dehumanizing. It is hurting and healing, being pushed, pulled, and prodded. It is channeling anger into productivity. It is substitutes and devices—straps, wheels, bars, tubes, bags—never as satisfactory as the real thing, but meeting a need. It is pills, suppositories, powders, lotions with side effects, cumulative effects, interactions, reactions. It is learning the mechanics of the body without becoming mechanical.

Rehabilitation is exuberance over small gains. It is banishing "has been" to replace it with the worth of being and becoming. It is negation of labels, because only pigeons fit pigeonholes.

Rehabilitation is teaching, learning. It is discovering teaching is good, learning better, but applying is best of all. It is continuing education of the teacher in each client. It is differentiating between "nice to know" and "need to know." It is bioethical dilemmas, the clarification of values.

Rehabilitation is advocacy, middlemanship, sometimes "caught-in-the-middlemanship"; a productive relationship is promoted for the client's sake. It is the cultivation of potential sources of help, with appreciation mixed with apprehension for volunteers and activists.

Rehabilitation is humanity in all its imperfection, but striving toward betterness [sic]. It is a daily lesson in our own humanity. It is an arena where we win the right to use the words describing coping, acceptance, equality, and caring to describe our behavior.*

The goals of rehabilitation are to maintain function through prevention of primary disability and containment of secondary disabilities, to restore optimum function in the performance of self-care activities, and to restore optimum function in the performance of social roles. Habilitation, a closely related term, refers to the development of functions never previously performed. Rehabilitation is viewed as a lifelong process carried out by the client, family, rehabilitation professionals, and society working together. The nature and type of clients served by rehabilitation professionals are described in the next section.

CLIENTS SERVED

A significant proportion of the United States population suffers from one or more chronic condi-

*From McEachron H: Personal philosophy of rehabilitation. Unpublished paper presented to graduate students in rehabilitation nursing, Buffalo, 1986, State University of New York School of Nursing.

tions and disabilities. Within this century, chronic diseases have replaced infectious diseases as the foremost public health problem. Limitations in the performance of major activities, that is, the ability to work, keep house, or engage in school or preschool activities, often accompany chronic conditions.

Statistics that specifically describe the magnitude of the problem of disability are difficult to obtain because of the substantial problems in quantifying disability. Many individuals having these diseases need rehabilitation services, yet only a small proportion receive them. A United Nations group of experts has estimated that at least 25 percent of any population consists of persons who are disabled and family members whose lives are affected by the deflection of time and energy required for assistance with their care.[1]

To obtain accurate and systematic information on illness and its impact in the United States, the National Health Survey, a nationwide household survey of noninstitutionalized persons, was initiated.[5] Begun in 1957, this survey monitors the incidence of accidental injuries, the prevalence of chronic diseases, the extent and causes of disability, and the medical problems of the aged. The Health Interview and Health Examination components of the survey are the largest and most comprehensive sources of data ever gathered about the health status of the United States population. Questions related to disability elicit information concerning demographic variables, restricted activity, bed disability days, time lost from work, and the existence of chronic conditions. Findings indicate that the number of noninstitutionalized civilians with activity limitations is growing.[15]

A dramatic increase in problems related to disability occurred between 1965 and 1976. Persons with some form of activity limitation increased by 25%. Restricted activity days increased an average of 13% to 18 days per person per year. Increases occurred in every age group, in both sexes, and in white and nonwhite races, although there were twice as many restricted activity days among nonwhites. Bed disability days increased from 6.4 to 8.8 days per year for nonwhites but remained relatively stable for whites. The only area where data showed a decrease was in the number of days lost from work. This 10% decline, however was limited entirely to white men. Members of lower income families (less than $3,000) experienced three times as many days of restricted activity and bed disability days and twice as many days lost from work as persons belonging to families with incomes of $15,000 or more. The greatest difference in disability according to income was apparent among persons 45 to 65 years of age.[5]

Information obtained by the National Center for Health Statistics showed that significant increases in the use of special aids, such as canes, leg or foot braces, walkers, wheelchairs, and crutches, occurred between 1969 and 1977. The use of all special aids, except crutches, was proportionately higher in 1977 than in 1969 among persons 65 years of age and over. In 1977 an estimated 358,000 persons reported absence of a leg, foot, arm, or hand. Of the persons using special aids, 42% used a cane or walking stick, 23% used special shoes, 22% used some type of brace, 11% used a walker, 10% used a wheelchair, and approximately 50% of those missing a lower extremity(ies) used an artificial leg(s)[5] (Table 1-1).

The most recent data from the National Health Survey show a slight increase in the numbers of persons experiencing restricted activity and bed disability. The greatest increases since 1971 in restricted activity days occurred among white men and persons living outside Standard Metropolitan Statistical Areas (SMSA) and in western states. The greatest increases in bed disability days are found among women, nonwhites, those living outside SMSA, and residents of north central states (Table 1-2).[15]

The number of days lost from work for each currently employed person declined as a whole slightly in 1980, but showed a small increase among nonwhites and residents of the Northeast (Table 1-3).[15] In 1980 currently employed workers residing in the Northeast had the highest rate of time lost from work among the four regions studied.

Some 10 million people in the United States receive a service or payment due to a disabling condition. The cost of disability has been estimated to run into the tens—even the hundreds—of billions of dollars. According to Coe,[4] "more than 7% of the gross national product is consumed by some 40 public and private disability systems." More alarming is the fact that since 1960 disability expenditures have been increasing one and a half times faster than the gross national product.

The disability insurance program, administered by the Social Security Administration, is the major agency protecting disabled workers and their families against financial disaster. As part of its responsibility, this agency devotes research resources to collection and analysis of data concerning the disabled. Economic, medical, and social consequences of disability have been a major focus of the national surveys conducted by the Social Security Administration in 1966, 1972, and 1978. At the end of February, 1980, data collected from noninstitutionalized civilians ages 18 to 64 indicated that 2.9 million disabled workers and 1.9 million of their dependents were receiving benefits. These figures represent a 60% increase from the 1972 survey when there were 3 million beneficiaries, half of whom were dependents. In 1978 more than 21 million working-age adults reported some limitation in their ability to work because of a chronic condition or impairment.[5]

Chronic disability is much greater in the elderly than among the young. Eighty-five percent of older people suffer from one or more chronic diseases; 46% of all noninstitutionalized elderly have some limitation in their activities, whereas 17% are unable to perform a major activity because of chronic illness.[15] Between 1900 and 1960 the proportion of the population age 65 and older doubled, and this number continues to increase, although at a slower rate.[5]

Although these statistics tell us very little about the institutionalized disabled population, they do indicate that the dependency of persons living outside institutions is increasing. Although only 5% of persons who are elderly reside in institutions, experts have estimated that one out of four will spend some time in a health care institution before death. In addition, many younger disabled persons will spend some time in institutions. For example, before World War II, few persons survived spinal cord injury. Today the mortality of the approximately 200,000 persons with spinal cord injury living in the United States has declined significantly, hospital stays are shorter, and readmission rates have decreased. Approximately 8,000 to 12,000 persons incur spinal cord injuries each year. As a result of improved care, these individuals will live longer and function at a higher level of independence. However, they will continue to require rehabilitation services for the rest of their lives.[7]

TABLE 1-1
Persons using special aids for getting around, by age and sex (civilian noninstitutionalized population, 1977)

Age and sex	Persons using one or more aids			Persons using specific mobility aids									Artificial limb		
	Total	One aid	Two or more	Cane, walking stick	Special shoes	Brace Leg, foot	Brace Other	Walker	Wheelchair	Crutches				Leg, foot	Arm, hand	Other aid
Thousands of persons using special aids	6,459	5,292	1,167	2,714	1,492	398	1,004	689	645	613				205	66	205
Sex																
Male	3,106	2,519	586	1,239	732	241	539	203	294	348				146	49	124
Female	3,353	2,773	581	1,475	760	157	465	486	351	265				60	16*	81
Age (years)																
Under 15	732	651	81	0*	572	76	51	22*	47	50				13*	6*	21*
15-44	1,067	906	161	153	265	133	296	26*	116	211				46	11*	36
45-64	1,674	1,333	342	550	401	119	460	93	148	202				82	26*	79
65 and over	2,985	2,401	584	2,011	253	70	196	549	334	151				64	22*	68
65-74	1,194	913	281	723	162	44	134	168	151	97				40	9*	32*
75 and over	1,791	1,488	303	1,287	92	27*	62	381	183	54				24*	13*	37
Number using aids per 1,000 population	30.4	24.9	5.5	12.8	7.0	1.9	4.7	3.2	3.0	2.9				1.0	0.3	1.0
Sex																
Male	30.3	24.6	5.7	12.1	7.2	2.4	5.3	2.0	2.9	3.4				1.4	0.5	1.2
Female	30.5	25.3	5.3	13.4	6.9	1.4	4.2	4.4	3.2	2.4				0.5	0.1*	0.7
Age (years)																
Under 15	14.2	12.6	1.6	0.0*	11.1	1.5	1.0	0.4*	0.9	1.0				0.3*	0.1*	0.4*
15-44	11.2	9.5	1.7	1.6	2.8	1.4	3.1	0.3*	1.2	2.2				0.5	0.1*	0.4
45-64	38.6	30.7	7.9	12.7	9.2	2.7	10.6	2.1	3.4	4.7				1.9	0.6*	1.8
65 and over	134.1	107.8	26.2	90.3	11.4	3.1	8.8	24.7	15.0	6.8				2.9	1.0*	3.1
65-74	83.7	64.0	19.7	50.7	11.4	3.1	9.4	11.8	10.6	6.8				2.8	0.6*	2.2*
75 and over	223.7	185.8	37.8	160.7	11.5	3.4*	7.7	47.6	22.9	6.7				3.0*	1.6*	4.6

From National Center for Health Statistics: Use of special aids: United States, 1977, Pub No 81-1563, series 10, no 135, Hyattsville, Md, 1980, US Department of Health and Human Services.

*Figure has low statistical reliability or precision (relative standard error exceeds 30%).

TABLE 1-2 _____

Unadjusted and age-adjusted days of restricted activity and bed disability per person per year, by selected characteristics (United States, 1971, 1975, and 1980)

Characteristic	Restricted activity*			Bed disability*		
	1980	1975	1971	1980	1975	1971
All persons						
Unadjusted rate	19.1	17.9	15.7	7.0	6.6	6.1
Age-adjusted rate	19.1	18.1	16.0	7.0	6.6	6.2
Sex						
Male						
Unadjusted rate	17.1	15.6	14.2	5.9	5.4	5.4
Age-adjusted rate	17.5	16.2	14.7	6.0	5.6	5.5
Female						
Unadjusted rate	21.0	20.0	17.0	8.0	7.6	6.8
Age-adjusted rate	20.5	19.0	17.1	7.8	7.6	6.8
Race						
White						
Unadjusted rate	18.7	17.5	15.4	6.6	6.2	5.9
Age-adjusted rate	18.5	17.5	15.5	6.5	6.2	5.9
All others						
Unadjusted rate	21.4	20.4	18.0	9.3	8.8	7.6
Age-adjusted rate	24.0	23.6	21.7	10.3	10.1	9.2
Place of residence						
SMSA						
Unadjusted rate	19.1	17.9	15.6	7.0	6.8	6.2
Age-adjusted rate	19.2	18.3	16.0	7.0	7.0	6.4
Outside SMSA						
Unadjusted rate	19.2	17.8	15.8	6.9	5.9	5.9
Age-adjusted rate	19.0	17.6	16.0	6.8	5.9	5.9
Geographic region						
Northeast						
Unadjusted rate	17.9	16.7	14.8	6.9	6.5	6.1
Age-adjusted rate	17.6	16.6	14.7	6.8	6.5	6.0
North central						
Unadjusted rate	17.2	15.9	14.2	6.3	5.8	5.3
Age-adjusted rate	17.2	16.1	14.5	6.3	5.8	5.3
South						
Unadjusted rate	19.8	18.7	16.6	7.5	7.1	6.8
Age-adjusted rate	19.9	19.2	17.3	7.6	7.3	7.1
West						
Unadjusted rate	22.0	20.8	17.6	7.0	6.8	6.3
Age-adjusted rate	22.3	21.3	18.1	7.1	6.9	6.3

From National Center for Health Statistics: Disability days: United States, 1980, Pub No 83-1571, series 10, no 143, Hyattsville, Md, 1983, US Department of Health and Human Services.
*Rates are age adjusted by the direct method to the age distribution of the 1980 total civilian noninstitutionalized population of the United States.

TABLE 1-3

Unadjusted and age-adjusted days lost from work per currently employed person 17 to 64 years of age per year, by selected characteristics (United States, 1971, 1975, and 1980)

Characteristic*	Work loss		
	1980	1975	1971
All persons			
Unadjusted rate	5.0	5.2	5.1
Age-adjusted rate	5.0	5.2	5.0
Sex			
Male			
Unadjusted rate	4.9	4.9	4.9
Age-adjusted rate	4.9	4.9	4.7
Female			
Unadjusted rate	5.1	5.8	5.5
Age-adjusted rate	5.1	5.7	5.5
Race			
White			
Unadjusted rate	4.7	5.0	4.8
Age-adjusted rate	4.7	5.0	4.7
All others			
Unadjusted rate	7.1	6.9	7.4
Age-adjusted rate	7.0	6.9	7.4
Place of residence			
SMSA			
Unadjusted rate	5.2	5.3	5.3
Age-adjusted rate	5.2	5.3	5.1
Outside SMSA			
Unadjusted rate	4.7	4.9	4.8
Age-adjusted rate	4.7	4.9	4.8
Geographic region			
Northeast			
Unadjusted rate	5.8	5.3	5.2
Age-adjusted rate	5.8	5.3	5.0
North central			
Unadjusted rate	4.8	4.8	4.8
Age-adjusted rate	4.8	4.7	4.7
South			
Unadjusted rate	4.9	5.1	5.4
Age-adjusted rate	4.9	5.1	5.4
West			
Unadjusted rate	4.5	6.1	4.8
Age-adjusted rate	4.5	6.1	4.8

From National Center for Health Statistics: Disability days: United States, 1980, Pub No 83-1571, series 10, no 143, Hyattsville, Md, 1983, US Department of Health and Human Services.
*Rates are age adjusted by the direct method to the age distribution of the 1980 total current employed population 17 to 64 years of age.

SUMMARY

The growing number of people living to an older age, the increase in chronic illnesses and disabilities, and the prolonged survival of persons with these problems will continue to place specific demands on nursing, medical, allied health, and social resources. With modern methods of rehabilitation and continued societal support of rehabilitation services, the activity limitations of disabled people can be substantially decreased, thus increasing the quality and the longevity of life. As rehabilitation nurses and team members, we must become more knowledgeable about and more active in the political and social arenas to assure the continued availability of services for persons who are disabled. The individual and social advantages of restoring function and meaning to the lives of this increasing segment of society through rehabilitation services has been demonstrated but, in light of decreasing health care resources, continues to require the vigilance of persons who are disabled and health care professionals.

REFERENCES

1. Acton N: The world's response to disability: evolution of a philosophy, Arch Phys Med Rehabil 63:145, April 1982.
2. Baldonado A and Stahl D: Cancer nursing, ed 2, New York, 1982, Medical Examination Publishing Co, Inc.
3. Buscaglia L: The disabled and their parents: a counseling challenge, rev ed, Thorofare, NJ, 1983, Slack, Inc.
4. Coe TC: Professionalism: a new challenge for rehabilitation, Arch Phys Med Rehabil 62:245, June 1981.
5. Congressional Research Service, Library of Congress: Digest of data on persons with disabilities, Washington, DC, June 1984, Mathematica Policy Research, Inc.
6. Dimond M and Jones SL: Chronic illness across the life span, Norwalk, Conn, 1983, Appleton-Century-Crofts.
7. Ditunno JF: Spinal cord injury. In Ruskin AP, editor: Current therapy in physiatry, Philadelphia, 1984, WB Saunders Co.
8. Garrett FJ and Levine ES, editors: Rehabilitation practices with the physically disabled, New York, 1973, Columbia University Press.
9. Granger CV: Health accounting—functional assessment of the long-term patient. In Kottke FJ, Stillwell GK, and Lehmann JF, editors: Krusen's handbook of physical medicine and rehabilitation, Philadelphia, 1982, WB Saunders Co.
10. Halstead LS and Grabois M: Medical rehabilitation, New York, 1985, Raven Press.

11. Hogstel MO, editor: Management of personnel in long-term care, Bowie, Md, 1983, Robert J Brady Co.

12. Lubkin IM: Chronic illness: impact and interventions, Boston, 1986, Jones & Bartlett Publishers, Inc.

13. Mayo L, editor: Guides to action on chronic illness, Commission on Chronic Illness, New York, 1956, National Health Council.

14. Nagi A: An epidemiology of disability among adults in the United States, Milbank Mem Fund Quart 54(4):439, 1976.

15. National Center for Health Statistics: Disability days: United States, 1980, Pub No 83-1571, series 10, no 143, Hyattsville, Md, 1983, US Department of Health and Human Services.

16. Rogers ES: Human ecology and health: introduction for administrators, New York, 1960, Macmillan Publishing Co, Inc.

17. Stotland E: The psychology of hope, San Francisco, 1969, Jossey-Bass Inc, Publishers.

18. Stryker RP: Rehabilitative aspects of acute and chronic illness, ed 2, Philadelphia, 1977, WB Saunders Co.

19. Trieschman RB: Spinal cord injuries, Elmsford, NY, 1980, Pergamon Press.

20. Twaddle AC and Hessler RM: A sociology of health, St Louis, 1977, The CV Mosby Co.

21. Wahlquist G: The family in rehabilitation, Rehabil Nurs 12:62, March/April 1987.

22. World Health Organization: International classification of impairments, disabilities, and handicaps, Geneva, 1980, The Organization.

23. Wright B: Physical disability: a psychological approach, ed 2, New York, 1983, Harper & Row, Publishers, Inc.

ADDITIONAL READINGS

American Nurses' Association and Association of Rehabilitation Nurses: Standards of rehabilitation nursing practice, Kansas City, MO, 1986, The Association.

Gillies DA: Family assessment and counseling by the rehabilitation nurse, Rehabil Nurs 12:65, March/April 1987.

Mumma CM, editor: Rehabilitation nursing: concepts and practice, a core curriculum, ed 2, Evanston, Ill, 1987, Rehabilitation Foundation.

Storlie FJ: The patient as colleague: a personal philosophy, Rehabil Nurs 6:16, July/Aug 1981.

Watson PG: Family participation in the rehabilitation process: the rehabilitators' perspective, Rehabil Nurs 12:70, March/April 1987.

Williams TF: Introduction—rehabilitation in the aging: philosophy and approaches. In Williams TF, editor: Rehabilitation in the aging, New York, 1985, Raven Press.

Theoretical Bases of Rehabilitation Nursing

Brenda P. Haughey
Sharon S. Dittmar

OBJECTIVES

After completing Chapter 2, the reader will be able to:

1. Define theory.
2. Identify the purposes of theory.
3. Describe the relationship between theory and nursing practice, education, and research.
4. Describe how theories from other disciplines relate to rehabilitation nursing.
5. Describe how nursing theories relate to rehabilitation nursing.
6. Determine the applicability of selected theories to rehabilitation nursing practice.

The nursing profession has only recently begun to recognize the relevance and importance of theory for practice, research, and education. Although theories help us understand everyday life, many nurses are still unfamiliar with their relationship to professional activities. The purpose of this chapter is to present a general overview of the meaning and purposes of theories and their applicability to nursing functions. Specific examples of theories that can be used to guide rehabilitation nursing practice, research, and education are presented. These include both theories from other disciplines and those developed by nursing theorists.

THE MEANING OF THEORY

The term theory has many meanings. "For some, theory may include ideas or hunches, whereas others believe that a theory must stand up to rigorous tests."[9] Theories are synonymously referred to in the nursing literature as theoretical frameworks and conceptual models.

According to Kerlinger,[15] a theory "is a set of interrelated constructs (concepts), definitions, and propositions that present a systematic view of phenomena by specifying relations among variables, with the purpose of explaining and predicting the phenomena." Similarly, theory is defined by Polit and Hungler[30] as "an abstract generalization that presents a systematic explanation about the relationships among phenomena" and by Seaman and Verhonick[35] as "an explanation for the interrelationships among facts, concepts, or propositions." More simply conceived, theories provide a framework for thinking about and interpreting reality.

Individuals tend to think of theories as "facts" or the "truth." However, as noted by Polit and Hungler,[30] "no theory, no matter what its subject matter, can ever be considered final and verified. . . . Today's successful theory may be relegated to tomorrow's intellectual garbage dump." Thus theories should be thought of as tentative explanations of phenomena that are subject to rejection or revision as new knowledge is gained.

THE PURPOSES OF THEORY

Theories serve a number of purposes, including the organization of what is known into a meaningful framework. They integrate findings from numerous research studies and thus contribute to the development and advancement of a body of scientific knowledge. Since theories provide explanations about the relationships between observed phenomena, they also afford the opportunity for prediction and control of events or outcomes.

In nursing, theories "assist nurses to understand, analyze, and interpret the client's complex health situations and apply knowledge while using the nursing process. . . . "[9] Theoretical perspectives provide a framework for assessing client problems, determining nursing diagnoses, and planning, implementing, and evaluating nursing care. Thus theories enhance professional growth and autonomy "by guiding the practice, education, and research functions of the profession."[20]

THE RELATIONSHIP BETWEEN THEORY AND NURSING PRACTICE, RESEARCH, AND EDUCATION

Theories are the major link between nursing practice, research, and education. "Ideas for nursing theory may develop in practice, be tested through research, and then serve to guide or explain practice."[9] Historically nurses have relied on knowledge derived from authority and tradition as a basis for their practice. However, as the use of

science in nursing has grown, we have begun to use theoretical approaches and knowledge to implement the nursing process. "Theoretical approaches provide broader frameworks that can integrate more aspects of the client's complex health situation than do facts and principles alone."[9] Thus theories facilitate the improvement of nursing practice. Nurses who participate in theory development contribute to unification of purpose, professional autonomy, and enhancement of communication.[4]

Theory also has a close relationship to nursing research. It stimulates and generates ideas for research; research in turn tests the validity of the theory and generates new data for theory development. Wilson[39] notes that for research findings to be incorporated into the scientific base of nursing knowledge, they "must be placed within a theoretical context or be designed to develop one." When a theoretical perspective is used for research, the investigator can "contribute the findings of even a small project to the larger theoretical perspective that uses the same theoretical frame of reference."[35]

As with practice and research, theoretical perspectives have relevance for nursing education. They are used, for example, "as the underlying rationale for each component in the nursing process."[9] Additionally, theories serve as organizing frameworks or themes for nursing curricula.

The development of nursing theories is a relatively recent undertaking. In the past, nurses relied heavily on theories "borrowed" from other disciplines. Many of these are useful frameworks to guide the practice of rehabilitation nurses. The following section of this chapter briefly describes selected perspectives that can be applied to rehabilitation nursing.

THEORIES FROM OTHER DISCIPLINES

Nurses have borrowed theories from other disciplines and applied them to nursing practice, education, and research. Among the theories borrowed have been those concerned with stress, human needs, social learning, and role.

Stress Theories

Stress is a complex phenomenon that has been variously conceptualized. In some theories, stress is viewed as a stimulus, whereas in others it is defined as a response or an intervening state.

Hans Selye made outstanding contributions to stress theory by elaborating the physiological responses to stress and explaining how and under what conditions these responses may become pathological. In Selye's view,[36] stress is "the state manifested by a specific syndrome which consists of all the nonspecifically induced changes within a biologic system." He defines the agents that produce stress as stressors and contends that all stressors, regardless of their pleasant or unpleasant nature, evoke essentially the same physiological response.[37] Stressors increase the demand on the body to readjust itself. The totality of the changes induced by stressors is manifested as the general adaptation syndrome (GAS).

The GAS has three stages. The first stage, the alarm reaction, includes a shock phase and a countershock phase. In the former, resistance is lowered; in the latter, defenses are activated. This is followed by a stage of resistance during which maximum adaptation occurs. The third stage, exhaustion, is reached if the stressor persists or defenses are inadequate. At this point, adaptive mechanisms collapse and disease or death may ensue.

Subsequent to Selye's work, theories on stress proliferated among a variety of disciplines. Each has enriched our understanding of the phenomenon of stress and the complexities involved in the development, testing, and application of stress theory. One of these theories, namely, that proposed by David Mechanic, has particular relevance for rehabilitation nursing practice. Other theories of stress are reviewed in the citations included in the additional reading list at the end of this chapter.

Mechanic[22] defines stress as "the discomforting responses of persons in particular situations." Furthermore, he states that "whether or not a person experiences stress will depend on the means, largely learned, that he has available to deal with his life situations. Thus stress is likely to become evident when the individual perceives these means as lacking or insufficient, or when they actually do become so."[22]

Adaptation, which includes both coping and defense, is the major focus of Mechanic's theory. Behavior that facilitates dealing with the situation is termed coping behavior. Defenses are part of the coping behavior and refer to the ways "in which a person manages his emotional and affec-

tive states when discomfort is aroused or anticipated."[23] Practice, experience, and familiarity with ways to handle a situation are all important to the adaptive process. A person who feels unprepared is likely to experience discomfort. Throughout his work, Mechanic emphasizes the importance of an individual's perception of the situation in determining the response to stress. This notion is particularly relevant to understanding individual reactions to disability and thus to implementing the nursing process.

As noted earlier, there are multiple perspectives within the larger framework of stress theory. The nursing implications, then, might vary according to the particular theoretical stance the nurse assumes. In general, however, stress theory suggests that an important role of the rehabilitation nurse would be to identify those factors which are stressful to the disabled client and to develop a care plan aimed at stress reduction and the promotion of coping and adaptation.

Maslow's Hierarchy of Needs

Maslow's hierarchy of needs is one of many theories of motivation that attempt to explain human behavior. As noted by Griffith-Kenney,[8] "advocates of human needs theory view individuals as integrated, whole beings who are motivated by internal and external needs that create tension. To reduce this tension, an individual seeks to meet specific needs through goal-directed behavior." According to Maslow,[21] "the single holistic principle that binds together the multiplicity of human motives is the tendency for a new and higher need to emerge as the lower need fulfills itself by being sufficiently gratified."

Maslow identifies five categories of needs: physiological, safety, love and belonging, esteem and recognition, and self-actualization. These needs are organized in a hierarchy of priority, with basic, physiological needs providing the foundation for all higher level needs (Figure 2-1). Self-actualization, the highest level in Maslow's hierarchy, is achieved through the process of successfully meeting the needs of all lower levels. For some individuals "the striving for self-actualization is lifelong; others may actually reach the self-actualized level at various points within the span of their adult years. Self-actualizing people tend to have a realistic orientation; to accept self and others; to be spontaneous, autonomous, and

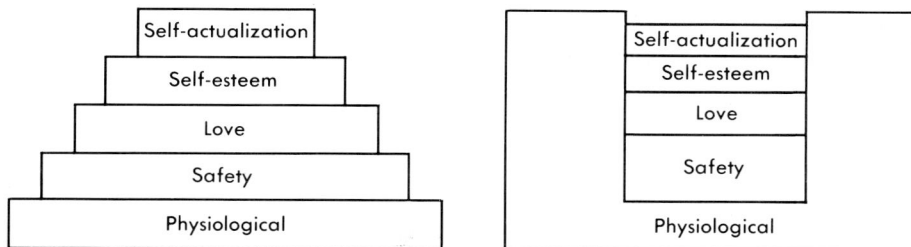

Figure 2-1
Hierarchy of needs. Basic needs form foundation upon which fulfillment of higher needs rests. If basic needs are not fully met, foundation for higher needs is not complete. Thus higher needs may be submerged or engulfed by lower level needs. *(From Mitchell PH: Concepts basic to nursing, New York, 1977, McGraw-Hill Book Co.)*

independent; to hold democratic attitudes and values; and to develop a limited number of deep and profound intimate relationships rather than numerous associations that are superficial."[10] Overall, self-actualizing individuals tend to feel satisfied with their life and accomplishments.

Griffith-Kenney[8] suggests that Maslow's theory "can be used to prioritize nursing diagnoses and can serve as a guide in assessing and analyzing data and in planning nursing implementation." It is particularly relevant in the rehabilitation setting in that disabled individuals must first learn to cope with issues of survival before they can move on to meeting higher level needs. Since the onset of disability may alter one's predominant need level, the rehabilitation nurse needs to carefully assess the client's status in the hierarchy in order to facilitate movement toward self-actualization and the achievement of the individual's maximum potential.

Social Learning Theory

Social learning theory provides another useful framework for rehabilitation nurses, particularly with regard to health education directed toward changing a disabled client's behavior. This perspective, which evolved from the well-known work of Pavlov and Skinner, builds upon the currently well-documented finding that "behavior is influenced by its consequences much of the time."[2] According to Bandura,[2] "outcomes change behavior in humans through the intervening influence of thought"; they also "motivate through their incentive value, as well as inform." Fur-

thermore, Bandura[2] notes that "many of the things we do are designed to gain anticipated benefits and to avert future trouble. Our choices of action are largely under anticipatory control."

In the social learning paradigm, "reinforcement can be used to change behavior *directly*, by directly providing the reinforcement; *vicariously*, by having the learner observe someone else be reinforced for a behavior (social modeling); or by *self-management*, by having the client or patient monitor and provide self-rewards."[26]

Baranowski[3] delineates four phases in the process of directing changes in behavior: pretraining, training, initial testing and continued performance. These are succinctly summarized in a recent article by Parcel and Baranowski. The pretraining phase "comes after the person realizes something needs to be done but before the formal attempt at directed behavior change."[26] A major task of the nurse in this phase is to find out "what beliefs a person has developed about the targeted health problem or need, what anxieties accompany these beliefs, and how the person decides to seek help."[26] The concepts of expectations, expectancies, and emotional coping are important here. In the view of social learning theorists, expectations, or one's anticipations about the behavior, "are learned from previous experiences with similar situations, observing others in similar situations, or learning from others about these situations."[26] Expectations are differentiated from expectancies, which refer to the values one has with regard to outcomes. Expectations function on the principle that individuals are likely to perform activities perceived as enhancing favorable outcomes while minimizing behaviors that are negative.[26] Emotional coping also plays a role in this stage. As noted by Parcel and Baranowski,[26] "Bandura recognized the implications of emotional arousal for learning and the fact that excessive emotional arousal inhibits performance." The onset of health problems may stimulate fear, anxiety, or emotional arousal. Successful coping with "these anxieties is prerequisite to implementing a behavior change program."[26]

The training phase incorporates the health educator's specification of what the new behaviors include and how they can be performed.[26] In other words, the focus is on developing the client's behavioral capability to perform the new activity and cope with problems encountered in attempting to do so.

In the testing phase, the client tries to perform the activities taught in the education program, "including testing these activities, and adapting a strategy to meet the needs of situations outside the health education program."[26] Self-efficacy is a relevant concept in this phase. Social learning theorists believe that "interventions promoting behavior change must develop within the person the self-perception of confidence in being able to perform certain tasks."[26] This can be facilitated by breaking down the behavior into the smaller components it comprises. "The small steps ensure that the person can perform the task, and each new success builds the person's perceived self-efficacy in doing this new task."[26]

In the final phase, continued performance, the client "has completed the learning and has developed a pattern of behaviors appropriate to the situation."[26] However, maintaining these changes is often difficult. Social learning theorists use the concept of self-control in reference to promoting long-term changes, such as those typically demanded in coping with disability. Parcel and Baranowski[26] refer to Kanfer's model of self-control in which there are five components for understanding and promoting self-control: "the unambiguous specification of a target behavior, the setting of some criterion of performance, the establishment of some mechanism for monitoring the performance, the establishment of mechanisms to evaluate one's monitored performance against the criterion, and the establishment of some mechanism of self-reward."

Health education, especially that which focuses on assisting disabled clients to make behavior changes, is a major component of the rehabilitation process. Social learning theory, as previously described, provides one perspective the rehabilitation nurse can use to devise health education strategies.

Role Theory

Rehabilitation nursing also can be implemented from the perspective of role theory. *Role* is defined as "a set of social norms that governs a person's behavior in a group and determines relationships to other group members."[19] Social roles provide guidelines or expectations for behavior for a particular social status, or position within society. "Status is the individual's fixed position in a group," whereas "role is the dynamic aspect that defines how the person who occupies the status should behave."[31] Most persons have numerous statuses and thus perform many roles, which at times may conflict with one another. For example, one's enactment of an occupational role may conflict with that of the parental role.

Throughout life individuals are required to make role transitions. The difficulties surrounding these transitions vary among individuals and according to the particular circumstances involved. "Often they are a rich source of new opportunities, challenges, and alluring rewards" and "can hold promise of heightened self-esteem."[31] Alternatively, they can "lead to a sense of failure and to hurt, defensiveness, and withdrawal."[31] For many reasons, the transition can be stressful and accompanied by feelings of inadequacy and insecurity.

Individual differences aside, two problems characterize role transitions. "One is the strain of learning: orienting to new roles, making myriad adjustments, resolving conflicts with the competitive demands of the other roles the person plays."[31] The second stems from the fact that the process has a dual nature: the taking on of new roles and the giving up of old ones. The latter requires learning, but it "also means relinquishing the former rewards and abandoning that portion of one's self that had become invested in the previous role."[31]

Clearly, role problems are not unique to persons with disabilities. The extent to which they create serious needs for adjustment in either a nondisabled or disabled individual depends upon the "entire complex of personal and environmental pressures in his life."[38] However, the onset of disability often imposes the requirement of immediate, unanticipated role transitions. Unlike role problems imposed by short-term illnesses, where recovery is expected, "the rewards for the disabled are not as immediate and dramatic; the disabled person may never again be able to fully resume the various activities in which he was once able to engage."[14]

Thomas[38] has identified five disability-related roles. The occurrence, pattern, and sequencing of these roles vary among individuals. Some may last longer than others and several may be present at once, but at least one of the following is part of the repertoire of all persons with a long-term disability:

1. *The disabled patient:* At some point, "the disabled individual is typically a patient, thereby exposing himself to a characteristic set of expectations."[38] For example, Parsons[27,28] identifies four aspects of institutionalized expectations and features of the role of the sick person:

   • The sick person is exempted from normal social role responsibilities, with the degree of exemption related to the nature and severity of the illness.

   • The sick person is seen as needing to be taken care of. The state of incapacity is viewed as beyond the person's control and the person is not held responsible for the condition.

   • The sick person's state is partially and conditionally legitimate. The person must view the state as undesirable and must want to get well.

   • The sick person is obligated to seek help and to cooperate in efforts to restore health. Thus legitimization depends on the person wanting to get well and doing everything possible to accomplish this goal.

2. *The handicapped performer:* Disablement is often accompanied by limitations of performance. The extent of functional impairment may range from minimal to complete loss of function. Regardless of the degree, impaired function has several ramifications, that is, "the disabled person may be less able to care for himself physically . . . , the impaired function may be one which is requisite to the performance of normal social roles . . . , the disablement may preclude the fulfillment of normal responsibilities to others . . . ," and "the disabled may simply hinder others."[38]

3. *The helped person:* Impaired individuals often require more help than normal, healthy persons. "The disabled is thus on the receiving end of helping acts; he must adjust, accommodate, and respond to being an object of aid."[38] In this sense, those with disabilities are deviant in a culture such as ours in which self-reliance and independence are so highly valued.

4. *Disability co-manager:* The disabled person "often becomes an active participant in the decisions and regimen of living attending his impairment and rehabilitation."[38]

5. *Public relations expert:* Usually, we do not have to explain our roles to one another. "The disabled, in contrast, typically have a particular impairment, the understanding of which is not provided for others by such a widely held common store of knowledge."[38] Thus the disabled must carry the burden of explanation and interpretation.

Numerous problems attend the expectations of these disability-related roles.[14] First, the individual must accept the disablement. However, "the prospect of disability can be so psychologically devastating that the defense mechanism of denial is used to cope."[14] Second, the person has to learn to be a "handicapped performer" and "losing hope of further improvement is itself a frequent problem encountered by those who develop a disability."[14] Third, the requirement that the individual actively participate in the rehabilitation process may be problematic in that denial may result in the development of a rehabilitation plan that is overly optimistic. Alternatively, the individual who is in a state of despair may simply give up and withdraw. Fourth, the person's need for assistance may give rise to "feelings of inferiority, excessive obligation to others, or guilt. . . . "[14] Finally, disabled persons must develop strategies for interacting with others who know little about their disabilities. Interactions may be strained because "most people are unsure about how to interact with someone who is visibly disabled."[14]

Nursing practice, based on the perspective of role theory, might logically be directed toward identifying and resolving role conflict and facilitating smooth role transitions. However, this framework suggests many other implications for rehabilitation nursing.

Understandably, nurses have recognized the need to use caution in applying theories from other disciplines because the reality they appear to represent in nonnursing situations may not be the reality that exists in nursing situations.[4] To help solve this dilemma, nurses began to develop their own theories in the late 1950s. This activity continued with a flourish through the 1960s and 1970s. Recent efforts have focused on testing these theories in specific areas of nursing practice.

THEORIES IN NURSING

Chapter 1 describes beliefs about the individual as a holistic being, an approach that is not without problems. The concept of holism in rehabilitation nursing dictates that no part can be analyzed in isolation of the whole.[7] Yet, in describing rehabilitation nursing practice, the client is reduced to discrete elements in order to analyze physical, social, psychological, vocational, and spiritual areas of function within these realms. Chinn and Jacobs[4] quote Newman's position as follows: "The study of nursing problems requires the identification of patterns that reflect the whole. For example, patterns of sleep, movement, or communication might be conceptualized as reflective of the whole person." Thus a theoretical base for rehabilitation nursing might begin by identifying patterns of client problems that reflect the whole.

A number of nurse theorists have contributed to the conception of what is uniquely rehabilitation nursing. Nurses generally agree on four concepts necessary for a nursing theoretical formulation: (1) humans, (2) health, (3) society, and (4) nursing.[10] Depending upon the individual theorist, theories have been derived from intuitive knowledge of nursing practice (for example, King[16]) or as an effort to revise and extend theories from other disciplines. For example, a physiologist-psychologist's work with adaptation to describe and explain function of the eye was used by Roy to develop adaptation theory in nursing. Other nurse theorists (for example, Rogers[32]) have formulated theory from a philosophical stance about nursing and the nature of health and human behavior. The concept of environment has been included as an element of society by some theorists and examined as a separate concept by others.

The purpose of developing and testing theories in rehabilitation nursing is to help describe, explain, predict, and control phenomena that affect rehabilitation nursing practice and client outcomes. Using a theory or theories as a basis for practice challenges thinking, provides new analytical skills, and helps all levels of practicing nurses become more purposeful in planning and implementing nursing actions. Selected nursing theories developed by Henderson, Hall, Orem, King, Roy, and Roper are described and the relevance of each theory for rehabilitation nursing is explained.

Virginia Henderson: Humanistic Nursing

Virginia Henderson did not set out to develop a theory of nursing, but rather to synthesize her own definition of nursing. Early in her career, she realized it was important to be clear about the functions of nurses. Her practice experience in rehabilitation nursing also strongly contributed to her conception of nursing.

Henderson[1] describes the role of the nurse in functional terms as follows:

> To assist the individual, sick or well, in the performance of those activities contributing to health and its recovery (or to a peaceful death) that he would perform unaided if he had the strength, will, or knowledge and . . . to help him gain independence as rapidly as possible.

She defines health as the client's ability to accomplish 14 basic needs, identified as the 14 components of nursing care: (1) breathing, (2) eating and drinking, (3) eliminating, (4) moving and maintaining posture, (5) sleeping and resting, (6) clothing (dressing and undressing), (7) maintaining body temperature, (8) cleaning and grooming the body and protecting the integument (9) avoiding environmental dangers and injury of others, (10) communicating, (11) worshipping, (12) working, (13) playing and participating in recreation, and (14) learning and discovery. These basic needs of clients correspond with those of Maslow's hierarchy of needs that were described earlier.

Henderson also described environment and the nurse-patient relationship. She does not give her own definition of environment but relies on the Webster's New Collegiate Dictionary (1961) definition of environment as "the aggregate of all the external conditions and influences affecting the life and development of an organism."[1] Influenced by Orlando and Deavers, she views the nurse-patient relationship as having three levels, ranging from dependence to independence:

1. The nurse as a substitute for the patient in the period of grave illness.

2. The nurse as a helper to the patient in the period of convalescence.

3. The nurse as a partner to the patient. Although not specified by Henderson, we assume this is the period of rehabilitation.

Henderson believes that the nurse must be able to assess client needs and pathological conditions altering need states. Needs, as determined by the nurse, must be validated with the client. Both the nurse and client are always working toward a goal, whether this be independence or peaceful death. The nurse's goals are to keep the client's day as normal as possible and to promote health.

Henderson has ideas about how the nurse functions in relation to the physician and to other health team members. She believes that nurses do not *follow* doctors' orders, but help carry out the total program of care. Although she believes the functions of the physician and nurse often overlap, she does think they have distinct roles. Nurses work interdependently with other health team members. The responsibilities of each team member depend upon the current needs of the client. Thus the responsibilities of team members vary according to (1) the problem of the patient, (2) the patient's self-help ability, and (3) help resources.[4] These ideas are consistent with approaches used by rehabilitation teams.

Her approach to client care is deliberative and involves decision making. The nurse uses a problem-solving process called the nursing process to gather data; develop a plan that integrates the work of all health team members; and implement an individualized plan that considers physiological principles, age, cultural background, emotional balance, and physical and intellectual capabilities of the client.

Henderson[12] incorporates beliefs about education and research in her definition of nursing: "In order for a nurse to practice as an expert in her own right and to use the scientific approach to the improvement of practice, the nurse needs the kind of education available only in colleges and universities." She supports the development of nurses in a research atmosphere and strongly believes that research is needed to evaluate and improve nursing practice. Her hope is that nurses will conduct research to improve practice rather than merely to satisfy an academic responsibility.[6]

It is clear that Henderson has a broad definition of nursing, and her delineation of 14 basic needs of clients is relevant to rehabilitation nursing practice. Although she never intended to develop a theory of nursing, since theory development was not in vogue at that time, her definition lays the groundwork for developing a theory of rehabilitation nursing. Her experience in rehabilitation nursing; mentors in physiology, psychology, and rehabilitation medicine; and attention to nursing theories of client-nurse interaction have influenced more recent nurse theorists.

Lydia Hall: Quality of Nursing Theory

Lydia Hall,[11] one of the earlier nursing theorists, had several beliefs about nursing and patients. She proposed that patients have three interacting parts: core, care, and cure.[29] The core of the patient was the person and responded to the therapeutic use of self aspect of nursing, the care of the patient related to the body and responded to the intimate body care aspects of nursing, and the cure related to the disease and responded to seeing the patient and family through the medical care aspects of nursing. She believed persons came to the hospital for care and cure. Cure activities were primary to care activities in a modern medical center. Lacking, however, was and often is help to see the person through the core of difficulties. She believed help in the core difficulties would come when nurses were prepared to teach and were committed to individual learning.

Hall[11] believed in two distinct phases of medical care: (1) "intensive, diagnostic, biologically critical medicine and (2) evaluation and follow-up care." The first phase could last from a few days to more than a week; the latter phase could take a much longer time.

Hall identified health care professionals who took care of specific tasks related to the three aspects of the patient. The physician was expert in pathology and treatment, the CURE; the psychiatrist, psychologist, sociologist, economist, social case worker, and religious person were responsible for the spiritual development of the patient, the CORE. Hall[11] concluded that the public and the nurse viewed and respected the nurse as the expert in body CARE, that is, expert in its techniques and also in modifications in light of the pathology, treatment, and personality of the patient. By body care, she meant such processes as bathing, feeding, toileting, dressing, undressing, positioning, and moving.

According to Hall,[11] the nurse is the nurturer: "Our intent when we lay hands on the patient in bodily care is to comfort. While the patient is being comforted, he feels close to the comforting one. At this time, the person talks out and acts out those things that concern him—good, bad, and indifferent. If nothing more is done with these, what the patient gets is ventilation, or catharsis. This may bring relief of anxiety and tension but not necessarily learning. If the individual who is in the comforting role can offer a teaching-learning experience around the client's need, he/she proceeds to something beyond—someone who fosters learning, someone who fosters growing up emotionally, someone who even fosters healing." However, she believed when patients were most receptive to teaching and learning (her phase II of medical care), their care was left primarily to practical nurses and aides, those least equipped by their education to provide the kind of care needed.

Hall's major contribution was to develop a theory that was testable in rehabilitation nursing practice. The Loeb Center, established at Montefiore Hospital, New York City, has supported the propositions in her theory. The philosophy of this unit demands that nurses direct the admission, rehabilitation, discharge, and follow-up care of clients. Furthermore, she encouraged the recognition of professional nursing's contribution to client outcome.[5] Her emphasis was on teaching and learning and physical care as a means of establishing rapport with the client. She perceived teaching and learning as a way to change behavior. Rehabilitation nurses use the teaching-learning principles discussed in Chapter 5 to teach clients new ways to perfom self-care and to live with a disability.

Dorothea Orem: Self-Care Deficit Theory

Dorothea Orem,[24,25] a more recent theorist, states that "self-care is the practice of activities that individuals initiate and perform on their own behalf in maintaining life, health, and well-being. . . ." It is an adult's "continuous contribution to his or her own continued existence."[25] She described three categories of self-care: (1) universal self-care activities that support the basic needs for air, water, and food; elimination; activity and rest; solitude and social interaction; hazards to life and well-being; and being normal; (2) developmental

self-care activities that promote developmental processes throughout life; and (3) health deviation self-care activities that result when there are obvious changes in human structure (edematous extremities, contractures, decubiti), physical functioning (difficulty breathing, limited movement of a joint), or in behavior and habits of daily living (extreme irritability in relations with others, sudden changes in mood, loss of interest in life) that focus a person's attention on self.[25]

Orem views the nurse's role as one of helping people "maintain continuously that amount and quality of self-care which is therapeutic in sustaining life and health, in recovering from disease or injury, or in coping with their effects."[2] She describes the action necessary when disease, injury, or disability occur as "(1) adjusting the ways of meeting universal self-care requirements, (2) establishing new ways of self-care, (3) modifying the self-image, (4) revising the routine of daily living, (5) developing a new life-style compatible with the effects of the health deviation, and (6) coping with the effects of the health deviation or the medical care used in the treatment of it. . . ."[24] These actions necessitate relationships with a number of health care workers. Nurses, she believed, have a unique role in helping individuals to manage the multitude of relationships necessary to meet self-care demands.

Nursing involves assisting clients in the design, provision, and management of self-care to improve human functioning. Nursing intervention is needed when qualitative or quantitative self-care deficits interfere with a client's ability to meet therapeutic self-care demands.

Orem also describes three categories of nursing intervention or "nursing systems": wholly compensatory, partially compensatory, and supportive-educative. Wholly compensatory systems occur when the client has no active role in performing self-care. In other words, the nurse acts for or does for the person who is unconscious or totally incapacitated. A partially compensatory system is used when "both the nurse and client perform care measures requiring manipulative tasks or ambulation."[25] The assistance given depends upon the client's actual physical or medically prescribed limitations, the scientific or technical knowledge of the nurse, and the psychosocial readiness of the client to care for self. For example, a person who must lie prone because of a sacral pressure sore can still inspect all areas of the body for redness, the nurse requires scientific or technical knowledge to measure circumference of both calves in order to detect deep vein thrombosis in the immobile client, and the client's psychosocial readiness determines readiness for inserting his or her own catheter. The supportive-educative system is used when "the patient is able to perform or can and should learn to perform required measures of externally or internally oriented therapeutic self-care but cannot do so without assistance."[25] When a self-care deficit is identified, the nursing system selected is based on "who can or should perform those self-care actions that require movement in space or manipulation."[25]

Knust and Quarn[18] suggest that "the key to utilizing self-care theory in rehabilitative nursing is a thorough assessment of each category of self-care (universal, developmental, and health deviation). The interrelationship among areas of the assessment indicates the uniqueness of the individual client and ultimately directs interventions that are holistic." They also identify some problems in the application of criteria Orem uses to determine the effective nursing system. Orem states that "patients with extensive action limitations may develop the capabilities needed to design and manage their own care and to guide and direct a helper. . . ."[25] However, her choice of the wholly compensatory nursing system focuses on physical disability while negating psychosocial ability. Knust and Quarn point out that "while a severely disabled person might be wholly dependent on others to perform the universal self-care requisites previously mentioned, the person may be 'wholly independent' in directing and taking responsibility for his own care."[2] Knust and Quarn believe all three nursing systems may be operational at the same time with the same client. Since the rehabilitation process is dynamic, the nursing systems must be dynamically applied.

Imogene King: Theory of Goal Attainment

Imogene King[16] initially identified social systems, perception, interpersonal relations, and health as a conceptual framework for nursing practice. Later she developed a theory of goal attainment from this conceptual framework.[17] She proposed an open systems model with three subsystems—the individual, groups, and social systems—all of which interact dynamically. Major concepts

within each of these subsystems are explained as substantive content for nursing and relate primarily to the interpersonal relationship between the patient and the nurse. She describes the nurse-patient interaction as two people who are usually strangers coming together "in a health care organization to help and to be helped to maintain a state of health that permits functioning in roles."[16]

The theory of goal attainment describes the nature of nurse-patient interactions. Perception, communication, transaction, role, growth and development, time, space, and stress are viewed as influences on the nature of the nurse-patient interaction. The intended consequences of the nurse-patient interaction are attainment of nurse and patient goals. If goals are to be attained, perceptual accuracy, transaction, mutual goal setting, communication leading to satisfaction, a decrease in stress and anxiety, an increase in patient learning and coping ability, and congruence in role expectation and role performance must occur.[16]

In King's perspective, the goal of nursing action is to interact purposefully with clients to mutually establish goals and means for achieving them. The focus of nursing action is the patient who is potentially stressed and unable to cope with changes in daily activities. The nurse's role is to help patient's attain, maintain, and restore health, and, when this is not possible, to help them die with dignity. Individuals experience difficulty when they cannot cope with changes in daily living.[17]

The nurse-patient interaction is the intervention focus. When transactions are made between the nurse and patient, goals are attained. King tested her theory to describe the elements in nurse-patient interactions that lead to transaction. She identified them as nurse-patient interactions, relationships between the elements that lead to transaction, and the essential variables in nurse-patient reactions that lead to transactions. In a small sample, she found that the following elements in nurse-patient interactions lead to transactions: identification of a problem, concern or disturbance in the patient environment; exploration of the situation, shared information, and mutually set goals; exploration of the means to resolve the problem and achievement of goals; and action by the patient and the nurse to implement a plan and attain a goal. Although she does not describe the findings, she identified accurate perceptions of the nurse and the patient, adequate communication, and mutual goal setting as the essential variables found in nurse-patient interactions that result in transaction.[17]

King describes a number of areas of concern for rehabilitation nurses. Her perspective is concerned with the client who experiences disturbances in ability to cope with changes in daily living. Her holistic view of the client includes body image, growth and development, stress, time, space, and role as a disabled individual, family member, and societal member. She recognizes that both the nurse and the client have concerns, needs, and values. The nurse uses the nursing process to assist the individual in coping with changes in daily living and return to social roles. The nurse must establish goals with the client and then measure client outcome based on accomplishment of these goals.

Sr. Callista Roy: Theory of Adaptation

Sr. Callista Roy formulated a theory of adaptation for nursing practice based on the work of Helson. According to Roy, "man, as a biopsychosocial being, is interacting constantly with his changing environment."[34] To cope with change, humans use innate and acquired mechanisms that are biological, psychological, and social in origin. At any given time, human health can be identified along a health-illness continuum and responds to a variety of environmental stimuli. A positive response requires adaptation. Since "nursing is concerned with man as a total being at some point along the health-illness continuum,"[34] the function of the nurse becomes one of supporting and promoting adaptation.

Roy identifies four modes of adaptation. The first involves basic physiological needs, including circulation, temperature regulation, oxygen, fluids, sleep, activity, elimination, and digestion. These needs must be kept in balance as humans respond to the environment. The occurrence of disability or chronic illness presents a severe threat to the maintenance of basic physiological needs.

The second mode of adaptation relates to one's self-concept. "Self-concept is a term which encompasses conscious and unconscious thoughts, beliefs, attitudes, and values that an individual has regarding himself and his world."[34] The concept of self changes continuously and is influenced

by one's own image, feedback from significant others, success in performing social roles and responsibilities, and location on the health-illness continuum.

In role mastery, Roy's third mode of adaptation, "man regulates his performance of duties according to his varying positions in society."[34] For example, when a man becomes disabled, he may no longer be able to perform prescribed family roles, such as breadwinner, father, or husband. Often those members of the family who are not disabled must change existing roles and responsibilities to accommodate the tasks previously assigned to the disabled family member.[34] This same man may not be able to fulfill his roles in the community as a scout leader, voter, and political party committee person.

The fourth mode of adaptation is interdependence. According to Roy, "the self-concept of a person and his role mastery interact with other persons in the environment in an interdependent way."[34] Essentially, a change in environment may threaten interdependence related to self-concept and role mastery. A person's needs are based on level of adaptation within the four modes, and any change in the environment can provide a threat to one or more of them. She recognizes that at any point on the health-illness continuum the individual who has a disability is bombarded with environmental stimuli that necessitate adaptation.

Roy's adaptation theory can be used as a framework for rehabilitation nursing practice. The disabled person experiences both overt and covert physiological changes that may affect self-concept negatively and hinder successful adaptation to a disability. Roy views the role of the nurse as assisting the client and family in achieving a positive response and thus adaptation to environmental stimuli, a role that is often enacted by rehabilitation nurses. She also identifies the nursing process as the method by which the nurse delivers nursing care.

Roper: Activities of Living

Roper,[33] a British nurse theorist, developed a model of living to conceptualize an "amalgam of activities," with activities of living as the criteria for the model. She defines activities of living as all things people do in everyday life and with which they need help when they are unable to

---

Activities of Daily Living

To sustain life
Breathing
Controlling body temperature
Eating and swallowing
Bladder elimination
Bowel elimination
Sleep and rest
Maintaining skin integrity

To participate in life
Personal hygiene and grooming
Communication
Movement
Sexuality and sexual function
Work and recreation
Accessing home and community
Coping

---

perform these activities independently.[33] Breathing, eliminating, controlling body temperature, eating, sleeping, washing, dressing, communicating, moving, maintaining a safe environment, expressing sexuality, and dying are examples of activities of living. Several dimensions and many specific activities may be involved in each activity of living. Compounding this complexity is the fact that all of these activities are interrelated and affect total function.[33] For example, for one individual, absence of movement of the lower extremities may affect relationships with friends, the ability to dress, and the ability to get to the bathroom, despite the availability of a wheelchair. In another individual with the same impairment, a wheelchair will allow independence in these same functions.

Performing self-care tasks, such as breathing, eating, controlling body temperature, eliminating, maintaining skin integrity, and obtaining sleep and comfort, enable a client to sustain life. Other activities of living, such as personal hygiene and dressing, communicating, moving about, engaging in work and play, establishing and maintaining intimate relationships, and coping, allow a client to participate in life. The self-care tasks shown in the box are addressed in parts II and III of this book.

Roper's client model of living contributes to her model of nursing by explaining the dependence-independence continuum experienced by clients and the circumstances that prevent movement toward maximum independence. These are identified as physical, psychological, and social environment; disability and disturbed physiology; degenerative or pathological tissue changes; and accidents.[33]

In Roper's model of nursing, nursing activities are described as prevention, comfort, and dependence of nursing in such areas as administration of prescribed medications and treatments. The focus on activities of living is also the focus of rehabilitation nurses, and Roper's components of nursing are similar to the activities described by Hall as relating to the core of the patient.

Roper's theory of nursing is similar to Henderson's definition of nursing. She addresses social and biological aspects of living, as well as stages of growth and development, as concepts. Her framework considers function in activities of daily living on a dependence-independence continuum. She also identifies the nursing process as the vehicle whereby the nurse delivers nursing care.

SUMMARY

Theory provides a framework for nursing practice, research, and education. Theory development and testing are essential to the advancement of nursing science overall and rehabilitation nursing practice in particular. This chapter provides a definition of theory and a description of its purposes. Selected theories "borrowed" from other disciplines and theories proposed by nursing theorists are presented and their relevance for rehabilitation nursing described. Although theory cannot be directly applied to daily rehabilitation nursing practice, knowledge of the concepts in the theories presented here can be used to guide rehabilitation nursing practice, stimulate thought about theory development applicable to rehabilitation nursing, design research studies to test hypotheses generated by these theories, and guide curriculum in teaching rehabilitation nursing to student nurses.

REFERENCES

1. Abdellah FG and Strachan EJ: Progressive patient care, Am J Nurs 59:5, May 1959.
2. Bandura A: Behavior theory and the models of man, Am Psychol 29:859, Dec 1974.
3. Baranowski T: A cognitive-emotional social learning theory approach to regimen compliance behavior. Paper presented at the meeting of the American Psychological Association, New York, Sept 1979.
4. Chinn PL and Jacobs MK: Theory and nursing: a systematic approach, ed 2, St Louis, 1987, The CV Mosby Co.
5. Choi EC: Evolution of nursing theory development. In Marriner A, editor: Nursing theorists and their work, St Louis, 1986, The CV Mosby Co.
6. DeMeester DW, Lauer T, and Neal SE: Virginia Henderson: definition of nursing. In Marriner A, editor: Nursing theorists and their work, St Louis, 1986, The CV Mosby Co.
7. Flaskerud JH and Halloran EJ: Areas of agreement in nursing theory development, Adv Nurs Sci 3(1):1, 1980.
8. Griffith-Kenney JW: Overview of selected theoretical approaches. In Griffith-Kenney JW and Christensen PJ, editors: Nursing process: application of theories, frameworks, and models, ed 2, St Louis, 1986, The CV Mosby Co.
9. Griffith-Kenney JW: Relevance of theoretical approaches. In Griffith-Kenney JW and Christensen PJ, editors: Nursing process: application of theories, frameworks, and models, ed 2, St Louis, 1986, The CV Mosby Co.
10. Hall CS and Lindzey G: Theories of personality, New York, 1957, John Wiley & Sons, Inc.
11. Hall LE: The Loeb Center for nursing and rehabilitation, Int J Nurs Stud 5:81, 1969.
12. Henderson V: The nature of nursing: a definition and its implications for practice, research, and education, New York, 1966, Macmillan Publishing Co, Inc.
13. Henderson V and Nite GA: The principles and practice of nursing, New York, 1978, Macmillan Publishing Co, Inc.
14. Hingson R and others: In sickness and in health: social dimensions of medical care, St Louis, 1981, The CV Mosby Co.
15. Kerlinger FN: Foundations of behavioral research, New York, 1973, Holt, Rinehart & Winston, Inc.
16. King IM: Toward a theory for nursing: general concepts of human behavior, New York, 1971, John Wiley & Sons, Inc.
17. King IM: A theory for nursing: systems, concepts, process, New York, 1981, John Wiley & Sons, Inc.
18. Knust SJ and Quarn JM: Integration of self-care theory with rehabilitation nursing, Rehabil Nurs 8:26, July/Aug 1983.
19. Leslie GR, Larson RF, and Gorman BL: Introductory sociology, ed 3, London, 1980, Oxford University Press, Inc.
20. Marriner A: Nursing theorists and their work, St Louis, 1986, The CV Mosby Co.
21. Maslow AH: Toward a psychology of being, ed 2, Princeton, NJ, 1968, D Van Nostrand Co, Inc.
22. Mechanic D: Students under stress, New York, 1962, The Free Press.
23. Mechanic D: Medical sociology, New York, 1968, The Free Press.
24. Orem DE: Nursng: concepts of practice, New York, 1971, McGraw-Hill Book Co.
25. Orem DE: Nursing: concepts of practice, ed 2, New York, 1980, McGraw-Hill Book Co.
26. Parcel GS and Baranowski T: Social learning theory and health education, Health Educ 12:14, May/June 1981.
27. Parsons T: Definitions of health and illness in light of American values and social structure. In Jaco EG, editor: Patients, physicians and illness, New York, 1972, The Free Press.
28. Parsons T: The social system, New York, 195_, The Free Press.
29. Pescoe KT and Gumm SB: Lydia E Hall: Core, care, and cure model. In Marriner A: Nursing theorists and their work, St Louis, 1986, The CV Mosby Co.
30. Polit DF and Hungler BP: Nursing research: principles and methods, ed 2, Philadelphia, 1983, JB Lippincott Co.
31. Riley MW and Waring J: Age and aging. In Merton RK and Nisbet R, editors: Contemporary social problems, New York, 1976, Harcourt, Brace, Jovanovich, Inc.
32. Rogers M: An introduction to the theoretical basis of nursing, Philadelphia, 1970, FA Davis Co.
33. Roper N, Logan WW, and Tierney AG: The elements of nursing, New York, 1980, Churchill Livingstone, Inc.
34. Roy C: The Roy adaptation model. In Riehl JP and Roy C, editors: Conceptual models for nursing practice, ed 2, New York, 1980, Appleton-Century-Crofts.
35. Seaman CC and Verhonick PJ: Research methods for undergraduate students in nursing, ed 2, New York, 1982, Appleton-Century-Crofts.
36. Selye H: The stress of life, New York, 1956, McGraw-Hill Book Co.
37. Selye H: Stress without distress, Philadelphia, 1974, JB Lippincott Co.
38. Thomas E: Problems of disability from the perspective of role theory, J Health Hum Behav 7:2, Spring 1966.
39. Wilson HS: Research in nursing, Menlo Park, Calif, 1985, Addison-Wesley Publishing Co, Inc.

ADDITIONAL READINGS

Chang BL: Evaluation of health care professionals in facilitating self-care: review of the literature and a conceptual model, Adv Nurs Sci 3(1):43, 1980.

Cox CL: An interaction model of client health behavior: theoretical prescription for nursing, Adv Nurs Sci 5(1):41, 1982.

Dohrenwend BS and Dohrenwend BP: Stressful life events: their nature and effects, New York, 1974, John Wiley & Sons, Inc.

Gambrill ED: Behavior modification, San Francisco, 1981, Jossey-Bass, Inc, Publishers.

King IM: Keynote address: translating research into practice, J Neurosci Nurs 19:44, Feb 1987.

Jaco EG, editor: Patients, physicians, and illness, New York, 1972, The Free Press.

Levine S and Scotch A: Social stress, Chicago, 1970, Aldine Publishing Co.

Monat A and Lazarus RS, editors: Stress and coping: an anthology, New York, 1977, Columbia University Press.

Moss GE: Illness, immunity and social interaction, New York, 1973, John Wiley & Sons, Inc.

Scott CW: A stress coping model, Adv Nurs Sci 3(1):9, 1980.

Silva MC and Rothbart D: An analysis of changing trends in philosophies of science on nursing theory development and testing, Adv Nurs Sci 6(2):1, 1984.

Stone GC and others: Health psychology—a handbook, San Francisco, 1979, Jossey-Bass, Inc, Publishers.

Wiggins SR: Lydia Hall's place in the development of theory in nursing, Image 12:10, Feb 1980.

CHAPTER 3

Rehabilitation Team

Sharon S. Dittmar

OBJECTIVES

After completing Chapter 3, the reader will be able to:

1. Define the concept "rehabilitation team."
2. Describe the rationale for development of the team approach.
3. Identify responsibilities of the rehabilitation team leader and rehabilitation team members.
4. Describe the roles and functions of individual rehabilitation team members.
5. Examine team processes: communication, collaboration, coordination, evaluation.
6. Recognize barriers to effective team function.

A holistic approach to rehabilitation of the individual who is disabled requires the expertise of a number of rehabilitation disciplines. Although there has been a paucity of research concerning the team approach, it has been the established practice of rehabilitation disciplines to work together to meet the physical, social, emotional, economic, and vocational needs of these individuals and their family members.

Although rehabilitation teams have been the modus operandum, it is not always easy to function as a team leader or team member. One main reason is that health care professionals receive little, if any, formal education on working with members of other disciplines in a collegial relationship. Thus, nurses and other rehabilitation team members often have little more than a superficial understanding of each other's roles and functions.

This chapter includes a definition of the re-

habilitation team, a rationale for the development of a team approach to rehabilitative care, a discussion of the responsibilities of the team leader and team members, an examination of roles and functions of individual team members, a description of team processes, and identification of barriers to effective team functioning.

DEFINITION OF TEAM CONCEPT

Webster's *Third New International Dictionary* (1979) defines team as "a number of persons associated together in work or activity: a group of specialists or scientists functioning as a collaborative unit." Teamwork is defined as "work done by a number of associates with usually each doing a clearly defined portion but all subordinating personal prominence to the efficiency of the whole."

This definition of team can be applied to a number of circumstances and situations. Disaster teams are composed of persons who specialize in working together in times of emergency to meet individual and community needs. Snow removal teams clear snow from clogged thoroughfares. Football teams compete to win a game. Members of these teams receive special training and practice long hours to give their best to the team effort.

In health care, there also are many types of teams. Multidisciplinary teams consist of people from a number of disciplines who may or may not meet together to coordinate efforts. In contrast, interdisciplinary teams meet and work together to coordinate the plan for rehabilitation and to meet the complex needs of individuals with disability and chronic illness. Hirschberg, Lewis, and Vaughan[11] emphasize that the team must be efficient and economic and point out that when team members vie for control of what each considers important, rehabilitation may be delayed. Thus the disabled person could be subjected to complicated but fragmented care.

Although there are many types of teams and varying definitions, certain commonalities define the term team. First, two or more persons who have regular communication for a common purpose are viewed as a team. Second, the communications of these persons are coordinated through an identified leader. Third, roles and functions of team members are clarified, agreed upon, and centered around a task. Finally, teams that function smoothly and effectively have either rules as norms or formalized procedure manuals.

The size and composition of the rehabilitation team are influenced by many factors. These include the geographic location of the rehabilitation setting, the typical needs of the clients served, the philosophy and concept of rehabilitation existing in the agency, the financial resources available for hiring personnel, the availability of personnel, and state and federally mandated policies and requirements.

The client and family are the core members of the rehabilitation team and the reasons for its existence. The constant rehabilitation team consists of a rehabilitation nurse, physical therapist, occupational therapist, speech language pathologist, nutritionist, psychologist, social worker, physiatrist, and vocational rehabilitation counselor. Other persons who may become members of the team, depending upon the client's particular

situation and needs, are the audiologist, biomedical engineer, prosthetist, orthotist, and cleric. At various stages of rehabilitation, representatives of community services, as well as equipment and supply houses, may become an integral part of the team.

During the acute stage of rehabilitation, the rehabilitation team also relies heavily on a number of medical specialists. A neurologist, orthopedist, surgeon, gastroenterologist, or urologist may be called upon for management of specific aspects of care or may act as the coordinator of care. Their involvement will vary according to specific client situations during the rehabilitation process.

The leader of the team during the acute stage is usually the physician. Leadership of the team is not confined to any one profession but may be assigned by team members according to client needs, by traditional practice in a facility, or by the organizational structure that exists in the agency. It is important that the client recognizes one person as the primary coordinator of the rehabilitation plan and that the team members recognize one person as the leader of the team in relation to goals and policies. These positions may be one and the same, or the coordinator of a client's care plan may be appointed by the team leader. Ideally, the client eventually becomes the team leader and coordinator of his or her own care plan, calling upon team members only when assistance is needed to solve problems.

The roles of the rehabilitation team members are identifiable by virtue of educational preparation and standards of practice. A rehabilitation team that operates effectively consists of members who understand and respect the educational backgrounds, professional attitudes, personalities, and approaches to client care used by each member of the team and can work together with the client and family members to contribute to one total rehabilitation plan. Although roles and functions may overlap and sometimes conflict, no one person on a team is prepared to assume all the roles of other team members.

Rehabilitation teams generally meet at specified intervals to coordinate the team plan of care and follow an established format for conduct and documentation of the conference. The client and family may attend all, some, or none of the meetings. Regardless of the manner in which the client and family participate, their input, feelings, and decisions about any proposed plan of care should be obtained before and during implementation of the rehabilitation plan. Goals are mutually established with the client and family. Without their participation in goal setting, implementing the plan, and evaluating the outcome, the rehabilitation process is doomed to failure.

The protocol for conduct and documentation of team conferences varies from agency to agency but usually involves the reports of each discipline on the client's short- and long-term goals, functional progress, discharge plans with a projected discharge date, and team plan for follow-up monitoring and maintenance care. Each discipline contributes professional expertise to the total rehabilitation plan, and the treatment plans are coordinated through the direction of the team leader. Written reports of the team meetings are recorded in the client's record and are available for review by all team members and by third-party payers.

RATIONALE FOR THE DEVELOPMENT OF A TEAM APPROACH

According to Rothberg,[18] "we in rehabilitation speak of 'team delivery' of services and care as though we had invented and perfected the concept." Such is not the case. The major factors that have been particularly relevant in the development of the team approach in rehabilitation are the concept of the client as a total person, the need for coordination of fragmented care, the needs of organizations, and external mandates from federal and state agencies.

The rehabilitation philosophy presented in Chapter 1 addressed the individual as a holistic being, a belief that has been adopted by most other health care disciplines. Early in this century, medicine and nursing were able to meet the needs of clients. As society evolved from an agrarian to an industrial orientation and then to an information society within a technological age, individual lives became more complex, expectations of quality of life changed, different health problems affected activities of daily living, and costs of maintaining and restoring abilities necessary for quality of life dramatically increased. Consequently, new health care professions emerged and proliferated, each with in-depth knowledge and expertise in a specific area of client need. When a number of health care disciplines serve the same

client, care can become fragmented. This places a burden on the client to relate to a number of health care professionals who may or may not communicate with one another in establishing a consistent plan of care. Thus a need existed to coordinate services of the growing number of health care disciplines so that the treatment plan of one discipline would not conflict with the plan implemented by other disciplines.[5] Theoretically, the collective expertise of these disciplines should equal more than the sum of a number of health care professionals delivering services to an individual and family.

As society became more complex, organizations grew in number and size. A need for clarifying communication to individual clients and for establishing channels of communication within and among organizations became apparent. The team approach was one method of facilitating communication and providing an information exchange among health professionals within the organization and between health professionals and the administrative officers of organizations.

Health care organizations also are controlled by external forces such as legislation, state and federal regulations, and requirements of third-party payers. The development of the team approach to care was one way of improving quality and professional accountability. Rehabilitation professionals were in the forefront in seeing the need for a team approach that is, in many instances, now imposed from outside forces.[5]

RESPONSIBILITIES OF THE REHABILITATION TEAM LEADER

Any team member with knowledge of small-group dynamics, organizational acumen, interpersonal skills, and commitment to excellence in rehabilitative care could function as the leader of the rehabilitation team. More often, leadership is assigned according to the ascribed status of a discipline or by team or organizational policies that delineate academic and professional background for the position. Professional background may or may not include previous preparation or experience in leadership positions. Conversely, research attempts to distinguish the characteristics that identify leaders from nonleaders has been disappointing. What has emerged is the conclusion that leaders must be able to perform certain functions to accomplish the goals of a group and be able to adapt to changing situations. This view of leadership stresses the characteristics of the group within the current situation, a view entirely consistent with the notion that leadership of the team can rotate as the needs of the client and of the team change.

Team leadership involves certain responsibilities. First, although certain leadership functions are shared with other members of the team, the leader must assume overall responsibility for the coordination of client care and for guiding the team in planning, implementing, and evaluating rehabilitation programs. The team leader must act as a role model for other potential leaders by consulting team members, respecting and listening to their professional advice, and involving them in administrative decisions of the agency that affect the team.

The team leader also must be able to identify the talents of team members and use those talents appropriately. Some group members may have particular talents for facilitating group process or coming up with creative ideas when others are blocked in their thought processes. Complimenting these abilities stimulates team members to work together toward accomplishment of team goals.

The primary functions of the team leader are to guide the team in establishing goals with the client and family and in implementing plans to meet these goals. As team members work on these tasks, the leader must be concerned with evaluation of the group process. When there is conflict between group members, the leader must objectively intervene by confronting the conflict with all members of the team, reflecting feelings, and interpreting behaviors in bringing the issue out in the open or diplomatically handling obvious conflicts. The leader must concentrate on the issues rather than the personalities of individual team members involved.

Sampson and Marthas[19] offered these suggestions for the management of conflict:

1. The leader should support the right of members to disagree and support the view that disagreement can be a healthy process.
2. The basis of the conflict should be clarified. The leader may wish to summarize the position taken by each party in the dispute and ask for validation or modification of this perception.
3. A compromise should be negotiated. All possible areas of agreement should be identified and explored. Using commonalities in the parties' perceptions, possibilities for compromise of the opposing perspectives should be explored and negotiated. The leader may wish to summarize the actions and changes required of each party in implementing the compromise.

In one team I participated in, the clinical nurse specialist was the leader. Although attempts were made to rotate team leadership of conferences, members, by group consensus, assigned the leadership of team meetings to her. Each team member, however, acted as a coordinator of care for clients whose needs could best be met by his or her discipline or because the client worked well with that particular team member. During the later stages of rehabilitation, the client often assumed the coordinator role and effectively solved problems with the assistance of other team members.

RESPONSIBILITIES OF REHABILITATION TEAM MEMBERS

Few health professionals are educationally or experientially prepared to assume collegial relationships with other team members to accomplish common tasks. Few disciplines have educational programs whereby students from different disciplines learn and work together on joint assignments, thus gaining experience in working as a team member. The nurse or other health care professional commonly has a first experience with team membership when it is required as a responsibility in the rehabilitation setting. Consequently, there may be little appreciation for the professional viewpoints of others and the interprofessional dynamics that are part of the team process.

To accept the point of view of another team member, an individual must recognize that[17]:

1. The perception of the task is influenced by personal experiences, previous educational preparation, and previous professional experience.
2. Perception is a primary determinant of behavior.
3. Subsequent behavior influences perception, which further influences behavior in a reciprocal fashion.
4. Behavior is reciprocal.

These forces are universal, expected, and often hidden from both the perceiver and the person being perceived. Often, judgments about the value and talents of other team members are made almost immediately. Often, these initial impressions are not accurate. Team members who work well together seek to discover how they appear to members of other disciplines, determine whether the cognitive and affective messages they are sending are interpreted correctly, and try to understand that opinions quickly made about others are time-limited hypotheses to be "tested" rather than set conclusions for which to gather support.[14]

As a group, team members have a common goal, that is, maintaining and enhancing client function. However, each member belongs to a different discipline with a separate and sometimes antagonistic identity. At times, role overlap can threaten the territory of another discipline. For example, when an occupational therapist working with one rehabilitation team wanted to learn more about intermittent catheterization, the nurse felt her territory was threatened. However, after further discussion with the therapist about a specific client's situation, the nurse discovered that the occupational therapist wanted to understand the catheterization schedule in order to plan for retraining in the kitchen and to design an adaptive device to assist the client in handling the catheter. Seeking further information enabled the nurse and occupational therapist to work together when each could have become angry because of perceived encroachment on professional territory.

To function effectively as a team member, team members accustomed to rehabilitation teamwork must act as role models for new team members and allow time for them to practice interacting as a team. This can be accomplished through formal inservice education programs in which communication, collaboration, territoriality, and managing conflict are discussed; through videotaping and analyzing team interaction; and through observation and critical analysis of team function. One of the best ways for new members to learn to work as a team is to be given assignments together that further the goals of the client and family, as well as the goals of the rehabilitation team and the organization.

Understanding and respecting the knowledge and skills of others is necessary to work as a team member. New members of the team should be welcomed and roles and functions of team members explained. Perspectives of the new team member should be given careful attention, since a new person often will offer better ideas and a fresh outlook in solving problems. Members of a team learn to respect each other through working together with the client and family in solving particularly difficult functional problems, suffering setbacks and disappointments together, and experiencing a sense of accomplishment when team efforts improve client and family function. When team members work together on such necessary projects as quality assurance, protocol manuals, and client and family education programs, they learn to appreciate and respect each other as individuals and as professionals.

According to Rothberg,[18] "we must develop clearer definitions of the roles and behaviors expected of team participants and lessen ambiguities regarding our expectations of others." One way to accomplish this task is to schedule retreats away from the agency so team members can review their roles and functions, state their wishes for team directions, evaluate their functions as team members and as a team, and plan ways to maintain, improve, eliminate, or expand their programs for the coming year. For example, at one such retreat a social reintegration program was planned. An occupational therapist, physical therapist, nurse, and psychologist volunteered to plan, implement, and evaluate a program that involved four sequential community social outings for clients. Each outing required progressively more social interaction. The sessions began with a visit to a zoo and ended with a night out to dinner at a local restaurant. Before and after each social outing, clients discussed their feelings about being disabled and reactions of able-bodied persons to their disability. Team members who had planned the program met during the week to develop criteria for acceptance of additional clients in the program, discuss the participation of each discipline, plan ways to finance the program, and determine directions for team research related to assisting individuals with social reintegration. This experience helped team members to better define professional roles and behaviors. Each member of the team contributed expertise to some aspect of the social reintegration program and worked together with other members in planning, implementing, and determining methods of evaluation.

ROLES AND FUNCTIONS OF INTERDISCIPLINARY REHABILITATION TEAM MEMBERS

A role is an expectation each team member has of another because of educational background, socioeconomic status, work experience, and personal background. Functions are those tasks expected of persons who fulfill expected roles on the rehabilitation team. No member works independently but contributes expertise to the total rehabilitation plan.

Core Members

Clients and their families are the core members of the team and must be included in goal setting and development of the plan of care, since there is no plan of care without their participation. To participate to the fullest extent, they must be able to obtain knowledge about the specific disability and practice care procedures with supervision until they can demonstrate safe performance. Clients and family members have a right to take charge of their own care and mobility, as well as to pursue work and play opportunities and gain expertise in accurately and appropriately directing their own care when unable to perform such care independently. (See Chapter 1.)

When clients are expected to be active participants and are the ultimate decision makers about their participation in a rehabilitation program, they play a major role in the development and implementation of the care plan. Clients also provide information about themselves, ask questions, and obtain knowledge needed to make informed decisions. Legislation mandates participation of clients and families receiving services from state and federal rehabilitation programs. The signature of the client receiving these services is required on the individualized written rehabilitation program.[5]

The family can share information and insights about the client with the rehabilitation team. Frequently, a family member will be the primary assistant in the rehabilitation program when the client returns to the community. Inclusion of appropriate family members in the planning and implementation of the rehabilitation program can contribute to the overall outcome of the plan. Family members also can support other families in the agency who are at different stages of adaptation to disablement of a family member.

Constant Members

The rehabilitation nurse, physical therapist, occupational therapist, speech language pathologist, nutritionist, psychologist, social worker, physiatrist, and vocational rehabilitation counselor are usually considered to be members of the rehabilitation team, regardless of whether rehabilitation services are delivered in an institution or in the community.

Rehabilitation nurse

Nurses working in community-based rehabilitation programs, freestanding rehabilitation facilities, and rehabilitation units within hospitals may receive their basic education in diploma, associate degree, or baccalaureate degree programs. Nurses prepared at the master's degree level function as clinical specialists in rehabilitation nursing. Some nurses working in rehabilitation settings are prepared at the doctoral level. These nurses often conduct research and function as teachers or administrators. Rehabilitation nurses prepared in any of these educational programs are licensed as registered professional nurses and also may take certification examinations and be certified by the Association of Rehabilitation Nurses.

Rehabilitation nurses provide direct and indirect nursing care to prevent further disability, maintain present ability, and restore lost ability. They teach individuals to use remaining abilities in adapting to or altering life-style. To accomplish these goals, they assess the client as a total being and plan, implement, and evaluate nursing care. As team members nurses share the nursing care plan and the client's responses with other team members, reinforce the care plans of other disciplines, and contribute to the rehabilitation team care plan. The functions of rehabilitation nurses are described throughout this book.

Physical therapist

A physical therapist must have a baccalaureate degree in physical therapy. Some physical therapists continue their education to obtain a master's degree. Master's degree programs for qualified physical therapists can be 1 to 2 years long. Professional programs in this discipline are accredited by the American Physical Therapy Association, and physical therapists are licensed by the state in which they practice.[10] By 1990 the American Physical Therapy Association expects that all physical therapists will hold a master's degree.

The responsibilities of physical therapists are to evaluate, prevent, and manage disorders of human motion.[10] They assist clients in regaining function and in preventing pain and disability following disease, injury, or loss of a body part. Physical therapists evaluate muscle strength, range of joint motion, posture and gait, limb length and circumference, activities of daily living, sensory and motor function, orthotic and prosthetic fit and function, reflexes and muscle tone, and sensorimotor performance.

Depending upon the needs of the client, a physical therapy program includes various modalities. Among the responsibilities of the physical therapist are the administration of hydrotherapy; shortwave or microwave diathermy; ultrasound, infrared, and ultraviolet radiation; and electrical stimulation (including transcutaneous electrical nerve stimulation for control of pain). Additionally, physical therapists perform massage and intermittent venous compression; set up cervical and lumbar spinal traction; assist clients in performing therapeutic exercises, reeducating muscles, and improving coordination; and teach relaxation techniques, use of biofeedback, and use of orthotic, prosthetic, and other assistive devices, including crutches, canes, walkers, and wheelchairs.[15]

Occupational therapist

Occupational therapists hold a baccalaureate degree in occupational therapy and are certified by the American Occupational Therapy Association. Occupational therapists average 6 to 9 months of clinical experience in a baccalaureate program. They may choose a specialty area of occupational therapy in a master's degree program after obtaining a baccalaureate degree in a related field. Occupational therapists collaborate with other disciplines and participate in the development of a team treatment program.

The goal of occupational therapists is to maintain and to restore the client's physical and psy-

chological ability to function in preparation for return to work, family, school, or community. They assess muscles that need strengthening and coordination and recommend practical activities to improve strength. They also assess age-appropriate tasks and roles in family and community, including activities of daily living, work activities, play activities, and driving capabilities. Sensory function, motor skill, and coordination of the client are assessed before involvement in a specific program. Occupational therapists must know the medical diagnosis, physical status, mental and emotional status, and general condition of the client in order to conduct their evaluations.

They may teach homemaking skills, energy conservation, and work simplification methods to improve work tolerance. In addition, occupational therapists may work with the client to improve communication skills, such as reading, writing, and using the telephone. They may redirect vocational, avocational, and social interests to accommodate the specific disability.[10]

Functional occupational therapy usually complements physical therapy. Functional or kinetic activities are used for mobilizing, coordinating, or strengthening muscle parts. This work is coordinated with work of other members of the rehabilitation team and with certain phases of training in self-help, transfers, and daily living activities taught by nurses and physical therapists.[15] Occupational therapists also design assistive and adaptive devices to help the client in activities of daily living. In some occupational therapy departments, splints are designed for preventing or controlling potential deformities of the hand for clients with arthritis or hemiplegia. Functional splints such as a tenodesis splint for a person with quadriplegia are fitted, with assistance and practice opportunities provided for use of these splints.

Speech-language pathologist

Speech-language pathologists must be certified by the American Speech and Hearing Association after successful completion of a national examination in speech pathology and audiology. Speech-language pathologists must have a baccalaureate degree, although most are educated at the master's or doctoral level in their specialty area.[10]

Speech-language pathologists evaluate and treat communication disorders secondary to disability, surgical procedures, and developmental disorders. They may administer psycholinguistic, auditory, and speech-language tests. Speech therapy is concerned with resolving speech, language, and hearing problems that may affect expression, reception, or both. Treatment techniques are designed to facilitate speech and language recovery and also prepare staff and family members to communicate effectively with a client who has a communication disorder.

Nutritionist

Nutritionists possess a bachelor's degree in nutrition. Many have been prepared at the master's level and a few are obtaining doctoral degrees.

Nutritionists provide for the nutritional needs of disabled clients. They determine ideal body weight and nutritional history, decide what foods will facilitate swallowing, plan and modify special and therapeutic diets, educate team members in basic and therapeutic nutrition, counsel clients and family members about dietary modifications to be made after discharge, and consult with the rehabilitation team on client care problems related to nutrition.[2] Ongoing evaluation is based on weight monitoring, the client's general health, and adherence to the foods recommended to provide adequate nutrition.

Psychologist

Psychologists are minimally prepared at the master's level, but most psychologists hold a doctor of philosophy degree. Psychiatrists, on the other hand, possess a medical degree. The law states that only physicians can prescribe medication and engage in highly sophisticated treatment such as electroshock therapy.

Although rehabilitation psychology has not been established as a specialty within psychology, this area of practice has had a long history of contributions to clinical and counseling psychology. The Rehabilitation Psychology Division of the American Psychological Association has made attempts to define the field and training required for rehabilitation psychologists. Although standards exist for psychologists, there are no minimum standards for specialty practice of rehabilitation psychologists.[13]

Psychologists predict what the client is likely to do in rehabilitation and in relevant situations in the future. In addition, they identify stimulus situations and reinforcers that are likely to be effective in influencing behavior. Psychometric as-

sessment contributes to analysis of the precise configuration of intellectual, cognitive, and emotional changes created by the disability.[6]

Psychologists counsel clients and families in institutions and communities, conduct research, and act at times as primary therapists. They consult with rehabilitation team members to facilitate goal setting and behavioral management. Psychologists also instruct clients, families, and staff about expectations of cognitively impaired individuals, emotional adaptations to disability, and behavioral management techniques. In a number of rehabilitation facilities, psychologists meet regularly with staff members to assist them with difficult client problems and suggest alternate coping strategies.

Psychologists monitor progress through observation, feedback, and reassessment. The treatment plan and follow-up are modified as appropriate.[16] They rely on other members of the rehabilitation team for information regarding the client's response to recommended psychotherapeutic techniques. During team conferences, psychologists also may help team members recognize feelings toward the client that could interfere with the rehabilitation process.

Social worker

Social workers hold a master's degree and in some states must be certified with the Department of Human Resources.[10] Some social workers may choose to specialize in medical or psychiatric social work.

Social workers assess family support systems and assist clients and families in alleviating or solving personal problems that surface when disability and chronic illness occur. These problems may be related to work, finance, living situations, social life, marriage, child care, and emotional state.[16]

Social workers assess social situations and help the rehabilitation team view the client in light of the effect of the disability on the social situation and the effect of the social situation on the disability. They diagnose the psychosocial situation and use the problem-solving process to help the client. This assistance consists of support and encouraging change, while at the same time providing services offered by rehabilitation agencies and referral to appropriate community agencies.[21] They assist the client and family in obtaining income replacement, medical coverage for rehabilitative care and equipment needs, home modifications, transportation, appropriate placement in extended care, and recreational resources.[16]

Information is shared with the client and family and with the rehabilitation team members. Social workers remain available along with other team members after discharge to assist in problem solving and to act as resource persons.

Physiatrist

Physiatrists hold a medical degree and have completed a 4-year approved residency in the specialty of physical medicine and rehabilitation. During the final year of the residency, physicians take a written examination as the first part of the certification requirement. After completing 1 year of practice or additional research in the specialty, candidates take an oral examination to be certified by the American Board of Physical Medicine and Rehabilitation.[8]

Physiatrists are generally responsible for medical management of rehabilitation clients and facilitate physician-to-physician communication, determine medical diagnoses, and prescribe medical therapy appropriate for the client's physical and functional status.

In collaboration with other rehabilitation team members, they develop a comprehensive rehabilitation plan. Activities and therapies prescribed for the client by physiatrists are based on scientific knowledge, expertise in the field of physical medicine and rehabilitation, and individual assessments performed by rehabilitation team members. Physiatrists may coordinate activities of the team to provide continuity of care between departments, although more often, nurses now perform this activity. Physiatrists prescribe or recommend therapeutic aids such as medication, exercise regimens, mechanical or motorized wheelchairs, and prosthetic and orthotic devices, according to the needs of the client. They also confer with the client and family and their primary physician, arranging for consultations with other physicians as the need arises.

Physiatrists are responsible for evaluation of functional progress, the continuous evaluation of the comprehensive rehabilitation process for each client, altering the medical treatment plan based on progress and prognosis, and follow-up and maintenance medical care in the outpatient clinic.

Vocational rehabilitation counselor

Vocational rehabilitation counselors are prepared as specialists at the master's degree level. They are certified by the Board for Rehabilitation Certification. In some states, licensure is required.[10] Their expertise is in assessment of disability, vocational evaluation, and planning and coordination of rehabilitation services. Many vocational rehabilitation counselors also are prepared as psychologists.[7]

Vocational rehabilitation counselors provide employment evaluation, treatment, training, placement, and follow-up evaluation for disabled persons. They obtain the client's educational and vocational history and match people to jobs for which they are suited based on education, aptitude, skill, experience, and physical and mental ability. Vocational rehabilitation counselors consider the client's material needs, self-esteem, respect for others, financial disincentives, and motivation to work when collaborating with the client to plan for vocational rehabilitation.[16]

Counseling, reevaluation, and reeducation are continuous processes for vocational rehabilitation counselors. As part of the treatment plan, counselors administer vocational interest inventories or achievement tests to assist in decision making, act as liaisons with various community agencies such as the Office of Vocational Rehabilitation and Department of Labor and Industries, and are responsible for job placement and referral of individuals to employment services.[16] Outside the medical setting, vocational rehabilitation counselors are often regarded as "captains of the rehabilitation team."[1]

The role and functions of vocational rehabilitation counselors overlap with those of other disciplines. For example, social workers and clinical psychologists share some of the counselors' interests in the client's family relationships and functional performance in social roles in the community. Although all of these disciplines are represented on the rehabilitation team, the counselor, social worker, and psychologist often work together as a subgroup to ensure that areas of overlap become a strength rather than a barrier to the rehabilitation process.

Vocational rehabilitation counselors monitor client progress in relation to job placement and coordinate rehabilitative services as necessary. In addition, they act as liaisons between client and employer, interpreting job abilities and expectations and evaluating job performance. Findings are communicated to rehabilitation team members.

Additional Rehabilitation Team Members

A number of other persons at some time become part of the rehabilitation team. A complete discussion of these professionals and the support members of the team in rehabilitation facilities and in the community is beyond the scope of this book. However, some professionals—the audiologist, biomedical engineer, prosthetist-orthotist, and a member of the clergy—frequently are considered members of the team.

Audiologist

Audiologists evaluate the client's ability to hear vocal sounds. The ability to hear, as well as the ability to use alternate systems to hear, is assessed through the use of pure-tone audiometry, which measures hearing sensitivity to selected frequencies. The results are displayed on an audiogram.[20]

Audiologists may recommend and prescribe hearing aids and also instruct the client, family, and staff in their use and care. Audiologists also teach lip-reading or alternate modes of communication when hearing ability is absent or poor and sign language when a client is mute and deaf. Referral is made to community resources as necessary.

Audiologists reassess clients for appropriate use of therapeutic aids and participate in team evaluation with regard to communication reception.

Biomedical engineer

Biomedical engineers must hold a baccalaureate degree in engineering. This degree is supplemented by on-the-job training in a laboratory or rehabilitation unit. Some universities offer specialized courses in the field.

The need for specialists in biomedical engineering is growing. These specialists apply scientific theory and technology to the development of new medical instruments such as sonar devices, miniature transistorized radio transmitters, laser beams, and biofeedback instruments. They also replace and repair rehabilitation devices, such as the battery-operated artificial forearm and hand

that is activated by nerves and residual muscles and wheelchairs operated by the eyes. In addition, they work with computers and data processors. Their research focus includes evaluating the effects of medications on internal organs, brain mapping, investigating the operations of other parts of the nervous system, simulating complex biological systems, and evaluating the effects of environmental conditions on body processes.[7]

Prosthetist and orthotist

In many cases, the responsibilities of prosthetists and orthotists overlap so these are addressed simultaneously. Both of these careers require manual and mechanical skill, as well as inventiveness, accuracy, patience, concern for the disabled, and the ability to communicate effectively with the client, family, and other members of the rehabilitation team. Several leading universities offer courses of 2 to 5 weeks' duration for individuals with practical experience. Although once one could prepare for these occupations through apprenticeships, most prosthetists and orthotists now must obtain a baccalaureate degree. To become certified, a candidate must have an associate degree in either of these fields and take the certification examination offered by the American Board for Certification in Orthotics and Prosthetics.

These fields complement each other. Prosthetists make and fit prostheses, whereas orthotists make and fit orthopedic braces to support or correct body parts weakened by injury or disease. Both need a physician's prescription for their work. After the limbs or braces are made and fitted, physical or occupational therapists help the client learn to use the devices.[7]

Clergy

Members of the clergy fulfill a vital function for the client, family, and rehabilitation team. A number of hospitals have chaplain training programs, and a cleric may be assigned to the rehabilitation service. These individuals help clients and families during crisis periods, assist them in reaffirming their beliefs, and frequently establish communication between a church group and the client and family. They frequently channel information, although not privileged information, to the rehabilitation team through the rehabilitation nurse.

TEAM PROCESSES

For effective team function, services of team members are delivered in a dynamic fashion by professionals who communicate regularly, integrate decisions and actions in relation to their separate goals, and coordinate the team plan to focus on the individual as a whole existing within the total environment and within the total problem.[10] Effective team functioning requires communication, collaboration, coordination, and evaluation.

Communication

Formal and informal channels exist for team communication.[3] Formal channels include team conferences, daily meetings, administrative meetings, and written communication. Informal channels include impromptu conversations, social gatherings, and the grapevine.

Team conferences

Most rehabilitation teams hold weekly conferences to review the progress of clients. During this meeting, short- and long-term goals for rehabilitation are established and reevaluated with each client and family, the length of stay in the rehabilitation program is estimated, functional progress is reviewed, and the total rehabilitation program is evaluated. Discharge plans are initiated when the client enters the rehabilitation program and are reviewed and evaluated for feasibility at the team conference. Each team member reports on client progress and participates in the development of the total plan of care. One or more clients may be reviewed at each team conference, but all clients are reviewed at least monthly.

Daily meetings

Some rehabilitation teams meet daily to share reports about client status. This can be accomplished at an early morning report so that plans can be made for the rest of the day.

Face-to-face interactions with other team members take place during daily rehabilitation therapy when more than one team member is involved in delivering rehabilitative care. For example, a nurse, physical therapist, occupational therapist, physiatrist, and social worker may work with a person who has multiple sclerosis and progressive decline in functional ability. Their evaluations are discussed with the client and family, and they are involved in determining the team plan of care. Client and family goals are validated and plans made with them to meet these goals.

Administrative meetings

Time must be set aside for administrative concerns when members of the team can review the structure of client-centered conferences and policies and procedures, evaluate team process, and determine future directions. Administrative support from boards of directors and administrators is necessary to obtain time, space, and financial resources for daily team operation and evaluation of team programs.

Administrative approval of all policies and procedures of the team should be sought, and the administrator should be closely involved with any plans for new programs. The ultimate responsibility for program planning, implementation, evaluation, and fiscal review lies with the administrator.

Team members also may communicate with each other at these meetings to determine strategies for financing new programs, obtaining administrative approval, and marketing programs. In addition, plans may be formulated for presenting programs to third-party payers, community groups, and students in medicine, nursing, and allied health professions within the rehabilitation agency and within local universities. Team members also may discuss prevention of disability at local high schools. Necessarily, any programs taking place outside an agency related to agency programs must be approved by administrators of the facility.

Written communication

Written communication takes a number of forms. First and foremost, results of team conferences should be documented and placed in the client's record. A team member or secretary may be appointed to coordinate the filing of written team plans and assure that these plans are kept up-to-date. The client also should have a copy of the plan, which then serves as a contract between all members of the team.

Rehabilitation plans also are used for interagency referral. Becoming familiar with key personnel in these agencies facilitates communication and services for the client and family. Knowing the structure of the organization, services offered, clients served, reputation, and reimbursement mechanisms of local community agencies that assist with rehabilitation can speed community reintegration. Verbal communication should always be reinforced with written communication when obtaining services from another agency.

Bulletin boards and newsletters can be used for other forms of written communication. Attractive bulletin boards, placed in areas that are easily seen, can be used to inform clients and families of services offered, explain roles of team members, describe successes of clients, and offer inspiring messages to clients and their families. Some team members can use their artistic talents to publish newsletters and design brochures that make agency personnel and the public aware of services available. Personnel in public relations or biomedical communications departments can be indispensable in helping the team increase the awareness of the public about disability prevention and services offered to the disabled. They also can assist team members in designing educational programs that can be used repeatedly.

Informal communication

Impromptu conversations between team members take place at lunch, in hallways, at desks, and on the way in and out of work. Planned social gatherings to celebrate the addition of new team members, picnics for clients and their families, retirement parties, and such gatherings as weddings, showers, and holiday parties provide opportunities for team members to get to know each other better as persons.

An informal communication network commonly referred to as "the grapevine" often circulates information faster than official channels of communication. This grapevine exists between clients, clients and family members, team members, clients and team members, families, and family and team members. It is the responsibility of the team leader and team members to use this grapevine in the service of team building and to intervene quickly when the grapevine is circulating inaccurate or potentially destructive information.[2]

Collaboration

Collaboration occurs when team members use communication channels to work together successfully and harmoniously. A successful team ef-

fort is like a fine orchestra, in which each instrument blends with other instruments to create an impressive symphony. At times one instrument may play solo, but all of the instruments are required to create a truly great performance.

Collaboration requires feedback among all team members. Mutual respect opens the door for feedback, be it honest praise or constructive criticism. Through feedback, team objectives and plans can be modified and revised.

Team members collaborate in designing each client's overall care plan, refining and modifying old programs, and developing new programs. They may collaborate in the search for new knowledge by attending conferences together, sharing articles at journal clubs, and conducting research and publishing findings.

Coordination

Without coordination of administrative policies and procedures and client and family plans of care, the team loses its usefulness and becomes only an amalgam of disciplines coming together without team assessment, plans, or evaluation.

The team leader either performs or delegates coordinating activities to individual team members. These activities may include but are not limited to distributing agendas for meetings in a timely fashion, arranging client and family meetings, coordinating reports of team meetings, distributing information regarding policies and procedures, evaluating new equipment and procedures, developing and reviewing protocols, establishing inservice education programs for staff, communicating with other departments within the agency or between agencies, dealing with problems of role overlap between team members, talking with media, arranging consultations, following appropriate channels of communication within an agency and the community, and obtaining feedback from team members, clients and families, and community agencies.

Evaluation

Functional evaluation forms are now used by rehabilitation teams in many facilities to evaluate client progress or lack of progress quantitatively and to determine client outcomes as a result of the team plan. These instruments are designed so that a team can evaluate a client's progress globally, according to a specific disease category or in a number of activities of daily living. Use of these instruments to observe and evaluate a client gives a numerical and objective measure of a client's functional progress. Evaluation also should address individual client benefits in relation to cost.[12] (See Chapter 25.)

The needs of the professional team member also can be evaluated. Answers to the following questions can be investigated: Is there an "efficient" use of time for the professional? What are the direct benefits in terms of professional satisfaction? Does the team approach enhance the professional's ability to provide better service?

The overall organization also has an interest in evaluation. From the organizational viewpoint, it is necessary to ascertain whether the team approach is meeting the broad organizational goals. The organization, as well as third-party payers, is interested in determining costs of care and keeping costs down.[12]

Ducanis and Golin[5] suggest four questions that should be addressed in team evaluation: "(1) How is team 'effectiveness' or 'success' to be measured? (2) Which elements of the team approach lead to more effective outcomes? (3) With which clients is the team approach most effective? (4) Under what conditions does the team operate most effectively?" They discuss formative and summative evaluation as approaches to team evaluation. Formative evaluation provides feedback for the team as various parts of the team approach develop. Summative evaluation, on the other hand, assesses the overall effectiveness of a program after it is in operation. Both approaches require development of measurement criteria and collection and analysis of data to determine future program direction. The formative evaluation often is an internal process, whereas the summative evaluation is conducted frequently by an outside, well-known, rehabilitation expert who is likely to give a more objective evaluation.

BARRIERS TO EFFECTIVE TEAM PERFORMANCE

Lack of an organizing framework for team operation can be one of the biggest stumbling blocks to a smoothly functioning team. Therefore it is important initially to spend time organizing an approach to team operation and then allot time for maintenance activities. Analysis and evalua-

tion of the team's performance and identification of possible solutions to recurring problems also should be included in this time allocation.

Professional territoriality, differing philosophies, lack of structure and organization, poor communication, and limited commitment or lack of commitment to the rehabilitation process are barriers to effective team performance. Others argue that organizational complexity rather than the factors previously mentioned influences the level of conflict across disciplines.[9] Poor communication among individual members should be identified quickly, confronted, and eliminated.[4] Coordination of information between all members helps to avoid confusion and conflicting messages. Team members can ensure that appropriate channels of communication exist among the disciplines, with the client and family, and among the client, family, and team. Approaches to team communication and collaboration were discussed in the sections addressing responsibilities of the team leader and team members.

Because most health professionals have not worked as colleagues with other health team members with different educational backgrounds and knowledge bases, it takes time to learn to trust the professional judgments of one another. A willingness to learn about the educational preparation, roles, and functions of other disciplines will contribute to smooth functioning of the team.[18]

When new team members have been accustomed to practicing independently, they may become frustrated working interdependently with other team members to accomplish goals, and the effectiveness of the team suffers. Conversely, those whose needs for dependence are high also may compromise the team function by making unreasonable demands on other team members. Education in teamwork as discussed previously and experiences as a team member may resolve these problems. At other times, however, such members may have to seek other positions that are more consistent with their approach.

"Role ambiguity is a large source of intrateam conflict."[18] Each team member has a perception of his or her role and function on the team. Each person may feel that his or her discipline is the most important or, because of varying degrees of experience, may feel that he or she knows better than others how a particular program should be planned, implemented, and evaluated. According to Rothberg,[18] "team members must understand and accept the content description of each other's roles and come to agreement regarding practice boundaries. Otherwise, role ambiguity will lead directly to territorial and domain disputes, since the range or scope of practice of any discipline may easily overlap the boundaries of another."

SUMMARY

The rehabilitation team is well established as an important aspect of rehabilitation. This combination of experts with in-depth knowledge and skill in a variety of areas is necessary to meet the client's total needs. Although each member contributes the expertise of a specific discipline, the sum of the individual disciplines is theoretically more effective than a number of health care professionals independently giving service to the same individual.

The ability to work as a team sometimes demands negotiation. Learning to respect one another for contributions to the team effort contributes to the ability to negotiate roles and functions. Communication, collaboration, coordination, and evaluation are necessary for effective team performance. Superficial understanding of roles and functions of other team members, coupled with inexperience in working with other health care professionals as colleagues, leads to barriers to team function. Thus it is important for each team member to learn the contributions that others can and do make to the rehabilitation process. The use of such knowledge facilitates effective team functioning and the delivery of quality rehabilitative care.

REFERENCES

1. Athelstan GT: Vocational assessment and management. In Kottke FJ, Stillwell GK, and Lehmann JF, editors: Krusen's handbook of physical medicine and rehabilitation, ed 3, Philadelphia, 1982, WB Saunders Co.
2. Browning MS: An interdisciplinary approach to long term care. In Hogstel MO, editor: Management of personnel in long term care, Bowie, Md, 1983, Robert J Brady Co.
3. Cartwright D and Zander A: Group dynamics, ed 3, New York, 1968, Harper & Row, Publishers, Inc.
4. Clark GS and Bray GP: Development of a rehabilitation plan. In Williams TF, editor: Rehabilitation in the aging, New York, 1984, Raven Press.
5. Ducanis AJ and Golin AK: The interdisciplinary health care team: a handbook, Germantown, Md, 1979, Aspen Systems Corporation.
6. Fordyce WE: Psychological assessment and management. In Kottke FJ, Stillwell GK, and Lehmann JF, editors: Krusen's handbook of physical medicine and rehabilitation, ed 3, Philadelphia, 1982, WB Saunders Co.
7. Goldenson RM, Dunham JR, and Dunham CS: Disability and rehabilitation handbook, New York, 1978, McGraw-Hill Book Co.
8. Gresham GE: Personal communication, 1986.
9. Guy ME: Interdisciplinary conflict and organizational complexity, Hosp Health Serv Admin 31:111, Jan/Feb 1986.
10. Halstead LS and Grabois M, editors: Medical rehabilitation, New York, 1985, Raven Press.
11. Hirschberg GG, Lewis L, and Vaughan P: Levels and places of rehabilitation. In Hirschberg GG, Lewis L, and Vaughan P: Rehabilitation—a manual of care for the disabled, Philadelphia, 1976, JB Lippincott Co.
12. Jacobs P: The economics of health and medical care, ed 2, Rockville, Md, 1987, Aspen Publishers, Inc.
13. Leung P: Training in rehabilitation psychology. In Golden CJ, editor: Current topics in rehabilitation psychology, New York, 1984, Grune & Stratton, Inc.
14. Margolis H and Fiorelli JS: An applied approach to facilitating interdisciplinary teamwork, J Rehabil 50:13, Jan/Feb/March 1984.
15. Martin GM: Prescribing physical and occupational therapy. In Kottke FJ, Stillwell GK, and Lehmann JF, editors: Krusen's handbook of physical medicine and rehabilitation, ed 3, Philadelphia, 1982, WB Saunders Co.
16. Rehabilitation nursing: concepts and practice, a core curriculum, Evanston, Ill, 1981, Rehabilitation Nursing Institute.
17. Ross AO: Family problems. In Smith RM and Neisworth JT, editors: The exceptional child, a functional approach, New York, 1975, McGraw-Hill Book Co.
18. Rothberg JS: The rehabilitation team: future direction, Arch Phys Med Rehabil 62:407, Aug 1981.
19. Sampson EE and Marthas MS: Group process for the health professions, New York, 1977, John Wiley & Sons, Inc.
20. Schein JD and Miller MH: Rehabilitation and management of auditory disorders. In Kottke FJ, Stillwell GK, and Lehmann JF, editors: Krusen's handbook of physical medicine and rehabilitation, ed 3, Philadelphia, 1982, WB Saunders Co.
21. Yesner HJ: Psychosocial diagnosis and social services—one aspect of the rehabilitation process. In Kottke FJ, Stillwell GK, and Lehmann JF, editors: Krusen's handbook of physical medicine and rehabilitation, ed 3, Philadelphia, 1982, WB Saunders Co.

ADDITIONAL READINGS

Cohen MH and Ross ME: Team building: a strategy for unit cohesiveness, J Nurs Admin 12:29, Jan 1984.

Halstead LS: Team care in chronic illness: a critical review of the literature of the past 25 years, Arch Phys Med Rehabil 57:507, Nov 1976.

Halstead LS and others: The innovative rehabilitation team: an experiment in team building, Arch Phys Med Rehabil 67:347, June 1986.

Leonard HS: Resolving differences within the rehabilitation team, Rehabil Nurs 9:22, March 1984.

Lloyd M: Baseball lessons for nurses, Nurs. Outlook 32:200, July/Aug 1984.

Palmer S and others: Psychosocial services in rehabilitation medicine: an interdisciplinary approach, Arch Phys Med Rehabil 66:690, Oct 1985.

CHAPTER 4

Nursing Process

Rita J. Boucher

OBJECTIVES

After completing Chapter 4, the reader will be able to:

1. Define rehabilitation and rehabilitation nursing practice.
2. Explain the components of the nursing process.
3. Describe nursing assessment.
4. Identify ways to formulate nursing diagnoses.
5. Describe goals and plans of care.
6. Discuss nursing interventions.
7. Describe outcome evaluations.
8. Identify a way to document the nursing process.

I believe that examining the nursing process in isolation from a sound philosophy of rehabilitation nursing practice is a futile effort. For many years nurses have articulated a philosophy of comprehensive nursing care, yet all too frequently, there is a gap between what we say we believe and what we demonstrate our beliefs to be. Boroch[3] states that "the philosophic framework operant within each individual is composed of basic values, beliefs, and attitudes learned through varying experiences throughout life. A philosophy, which is expressed in behavior patterns, governs abilities and establishes the boundaries for coping with new and unusual situations, observing with objectivity, making decisions, relating to others as persons, seeing another's point of view, and providing learning opportunities for self and others."

In an effort to operationalize the philosophy of nursing presented in Chapter 1, this chapter ex-amines the nursing process and presents a method for its implementation.

DEFINITIONS

Krusen, Kottke, and Ellwood[11] define rehabilitation as "a creative procedure which includes the cooperative efforts of various medical specialties and their associates in other health fields to improve the mental, physical, social, and vocational aptitudes of persons who are handicapped, with the objective of preserving their ability to live happily and productively on the same level with the same opportunities as their neighbors." The major objective of rehabilitation is to add quality to the life of any person who has a chronic disease or disability.

The American Nurses' Association, Division of Medical-Surgical Nursing Practice, and the Association of Rehabilitation Nurses define rehabilitation nursing practice as "the diagnosis and treatment of human responses of individuals and groups to actual or potential health problems with the characteristics of altered functional ability and altered life-style."[1]

Concepts of rehabilitation nursing are applicable in a variety of health care settings. Specialized knowledge, however, is necessary for the practice of rehabilitation nursing in a specialized rehabilitation setting. The entire rehabilitation team is concerned with three basic goals of rehabilitation, namely, prevention of further disability, maintenance of remaining abilities, and restoration of as much function as possible in activities of daily living and in social roles. Additionally, rehabilitation nursing involves teaching the client and family to adapt to previous or new life-styles so that high-level wellness may be achieved. If these goals are ignored, the client may succumb to preventable secondary complications such as contractures, pressure ulcers, depression, loss of morale, and even death. The lack of a rehabilitation plan will deprive the client of opportunities to maintain existing abilities and will prevent the individual with a disability from realizing full potential and a satisfying future.

COMPONENTS OF NURSING PROCESS

Implementation of a philosophical orientation and accomplishment of the goals of rehabilitation are achieved by using nursing process. Nursing process is the application of scientific problem solving to nursing practice. It is used to identify client health concerns, to systematically plan and implement nursing care, and to evaluate the results of that care.[13]

Nursing process involves a series of actions in an ongoing cycle of related steps that occur with order and definition. Although different conceptualizations of these steps exist, components of nursing process are commonly identified as assessment, diagnosis, establishing goals, planning, intervention, and outcome evaluation. Assessment involves collection of data and identification of nursing diagnoses. Establishing goals requires mutual collaboration between the nurse and client and those who may become responsible for assisting with care. Planning includes setting priorities. Intervention requires the nurse to carry out

the plans. Outcome evaluation refers to the examination of the results of the plan to determine whether nursing interventions were effective in achieving the goal and whether the client's health concerns were alleviated.

The application of the nursing process requires the integrated use of cognitive, psychomotor, and affective or interpersonal skills. It is a logical and rational way for the nurse to organize information so that the care delivered is appropriate, efficient, and effective.[12] To a large extent, the nurse's philosophical and theoretical orientations influence the application of the nursing process.

Assessment

Nursing assessment is defined as the deliberate, systematic collection of data, which leads to the identification of the client's health status, including health concerns, strengths, and limitations. Assessment takes place when the client first receives rehabilitative nursing care and continues as long as actual or potential health concerns exist.

Assessment is guided by models and theories in nursing and related disciplines. Since the client's state of health and ability to cope with impairment are influenced by physical, functional, psychosocial, economic-vocational, and spiritual concerns, these five categories are used as guidelines for data collection in the examples given in this chapter (Figure 4-1).

Physical status is a description of the client's organic condition. The client's physical status depends on the control of disease, extent of joint limitation, and neurological involvement. Functional status describes how clients function with the organic equipment they possess. Briefly, functional status refers to the level of dependence or independence in activities of daily living.[2] Psychosocial status refers to the marital status, number of children, housing, home life, relationships with others, interests and hobbies, education, habits, and coping abilities. Economic-vocational status refers to clients' financial resources and past and present occupation. Although spiritual status is regarded frequently as synonymous with religious practices, spiritual status in this text also refers to the client's realm of basic needs, such as need to belong, to feel attachment to a person or group, to reach out beyond one's self, to have a meaningful life, and to be creative.[4] The initial

Text continued on p. 52.

Client's name _____ Date of birth _____ Age _____

ID number _____ Race/ethnic origin _____

Date of admission _____ Date of initial assessment _____

Medical diagnosis: Primary _____ Secondary _____

Attending physician _____ Primary nurse _____

Rehabilitation team members _____

Informant: Client _____ Family member _____

Reliability of historian: Good _____ Fair _____ Poor _____

PHYSICAL/FUNCTIONAL HISTORY

1. How would you describe your general health? Excellent _____ Very good _____ Good _____
   Fair _____ Poor _____
2. Breathing
   a. Have you had any difficulty breathing before or with this admission? No _____ Yes _____
      If yes, describe the difficulty _____
   b. What can be done during your rehabilitation to make breathing easier for you? _____
      _____
   c. Do you expect any difficulties in breathing when you return home? _____
      _____
3. Nutrition
   a. How would you describe your nutrition? Excellent _____ Very good _____ Good _____
      Fair _____ Poor _____
   b. Describe a typical day's food intake _____
      _____
      _____
   c. What is your weight? _____
   d. What foods do you like the best? _____
      _____
   e. What foods do you like the least? _____
      _____
   f. Are you now or have you ever been on a special diet? No _____ Yes _____
      If yes, what was the diet? _____
   g. At what times do you usually eat?
   h. Have you needed any assistance to eat? No _____ Yes _____
      If yes, what types of assistance? _____
   i. What is the condition of your mouth? Good _____ Cavities _____ Gum disease _____
      Other _____ Specify other _____
   j. Do you wear dentures? No _____ Yes _____ Upper _____ Lower _____ Partial _____
4. Elimination
   a. Bladder
      (1) Have you had any difficulty passing urine? No _____ Yes _____
          If yes, what was the problem? _____
             what did you do about it? _____
             what treatment, if any, did you receive? _____
             _____

      (2) Do you frequently experience any of the following symptoms?
          Incontinence   _____   Foul-smelling urine   _____
          Urgency   _____   Cloudy urine   _____
          Frequency   _____   Burning on urination _____
          Pain on urination _____   Bloody urine   _____
          If yes, to any of the above problems, what was done about it? _____
          _____

Figure 4-1
Guidelines for recording health history.   *Continued.*

PHYSICAL/FUNCTIONAL HISTORY—cont'd

  (3) Do you need any assistance with bladder elimination? No _____ Yes _____
      If yes, what type of assistance do you need? _____
  b. Bowel
  (1) How would you describe your bowel habits? Regular_____ Irregular _____
  (2) How often do you usually have a bowel movement? Every day_____ Every other day _____
      Twice a week _____ Once a week _____ Other _____
  (3) What time of day do you usually have a bowel movement? Morning _____ Afternoon _____
      Evening _____
  (4) Tell me if you do any of the following things to assist you in having a bowel movement:
      Eat certain foods _____ Specify _____
      Drink certain fluids _____ Specify _____
      Take medications _____ Specify _____
      Insert suppositories _____ Specify _____
      Perform digital stimulation _____ Perform Valsalva maneuver _____
      Specify other _____
  (5) Do you frequently experience any of the following problems?
      Diarrhea _____   Impaction _____
      Constipation _____   Incontinence _____
      Specify other _____
      If yes to any of the above, what did you do about the problem? _____
      _____
      What treatment, if any, did you receive? _____
      _____
  (6) Do you need any assistance in getting to the bathroom? No _____ Yes _____
      If yes, what type of assistance? _____
5. Skin integrity
  a. How would you describe the condition of your skin? Excellent _____ Very good _____
     Good _____ Fair _____ Poor _____
  b. Do you bruise easily? No _____ Yes _____
  c. Have you ever had open sores or ulcers that are slow to heal? No _____ Yes _____
  d. Have you ever had rashes? No _____ Yes _____
  e. Have you ever had moles that have grown? No _____ Yes _____
  f. Do you sweat easily? No _____ Yes _____
  g. Have you ever had itchy skin? No _____ Yes _____
  h. If yes to any of the above problems, describe the circumstances and what you did about the problem? _____
     _____
     _____
6. Rest/comfort
  a. Rest
  (1) How would you describe the amount of rest you get? Always enough _____ Enough _____
      Sometimes enough _____ Never enough _____
  (2) What time do you usually go to bed? _____ Get up in the morning? _____
  (3) Do you have any difficulty going to sleep at night? Always _____ Usually _____
      Sometimes _____ Never _____
  (4) Do you awaken during the night? Always _____ Usually _____ Sometimes _____
      Never _____
  (5) Do you take naps? No _____ Yes _____ If yes, when? _____
  (6) What aids, if any, do you use to go to sleep at night?
      Drink warm liquids _____   Read _____
      Take an alcoholic beverage _____   Turn night light on in room _____
      Watch television _____   Take sleeping pills _____

Figure 4-1, cont'd
Guidelines for recording health history.

PHYSICAL/FUNCTIONAL HISTORY—cont'd

    b. Comfort

       (1) How would you describe your physical comfort? Always very comfortable _____
           Usually comfortable _____ Sometimes comfortable _____ Never comfortable _____

       (2) Have you experienced discomfort in the past? No _____ Yes _____
           If yes, describe _____
           _____
           What did you do about it? _____
           Did it help? No _____ Yes _____ Partially _____

       (3) If you have discomfort during your rehabilitation program, what would you like the nurse or therapists
           to do about it? _____
           _____

7. Personal hygiene/grooming

    a. Have you needed the help of another person with:

      Bathing _____   Shaving _____
      Brushing/combing your hair _____   Applying makeup _____
      Brushing your teeth _____   Feminine hygiene _____
      Applying deodorant _____   Dressing: Uppers _____ Lowers _____ Both _____

    b. Have you used any adaptive aids to assist with any personal hygiene or grooming activities?
      No _____ Yes _____
      If yes, specify _____

8. Communication

    a. Vision

       (1) How would you describe your vision? Excellent _____ Very good _____ Good _____
           Fair _____ Poor _____

       (2) Do you wear glasses? All the time _____ For reading _____ Never _____

       (3) Do you wear contact lenses? All the time _____ While awake _____ Sometimes _____
           Never _____

    b. Hearing

       (1) How would you describe your hearing?
           Right ear: Excellent _____ Very good _____ Good _____ Fair _____ Poor _____
           Left ear: Excellent _____ Very good _____ Good _____ Fair _____ Poor _____

       (2) Have you ever had pain in either ear? No _____ Yes _____

       (3) Have you ever had ringing in your ears? No _____ Yes _____

       (4) Have you ever had a discharge from either ear? No _____ Yes _____

       (5) If yes to any of these problems, describe _____
           _____
           What did you do about it? _____
           What treatment, if any, did you receive? _____
           _____

    c. Sensation/perception

       (1) Do you have any difficulties with feeling pain? No _____ Yes _____
           With feeling temperature? No _____ Yes _____

       (2) Do you have any intolerance to temperature? No _____ Yes _____

       (3) If yes to 1 or 2, describe _____
           _____
           What do you do about the problem? _____

    d. Speech/language

       (1) How would you describe your ability to express yourself? Excellent _____ Very good _____
           Good _____ Fair _____ Poor _____

       (2) How would you describe your ability to understand others? Excellent _____ Very good _____
           Good _____ Fair _____ Poor _____

Figure 4-1, cont'd
Guidelines for recording health history.   *Continued.*

PHYSICAL/FUNCTIONAL HISTORY—cont'd

      (3) Have you ever had difficulty expressing yourself? No _____ Yes _____
           If yes, describe the circumstances _____

      (4) Have you ever had difficulty understanding others? No _____ Yes _____
           If yes, describe the circumstances _____

9. Mobility (ask questions appropriate to client's mobility status)
    a. How would you describe your ability to get out of or into a bed or chair? Excellent _____
       Very good _____ Good _____ Fair _____ Poor _____
    b. How would you describe your ability to get into the bathtub? Excellent _____ Very good _____
       Good _____ Fair _____ Poor _____
    c. How would you describe your ability to walk/navigate a wheelchair? Excellent _____
       Very good _____ Good _____ Fair _____ Poor _____
    d. Have you ever had difficulty moving about? No _____ Yes _____
       If yes, describe the difficulty_____
       How did you manage?_____
    e. Do you expect to have any difficulty getting around when you leave the rehabilitation unit?
       No _____ Yes _____
       If yes, what do you expect to do about it? _____

10. Sexuality (ask questions according to client's marital status)
    a. How would you describe your sex life? Very satisfactory _____ Satisfactory _____
       Not very satisfactory _____
    b. Has there been or do you expect differences in your ability to be a:
       Husband   No _____ Yes _____
       Father   No _____ Yes _____
       Wife   No _____ Yes _____
       Mother   No _____ Yes _____
       Significant other No _____ Yes _____
       If yes, describe what you expect the differences to be _____
       _____
    c. Do you expect your sexual functioning to be changed in any way after your rehabilitation?
       No _____ Yes _____
       If yes, describe expected changes _____
       _____
    d. Do you want the nurse to obtain more information about sexual function for you?
       No _____ Yes _____
       If yes, specify interests _____
       Refer you to a sex counselor? No _____ Yes _____

PSYCHOSOCIAL HISTORY

1. What is your marital status? Married _____ Divorced _____ Separated _____
    Widowed _____ Never married _____
2. Do you have any children? No _____ Yes _____
    If yes, how many?_____ What are their ages?_____
3. What type of housing do you live in? Upper apartment _____ Lower apartment _____
    Ranch _____ Two or more story dwelling _____
4. How many people live in your home?   _____
5. Where do you sleep? _____
6. Where is the bathroom located? _____
7. How would you describe your relationships with others living in your home? Excellent _____
    Very good _____ Good _____ Fair _____ Poor _____
    If fair or poor, would you like to tell me anything about these relationships? _____
    _____

Figure 4-1, cont'd
Guidelines for recording health history.

PSYCHOSOCIAL HISTORY—cont'd

8. Do you have any interests or hobbies? No _____ Yes _____
   If yes, describe _____

9. How far did you go in school?

   Grammar school _____   College graduate _____
   Some high school _____   Some graduate school _____
   High school graduate _____   Graduate school degree _____
   Some college _____

10. What are your habits?

    Smoking _____ How long? _____ How many packs/day? _____
    Drinking _____ How long? _____ How much? _____
    Drugs _____ How long? _____ How much? _____
    Coffee _____ How many cups/day? _____
    Exercise _____ Type? _____ How often? _____ How long? _____

11. Coping
    a. How would you describe your coping abilities? Excellent _____ Very good _____ Good _____
       Fair _____ Poor _____
    b. What do you do when you are upset? _____
       _____
    c. Does it help? No _____ Yes _____

12. Relationships
    a. Who is the most important person to you? _____
    b. How many close friends do you have? _____
    c. What affect has your disability had on your family and friends? _____
       _____
    d. Do you expect your family and friends to visit during your rehabilitation program? _____
    e. Who of your friends or family would you most like to assist with your rehabilitation program? _____
       _____
    f. Who should be notified in case of an emergency? _____
       Telephone number _____
       Address _____

ECONOMIC/VOCATIONAL HISTORY

1. What is your occupation? Present _____ Past _____
   Unemployed _____ If unemployed, are you retired? No _____ Yes _____
2. How would you describe your financial resources? Excellent _____ Very good _____ Good _____
   Fair _____ Poor _____
3. How will you pay for your rehabilitation program?

   Self, family _____   Vocational rehabilitation agency _____
   Insurance plan _____   Medicaid _____
   Worker's compensation _____ Medicare _____
   Specify other _____

SPIRITUAL HISTORY

1. Do you practice a religion? No _____ Yes _____
   If yes, what denomination? Catholic _____ Protestant _____ Jewish _____
   Specify other _____
   a. Do you attend a place of worship regularly? No _____ Yes _____
   b. Do you have any dietary restrictions as part of your religious practices? No _____ Yes _____
   c. Would you like to see a chaplain while you are here? No _____ Yes _____
2. Do you feel your spiritual needs are met? Yes _____ No _____
   If no, is there anything the nurse can do to assist you in meeting your spiritual needs? _____
   _____

Figure 4-1, cont'd
Guidelines for recording health history.   *Continued.*

OTHER

1. What do you know about your current health concerns? _____
_____
_____
_____
_____

2. Do you have any questions right now about your current health concerns? _____
_____
_____
_____

Thank you for answering all my questions. I will be back later to see if we agree on your major health concerns and sit down to establish goals with you for your rehabilitation program.

Figure 4-1, cont'd
Guidelines for recording health history.

assessment identifies strengths, limitations, and health concerns. When a health concern exists, further information is required.

Regardless of the framework used to guide data collection, data obtained must be assembled, analyzed, and synthesized. To accomplish these tasks, nurses rely on theoretical orientation and empirical knowledge to draw conclusions and formulate nursing diagnoses. For example, when Orem's self-care theory is used as a theoretical orientation, nurses would identify universal, developmental, and health deviations. They might then plan the type of nursing system—wholly compensatory, partially compensatory, or supportive-educative—the client needs. Previous experiences with similar clients in similar situations will help nurses choose and adjust interventions that were successful before.

Sources of data

Clients are the primary source of data. The way in which they present data and the way in which nurses perceive the information influence the data collection process. Each participant in the interaction brings beliefs, values, and attitudes developed over a long period of time within one's own family and culture. When nurses are aware of their own perceptions, they are better able to develop a reliable basis from which to judge the experiences of others.[18]

When the client is an unreliable historian, other sources, such as family, rehabilitation team members, and health and social records may be used. Nurses' notes, nursing conferences, nursing rounds, change of shift reports, Kardexes, and referral forms to community agencies also may be used as sources of data. The nurse must maintain an objective approach to data collection and refrain from making premature conclusions about the client's health concerns until enough objective data are obtained to make informed and knowledgeable clinical judgments leading to a nursing diagnostic statement.

Assessment skills

The nurse must possess excellent interviewing and health assessment skills in order to elicit objective data. Often the nurse will have two purposes when obtaining a health history: to obtain data about health concerns and to build rapport. Thus the nurse may start with open-ended questions after explaining the purposes of the interaction. Such questions as "How have you been feeling lately?" help establish rapport and comfort. Gradually, questions become more specific in order to elicit information that has not surfaced. Since the health history is a crucial component of the assessment, interviewing skills are extremely vital.[14]

Skills in health assessment, including observation, auscultation, palpation, and percussion should be part of the nurse's repertoire. Health assessment skills enrich the data base and enable the nurse to monitor the effectiveness of nursing interventions during reassessments. Furthermore, these skills assist the nurse in validating observations and in making clinical judgments.

Following the necessary data collection, the nurse analyzes the data by classifying and examining relationships among categories. The nurse then draws conclusions and formulates nursing diagnoses.

Nursing Diagnosis

Bonney and Rothberg[2] define a nursing diagnosis "as an evaluation within the framework of current knowledge, of the patient's condition as a total human being, including physical, physiological, and behavioral facets." More recently, Gordon[8] states that the nursing diagnosis contains three essential components referred to as the *PES format*. These three components "are the health problem *(P)*, the etiological or related factors *(E)*, and the defining characteristics, or cluster of signs and symptoms *(S)*." For example, a client may be diagnosed with "alteration in patterns of urinary elimination related to uninhibited neurogenic bladder manifested by urgency and frequency." She also defines nursing diagnosis as the process by which nurses arrive at clinical judgments.

The nursing diagnostic statement reflects the client's needs. Needs are concerned with the client's life processes and responses to the environment. Maslow has identified a hierarchy of needs (Chapter 2). Identifying and classifying human needs and then formulating a nursing diagnostic statement about each need requires objectivity, critical thinking, and application of sound judgment. The resultant nursing diagnostic statement should be clear, specific, accurate, and client centered. Such a statement provides direction and serves as a basis for goals, planning, and nursing interventions. The statement should reflect the client's actual and potential health concerns and be validated with the client, family, and other rehabilitation team members.[16]

Potential or actual family problems may occur when illness and disability lead to conflicts that interfere with an individual's ability to perform self-care activities and carry out social roles. Thus the client's roles and responsibilities within the family structure must be considered in relation to action or potential needs. Often the family must assist the client with continuation of the rehabilitation process in the community.

There are many advantages to using nursing diagnoses, including the development of a common language for professional nursing; identification, validation, and response to a client's actual or potential health concerns; and detection of areas for nursing research. A national task group of nurses representing education, practice, and research was formed in 1973 to develop a taxonomy of nursing diagnoses. Six additional conferences have been held since that time. NANDA, the North American Nursing Diagnosis Association, accepted 61 diagnostic categories and subcategories for clinical testing at the sixth conference.[10] The list was expanded to 74 diagnostic categories at the seventh conference.[15] In 1988 additional categories were approved (see box) and guide the wording of nursing diagnoses used in this text.

Gordon[8] points out that "nursing diagnoses are not established in isolation and because nurses need to increase their participation in joint planning, an appreciation of other professions is needed." This view is particularly appropriate in rehabilitation nursing because nurses routinely work with other rehabilitation team members to develop the client's rehabilitation plan. When needs are identified and translated into nursing diagnoses, the nurse is prepared to recommend actions designed to influence the client's level of independence.

Establishing Goals

Immediate, short-term, and long-term goals are identified. A goal statement describes a broad or abstract intent, state, or condition and reflects the outcome.[13] Goals—sometimes referred to as outcome projections[8]—flow directly from the nursing diagnoses and should be mutually established with the client, family, and other members of the rehabilitation team. Immediate goals are formulated when there are life-threatening situations. Short-term goals can be accomplished within a relatively short period of time, such as a week. For example, the client diagnosed with "impaired

NANDA-Approved Nursing Diagnoses

Activity intolerance
Altered family processes
Altered growth and development
Altered health maintenance
Altered nutrition: less than body requirements
Altered nutrition: more than body requirements
Altered nutrition: potential for more than body requirements
Altered oral mucous membrane
Altered parenting
Altered patterns of urinary elimination
Altered role performance
Altered sexuality patterns
Altered thought processes
Altered (specify type) tissue perfusion, (cerebral, cardiopulmonary, renal, gastrointestinal, peripheral)
Anticipatory grieving
Anxiety
Bathing/hygiene self-care deficit
Body-image disturbance
Bowel incontinence
Chronic low self-esteem*
Chronic pain
Colonic constipation*
Constipation
Decisional conflict (specify)*
Decreased cardiac output
Defensive coping*
Diarrhea
Dressing/grooming self-care deficit
Dysfunctional grieving
Dysreflexia*
Family coping: potential for growth
Fatigue*
Fear
Feeding self-care deficit
Fluid volume deficit (1)
Fluid volume deficit (2)
Fluid volume excess
Functional incontinence
Health seeking behaviors (specify) or desire for high-level wellness (specify)*
Hopelessness
Hyperthermia
Hypothermia
Impaired adjustment
Impaired gas exchange
Impaired home maintenance management
Impaired physical mobility
Impaired skin integrity

Impaired social interaction
Impaired swallowing
Impaired tissue integrity
Impaired verbal communication
Ineffective airway clearance
Ineffective breastfeeding*
Ineffective breathing pattern
Ineffective denial*
Ineffective family coping: compromised
Ineffective family coping: disabled
Ineffective individual coping
Ineffective thermoregulation
Knowledge deficit (specify)
Noncompliance (specify)
Pain
Parental role conflict*
Perceived constipation*
Personal identity disturbance
Post-trauma response
Potential activity intolerance
Potential altered body temperature
Potential fluid volume deficit
Potential for aspiration*
Potential for disuse syndrome*
Potential for infection
Potential for injury
Potential for poisoning
Potential for suffocating
Potential for trauma
Potential for violence: self-directed or directed at others
Potential impaired skin integrity
Powerlessness
Rape-trauma syndrome
Rape-trauma syndrome: compound reaction
Rape-trauma syndrome: silent reaction
Reflex incontinence
Self-esteem disturbance*
Sensory/perceptual alterations (specify) (auditory, gustatory, kinesthetic, olfactory, tactile, visual)
Sexual dysfunction
Situational low self-esteem*
Sleep pattern disturbance
Social isolation
Spiritual distress (distress of the human spirit)
Stress incontinence
Toileting self-care deficit
Total incontinence
Unilateral neglect
Urge incontinence
Urinary retention

* Diagnosis accepted in 1988.

mobility related to right-side hemiplegia" may have a short-term goal to "transfer independently from bed to wheelchair." This same client may have a long-term goal to function independently at home. Thus a series of short-term goals can help the client meet the long-term goal.[5]

Planning

Individualized rehabilitation plans are developed for each disabled client after the nursing diagnoses have been assigned priorities and goals have been established. Rehabilitation nurses can then begin to intervene.

The client and family are ultimately responsible for implementing the plan, so they should be key decision makers in determining priorities and establishing the goals and plan for rehabilitation. Plans for discharge should be incorporated at the outset and goals established for learning, performing care, maintaining and restoring abilities, and dealing with crises.

Interventions

Bulechek and McCloskey[5] define nursing intervention as "an autonomous action based on scientific rationale that is executed to benefit the client in a predicted way related to the nursing diagnosis and the stated goals."

Nursing interventions encompass such activities as establishment of a therapeutic environment, physical care, application of rehabilitation nursing techniques for restoration, client and family education, client and family counseling, psychological support, consultation and referral to other rehabilitation team members, administration of prescribed medical therapies, reinforcement of activities taught by other members of the rehabilitation team, prevention of complications, maintenance, discharge planning, and follow-up. The client's priority of needs determines the type, level, and speed of intervention. Nursing interventions are determined by the nurse and are based on the characteristics of the nursing diagnosis, research base associated with the intervention, potential for successful implementation, acceptability of the intervention to the client, and capability of the nurse.[5]

Specific interventions are planned to assist the client in accomplishing a goal. An example of a specific intervention for the client with a short-term goal for independent transfer could be "Instruct Mr. Jones to pull himself to the side of the bed at 9 AM, for 2 consecutive days. Instruct him to use his left arm and leg to assist with his right arm and leg."

Outcome Evaluation

The question to be answered in the evaluation process is: Was the rehabilitation nursing plan effective in facilitating the client's achievement of goals? Evaluation is the "planned, systematic comparison of the client's health status with defined goals and objectives. It is an ongoing activity involving the client, nurse, and other health care team members."[9] Evaluation is used to determine if the goal established for the nursing diagnosis was accomplished by the nursing intervention. Evaluation often leads to an additional nursing diagnosis.

Evaluation of structure, process, and outcome should take place. Structure focuses on the physical facilities, equipment, and administrative patterns of an organization offering rehabilitative services. Process focuses on the activities of the rehabilitation nurse's performance and helps to determine whether rehabilitation nursing techniques were properly performed. Outcome focuses on the change in the client's performance of self-care activities and social roles. Criteria are developed to measure qualities, attributes, or characteristics that specify skills, knowledge, or health status.[7]

Evaluation can be performed either retrospectively or concurrently. A retrospective evaluation is performed after a client is discharged by means of chart reviews or audits to determine the structure, process, and client outcome. A concurrent review evaluates structure, process, and outcome as it takes place.[9]

As a group, nurses are in the beginning stage of developing outcome criteria that are nursing specific. It is difficult to isolate those outcomes which are specifically the result of nursing intervention because a number of rehabilitation team members contribute to the ultimate client outcomes. Nurses continue to work on and refine nursing-specific outcome criteria, as well as work with other rehabilitation team members to determine outcomes that are the result of a specific rehabilitation team plan.

Since the nursing process is cyclical, reassessment follows evaluation as long as client health concerns exist or when actual or potential new concerns appear. Data must be constantly gathered, analyzed, and synthesized. Conclusions are continuously drawn and new information regarding client status recorded. If nurses are to provide humanitarian, scientific, holistic, and personalized care to clients and their families, the nursing process must be used consistently in practice. Although the labels attached to the components of the process may vary, the steps by which the nurse proceeds to effect client care have the support of the nursing profession.[18]

DOCUMENTATION OF THE NURSING PROCESS

To document the nursing process in rehabilitation settings, a number of forms may be used. Most rehabilitation agencies have prescribed forms developed by nurses who have served on policy and procedure committees. Regardless of the format used, the nurse should document the assessment, including the health history and physical examination; nursing diagnoses; goals and plan of care; nursing interventions; and outcome evaluation of the plan of care in relation to alleviating the client's health concerns in the client's record.

Health History

A health history is the first element of the data base because it is the single most important element in establishing the client's functional strengths and limitations. A comprehensive history should give the examiner a picture of the person, knowledge of current and past health problems, and information about the individual as a total being in his or her environment. The medical history includes the chief complaint, history of present illness, past history of client and family health problems, and a review of systems. The nurse obtains a history of the client's perception, knowledge, and performance in several areas of daily living.

Figure 4-1 presents a form for recording the client's health history. It is only one of many forms that may be used. The nurse skilled in interviewing techniques will be able to use any form that suits the purpose to obtain vital data from which

client strengths, limitations, and health concerns may be identified and subsequent nursing diagnoses formulated.

Physical Examination

The second phase of the health assessment consists of the physical examination. The purpose of the physical examination is to detect variations from normal. This information becomes the second part of the data base.

The physical examination used in rehabilitation settings contains all essential elements of the examination used in routine clinical nursing practice. The guiding principle in the physical examination of a client with a disability is that, in addition to the conventional and pathological data, all information concerning the client's functional ability must be obtained. The fundamentals of the physical examination include general appearance, examination of the head and neck and examination of the cardiopulmonary, gastrointestinal, genitourinary, neuromuscular, and locomotor systems.[17] The physical evaluation will yield an estimate of the client's physical disabilities or limitations, physical assets, and activities of daily living (ADL) capabilities.

Functional Assessment

The functional assessment elicits information regarding how the client performs self-care activities and social roles based on physical status. When evaluating the client's ADL performance, the primary focus is mobility and self-care. The nurse must determine the extent to which the client is independent in daily activities, dependent, or needs assistance or supervision.

Table 4-1 presents an assessment instrument for determining ADL performance of a gentleman with right-side hemiparesis. This assessment was performed 1 week after his cerebrovascular accident. Special needs, such as assistive devices or human assistance, are identified when the client has some degree of dependence.

This client is independent in bed activities and positioning in the supine, side, and prone position by using siderails to manipulate the turns. However, a turning schedule is to be posted at the bedside, and he needs assistance in turning to the left side. The client also needs help in bathing the back and feet during a bed bath, but is totally independent in washing his face, neck, chest, and legs. The functional assessment also yields information that the client can shave himself with an electric razor, provided the razor is plugged in, and can comb his hair with a long-handled comb. He has some independence in dressing. He can come to a sitting position, lower himself to the wheelchair, and relieve pressure every 15 minutes, but needs assistance for transfer and frequent reminders to relieve pressure. He can use a three-point gait with a brace on the right leg, quad cane, and supervision. When the client eats, he is totally independent, except for opening milk cartons, and can eat at the table. Special needs for elimination, managing stairs, and traveling also are identified. The miscellaneous category includes any activity not noted. It helps to personalize notations that are unique to the individual. For example, the client uses a robot to smoke and uses a cardholder while playing cards.

A functional assessment should be considered an important part of the data base, and reassessments of ADL should be scheduled at predetermined intervals to quantify progress over time. A functional assessment assists the nurse in identifying areas of dependence and independence in

TABLE 4-1
Activities of daily living: initial functional assessment of a man with right-side hemiplegia

Activity	Location	Special needs	Independent areas
Mobility			
Bed	Room	Bedside turning schedule: q2h Siderails Assist in turning to left side	Turns to supine, lateral semi-prone positions
Wheelchair*	Room Hallways	One-person assist with pivot transfer Frequent reminders to shift weight	Comes to sitting position; lowers self to chair; relieves pressure on buttocks q15 min by lifting
Ambulation*	Room	Brace on right leg Quad cane Supervise	Three-point gait
Elevation*	Stairwell	Quad cane Supervise	Grabs railing with left hand Places unaffected leg first on step going up Follows with cane and affected leg Places affected leg first on step going down; follows with cane and then unaffected leg
Traveling*	Private car Public transportation	Supervise pivot transfer Quad cane	Not attempted as yet Not attempted as yet
Hygiene			
Bathing	Tub in bathroom	Assist with transfer Assemble bathing equipment Mit washcloth Wash back, feet	Washes face, neck, chest, legs
Grooming	Bathroom	Provide electric razor and plug in Provide long-handled comb	Shaves with left hand Combs hair with left hand
Dressing*	Bedside	Slip feet into underpants, trousers Pull to knees Velcro to shirt and pant closures Zipper pull to pants	Pulls up underpants, trousers Dons shirt Fastens closures on pants, shirt Pulls up zipper

*Specific client activity needing more teaching and guidance.   *Continued*.

TABLE 4-1 _____

Activities of daily living: initial functional assessment of a man with right-side hemiplegia—cont'd

Activity	Location	Special needs	Independent areas
Elimination			
Bladder	Bathroom	Assist with transfer to and from toilet Guardrails on wall by toilet, obliquely angled Elevated toilet seat Stay with client	Wipes self; flushes toilet
Bowel	Bathroom	Glycerin suppository High-fiber diet Other aids used for bladder elimination as above	Same as above
Nutrition			
Eating	Wheelchair	Table Open cartons Cut meats Stabilize dishes with suction cup or wet washcloth Plate guard	Eats all foods
Miscellaneous			
Smoking	Room	Light cigarette Supervise	Smokes using left hand
Plays cards	Room	Cardholder	Plays cards using left hand

ADL. Forms currently used to quantify functional status are described in Chapter 23.

Client problems identified from the physical examination and functional assessment should be translated into nursing diagnoses and documented in the client's progress record. Goals and nursing interventions are then established for each nursing diagnosis.

Documentation of Ongoing Progress

The nursing process applied without a systematic means of recording findings is a totally wasteful effort. Since the nursing record reflects nursing practice, it should be comprehensive and up-to-date in all areas. Record keeping facilitates nursing care among nursing personnel in hospitals, long-term care facilities, community agencies, and homes and publicly documents the rehabilitation nurse's contribution and accountability to the client's welfare.

Since the rehabilitation process reflects a team effort, the activities of the various disciplines

TABLE 4-2 _____

Prescribed therapies

Therapy	Time	Prescribed activities
Occupational therapy	9 AM daily	Dressing activities, with emphasis on lower extremities
Physical therapy	10:30 AM daily	Ambulation with quad cane using three-point gait Stair climbing
Speech therapy	2 PM daily	Repetitive presentation of pictures and corresponding words
Other therapies	3 PM two times/wk	Psychological counseling

should be noted so that these activities do not exist in isolation but may be incorporated into the nursing plan of care. Table 4-2 demonstrates a method to record the activities of other disciplines. By reinforcing procedures carried out by

TABLE 4-3

Initial assessment and ongoing progress record

Date/time	Nursing diagnosis	Goals	Nursing interventions	Outcome evaluation
5/23/85 2 PM	Impaired verbal communication related to left-hemisphere cerebrovascular accident	To establish adequate means of communication	1. Approach client in calm, relaxed manner. 2. Control environment for extraneous and confusing stimuli. 3. Evaluate what language skills are intact. 4. Speak to client in clear, simple sentences; use gestures as necessary. 5. Allow time for client to respond. 6. Make effort to understand client's gestures, syllables, words, phrases. 7. When handling object, name object. 8. Point to written names of objects and repeat name of object. 9. Ask client to write words and simple sentences. 10. List words that client can express in room; add to list of client's vocabulary. 11. Consult with speech-language pathologist (scheduled for 5/24/85).	5/23 Client can express needs by using gestures; can say "yes," "no," provided room is quiet and there are no distractions. 5/23 Client writes words and simple sentences.

5/23/85	Impaired mobility related to right-side paresis, potential heel cord tightening	To ambulate independently	1. Reposition q2h; post schedule at bedside.
			   a. Trochanter roll to prevent external rotation of right hip.
			   b. Flat pillow for head.
			   c. Anticipate areas of contracture and position to prevent development.
			 2. Posey footboard angled at 120 degrees.
			 3. Passive range of joint motion on affected side qid.
			 4. Active range of joint motion on unaffected side qid.
				5/24 Client lifts right leg 2 inches.
				
				 5/23 Client has full range of joint motion in both upper extremities and both lower extremities.

Continued.

TABLE 4-3
Initial assessment and ongoing progress record—cont'd

Date/time	Nursing diagnosis	Goals	Nursing interventions	Outcome evaluation
			5. Isometric exercises: quadriceps, gluteal, abdominal muscles qid.	5/23 Client has minimum strength in these muscles.
			6. Heel cord stretching of affected heel qid.	5/24 Client has slight heel cord tightening
			7. Balancing exercises at bedside qid.	5/24 Client is able to balance self for 5 sec.
			8. Consult with physical therapist.	5/24 Muscle strength +2 on right side
5/23/85	Potential skin integrity impairment related to immobility, sensory loss	Maintain skin integrity	1. Reposition q2h; position for 30 min only on affected side. 2. Monitor skin areas for redness after each turn. 3. Gentle massage to back and bony prominences bid. 4. Protect elbows and heels with sheepskin pads. 5. Cushion to wheelchair. 6. Reposition q30 min while in wheelchair. 7. Teach client to inspect skin. 8. Teach family to inspect skin. 9. Keep skin clean and dry.	5/24 Client has no breakdown in skin; he has difficulty remembering to routinely inspect skin with mirror and requires frequent reminders.

5/25 Family understands importance of inspecting skin and reminding client to inspect skin. |

Week of: May 21, 1985

Vital signs stable. Client continues to be unable to communicate verbally. Responds well to verbal orders. Skin in

good condition. Full range of all joints with exception of ankle. Slight tightening of heel cord. No change in

rehabilitation nursing care plan.

Figure 4-2
Weekly nursing progress notes.

other rehabilitation disciplines, the progress of many clients will be accelerated.

Table 4-3 shows my format for recording the ongoing nursing process. This format identifies the time and date the nursing diagnosis was made and recorded. For example, the client has impaired verbal communication related to cerebrovascular accident and is unable to express himself. The client and nurse goals are documented. Nursing interventions for each nursing diagnosis are listed. A number of nursing interventions for this client's problem are shown. This format provides a column for evaluation of client outcome where the degree to which the problem has been resolved is recorded. The evaluation column also allows for ongoing evaluations of referrals in the various disciplines.

A second nursing diagnosis identified is impaired mobility related to right-side paralysis with flaccidity. The subsequent nursing interventions consist of changing positions every 2 hours, with the schedule posted at bedside, a Posey footboard at a 120-degree angle, passive range of joint motion to the affected side, active range of joint motion to the unaffected side, isometric exercises, heel cord stretching, balancing exercises, and a consultation with a physical therapist.

A third nursing diagnosis is noted as potential for impaired skin integrity related to immobility and sensory loss. Again, a number of nursing interventions are identified. Additional nursing diagnoses derived from physical, functional, psychosocial, economic-vocational, and spiritual assessment areas will be identified by the rehabilitation nurse for this client.

A weekly summary of the client's status should be provided (Figure 4-2). The weekly progress notes also should be part of the client record.

SUMMARY

The nursing process facilitates the identification of client health concerns, strengths, and limitations and ensures personalized, rehabilitation nursing care. Furthermore, it assists the nurse by providing a framework and method of implementing professional nursing practice. This cyclical method assists the nurse in exercising clinical judgment, prioritizing client concerns, translating client needs to mutual client and nurse goals, establishing nursing interventions to meet these goals, and ensuring continuity of the rehabilitation plan. In addition, the nursing process facilitates evaluation of client progress in relation to the nursing diagnosis, goals, and nursing interventions. Last, documentation of the nursing process facilitates communication among nurses, as well as between nurses and members of other disciplines.

REFERENCES

1. American Nurses' Association, Division of Medical-Surgical Nursing Practice, and the Association of Rehabilitation Nurses: Standards of nursing practice, Kansas City, MO, 1986, The Association.
2. Bonney V and Rothberg J: Nursing diagnosis and therapy: an instrument for evaluation and measurement, New York, 1963, National League for Nursing.
3. Boroch RM: Elements of rehabilitation in nursing, St Louis, 1976, The CV Mosby Co.
4. Bowers CC: Spiritual dimensions of the rehabilitation journey, Rehabil Nurs 12:90, March/April 1987.
5. Bulechek GM and McCloskey JC: Nursing interventions: treatments for nursing diagnoses, Philadelphia, 1985, WB Saunders Co.
6. Christensen PJ: Planning: priorities, goals, and objectives. In Griffith-Kenney JW and Christensen PJ, editors: Nursing process: application of theories, frame-

works, and models, ed 2, St Louis, 1986, The CV Mosby Co.

7. Christensen PJ and Fayram ES: Planning: strategies and nursing orders. In Griffith-Kenney JW and Christensen PJ, editors: Nursing process: application of theories, frameworks, and models, ed 2, St Louis, 1986, The CV Mosby Co.

8. Gordon M: Nursing diagnosis: process and application, ed 2, New York, 1987, McGraw-Hill Book Co.

9. Griffith-Kenney JW: Evaluation. In Griffith-Kenney JW and Christensen PJ, editors: Nursing process: application of theories, frameworks, and models, ed 2, St Louis, 1986, The CV Mosby Co.

10. Hurley M, editor: Classification of nursing diagnoses: proceedings of the sixth conference, St. Louis, 1986, The CV Mosby Co.

11. Krusen FH, Kottke FV, and Ellwood PM, editors: Handbook of physical medicine and rehabilitation, ed 2, Philadelphia, 1971, WB Saunders Co.

12. Leddy S and Pepper MJ: Conceptual bases of professional nursing, Philadelphia, 1985, JB Lippincott Co.

13. Mager RF: Goal analysis, Belmont, Calif, 1972, Fearon Publishers, Inc.

14. Marriner A: The nursing process: a scientific approach to nursing care, ed 3, St Louis, 1983, The CV Mosby Co.

15. McLane A, editor: Classification of nursing diagnoses: proceedings of the seventh conference, St Louis, 1987, The CV Mosby Co.

16. Risner PB: Diagnosis: diagnostic statements. In Griffith-Kenney JW and Christensen PJ, editors: Nursing process: application of theories, frameworks, and models, ed 2, St Louis, 1986, The CV Mosby Co.

17. Sherman JL and Fields SK: Guide to patient evaluation, ed 2, Flushing, NY, 1976, Medical Examination Publishing Co., Inc.

18. Yura H and Walsh MB: The nursing process, Norwalk, Conn, 1983, Appleton-Century-Crofts.

ADDITIONAL READINGS

Carnevali D: Nursing care planning: diagnosis and management, ed 3, Philadelphia, 1983, JB Lippincott Co.

Carpenito L: Handbook of nursing diagnosis, Philadelphia, 1984, JB Lippincott Co.

Duke University Hospital Nursing Services, Durham, NC: Guidelines for nursing care: process and outcomes, Philadelphia, 1983, JB Lippincott Co.

Gordon M: Manual of nursing diagnosis, New York, 1985, McGraw-Hill Book Co.

Joint Commission on the Accreditation of Hospitals: Accreditation manual for hospitals, Chicago, 1985, The Commission.

Murray R and Zentner J: Nursing assessment and health promotion through the life span, ed 3, Englewood Cliffs, NJ, 1985, Prentice Hall, Inc.

Sundeen SJ and others: Nurse-client interaction: implementing the nursing process, ed 3, St Louis, 1985, The CV Mosby Co.

CHAPTER 5

Teaching-Learning Process

Barbara G. White

OBJECTIVES

After completing Chapter 5, the reader will be able to:

1. Identify three prerequisites to learning.

2. Describe the impact that a family's readiness to learn has on a client's potential for rehabilitation.

3. List the three domains in which learning occurs and give a description and examples of action verbs for each domain.

4. Briefly discuss the five learning principles related to establishing a learning climate.

5. Describe each of the four steps of the teaching-learning process.

6. Identify the advantages of the group versus the individual learning environment

Teaching and learning occur any time health care is rendered. In the rehabilitation setting, the process focuses on the individual's need to incorporate adaptive behavior into the life-style. The ultimate goal of the process is to assist the disabled individual to reach a maximum level of functioning. It is the responsibility of each member of an interdisciplinary health care team to be knowledgeable in both rehabilitation techniques and the teaching-learning process in order to provide appropriate learning experiences for a client. To be an effective member of the instructional team, the nurse-teacher must have a conceptual background in principles of learning theory.[13] The intent in this chapter is to explore specific learning principles that, when applied to the rehabilitation process, enhance the adaptive responses* of the client. The principles of learning include the following:

1. "Learning is more effective when the content is relevant to the patient's concerns."[18]

2. "Learning is most effective when an indi-

The author acknowledges the Veterans Administration Medical Center, Salisbury, NC, for use of their educational facilities.

*Adaptive behavior is new behavior "used to adjust to changes in internal or external environments."[5]

vidual is ready to learn, that is, when he feels a need to know something."[16]

3. Participation by the client in goal setting enhances learning.[18]

4. Content should be broken down into "meaningful parts."[14]

5. Learners have different capabilities for moving through the cognitive, psychomotor, and affective domains.[14]

6. Content should build on the knowledge and skills previously acquired by the learner, that is, move from the familiar to the unfamiliar.[25]

7. "Distractions reduce the efficiency of teaching and learning."[16]

8. "Learning is more effective if carried out over a period of time."[18]

9. "The environment can be used to focus the patient's attention on what he is to learn."[15]

10. "Satisfaction reinforces learning."[15]

11. "Because it requires change in beliefs and behavior, learning normally produces a mild level of anxiety, which is useful in motivating the individual; however, severe anxiety is incapacitating."[16]

DESCRIPTION

The teaching-learning process is defined as a cooperative effort between the teacher and the learner designed to effect change in the learner's knowledge, skills, and attitudes. The teacher is anyone who provides health care. Every time care is rendered, teaching occurs. For example, teaching occurs when knowledge is shared or a procedure is explained. Teaching also occurs through the attitude expressed toward the client.[13] The learner is most often the client. However, a spouse or significant other also may be a learner.[22] Sometimes clients may want others to learn with them in order to supplement their own learning. If clients cannot learn what is necessary because of a cognitive impairment or stage of adaptation, the active participation by individuals who will be assisting the clients after the instruction is essential.

The teaching-learning process consists of four steps: assessment, planning, implementation, and evaluation. These four steps are easily recognized as the same four steps of the nursing process[22] and are described as follows:

1. In assessment, data relevant to establishing nursing diagnoses requiring learning interventions are collected. These diagnoses reflect learning needs in the cognitive, psychomotor, and affective domains. Levels of functioning in the three domains should be assessed for both predisability and present disability states. By examining how the client functioned before the disabling event, realistic learning needs can be determined in light of present disabilities. Should the need arise for discussing clients' learning needs with family members or significant others, the clients' permission to do so must be obtained unless they are physically or mentally unable to do so. This right of the client is supported by the Patient's Bill of Rights adopted by the American Hospital Association in 1972.[22]

2. The planning step begins by establishing priorities of learning needs. Based on the needs identified during the assessment, the desired adaptive behaviors* for learning are behaviorally defined using measurable terms. The teaching-learning activities selected are based on the objective to be achieved. A target date for achievement is established for each behavior.

3. Implementation is the instructional phase of the process in which the predetermined adaptive behaviors are taught and learned. Target dates established during planning keep the process moving at a prescribed rate.

4. The final step is evaluation of the teaching-learning process. The effectiveness of the process is measured in terms of whether the adaptive behaviors have been achieved. Since the behaviors are described in measurable terms, there should be no doubt as to their achievement.

ASSESSMENT

Assessment involves identifying learner needs, determining the client's readiness to learn, and establishing family readiness to learn. The first and second principles relate to assessment

---

*Desired adaptive behaviors defined in measurable terms are the objectives for the teaching-learning process and the basis for evaluation.

Identifying Learning Needs

Principle 1. "Learning is more effective when the content is relevant to the patient's concerns."[18]

The clue to identifying the learning needs of the client is to remember that "disability means lost functions."[10] Learning needs are identified in many ways. Evidence of the need might be brought to the nurse-teacher's attention by the client, a family member, friend, member of the health team, or a number of other individuals. The need might be made obvious through a direct request or through observation of the individual's physical and emotional states. Many times the needs are identified in the assessment phase of the nursing process.[16]

Four categories of potential problems should be assessed for learning needs. The first category focuses on the client's physical functioning with regard to the present illness and any limitations from a previous illness. Essentially, the basic activities that should be assessed in terms of present and past physical functioning are ambulation, transfer activities, dressing, eating, elimination, and personal hygiene. Such questions as "Which hand do you eat with?" or "Do you normally walk without any kind of assistance?" will give the nurse-teacher clues to the adaptive behavior to be learned.[10]

The second category has to do with social needs. How much the learner and the family have been compromised by the disability must be determined. For example, if the learner provided total financial support of the family before the disability, major adjustment problems for the client and each family member can result in changes in both finances and future plans. The type of living arrangements (whether the client rents or owns) and the structural arrangement of the home are significant. Do clients have to climb stairs to enter the home or to get to the bedroom? Who will be at home with them? Are they married? Do they have children? These and many other questions must be answered to determine social learning needs.[10]

The third category encompasses psychological needs, which should be assessed for a number of reasons. The stress imposed by disease and disability can be of such magnitude that psychological counseling is needed before learning can take place. The need for counseling might be manifested in clients' self-esteem and perceived ability

to control the learning outcomes. If they believe participation in the learning process will have little or no influence over the outcomes, clients' potential for learning will be greatly diminished.[21] In addition, intellectual functioning may be impaired because of brain trauma or deterioration from disease. An understanding of psychological functioning is essential if learning is to occur.

The fourth and last category focuses on vocational problems. The disability might have produced unemployment and loss of all job-related skills. Vocational counseling and training may be determined as a need of the client or family member.[10,26]

When the learning needs of the client are assessed in these four functional categories and considered in light of the goals of rehabilitation,* appropriate goals are determined jointly by the client, family member, and nurse-teacher. Obviously, some of the needs identified in the four categories cannot and are not intended to be met by the nurse-teacher. However, the nurse must know what has and is being taught by other members of the interdisciplinary instructional team.

Assessing a Rehabilitation Client's Readiness to Learn

Principle 2. "Learning is most effective when an individual is ready to learn, that is, when he feels a need to know something."[16]

Readiness for learning can be defined as the capability to expend energy and focus attention for a given purpose. This definition implies three elements necessary for learning. First, clients must be physiologically capable of participating in a learning experience. Second, the purpose of the learning experience must be such that intellectually clients can see its relevance to their needs. Third, the purpose also must have emotional appeal so clients are willing to actively participate.

The physiological capacity to learn depends not only on neuromuscular functioning, but also on limitations from previous illness or injury.[10,14] Any limitations that impair clients' capacity to learn adaptive behaviors are significant. Examples of

---

*"Three goals are sought in rehabilitative care: the prevention of complications arising from inactivity, the restoration of functions disturbed by the illness to their maximum potential, and the maintenance of functions unaffected by the illness."[25]

such limitations include joint stiffness from arthritis, diminished visual and auditory acuity, and
decreased cardiac reserve because of myocardial
hypertrophy. Acute needs such as relief from pain
or anxiety always take priority over learning
needs.[3,13]

Intellectually, the learner must have the cognitive ability to understand the relationship between learning and future well-being. Sometimes
helping clients, through increased self-confidence, to accept the reality that they can learn is
a giant step toward helping them learn.[22]

Emotional readiness to participate actively in
the learning process is greatly enhanced by positive life experiences, beliefs, and values. This
readiness can be impaired by hopelessness, negative beliefs about the disease process or injury,
or unpleasant past experiences with the same or
similar disease state. Lack of readiness to learn
also might be due to the clients' stage of adaptation to loss. Information given at properly timed
intervals can support clients' move to the later
stages in which they can begin to reassess needs
and deal with dependence.[6,16]

To determine the impact each of the three elements has on learning, the nurse-teacher should
assess four major sources of information: the
learner, the learner's significant others, the
nurse's own observations, and observations of
other members of the interdisciplinary team.[14]
From each of these sources, insights can be gained
into the following:

- Life experiences that have an impact on
  learning
- Responses of the client and family (both
  physiological and emotional) to previous ill-
  nesses
- Psychosocial adaptation to a dysfunctional
  state
- Normal daily activities prior to the disabling
  event
- Willingness to achieve rehabilitation
- Perception of rehabilitation potential
- Beliefs about health and health care

Data collected from the four sources not only
reflect the client's readiness to learn, but also
serve as the basis for developing the teaching-
learning plan. During the same process, the
nurse also can provide information needed to
rid the client and significant others of misunderstandings related to disability and rehabilitation.[4]

Assessing a Family's Readiness to Learn

Readiness of the family to participate actively in
the learning process enhances the learner's potential for rehabilitation. Information gleaned
from family members related to family relationships and attitudes before the onset of disability
provides a clue to clients' support systems. Evidence suggests that families with close relationships tend to have supportive attitudes and behavior toward disabled family members, enhancing clients' prospects for rehabilitation and
returning home. Conversely, in families where
hostility, alienation, or other negative attitudes
prevail, the support system is less effective. Additionally, the expectations for clients to return
home are greatly diminished.[8] In assessing a family's readiness to learn, learners should be chosen
with the realization that they will serve as backup
to the primary learner. From the very beginning,
it is essential that backup learners understand
they provide assistance only with activities the
learner is unable to perform. Another important
factor in the selection process is how the learner
feels toward the family member(s) designated as
the backup learner. There must be compatibility
between or among the individuals.[13]

Knowledge and understanding of the illness or
disability by the family tend to increase their supportive behavior. The nurse who provides information relating to both the illness or disability,
as well as the recovery and learning process, enhances the participative efforts of family members. Through continuous and open communication, much of the family's anxiety can be anticipated and allayed. As a result, more energies on
the part of family members are available to support the disabled individual and the learning endeavor.

PLANNING THE LEARNING EXPERIENCE

Planning the learning experience involves developing goals and objectives, identifying resources,
and writing the plan. Principles 3 through 6 are
concerned with this process.

Developing Goals and Objectives

Principle 3. Participation by the client in goal setting enhances learning.[18]

Since the learning experience is designed to

assist the client to develop adaptive behavior and to function at maximum potential, the learner must actively participate in determining both the goals and the objectives to be achieved. Learners who do not clearly understand that the objectives lead to the achievement of the goal(s) will have difficulty complying with the instruction.[7] For example, "applies (unassisted) a straight leg brace" is a behavioral objective that can help achieve the goal of "ambulates independently."

The family should also play a major role in identifying the goal(s) and objectives. "Family theory"[17] indicates that "stress or change affecting one family member, affects other family members as well."[19] Trieschmann[23] maintains that failure of the disabled individual to rehabilitate "may often be traced to lack of family involvement in the rehabilitation process." Consequently, family involvement in planning the learning experience enhances the client's potential for rehabilitation and helps to assure that the goal(s)—that is the overall purpose of the learning experience—is realistic.

Before appropriate goals and objectives can be established, the nurse-teacher should first determine the domain in which learning needs to occur and whether impairment exists in the domain. Learning that is reflected in human behavior occurs in three domains.[12] The cognitive domain activates thought processes, enabling the client to recognize the need for retraining, as well as to grasp the concepts (mental constructs) relative to the disability and life-style.[1] The ability to conceptualize is basic to problem solving, and the learning process leading to rehabilitation is a problem-solving process.

The motor domain concerns clients' ability to perform physical skills within the parameters set by the state of their neuromuscular systems. In addition, learning to perform a skill depends upon the ability to envision mentally how the skill is performed.[1,16]

The affective domain involves attitudes, feelings, values, and emotions.[1] Expressions of this domain permeate all client behaviors and must be incorporated into the learning process.[14] It is activity in this domain that has a heavy impact on readiness to learn.

Upon determining the domain or domains in which learning is to occur, the nurse-teacher and client are ready to establish the goal(s) that should be achieved by the learning. These goals are bro-

ken down into behavioral objectives,* using action verbs that enable the observer to measure whether the objective has been accomplished.[16] Examples of verbs suggested by Mager[11] include the following:

Cognitive verbs	Affective verbs	Psychomotor verbs
Recognize	Select	Use
State	React to	Write
Identify	Solve	Operate
Organize	Choose	Perform

By using Mager's principles for preparing instructional objectives, the objectives will be stated in behavioral terms and can be clearly understood by the learner, family members, and each member of the instructional team.

Identifying Resources

Principle 4. Content should be broken down into "meaningful parts."[14]

When selecting resources for the teaching-learning process, a number of factors must be considered:
- The objectives to be achieved by the process
- The functional senses of the client capable of participating in the learning experience
- The client's intellectual capability, including reading ability

The objectives to be achieved by the process dictate, to a large measure, the resources appropriate for the experience. The learning required for each objective should be broken down into small units. Based on the small units, resources for learning can be selected. For example, an objective that involves knowledge acquisition (cognitive domain) would be met primarily through the use of media, whereas a skill might be taught more effectively through demonstrations.[16] In making the selections, the nurse-teacher must consider not only the domain in which learning is to occur but other factors as well. If reading is required in the learning process, then reading level† (ability) must be assessed to ensure that the teaching aid is appropriate. Media requiring

---

*A behavioral objective is an activity defined in observable and measurable terms.
†The Gunning formula enables the nurse-teacher to determine the reading level of written material.[13]

the sense of sight are ineffective for the visually impaired individual unless alterations, such as enlarging print, can be made. Likewise, audiovisuals require adequate sight and hearing. All senses of the client capable of actively participating in the learning process should be stimulated to do so.

Principle 5. Learners have different capabilities for moving through the cognitive, psychomotor, and affective domains.[14]

Not all clients need or are able to learn in all three domains. The cooperation and active participation of a learner in the learning process are contingent upon the ability to comprehend, remember, and organize behavior. Interference with one or more of these processes affects the resources to be used and dictates levels of learning achieved.[14]

If the learning process is to result in compliance with the prescribed regimen, clients must have access to resources outside the health care setting specific to their living environment. Clients should be acquainted with appropriate resources as a part of the learning process.

Members of the interdisciplinary team are excellent resources for determining what is available and appropriate for learners. The social worker is usually the most knowledgeable about community resources. Nursing referrals for home care and home visits can be arranged by the discharge planning nurse in collaboration with the social worker.

Public libraries also have collections of medical information available from governmental agencies and organizations for the disabled. Informal networking with other professionals and clients also provides an extremely effective means for learning about resources.[7] (See Appendixes D to F for additional equipment resources, organizations, and publications for the disabled.)

Writing the Plan

Principle 6. Content should build on the knowledge and skills previously acquired by the learner, that is, move from the familiar to the unfamiliar.[25]

Essentially, once the learning need is identified, the following six elements are included in the written teaching-learning plan:

- Goal(s) of the total experience
- Description of the target population
- Behavioral objectives
- Content
- Learning activities
- Method(s) of evaluation

In formulating the actual teaching-learning plan, the format for writing the plan must be determined. Any number of different formats can be used; however, the format chosen should show clearly the interdependency of the parts: the goal(s) and objectives depend on learner needs and content, and learning activities depend on goal(s) and objectives.[16]

The plan should begin with a statement of the overall goal(s) of the learning process. Following the goal statement, the target population for whom the plan is designed should be described explicitly. Next, behavioral objectives are identified. Based on the goal(s) and behavioral objectives, the tasks required to achieve each objective should be analyzed, that is, each task to be learned is broken down into logical steps. The steps should proceed from the simplest part of the task to the most complex.[24]

To analyze the task, the nurse should ask the following question related to the objective: What does the learner have to do or know to accomplish the objective. In this manner, specific tasks can be identified. From the historical data available, the nurse can determine if the specific behaviors required to perform the task have been previously learned by the client. If they have not been learned, the task is broken down until a known behavior is reached.[24]

The tasks that must be learned to achieve each objective are then broken down into content, that is, the steps necessary to accomplish the task. For example, learning the names of specific objects is a cognitive learning skill. An appropriate activity for this type of learning would be to have the client repeat the names of the objects while looking at the objects. To learn a skill such as handwriting, on the other hand, an appropriate activity might be to practice each subtask until the client can perform it without difficulty. From the content the nurse-teacher should determine the domain from which the learning will occur. Based on the content and the domain, learning activities are determined, and a target date for achieving each objective is established. Breaking tasks down into content is extremely important because it determines the appropriate activities. Omission of this step can result in failure of the client to learn.[24]

The method for evaluating how successfully each objective has been achieved also should be stipulated. Since the behavioral objectives are stated using action verbs, they can be used in the evaluation. Simply ask the learner to do whatever the behavioral objective states he or she should do.

The plan should sequence all activities according to priority of learning needs. Generally, a learning plan can be ordered according to the following types of needs[14]:

acute learning needs Knowledge, skill, or attitudes needed to avoid danger (for example, a client requiring insulin).

preventive learning needs Knowledge, skill, or attitudes needed to alleviate or diminish the potential for disease and injury (for example, foot care for the diabetic client).

maintenance learning needs Knowledge, skill, or attitudes needed to adapt to changes in normal functioning (for example, a client with compensated congestive heart failure).

IMPLEMENTING THE PLAN

When implementing the written plan, consideration is given to the establishment of a learning climate and the benefits of group versus individual instruction. Principles 7 through 11 are concerned with implementing the plan.

Establishing the Learning Climate

Principle 7. "Distractions reduce the efficiency of teaching and learning."[16]

The teaching-learning process can take place in any setting; however, the setting should be such that distractions of any type are kept to a minimum. Distractions impair the learner's ability to concentrate on the learning task. To prevent distractions, learning should take place in a self-contained area in which other clients, visitors, or personnel are limited.

The learning climate also should be comfortable. Seats should allow for appropriate positioning and flexibility in movement. Lighting should be indirect, if possible, to avoid glare. Room temperature must be adjusted according to amount of physical activity involved in the learning activities. The color and texture of walls and other surfaces should be "coordinated to assist in differentiation between surfaces and fixtures."[2]

Principle 8. "Learning is more effective if carried out over a period of time."[18]

Time is another important element to consider

in implementing learning experiences.[13] The length of time the learner can concentrate attention on a given activity is a major factor in determining the time of day, length, and frequency of the learning sessions. Clients who have diminished physical strength and energies might learn more efficiently early in the day or following a rest period. It also is important to recognize that time between sessions is needed to assimilate what has been learned. Without time for assimilation, the learner's endeavors are more likely to lead to failures rather than successes. Such an error in implementation can result in loss of desire to continue the learning process.

Principle 9. "The environment can be used to focus the patient's attention on what he is to learn."[16]

The use of different types of learning media in the environment, such as posters, booklets, and practice equipment, tends to gain the attention of the learner and lead to the exploration of the meaning and significance of the aids.[9] The visibility of assistive devices, such as a bathtub seat, utensil holder, or hygiene and grooming aids, can be just enough to not only stimulate learning but hopefulness as well.

The environment can be arranged to provide appropriate facilities for learners to practice relearned skills, such as dressing and shaving, at a time of their own choosing. The nurse-teacher is available if needed. Such an arrangement encourages independence and reestablishes routines for the learner.

Principle 10. "Satisfaction reinforces learning."[15]

The learning environment should provide positive reinforcement (reward) for new behaviors to encourage learners to repeat the behaviors. Initially the reinforcement should follow each time the behavior is performed until the behavior is learned well. Reinforcement should then be given intermittently.[7]

Rewards can take many forms. Perhaps the most common is praising the learner. Other incentives, such as special outings or food treats, unless medically contraindicated, provide variety. Each learner responds differently to different rewards. The nurse-teacher should identify which reward provides the most incentive to the learner.

Principle 11. "Because it requires change in beliefs and behavior, learning normally produces a mild level of anxiety, which is useful in motivating the individual; however, severe anxiety is incapacitating."[16]

An atmosphere that conveys warmth and acceptance promotes a positive attitude and a desire to learn. An equally important quality of the atmosphere is an attitude that encourages learners to begin at their level of need and progress at a comfortable rate to learn what they want to learn. Such an attitude promotes success.[7,16] As learners are guided to new achievements, they gain greater self-confidence and become more self-motivating.[9,16] Anxieties decrease as the fear of failure is diminished. Through interactions with the nurse-teacher and the environment and through increased self-motivation, learners develop positive feelings about their self-worth.

Group Versus Individual Client Learning Environment

Group learning provides an opportunity for clients to interact with other learners. This learning environment helps to avoid feelings of isolation. Such a climate also encourages learners to maintain contact with reality. Opportunity for sharing information on common mutual problems with others provides a supportive atmosphere. The stimulation derived from group concern can bring hope and encouragement to strive toward skillful performance of the adaptive behaviors. The experience of finding others willing to relate to the disabled individual often helps to improve social skills needed after the learning period.[19]

The group learning environment should be arranged to enable the teacher to provide guidance, demonstrations, and reinforcements to individual learners without interfering with the activities of the other learners. Such an arrangement provides for the ideal teaching-learning experience to occur.

EVALUATING LEARNING

The purpose of evaluation is to determine the effectiveness of the teaching-learning process. Evaluating the process is accomplished by determining if the goal(s) has been achieved by comparing and measuring behavioral outcomes that have been stated as objectives. If clients can perform the activities stated as objectives, then the process was effective and the goal(s) was achieved.

If they cannot, then the nurse-teacher should ask and answer each of these questions:

- Was the goal(s) realistic?
- If not, how should the goal be altered to become realistic?
- Were the learning activities appropriate for clients' learning abilities?
- Should the content be retaught?

Any time that evidence suggests the teaching plan is not working, the plan should be reviewed for deficiencies and appropriate corrections made. Evaluation of the plan is continued informally throughout all phases of the teaching-learning process.

Methods of evaluation are determined by the type of learning. For example, motor skills are readily evaluated through observation. The subtasks identified in the task analysis can be used to develop a checklist or scale for rating the behavior. Each component of the rating tool identifies a specific behavior that culminates in the achievement of the desired objective. Cognitive skill, on the other hand, cannot always be observed and might require evaluation through verbal or written responses to questions. Again, the subtasks identified in the task analysis can be used as the basis for oral or written questions.[3] Behavior in the affective domain is probably the most difficult to measure simply because learners can choose not to express their true feelings. Learning in this domain is best observed when learners are unaware of the evaluation being made.[16]

The evaluation process is twofold. It should include both teachers' and clients' evaluations of the clients' progress and the teachers' and clients' evaluation of the teaching plan. Results of the evaluation should be used in future learning processes designed for the same learners, as well as for different learners.

Documentation

Documentation of the teaching-learning process consists of two parts: (1) the teaching plan and (2) objective and measurable data describing movement of the client toward goal achievement. When the plan to be implemented is determined, it should become a part of the client's permanent record and conveyed to all members of the treatment-instructional team. Knowledge and availability of the plan encourages all team members to support the development of behaviors leading to the predetermined goal(s).

Progress notes describing the client's behavior in measurable terms enable team members to track progress and continuously evaluate the effectiveness of the teaching plan. Notes should include descriptions of behavior demonstrating change in all domains: cognitive, psychomotor, and affective.

SUMMARY

The beginning of the teaching-learning process is marked by the identification of learning needs. Since learning can occur any time health care is provided, every member of the rehabilitation team has the responsibility to be knowledgeable and skillful in both rehabilitative techniques and learning principles. Through the application of learning principles, the learner's potential for rehabilitation can be enhanced.

The steps of the teaching-learning process are the same as the four steps of the nursing process: assessment, planning, intervention, and evaluation. Specific learning principles relate to each step of the process and should be applied appropriately throughout the experience.

The format chosen for developing the teaching-learning process should show clearly the relationship and interdependency of the parts. It is usually the primary teacher who selects the format to be followed. Unlike the selection of the format, goals are cooperatively determined by the teacher and the learner with input from the family. Should discussion of the client's learning needs with the family be required, permission must be given by the client. Sometimes a family member accompanies the client through the learning experiences. It is essential that family members understand they are only to assist with activities the client is unable to perform independently.

When developing objectives for the learning experience, the objectives should be stated in behavioral terms (action verbs), such as those suggested by Mager.[11] The use of behavioral terms enables the learner and each member of the instructional team to know exactly what is expected from the learning experiences. Thus the terms also serve as the basis for evaluation of the process.

The teaching-learning process is a dynamic experience in which the behavior of both teacher and learner play a crucial role in the outcome. The application of learning principles by the teacher ensures that the teaching plan and the environment support the development of adaptive behaviors by the learner. Readiness of the client to accept the opportunity to learn is paramount to the successful learning of adaptive behaviors and subsequent rehabilitation.

REFERENCES

1. Bloom BS, editor: Taxonomy of educational objectives: the classification of educational goals. Handbook I: Cognitive domain, New York, 1956, David McKay Co, Inc.
2. Brever JM: A handbook of assistive devices for the handicapped elderly: new help for independent living, New York, 1982, The Haworth Press, Inc.
3. Brunner LS and Suddarth DS: Textbook of medical-surgical nursing, ed 3, Philadelphia, 1982, JB Lippincott Co.
4. Burke LE: Learning and retention in the acute care setting, Crit Care Q 4:67, Dec 1981.
5. Byrne ML and Thompson LF: Key concepts for the study and practice of nursing, St. Louis, 1972, The CV Mosby Co.
6. Crate MA: Nursing functions in adaptations to chronic illness, Am J Nurs 65:72, Oct 1965.
7. Grief E and Mataruzzo RG: Behavioral approaches to rehabilitation: coping with change, New York, 1982, Springer Publishing Co, Inc.
8. Hirschberg GG, Lewis L, and Vaughan P: Rehabilitation: a manual for the care of the disabled and elderly, Philadelphia, 1976, JB Lippincott Co.
9. Klausmeier HJ and Ripple R: Learning and human abilities: educational psychology, ed 4, New York, 1975, Harper & Row Publishers Inc.
10. Kottke FJ, Stillwell GK, and Lehmann JF, editors: Krusen's handbook of physical medicine and rehabilitation, ed 3, Philadelphia, 1982, WB Saunders Co.
11. Mager RF: Preparing instructional objectives, ed 2, Belmont, Calif, 1975, Fearon Publishers.
12. Magill RA: Motor learning concepts and applications, Dubuque, Ia, 1980, Wm C Brown Co.
13. McCormick RD and Parkevich TG: Patient and family education, New York, 1979, John Wiley & Sons, Inc.
14. Mumma CM, editor: Rehabilitation nursing: concepts and practice, a core curriculum, ed 2, Evanston, Ill, 1987, Rehabilitation Nursing Foundation.
15. Nursing Education Committee: MI: guidelines for patient and family teaching, Seattle, 1974, Washington Heart Association.
16. Redman BK: The process of patient education, ed 5, St. Louis, 1984, The CV Mosby Co.
17. Satir VM: Conjoint family therapy: guide to theory and technique, Palo Alto, Calif, 1967, Science & Behavior Books.

18. Scalzi CC, Burke LE, and Greenland S: Evaluation of an inpatient educational program for coronary patients and families, Heart/Lung 9:846, 1980.
19. Smith DW and Germain CPH: Care of the adult patient: medical-surgical nursing, ed 4, Philadelphia, 1975, JB Lippincott Co.
20. Speigel AD and Podair S: Rehabilitating people with disabilities into the mainstream of society, Park Ridge, NJ, 1981, Noyes Publications.
21. Stuart RB, editor: Adherence, compliance, and generalization in behavioral medicine, New York, 1982, Brunner/Mazel, Inc.
22. Toth S: Patient teaching: a nursing process approach, Philadelphia, 1983, JB Lippincott Co.
23. Trieschmann RB: Coping with disability: sliding scale of goals, Arch Phys Med Rehabil 55:556, 1974.
24. Watson PM: Patient education: the adult with cancer, Nurs Clin North Am 17(4):739, 1982.
25. White BG: Competency development for nursing personnel: specifications and evaluation, Raleigh, NC, 1983, North Carolina State University.
26. Wright GN: Total rehabilitation, Boston, 1980, Little Brown & Co.

ADDITIONAL READINGS

Bille DA, editor: Practical approaches to patient teaching, Boston, 1981, Little, Brown & Co.
Bleiberg J and Merbitz C: Learning goals during initial rehabilitation hospitalization, Arch Phys Med Rehabil 64:448, 1983.
Cooper SS: Principles of adult learning, Occup Nurs 31;17, June 1983.
Cross, KP: Adults as learners, San Francisco, 1981, Jossey-Bass, Inc, Publishers.
Hale G: The sourcebook for the disabled: an illustrated guide to easier, more independent living for physically disabled people, their families, and their friends, New York, 1979, Paddington Press Ltd.
Knowles MS: The adult learner: a neglected species, ed 2, Houston, 1978, Gulf Publishing Co.
Lindberg J and others: Introduction to person-centered nursing, Philadelphia, 1983, JB Lippincott Co.
Nichols JR, editor: Rehabilitation medicine: the management of physical disabilities, ed 2, London, 1980, Butterworths & Co, Ltd.
Rankin SH and Duffy KL: Fifteen problems in patient education and their solutions, Nursing 14(4):67, 1984.
Rankin SH and Duffy KL: Patient education: issues, principles, and guidelines, Philadelphia, 1983, JB Lippincott Co.
Stanton MP: Teaching patients: some basic lessons for nurse educators, Nurs Management 16(10):59, 1985.

Professional Practice of Rehabilitation Nursing

Denise Hanlon

Elizabeth L. Sharkey

OBJECTIVES

After completing Chapter 6, the reader will be able to:

1. Describe the roles and levels of practice of rehabilitation nurses.

2. Explain the educational levels of the rehabilitation nurse.

3. Describe the accomplishments of the professional organization for rehabilitation nurses, including standards of practice, core curriculum, and certification.

4. Identify settings for rehabilitation nursing practice.

The direction for this chapter evolved through our own practice and through review of the literature. We asked ourselves: How do we practice in our own individual settings (a general hospital and a university) and how is our practice as rehabilitation nurses different from that of other nurses? There was never any doubt in our minds that our practice was unique. We suppose, though, that any nurse committed to a specialized area of practice has the same belief. Our goal in writing this chapter is to convey to the reader the knowledge, attitudes, and skills of rehabilitation nursing and the roles of rehabilitation nurses. Additionally, levels of practice, educational preparation, professional organizations, standards of practice, core curriculum, certification, and settings for rehabilitation nursing practice are discussed.

ESSENCE OF REHABILITATION NURSING

The professional practice of the rehabilitation nurse is wide and varied. Professional responsibilities depend on the educational preparation of the nurse, as well as the work setting. Regardless of the practice setting and level of educational preparation, the practice of rehabilitation nursing requires special knowledge, attitudes, and skills. According to Hennig,[8] the attitudes of those involved in rehabilitation exhibit a dynamic influence on the client and on the rehabilitation process. Sensitivity, responsiveness, flexibility, creativity, and assertiveness are hallmarks of the rehabilitation nurse.

For rehabilitation nurses to effectively help clients meet goals, they must be sensitive to the clients' needs and feelings and be able to be firm, instill confidence, and foster self-esteem. Nurses must examine their own attitudes toward disability and determine if any negative attitudes exist that might create an obstacle in assuring a therapeutic environment. Attitudes are developed according to the individual nurse's personality. Not all nurses can work in specialized rehabilitation settings; some prefer the fast pace and drama of intensive care units or the type of client who gets better and goes home quickly.

In rehabilitation nursing, the nurse interacts therapeutically with the whole person over long periods of time.[12] Many clients and family members become lifelong friends and require intermittent therapeutic intervention despite their successful rehabilitation. Often, emotional involvement with clients exists to a greater degree than with those clients who enter the nurse's life for very brief periods.

Rehabilitation nursing takes place during all phases of illness and recovery. It begins when the client is admitted to a health care facility and continues throughout the client's rehabilitation process. Continual assessment and reassessment are of prime concern to the rehabilitation nurse. All components of the nursing process must be given attention in relation to the client's life situation and future plans and expectations. The nurse can give immediate feedback to questions and concerns as the client begins the process of community reintegration. The client must rely heavily on the knowledge learned and skills acquired. Thus the nurse also must involve the client's support systems—family, friends, neighbors, community services—in the reeducation process and be creative in solving problems with the client.

Roles of the Rehabilitation Nurse

The rehabilitation nurse fulfills the following roles:

1. *Caregiver:* Provides direct care to the client and family until they develop the necessary skills for self-care and role performance. As caregiver, the rehabilitation nurse establishes a therapeutic environment in which hope is present, encouragement and positive reinforcement are provided, and opportunities to test social skills are incorporated. Rehabilitation techniques are implemented to restore and maintain function and

to prevent the development of secondary complications.

2. *Coordinator:* Helps the client integrate activities and skills learned in therapy in order to achieve a balance and sequence appropriate to the client's specific needs. Consideration is given to timing, endurance, energy level, and the impact of psychosocial problems of disability on function. Additionally, the nurse conveys information to team members regarding the client's adaptation to disability and reports client progress in developing new skills so that team members can adjust the treatment plan accordingly. The rehabilitation nurse functions as a coordinator to give harmony and smoothness to the concerted efforts of the team and client.

3. *Educator:* Promotes the analysis and synthesis of information, validates information provided by others, and serves as a resource for information and clarification. The rehabilitation nurse helps the client and family to use new skills on a continuous basis and assists them in transferring these skills to different situations. Basic skills that require a lifetime for refinement are vitally important to one's existence but are rarely appreciated until disability occurs. Such human functions as walking and eating are taken for granted. When these functions must be relearned, the teacher becomes a prominent figure in the life of the person with a disability. Activities of daily living (ADL) skills are not as easy to relearn as adults as they were to learn when we were children. The emotional response to the disabling condition can present a block to learning. The rehabilitation nurse must be skilled in dealing with the emotional stress of the disability while assisting the client to relearn old and develop new skills. Adults do not usually recall how such ADL skills were learned—these skills have become habit. Most of us do not realize the number of steps involved in accomplishing ADL tasks until these abilities are impaired or lost. In addition, the rehabilitation nurse teaches nursing staff members the importance of and performance of rehabilitation nursing techniques and reinforces the teaching done by other rehabilitation team members.

4. *Advocate/case manager:* Supports the client in the restorative process in the health care facility and in the community. This activity includes assisting the client in adapting to or re-

solving problems presented by existing or potential barriers. Most often, the rehabilitation nurse acts as a liaison for the client when others are having difficulty understanding the client's responses. The rehabilitation nurse offers insight not only to others but to clients regarding others' responses to them and to their specific disability. The nurse initiates and supports community and legislative activities that promote the civil rights and community reintegration of the disabled.

5. *Leader:* Influences the client and team toward attainment of common goals. The rehabilitation nurse may function as the recognized or unrecognized leader, but in either position gives direction to the client and to team members.

6. *Collaborator:* Works jointly with team members, especially the client, to achieve common goals. Successful collaboration takes place only in an atmosphere of cooperation and respect, and its absence among team members is easily recognized by the client. A lack of collaboration can have deleterious effects on client functional outcomes.

7. *Facilitator:* Assists clients in accomplishing goals in a timely fashion. If the restorative process is more difficult than clients expect, they may become frustrated and possibly defeated. The importance of performing ADL tasks with optimum independence is emphasized, without creating anxiety in the client.

8. *Liaison:* Serves as a vital link for referral to other team members in the institution and in the community.

9. *Consultant:* Acts as a resource for information for clients and their families, nursing staff members, rehabilitation team members, and community agencies.

10. *Discharge planner:* Orchestrates the client's discharge from a rehabilitation program. Discharge often involves referring to multiple services in the community, facilitating the purchase of assistive and adaptive equipment, assisting the client to obtain supplies, adapting the environment, referring to vocational rehabilitation, and assisting the client in social skills and recreational activities.

11. *Researcher:* Uses and contributes to rehabilitation team and rehabilitation nursing research to benefit the client and family affected by disability. The clinical nurse specialist in rehabilitation nursing initiates rehabilitation nursing research and shares findings with other rehabilitation nurses and team members.

Levels of Practice

Since basic nursing education rarely offers a separate course in rehabilitation nursing, nurses specializing in rehabilitation often must be self-directed in obtaining specialized knowledge and skills. Methods of accomplishing this may be on-the-job experience, attendance at workshops and seminars on rehabilitation nursing, or preparation as a clinical specialist in graduate school. We have identified three levels of practice based upon acquired knowledge and skill:

Level I rehabilitation nurses: Nurses in this level practice in a rehabilitation setting and have acquired basic knowledge and skills through formal and informal education and on-the-job experience. They hold a diploma or associate degree in nursing.

Level II rehabilitation nurse specialists: These nurses practice in a rehabilitation setting and have acquired intermediate to advanced skills through formal education, self-education, continuing education, and on-the-job experience. They usually hold a baccalaureate degree in nursing.

Level III rehabilitation clinical nurse specialists: Level III nurses hold a master's degree in rehabilitation nursing and apply advanced knowledge and skills in the rehabilitation setting, participate in or initiate nursing research, act as change agents to improve client and family rehabilitative care, and teach clients, families, and staff members. They make nursing judgments and carry out nursing actions beyond levels I and II.[7]

Regardless of practice level, all rehabilitation nurses function in the roles previously mentioned. The degree of sophistication and ability to carry out these roles depends upon the nurse's educational level and professional growth. The rehabilitation nurse must recognize limitations of practice in the specialty area according to education, interest, and experience. Additionally, nurses in general practice or in other nursing specialties use rehabilitation nursing techniques. For example, critical care nurses frequently employ such rehabilitation nursing measures as positioning, splinting, and range of joint motion exercises.

Rehabilitation nurses focus on the client as a holistic being. They implement the rehabilitation philosophy, incorporate rehabilitation principles in practice, and apply rehabilitation nursing knowledge and skills within the framework of the nursing process. It is the application of the nursing process and the special knowledge, attitudes, and skills of rehabilitation nurses that help the client achieve an optimum level of physical, functional, psychosocial, economic-vocational, and spiritual function and eventual return to social roles within the community.

EDUCATIONAL PREPARATION

Rehabilitation nurses are prepared at the diploma, associate degree, baccalaureate degree, master's degree, and doctoral degree levels.

Basic Preparation

Rehabilitation nurses, whether prepared in a diploma, associate degree, or baccalaureate degree nursing program, need a sound foundation in anatomy and physiology, especially of the neurological, musculoskeletal, gastrointestinal, and urological systems; knowledge of growth and development; and an understanding of the aging process. They must understand functional assessment, kinesiology, interpersonal group dynamics, and teaching-learning principles. They must understand the grief response to loss and impairment and the ramifications of this response for both the client and family members during the rehabilitation process. In addition, rehabilitation nurses must be able to use manual skills to accomplish position change, range of joint motion exercise, transfer, ambulation, and ADL tasks with the client.

According to the American Nurses' Association (ANA), nursing education should take place in institutions of higher learning.[8] This goal is not so easily achieved, since many schools of nursing do not offer a specialized course and clinical experience in specialized rehabilitation agencies. It is common for students to lack opportunity for participation in a comprehensive rehabilitation team approach to care. More often, rehabilitation philosophy, principles, and techniques are integrated within the curriculum and within the adult health nursing clinical experiences.

TABLE 6-1

Master's degree programs in rehabilitation nursing

School	Curriculum offered
Rush-Presbyterian-St. Luke's Medical Center, Chicago	Rehabilitation nursing graduate program
State University of New York, Buffalo	Adult health with clinical specialist option in rehabilitation nursing
Thomas Jefferson University, Philadelphia	Clinical specialist in rehabilitation nursing
University of Alabama, Birmingham	Adult health with clinical specialist option in rehabilitation nursing
University of Texas, Arlington	Rehabilitation nursing Teaching Administration Clinical specialization Primary care

Continuing Education

The agency in which the nurse works must often assume responsibility for educating the new graduate in the art and science of rehabilitation nursing. The major sources of expanding knowledge on rehabilitation nursing are on-the-job experience, inservice education, and continuing education conferences within the health care facility and at local colleges and universities.

Graduate Preparation

Currently five graduate programs offer advanced nursing practice to prepare clinical specialists in rehabilitation nursing (Table 6-1).[11] The clinical specialist functions as an expert in the clinical practice of rehabilitation nursing; a client, family, and staff educator; a change agent and consultant; and a researcher. Nurses prepared at the graduate level in the specialty area often occupy leadership positions in the delivery of rehabilitation nursing and offer support, education, and assistance in planned change strategies to the nursing staff. These nurses also assist the nursing staff in conducting clinical nursing research designed to improve the quality of care. The clinical specialist is often in an advantageous position to identify clinical practices that could be improved when research findings are used. Mikulic[9] attributes the nursing staff's improved work satisfaction and commitment to a rehabilitation program to the contributions of a clinical specialist holding a joint appointment between a hospital and university.

PROFESSIONAL ORGANIZATIONS

The primary purpose of any professional organization is to foster high standards.[4] The methodology used includes (1) definition of the scope of specialty practice, (2) development and implementation of standards, and (3) quality assurance. According to Styles,[14] "organizations [are] vehicles for defining and achieving objectives of the professions and its members. . . ." She stresses that synchronization of functions is essential for preservation and development. These functions include (1) successful self-regulation, (2) common language, and (3) development and dissemination of science, skill, education, credentialing, and practice components.[14]

The rehabilitation nurse has the choice of belonging to one or more professional organizations devoted to rehabilitation. (See Appendix G.) The only organization developed to meet the specific needs of rehabilitation nurses, however, is the Association of Rehabilitation Nurses (ARN). This organization was founded in 1974 by a small group of rehabilitation nurses who recognized the need for a professional nursing organization specifically concerned with the professional and educational needs of rehabilitation nurses.

ARN is organized according to national, regional, and state levels of operation. The many accomplishments of this organization include the following:

1974 Founded

1975 *ARN Journal* published (name changed to *Rehabilitation Nursing* in 1980)

1976 Rehabilitation Nursing Institute established (name changed to Rehabilitation Nursing Foundation in 1986) (The primary responsibilities of this nonprofit educational and research foundation of the ARN are to provide opportunities for nurses to update knowledge on relevant areas of rehabilitation nursing practice and to carry out research activities of ARN.)

ARN accepted into the National Federation of Specialty Nursing Organizations and the ANA

1977 *Standards of Rehabilitation Nursing Practice* published with the ANA

1981 *Rehabilitation Nursing: Concepts and Practice, a Core Curriculum* published

1984 First certification examination administered[3]

1986 Revised *Standards of Rehabilitation Nursing Practice* published with the ANA

1987 Rehabilitation Nurses' Research Fund established (In 1988 and each succeeding year, the Research Committee will solicit and review proposals submitted by rehabilitation nurses. The goal of the research fund is to improve the quality of rehabilitation nursing care through nursing research and use of findings in delivery of care.)

Second edition *Core Curriculum* published

As these accomplishments show, the basic criteria for a professional organization have been met. In the course of 13 years, ARN has clearly defined the scope of practice, developed standards, and identified a common body of knowledge that forms the basis for practice in rehabilitation nursing. In addition, ARN has recognized the need for education and research and, under the leadership of the Rehabilitation Nursing Foundation, has been sponsoring conferences on both national and regional levels.

Other professional organizations are available to the rehabilitation nurse. Membership in these organizations is usually open to most members of the interdisciplinary team. Within these organizations, the rehabilitation nurse has the opportunity to share and exchange information and ideas on a national level at conferences and meetings with other members of the rehabilitation team. Nurses belonging to these organizations can gain knowledge and network, as well as educate other health care professionals about the vital role of rehabilitation nursing. Dr. June Rothberg, a leader in rehabilitation nursing and former dean of the school of nursing and vice-provost of Adelphi University, Garden City, New York, has been recognized by the American Congress of Rehabilitation Medicine (ACRM) as a leader in the field of rehabilitation. She was the first nurse to serve as president of this interdisciplinary organization and has been awarded the Gold Key by the ACRM, an honor recognizing "meritorious service to the cause of persons with physical disabilities."[2]

Standards of Practice

Standards are crucial to quality rehabilitative care and are intimately involved with the nursing process. Standards are used to measure quality by determining how well the nurse complies with the standards. Professional growth for the individual nurse and the specialty as a whole can be achieved and identification as a profession can be facilitated when standards of practice are used.

According to Donabedian,[5] standards are "operationalized definitions of the quality of care" developed by recognized leaders and experts in the field. The use of standards by the individual nurse requires a conscious decision and continuous level of awareness of the client's actual or potential problems. The nurse's assessment and validation of clinical competence are important. Standards facilitate nursing care delivery by maximizing continuity and consistency and providing an effective problem-solving approach.[2]

The development of standards was recognized by the ARN as one of the initial tasks of the organization. The draft of the standards, written by rehabilitation nursing leaders, was circulated to the entire membership for review and comment. A booklet entitled "Standards of Rehabilitation Nursing Practice" (Appendix A) was published with the ANA in 1977 and revised in 1986.[1] As recommended by Donabedian, the rehabilitation nursing standards truly represent the leadership and membership of the ARN.

Core Curriculum

Specialty groups must have a recognized common body of knowledge that clearly defines and delineates the scope of practice. This body of knowledge was defined by the ARN, published in 1981, and again in 1987. The entire ARN membership was involved in developing and responding to the content. A conceptual approach based upon functional status rather than a disease-oriented approach was chosen as the framework for describing common knowledge. Emphasis on function is a logical approach, since it is the aim of rehabil-

itation to restore the client to an optimum functional level, whereas the disease-oriented approach tends to focus on the pathological condition.[10]

Certification

Certification is a process undertaken to acknowledge and validate an individual's knowledge and clinical competence in a specific area of nursing. It is based on standards of practice and is usually awarded based on the results of a written examination. The responsibility for the certification procedure rests with the professional organization. Thus ARN offered the first certification examination in December, 1984. Upon successful completion of the examination, the rehabilitation nurse is entitled to use the designation *certified rehabilitation registered nurse* (CRRN). This examination was based upon the "Standards of Rehabilitation Nursing Practice" and the content delineated in *Rehabilitation Nursing: Concepts and Practice, a Core Curriculum*. According to Drew,[6] former chairperson of the ARN Certification Board, this examination certifies generalists who concentrate their practice in rehabilitation. Drew further states that the intent of the CRRN examination is to give nurses without available graduate education an opportunity to have their knowledge in rehabilitation nursing recognized.

The certification examination offered by the ARN is not the only certification opportunity available to rehabilitation nurses, but it is the *only* certification examination specifically addressing rehabilitation nursing practice. The other examination qualifies rehabilitation nurses as *certified insurance rehabilitation specialists*. This examination regulates practice within the insurance industry as it relates to rehabilitation and is open to any professional practicing in the insurance field. The content usually includes some nursing, but the ARN has not officially become involved in content development. Many rehabilitation nurses hold this certification.

SETTINGS FOR REHABILITATION NURSING PRACTICE

Rehabilitation nurses have the advantage of applying their skills and knowledge in a diverse range of settings. The philosophy and goals of the rehabilitation nursing process are the same, regardless of the setting.[13] Demand for rehabilitation nursing expertise and services is increasing, especially in the burgeoning home health care industry, and will continue to expand as the proportion of individuals affected by disability in our population increases.

Rehabilitation nurses practice in freestanding rehabilitation centers or rehabilitation units in general hospitals, as consultants in acute care units within general hospitals and in private homes, extended care facilities, schools, centers for independent living, the insurance industry, clinics, physicians' offices, and the community. Because the goals of rehabilitation are the same, the nurse can adjust with relative ease to any setting.

SUMMARY

Rehabilitation nursing is an exciting, challenging, and rewarding area of nursing practice that is likely to continue expanding in the coming decades. The aging population and increasing numbers of physically disabled and chronically ill persons will increase demands for rehabilitative services and for knowledgeable rehabilitation nurses. Rehabilitation nurses who collaborate effectively with other members of health and social disciplines to bring clients to their full functional potential will see an increasing demand for their services.

REFERENCES

1. American Nurses' Association, Division of Medical/Surgical Nursing Practice, and the Association of Rehabilitation Nurses: Standards of rehabilitation nursing practice, Kansas City, Mo, 1986, The Association.
2. Arch Phys Med Rehabil 66(2):127, 1985.
3. ARN Historian Committee: Association of Rehabilitation Nurses: the first ten years, Evanston, Ill, 1984, Association of Rehabilitation Nurses.
4. Boroch RM: Future confluence: the rehabilitation nurse and the profession. In Walsh A, editor: The expanded role of the rehabilitation nurse, Thorofare, NJ, 1980, Charles B Slack, Inc.
5. Donabedian A: Promoting quality through evaluating the process of patient care, Med Care 6(3):182, 1968.
6. Drew JW: Certification in rehabilitation nursing, Rehabil Nurs 10:20, March/April 1985.
7. Fanslow CA: The rehabilitation clinical nurse specialist. In Murray R and Kijek J, editors: Current perspectives in rehabilitation nursing, St. Louis, 1979, The CV Mosby Co.
8. Hennig LM: The rehabilitation nurse. In Nickel VL, editor: Orthopedic rehabilitation, New York, 1982, Churchill Livingstone, Inc.
9. Mikulic MA: The development of a rehabilitation program through a triple appointment, ARNJ 3:9, July/Aug 1978.
10. Mumma CM, editor: Rehabilitation nursing: concepts and practice, a core curriculum, Evanston, Ill, 1987, Rehabilitation Nursing Foundation.
11. National League for Nursing, Council of Baccalaureate and Higher Degree Programs: Baccalaureate and master's degree programs in nursing accredited by NLN, Pub No 15-1310, New York, 1987, The League.
12. Payne ME: The nurse as patient advocate in the rehabilitation setting, ARNJ 4:9, Sept/Oct 1979.
13. Rothberg JS: The challenges for rehabilitative nursing. Nurs Outlook 17:37, Nov 1969.
14. Styles MM: The anatomy of a profession, Rehabil Nurs 8:10, Sept/Oct 1983.

ADDITIONAL READINGS

Berrol S: An affirmative action course for rehabilitation nursing. In Walsh A, editor: The expanded role of the rehabilitation nurse, Thorofare, NJ, 1980, Charles B Slack, Inc.

Kraning MJ and Mumma C: The implementation of holistic/humanistic concepts in a rehabilitation setting, ARNJ 3:12, Nov/Dec 1978.

Kwan KL and Loo SYS: The rehabilitation nurse, ARNJ 1:5, March/April 1976.

Latus MJ: The role of the insurance rehabilitation nurse, Rehabil Nurs 7:26, May/June 1982.

Merton R: The functions of the professional association, Am J Nurs 58:50, Jan 1958.

Reeves R: Nurse, what are you all about? ARNJ 5:22, July/Aug 1980.

Watson PG: Components of rehabilitation nursing practice advancement, Rehabil Nurs 10:28, Sept/Oct 1985.

Wiener SM: Rehabilitation nursing in the private sector, Rehabil Nurs 8:31, March/April 1983.

Wunder SC and Glenn MJ: Rehabilitation nursing in action: O'Donoghue Screening Clinic, Rehabil Nurs 9:22, May/June 1984.

PART II

Promotion of Client Function in Activities of Daily Living Necessary for Sustaining Life

CHAPTER 7

Breathing

Elizabeth A. Moody-Szymanski
Yvonne Krall Scherer

OBJECTIVES

After completing Chapter 7, the reader will be able to:

1. Describe the structures of the respiratory system.
2. Discuss automatic and involuntary control of breathing.
3. Describe the chest bellows apparatus.
4. Explain the structure and function of the upper and lower airways.
5. Explain the significance of the alveolar-capillary unit.
6. Identify complications associated with impaired respiratory function.
7. Conduct a nursing assessment specific to the client with impaired breathing.
8. List common nursing diagnoses related to the client with respiratory impairment.
9. Identify pulmonary rehabilitation goals.
10. Discuss nursing interventions indicated for the client with impaired respiratory function.
11. Demonstrate methods of physical conditioning that may be indicated for the client with respiratory impairment.
12. Discuss modalities of respiratory therapy used to maintain adequate gas exchange.
13. Identify information and skills necessary for the education of clients and families affected by respiratory impairment.
14. Discuss the responsibilities of selected rehabilitation team members involved in assisting the client with impaired respiration to function at an optimum level.
15. List outcome criteria used as a basis for evaluating a rehabilitation plan for the client with impaired respiratory function.

Breathing can be described as the mechanical output required to deliver oxygen to the cells and remove carbon dioxide from the body. Normally this system is highly efficient, and breathing is performed unconsciously to meet a wide range of metabolic demands.

Respiratory disability can have a considerable physical, psychosocial, and financial impact on the client, family, and society. The client with pulmonary compromise presents a complex and difficult problem to the rehabilitation team. To develop an adequate plan of care, the multidimensional nature of impaired breathing must be understood. In addition to exercise intolerance, limitations may exist in many other activities of daily living. Clients may experience shortness of breath each time they eat or may have difficulty swallowing or chewing. The inability to cough or remove secretions may become a problem. Disruption of sleep patterns can change and contribute to decreased alertness and altered personality. Medications to improve breathing function frequently have numerous undesirable side effects. Environmental factors and atmospheric conditions often contribute to discomfort. The ability of the client and family to adjust will influence behavior patterns and social relationships.

Early diagnosis and prevention of respiratory problems may reduce the risk of chronic impairment. Consistent planning and intervention can often alleviate symptoms and prevent extension of existing problems. The rehabilitation team plays a vital role in improving the quality of life for persons with potential or real pulmonary compromise.

STRUCTURE AND FUNCTION OF THE RESPIRATORY SYSTEM

Respiration is the total process by which the body acquires oxygen, performs metabolic work, and eliminates carbon dioxide. Normally the respiratory system is efficient and accommodates a twentyfold increase in oxygen consumption or carbon dioxide production.[21] This gas transport and exchange system depends upon the integrated performance of the pulmonary, hematological, circulatory, and nervous systems. Dysfunction of any of these systems can result in respiratory compromise and lead to acute or chronic failure.

Ventilation is the process by which oxygen is delivered to and carbon dioxide eliminated from the alveolus, the principal site of gas exchange in the lungs. Normal ventilation is a rhythmic act dependent upon four separate but interrelated components: (1) nervous system control, (2) the chest bellows apparatus, (3) airways, and (4) the alveolar-capillary unit (Figure 7-1).

Nervous System Control

The central nervous system adjusts ventilation to meet the metabolic demands of the body so that oxygen (O_2), carbon dioxide (CO_2), and pH levels remain within normal limits. Appropriate interaction between central and peripheral neuronal networks is essential for transmission of information, allowing for critical adjustments to maintain homeostasis. Three principal interconnected parts of these networks can be described as controllers, effectors, and sensors (Figure 7-2).

Controllers

Breathing can be modified both automatically and voluntarily. Automatic control of breathing depends upon chemical stimulation and changes in lung inflation, whereas voluntary control responds to behavioral signals.

Automatic control. Interconnected neurons located bilaterally in the reticular substance of the medulla and pons form the respiratory center. The basic spontaneous rhythm of breathing is established here. Chemoreceptors, proprioceptors, and the vagus nerve send afferent input to the brainstem. Neurons in the spinal cord integrate efferent impulses arriving from the brainstem and send signals to the respiratory muscles.

The medullary center establishes the basic rhythm of respiration and is primarily responsible for initiating and maintaining the sequence and duration of inspiratory respiratory activity. Aggregates of neurons located in the pons modulate respiratory activity by action on the medulla. The pneumotaxic center in the upper pons regulates the volume and the rate of respiration, promoting a regular pattern of breathing. The apneustic center in the lower pons appears to have an inspiratory inhibitory mechanism. Sustained inspiration (apneusis) occurs with lesions affecting this area and can be seen as irregular, gasping respirations.

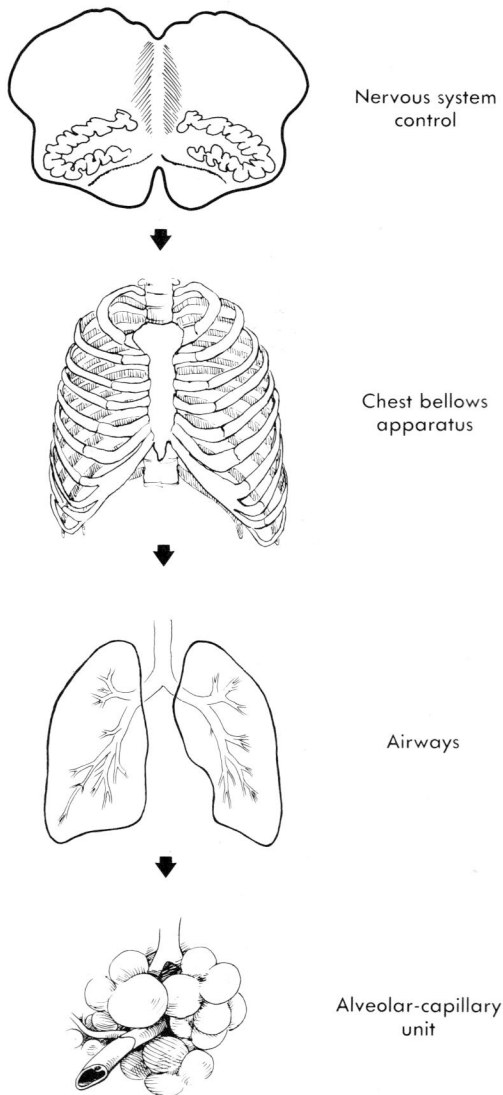

Figure 7-1
Respiratory system and its components. *(From Lankin PN: Weaning from mechanical ventilation. In Fishman AP, editor: Update: pulmonary diseases and disorders, New York, 1982, McGraw-Hill Book Co.)*

Voluntary control. Voluntary (behavioral) control of respiration is regulated by the cerebral cortex and modifies automatic mechanisms or partially bypasses them.[5] Activities that rely on voluntary control of breathing include talking, laughing, crying, and swallowing. The ability to increase breathing during exercise also involves the voluntary control system.

The voluntary conducting pathways in the spinal cord are distinct from those involved in automatic regulation. Automatic fibers can be injured while voluntary pathways remain intact and vice versa. Activity of the voluntary control system depends upon the state of wakefulness. If there is dysfunction of the automatic system but voluntary control is maintained, apnea and blood gas deterioration may occur during sleep, but normal breathing resumes when a person is awake. Conversely, voluntary control may be impaired but automatic function maintained. In such a situation, the person would respond normally to chemical and reflex stimuli but would be unable to perform consciously controlled respiratory maneuvers.[8]

Effectors

The muscles of respiration are the primary effectors of breathing and include the diaphragm, intercostal, and accessory muscles. These muscles possess no inherent rhythm, but depend upon the signals received from the controller. Efferents include the phrenic nerve (C3 to C5), which activates the diaphragm, and segments of the upper thoracic cord, which stimulate the intercostal muscles. Other effector pathways regulate smooth muscle and mucous gland response in the tracheobronchial tree and skeletal muscle activity in the upper airway.[32]

Sensors

Sensors acquire knowledge about certain features of the internal or external environment, send messages to the controlling system for interpretation, and monitor efficacy of compensatory mechanisms. The primary sensors within the respiratory system are chemoreceptors and pulmonary mechanoreceptors.

The respiratory system is highly sensitive to even slight changes in hydrogen ion (H^+), carbon dioxide (Pco_2), and oxygen (Po_2) tensions in the blood, extracellular fluid, and cerebrospinal fluid. There are two primary chemoreceptor areas, one central and the other peripheral.

Central chemoreceptors. Central chemoreceptors are aggregates of cells in bilateral areas of the medulla that are distinct from brainstem respiratory neurons. Activity of these receptors fluc-

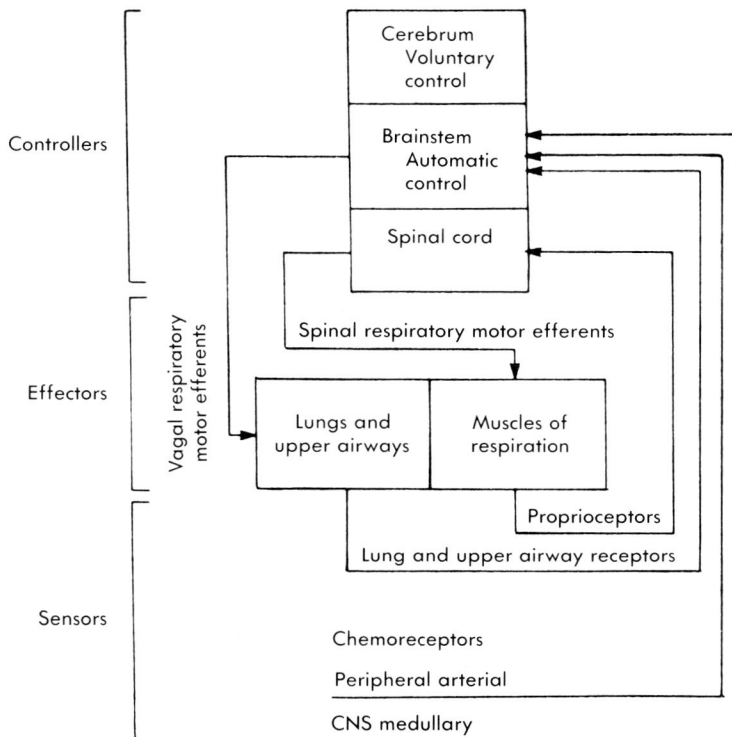

Figure 7-2
Schematic representation of respiratory control system. Interrelationships among central nervous system controllers, effectors, and sensors and connections among these components are shown. (*Modified from Berger AJ and others: N Engl J Med 297:93, 1977. Reprinted by permission of the* New England Journal of Medicine.)

tuates with changes in PCO_2 or H^+ in the surrounding extracellular fluid. Increased H^+ parallels increased PCO_2, lowers the pH, and stimulates the chemoreceptors to increase ventilation. The stimulant effect of PCO_2 on the central respiratory centers accounts for 80% of the total chemoreceptor response to that gas.[46] Blunting of this central drive to breathe leads to hypercapnia (an excess of CO_2 in the blood) and dependency on the peripheral chemoreceptors to maintain adequate alveolar ventilation.

Peripheral chemoreceptors. Chemoreceptors in the peripheral system, located at the bifurcation of the common carotid arteries (carotid bodies) and along the arch of the aorta (aortic bodies), produce essentially all of the changes associated with hypoxemia and approximately 20% of the ventilatory response to hypercapnia. In humans the carotid bodies play a far more important role than the aortic bodies as chemoreceptors.

The carotid bodies are well vascularized and have a high metabolic rate. They are stimulated by a fall in PO_2, elevation in PCO_2, or decrease in pH in arterial blood. Hypoxemia has no direct stimulatory effect on the respiratory center, but the peripheral chemoreceptors are highly sensitive and quickly transmit the information to the controller to increase ventilation. A fall in arterial PO_2, especially below 60, is a powerful stimulus that is further potentiated when combined with hypercapnia or acidosis. Peripheral chemoreceptors respond much more quickly to acute changes in acid-base balance than the central chemoreceptors, allowing for a dual-center mechanism that provides both prompt and delayed central response.[5]

Pulmonary mechanoreceptors. Pulmonary mechanoreceptors, sensory receptors within the airways and lungs, transmit signals to the central nervous system through the vagus nerve. Three groups of receptors have been defined: (1) stretch receptors, (2) irritant receptors, and (3) juxtacapillary receptors.

Stretch receptors in the smooth muscle of the airway are primarily sensitive to transmural or distending pressure. These receptors have an inspiratory-inhibiting effect by increasing expiratory muscle activity as lung volume increases, thereby assisting the return to a steady state. The main reflex effect is a slowing of respiratory rate by increasing expiratory time. By terminating inspiration, respiratory frequency also can be regulated in response to exercise or increased metabolic work.[5]

Irritant receptors line the epithelial layer of the airways and respond to a variety of stimuli, including chemical or mechanical stimulation or rapid inflation of the lung. These receptors are not active during normal breathing but, together with stretch receptors, play an important role in defense of the lung, coughing and sneezing, regulation of airway muscle tone and caliber, and regulation of the quantity and composition of mucous secretions.[32]

Juxtacapillary receptors (J-receptors) are located in alveolar walls close to the capillary network. J-receptors consist of the terminal branches of unmyelinated afferent nerve fibers and do not play an active role in normal breathing. Much of the dyspnea and rapid shallow breathing seen in persons with pulmonary congestion or interstitial lung disease may be attributed to activation of J-receptors.

Mechanoreceptor activity in the thoracic wall controls the movement and strength of respiratory muscle contraction, allowing for critical adjustments to improve muscle efficiency and maintain adequate alveolar ventilation.

Chest Bellows Apparatus

Mechanical performance of the chest bellows apparatus plays a crucial role in maintaining respiratory homeostasis. The bony thorax and muscles of respiration comprise this "ventilatory pump." Efferent impulses are sent from the central nervous system by peripheral pathways to inspiratory muscles, which then contract, causing the chest to expand and lungs to inflate.

Because of their elastic properties, the lungs have a natural tendency to contract while the chest wall expands. The opposing recoil creates a negative pressure within the pleural space. Expansion of the thorax during inspiration creates a further drop in intrapleural pressure and establishes a pressure gradient between the mouth (atmospheric pressure) and alveoli (subatmospheric pressure), causing the lungs to inflate with air. Expiration is normally accomplished passively as elastic recoil returns the lungs and chest wall to a resting position.

Coordination of these movements allows for appropriate levels of ventilation. Interruption of the systems by either failure in the transmission of signals along neural pathways or interference in the mechanics of breathing may lead to dyspnea, hypoventilation, and eventually respiratory failure.

The thoracic cage

The thoracic cage includes the chest wall, thoracic spine, and diaphragm and functions to (1) protect the contents of the thoracic cavity and (2) produce the changes in intrathoracic pressure that enable alveolar ventilation.

The diaphragm

Movement of the diaphragm, the primary muscle of inspiration, accounts for greater than two thirds of the air volume entering the lungs during tidal breathing.[2] This musculotendinous sheath separates the abdomen from the thorax, with peripheral insertions into the lower rib cage. Neural input to the diaphragm is transmitted via the phrenic nerve arising from spinal cord roots at C3, C4, and C5, with a lesser component from the lower thoracic nerves.[7]

When the diaphragm contracts, the abdominal viscera are displaced downward, causing increased abdominal pressure and protrusion of the abdomen outward. At the same time, the rib cage expands upward and outward, enlarging the thorax and creating more negative intrapleural pressure. This establishes a transdiaphragmatic pressure gradient that reflects the amount of work performed by the diaphragm (Figure 7-3). Although expiration is normally passive, the diaphragm can contribute an expiratory action when

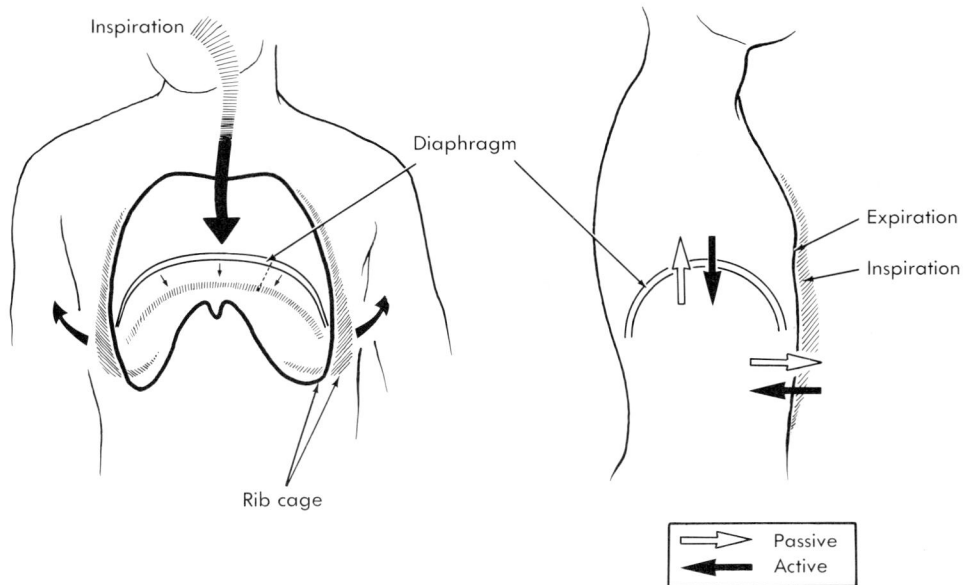

Figure 7-3
On inspiration, dome-shaped diaphragm contracts, abdominal contents are forced down and forward, and rib cage is lifted. Both increase volume of thorax. On forced expiration, abdominal muscles contract and push diaphragm up. *(From West JB: Respiratory physiology: the essentials, ed 3, Baltimore, 1985, The Williams & Wilkins Co.)*

its normal dome shape becomes flattened, as seen with hyperinflation or high lung volumes.[28]

Intercostal and accessory muscles

External intercostal and parasternal internal intercostal muscles are active during inspiration, whereas the internal interosseus intercostals contract only during expiration.[13] Together with the accessory muscles (scalenes, sternocleidomastoids, trapezius), the intercostal muscles stabilize the chest wall structures and are recruited to increase their activity during times of increased work of breathing.

Abdominal muscles

The abdominal muscles (rectus and transverse abdominis, internal and external obliques) facilitate inspiration by contributing to transdiaphragmatic pressure, thereby improving the mechanical action and efficiency of the diaphragm.[38] On expiration, contraction of the abdominal muscles causes an increase in intraabdominal pressure and

displacement of the diaphragm into the thorax, contributing to the elastic recoil of the lungs and chest wall. For this reason, the abdominals are usually considered expiratory muscles. Such actions as coughing, sneezing, vomiting, and the Valsalva maneuver are all facilitated through use of the abdominal muscles.[30]

Respiratory muscle function

The work of breathing is determined by the level of force required by the muscles to generate enough pressure to establish airflow. Usually this work is minimal and done almost entirely by the inspiratory muscles. Obstruction or resistance to flow and a decrease in elasticity (compliance) of the lungs or chest wall will increase the work of breathing. Signals originating in the respiratory muscles increase to maintain an appropriate level of ventilation and are considered a primary source leading to the sensation of breathlessness.[1]

The maximum force a muscle can generate is

a function of the initial fiber length before contraction; the longer the length, the greater the force. The fiber length of inspiratory muscles depends on lung volume. As volume increases, fiber length shortens and the muscle weakens. Therefore persons breathing at high lung volumes are predisposed to respiratory muscle fatigue. Consequently, hyperinflation often may cause a person to assume postures (leaning forward while sitting) that enhance function of the diaphragm by improving the length-tension relationship.[29]

Respiratory muscle strength also depends upon such factors as age, sex, nutritional status, and physical conditioning. For any given level of alveolar ventilation, there is an optimum tidal volume and respiratory rate that results in the minimum amount of work for the respiratory muscles. Deviation from this pattern results in increased work of breathing.[39]

The first sign of respiratory muscle fatigue is usually an increase in respiratory rate. With increasing fatigue, alternate use of the intercostal and accessory muscles with diaphragmatic breathing (discoordinate breathing) becomes apparent. Paradoxical breathing (inward displacement of the abdomen with inspiration) is seen as the diaphragm weakens, and action is necessary to identify and correct the cause before respiratory failure ensues.

The strength of the contraction depends on the intensity of the stimulus reaching the muscle, as well as the intrinsic properties of the muscle itself. Power insufficiency then can be of central origin from inadequate neural conduction, blockage of neural input at the myoneural junction, or peripheral failure from muscle weakness. Energy supply to the muscle must at least equal energy demands imposed by the work of breathing.

The following clinical conditions predispose a person to respiratory muscle fatigue:

Neurological conduction disorders
- Injury to cervical spinal cord
- Amyotrophic lateral sclerosis
- Poliomyelitis
- Acute intermittent porphyria
- Guillain-Barré syndrome
- Paralytic shellfish poisoning
- Phrenic nerve dysfunction

Myoneural junction disorders
- Myasthenia gravis
- Myasthenia-like disorders associated with neoplasia or pharmacological agents
- Tetanus

- *Clostridium botulinum* poisoning
- Fish poisoning (ciguatera)

Respiratory muscle dysfunction
- Hypoxia, low cardiac output
- Nutritional deficiency
- Congenital or acquired biochemical deficiencies (acid maltase deficiency, hypokalemia, hypophosphatemia)
- Muscular dystrophies
- Myopathies
- Atrophy
- Connective tissue disorders (polymyositis, systemic lupus erythematosus scleroderma)

Neuromuscular disease generally causes diffuse muscle weakness, including the muscles of respiration. Complaints of dyspnea, exertional fatigue, excessive somnolence, or recurrent headaches should be thoroughly evaluated for evidence of respiratory muscle dysfunction. Early identification and treatment of pulmonary problems can greatly reduce the threat of complications and prevent development of chronic respiratory insufficiency.

Central neural mechanisms also regulate the contribution of skeletal muscles in the upper airway to the breathing process. Those muscles must contract in synchrony with the inspiratory muscles to open the airway and allow air to flow. Interference with normal function can contribute to ineffective coughing, sneezing, and swallowing, predisposing to frequent infection and respiratory complications.

Paralysis of the diaphragm can occur with damage to the phrenic nerve from neurological disease, tumor, infection, trauma, surgery, or unknown causes. It can be either unilateral or bilateral, temporary or permanent. The degree of impairment depends upon the ability to maintain adequate alveolar ventilation to meet ventilatory requirements. Total loss of diaphragmatic function requires the intercostal and accessory muscles to assume responsibility for the work of breathing. As previously discussed, this is an inefficient way to breathe and may quickly progress to respiratory fatigue and failure.

Paradoxical movement of the abdomen on inspiration becomes especially pronounced in the supine position because the diaphragm cannot fall passively. Clients characteristically complain of shortness of breath that becomes accentuated when lying supine. Sleep can be particularly dangerous because increasing hypoxemia and hypercapnia are common. Treatment is focused on the underlying cause and efforts to reduce the work of breathing. The upright position should be maintained as much as possible. Mechanical ventilation with positive or negative respirators may be indicated, particularly at night. Use of a rocking bed to assist motion of the abdominal contents and thereby diaphragmatic excursion, may be helpful. Also, a pneumobelt, which compresses the abdomen intermittently and pushes the diaphragm into the thorax, can be used.[29]

A somewhat different situation exists in the client who is quadriplegic with a cervical lesion below C4-5. The lower intercostal and abdominal muscles are impaired, but diaphragmatic function is maintained. Respiratory mechanics are compromised by paradoxical motion of the upper thorax during inspiration and the inability to achieve residual volume during expiration. Marked expiratory muscle weakness impairs the ability to cough effectively. For those reasons, this client is often more comfortable in the supine position, because pressure from the abdominal contents can give the diaphragm a mechanical advantage and improved efficiency.[29] These persons may be highly susceptible to diaphragmatic fatigue, retained secretions, and atelectasis. Abdominal binding in the sitting position may be helpful. Respiratory therapy maneuvers to assist lung inflation and promote coughing are essential to prevent respiratory complications and improve the quality of breathing.

Airways

The airways of the pulmonary circuit deliver air from the environment to the alveoli for gas exchange and remove CO_2 from the system. Inspired air must be properly prepared for exposure to the alveolus, be able to flow with minimum resistance, and be evenly distributed for adequate exchange. Normally this transport system is highly efficient, allowing for daily traffic of greater than 10,000 L of air.[14] Effectiveness will depend on the proper structure and function of both the upper and lower airways.

Upper airway

The upper airway includes structures from the nose to the trachea and functions to warm, humidify, and filter environmental air. The nose is the preferred route for inhalation and contributes the most toward the "air-conditioning" function because of the pattern of airflow over the large surface area of the nasal mucosa. The mucosa is well vascularized and secretory, enabling inspired air to be heated to body temperature and humidified for presentation to the lower airways. Turbulent flow through the convoluted passages causes large particles of inhaled elements to stick to the mucosal surface. Combined with filtration by hair follicles in the anterior nares, ciliated epithelium, secretions with antibacterial properties, and extensive lymph drainage, this turbulent flow provides a major line of defense against noxious inhalants.[9] If the nasal passageway is bypassed or obstructed or if ventilatory demand exceeds the maximum airflow through the nose and mouth breathing becomes necessary, the inspired air may reach the trachea with little or no change from its initial ambient properties. When this happens, the lower airway soon becomes dry, ciliary function is impaired, and the threat of contamination from noxious or infectious agents increases.

The larynx extends from the pharynx to the trachea and includes the vocal cords, which allow phonation. The epiglottis, located at the entrance to the larynx, serves as a valve interposed in the airway and separates the alimentary pathway from the respiratory tract. Closure of the epiglottis protects the airway from aspiration during swallowing and allows for the development of the intrathoracic or intraabdominal pressure necessary for effective coughing or the Valsalva maneuver. The normal cough sequence depends on tight closure of the epiglottis and vocal cords to trap air in the chest after a deep breath and sudden release to permit forceful exhalation or cough. If vocal cord paralysis occurs for any reason, the explosive element of cough is lost.

Sensory fibers are located throughout the larynx and are sensitive to stimulation by mechanical irritants. The brain is signaled via the superior laryngeal nerve to initiate cough. Cold air and dryness of the mucous membranes can also stimulate the cough response. The cough reflex can be depressed with neurological dysfunction, unconsciousness, or anesthesia and seems to be less sensitive with age, increasing the risk of infection of the upper respiratory tract.[22]

Upper airway dysfunction. Significant obstruction may occur in the laryngotracheal area for a variety of reasons. Acute causes of airway obstruction are infection, thermal injury, aspiration of a foreign body or laryngeal edema from an allergic reaction.[49] Strictures of the trachea may occur after instrumentation or manipulation and can develop into chronic airway obstruction.

Early identification and treatment of upper airway dysfunction may alleviate symptoms of dyspnea and prevent progressive physiological impairment. Although the symptoms may be similar, upper airway abnormalities must be differentiated from lower airway abnormalities because treatment may vary considerably.

Lower airway

The lower airway begins at the trachea and continues to the alveolar level where gas is exchanged. The trachea extends from the larynx to a bifurcation (carina) in the mediastinum. Here the airway divides into right and left mainstem bronchi. Generally the right bronchus is shorter, wider, and in more direct line with the trachea. Thus the right lung is at greater risk for aspiration.

The mainstem bronchi further divide into lobar then segmental bronchi, supplying ventilation to corresponding areas of the lungs. The right lung has ten bronchopulmonary segments and the left lung has eight. The location of the bronchopulmonary segments becomes particularly important when positioning a client for chest physical therapy.

The trachea, bronchi, and bronchioles to the level of the terminal bronchioles constitute the conducting zone and transport air to the gas-exchanging airways. The terminal respiratory unit, or acinus, begins beyond the terminal bronchiole and consists of respiratory bronchioles, alveolar ducts, and alveolar sacs, and finally the alveoli, the basic units of gas exchange (Figure 7-4). Alveoli begin to appear as outgrowths of the bronchial wall in the smaller bronchioles and increase in number along successive generations. They comprise the respiratory zone or the sites of gas exchange and make up the greatest proportion of the lung itself, with a normal volume of approximately 3,000 ml.[50]

Secretions from the tracheobronchial tree consist of mucus from bronchial mucous glands and goblet cells, tissue fluid transudate, saliva, cellular debris, enzymes, and immunoglobulins. These secretions are viscoelastic and range from 10 to 100 ml a day in a normal adult.[33]

Lower airway dysfunction. Normal function can be impaired by either interference with ciliary action or change in the composition of the mucous layers. For example, change in the character of mucus may occur with infection or chronic bronchitis, making it difficult for the cilia to move within the surrounding mucous blanket. If the volume of secretions increases, the transport system may become overloaded and inefficient. Certain inhaled toxins, including cigarette smoke, may interfere with ciliary movement. Consequently, chronic mucous plugging and retention of secretions, frequent infections, and impairment of airway dynamics can result.

Inspired air travels down the conducting system to the respiratory unit by the generation of a pressure difference between the mouth and the alveoli. The pressure required for airflow must overcome compliance of the lungs and thoracic cage and frictional resistance of pulmonary tissues and the airways. The site of greatest airway resistance is at the level of the medium-size bronchi.[49]

The irregular construction of the tracheobronchial system creates turbulent airflow, particularly in the larger airways. This turbulence further adds to airway resistance, especially at high flow rates. Laminar flow is generally found in the smaller airways. Even small decreases in airway diameter at this level can greatly increase resistance. Because of their elastic properties, the airways can be either compressed or distended. Changes in transpulmonary pressures and in lung volumes can affect airway resistance. Large bronchi that contain cartilage are primarily affected by transpulmonary pressure change. The cartilage lends support, preventing overdistention or collapse of the airway during normal breathing. In contrast, bronchioles are tightly connected with surrounding pulmonary parenchyma and are significantly influenced by change in lung volume.[33] As volume increases, elastic recoil increases, applying traction to the walls of the intrathoracic airways, enlarging their lumen, and decreasing resistance. As lung volume decreases during exhalation, intrapleural pressure becomes less negative and resistance in the bronchi and bronchioles increases. If pleural pressure becomes positive, as with forced expiration, the airway becomes compressed but normally remains open because of counteracting internal airway pressure.

A variety of stimuli, many unknown, can trigger contraction of airway smooth muscle, decreasing the lumen and distensibility of bronchial walls. Expiration is prolonged, and air is trapped at the alveolar level, causing hyperinflation. Edema of bronchial walls and mucous plugging compound already elevated airway resistance and

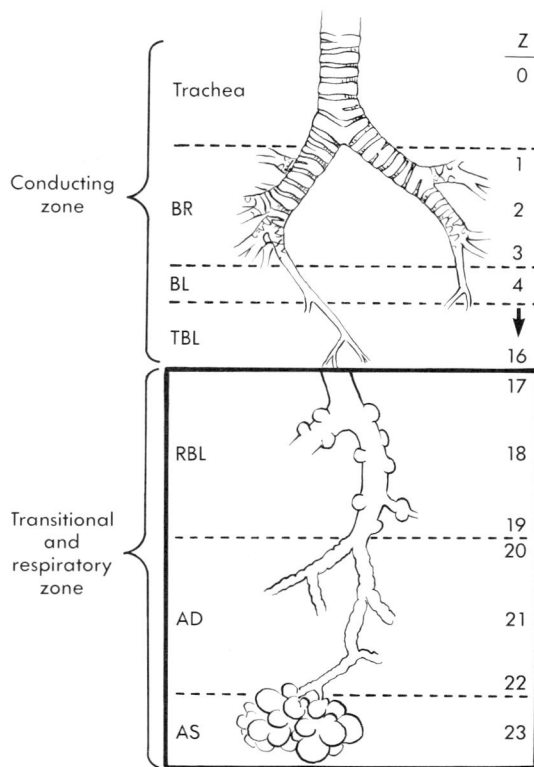

Figure 7-4
Idealization of airways. Note that first 16 generations make up conducting airways and last 7 make up respiratory zone (or transitional and respiratory zone). *BR*, Bronchus; *BL*, bronchioles; *TBL*, terminal bronchioles; *RBL*, respiratory bronchioles; *AD*, alveolar ducts; *AS*, alveolar sacs. *(Modified from Weibel ER: Morphometry of the human lung, Berlin, 1963, Springer-Verlag.)*

increase the work of breathing. The severity of response varies among people and even in the same individual from time to time. The situation may reverse spontaneously but often requires treatment. Pharmacological management is a major aspect of therapy and may include drugs that either relax airway smooth muscle tone or inhibit chemical mediator release.

Alveolar-Capillary Unit

Mature lung parenchyma is largely composed of alveoli connected to alveolar ducts and separated from each other by thin alveolar septa.[48] The alveolar ducts provide a supporting framework of connective tissue fibers and smooth muscle cells interspersed between closely packed alveoli.[32]

Alveoli constitute an enormous surface area, about the size of a tennis court, for gas exchange. The major portion is covered with capillary blood. The average diameter of an alveolus is estimated to be 200 to 300 μm, and although the number varies, approximately 300 million alveoli are found in adults.[48]

A continuous layer of epithelial cells lines the surface of alveolar walls. The alveolar capillary endothelium is composed of a single layer of squamous epithelial cells that have thin cytoplasmic extensions. The capillary endothelial cells are separated by clefts that form "open" junctions at irregular intervals and permit the passage of low–molecular weight proteins across the endothelial wall, thereby providing the major site for liquid and solute exchange.

The alveolar epithelial and capillary endothelial cells rest on separate basement membranes. These membranes appear to be fused at some points so that nothing else stands between the endothelial and epithelial cells. Diffusion of gases occurs at this "thin" portion of the alveolar-capillary septum.

The "thick" portion of the membrane refers to the areas where the basement membranes are separated by an interstitial space containing collagen and elastin, some nerve endings, and fibroblast-like cells.[49] Liquid and solute exchange takes place primarily across this thick portion. The spatial separation of the two basement membranes accommodates some excess fluid without necessarily impairing gas exchange. Interstitial tissue is also found in perivascular and peribronchial spaces around the larger blood vessels and airways and in the interlobular septa.[50] The interstitium at the alveolar level is continuous with these spaces and excess fluid normally drains to the lymphatics via this route, protecting the alveolus from edema formation. If fluid accumulates faster than the lymphatics can remove it, pulmonary edema results.

Gas Exchange

The exchange of O_2 and CO_2 between the alveolus and blood depends upon the passive movement of these gases from an area of greater partial pressure to one of lesser partial pressure.[31] Diffusing capacity depends on the properties of the gas, such as weight and solubility, and the resistances met along the pathway between the alveolus and the red blood cell (RBC).

Oxygen transport

The difference in partial pressures establishes a gradient for O_2 to cross the alveolar-capillary membrane and bind to hemoglobin (Hb) for transport to the body via the circulatory system. The flow of O_2 from ambient air therefore depends upon diffusion within the spaces of the terminal respiratory units, across the air-blood barrier, through a plasma layer of variable thickness and finally across the membrane and interior of the RBC for chemical combination with Hb.

The supply of O_2 to the tissues depends critically on the affinity of Hb for O_2. O_2 saturation

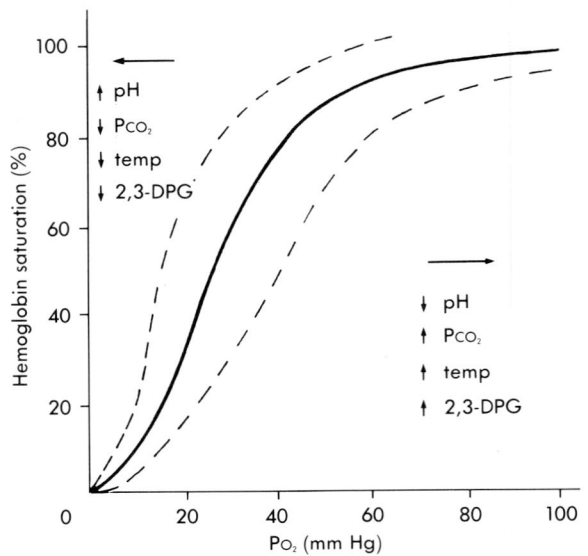

Figure 7-5
Oxyhemoglobin dissociation curve relating percentage of Hb saturation and Po_2. Solid line depicts normal curve. Dotted lines represent shift to left or right.

measures the amount of O_2 bound to Hb compared to the maximum amount that could be carried. The percentage of O_2 saturation is a function of the partial pressure of O_2 (Po_2), as described by the sigmoid-shaped oxyhemoglobin dissociation curve (Figure 7-5).

Normal Hb becomes almost fully saturated with O_2 at a Po_2 of 60 mm Hg. Increments above 60 mm Hg do not add appreciably to further O_2 uptake. Once the Po_2 drops below 60 mm Hg, however, there is an abrupt decrease in O_2 saturation and a decrease in tissue O_2 availability.

Factors that shift the position of the curve change the affinity of Hb for O_2. A right-shifted curve decreases Hb O_2 uptake but enhances the release of O_2 at the tissue level. A shift of the curve to the left increases Hb O_2 affinity but reduces tissue O_2 extraction.

Po_2 is not the only determinant of O_2 content and use. The presence of normal Hb in sufficient amounts is crucial. Delivery at the tissue level also requires adequate cardiac output and the physiological conditions to allow for diffusion and release of O_2 at the cellular level.

Carbon dioxide transport

CO_2 also moves by diffusion but in the opposite direction, from plasma to the alveolus. Several chemical reactions enable the transport of CO_2 from the tissues to the lungs. CO_2 is continually produced by cells throughout the body as an end-product of metabolism. The amount of CO_2 produced depends on the energy requirements of the body and also on the fuel being burned. A small amount is carried physically dissolved in plasma. An additional 10% to 20% combines reversibly with Hb to form carbamino compounds. Deoxygenated Hb has a greater affinity for CO_2 than oxygenated Hb. As blood in the pulmonary capillaries becomes oxygenated, the ability to bind CO_2 decreases and CO_2 elimination is enhanced.[49] The third and major means of CO_2 transport is in the form of bicarbonate (HCO_3^-). When CO_2 joins with water, it forms carbonic acid, which is then catalyzed by the enzyme carbonic anhydrase and dissociates into hydrogen ions (H^+) and HCO_3^-. In the pulmonary capillaries the chemical reactions that occurred at the tissue level proceed in reverse direction. Elimination from the system depends on the level of ventilation present.

Diffusion

Diffusion is directly proportional to the cross-sectional area of the alveolar-capillary membrane and inversely proportional to the thickness of the barrier membrane. Among humans diffusing capacity varies according to body build and correlates with height, weight, and alveolar volume.[32] Diffusing capacity also increases during growth until maturity and then gradually declines with age.

Lengthening of the diffusion pathway—such as occurs in interstitial fibrosis, decreased blood flow transit time commonly seen during exercise, and reduced driving pressure of O_2—may lead to a reduction in diffusion capacity. However, it appears that at least two factors must be present to impair gas exchange on the basis of true diffusion defect.[12]

Air volumes

The volume of air distributed to the respiratory units must be sufficient to provide O_2 and remove CO_2. At rest a person breathes approximately 500 ml of air with each breath (tidal volume), at a rate of 12 to 16 respirations per minute, for a total minute volume of 6 to 8 L.[49]

A portion of each breath stays in the conducting airways and does not contribute to gas exchange. This "wasted" ventilation is anatomical dead space and amounts to approximately 150 ml in the average-size adult. The remaining portion of the tidal volume that actually reaches the gas-exchange units is the alveolar volume. Anatomical dead space remains constant with each breath, whereas alveolar volume changes in direct proportion to tidal volume. In other words, if tidal volume decreases from 500 to 300 ml, 150 ml will still be dead space, but alveolar volume will decline from 350 to 150 ml. A decrease in respiratory depth can therefore significantly alter effective alveolar volume.

An additional component of dead space may be found at the alveolar level. For gas exchange to take place, ventilation must occur in opposition to perfusion. If an area of the lung is ventilated but lacks perfusion, the ventilation is once again "wasted" and becomes additional dead space volume. In a normal person dead space is generally not a significant problem. However, many persons with lung disease have associated destruction or occlusion of the pulmonary capillary bed, and dead space ventilation contributes greatly to abnormal gas exchange. As the proportion of dead space ventilation increases, effective alveolar volume decreases.

Alveolar ventilation is the total volume of gas moving in and out of "functioning" respiratory units during a given period of time. It is the product of alveolar volume times respiratory frequency and directly affects the amount of CO_2 eliminated from the body. Serum P_{CO_2} is inversely proportional to alveolar ventilation so that as alveolar ventilation decreases, P_{CO_2} rises.

Persons with increased CO_2 production or retention must be able to increase alveolar ventilation in order to exhale the excess CO_2. Hypoventilation can be defined as a level of alveolar ventilation that is inadequate to maintain P_{CO_2} at a normal level for a given metabolic rate.[12] Usually P_{CO_2} is tightly controlled by central and peripheral chemoreceptors that change minute ventilation at a level appropriate to maintain a normal P_{CO_2}. Pure hypoventilation is fairly uncommon but does occur if ventilatory drive is blunted from a central respiratory disorder, as seen with central nervous system depression from anesthesia or sedation. Chronic hypercapnia can also diminish the ventilatory response to CO_2.[49] Hypercapnia solely on the basis of hypoventilation also may be seen in persons with neuromuscular or skeletal abnormalities, resulting in weakness or dysfunction of the respiratory muscles.

Ventilation and perfusion

Ventilation and perfusion are not evenly distributed throughout the lungs. Regional variation in ventilation occurs as a result of the anatomy of the tracheobronchial tree and the vertical gradient of pleural pressures and the lung volumes present at the initiation of inspiration.[32] Generally the lower lung bases receive the greatest amount of ventilation, particularly in the upright position with normal use of the diaphragm. Conversely, persons who ordinarily use intercostal and accessory muscles to breathe may have the greatest portion of ventilation shifted toward the apices.[40]

Blood flow through the lungs is largely determined by gravity and hydrostatic forces, the greater flow going to the most dependent portions of the lung. Although both ventilation and perfusion are influenced by gravity, the effect on perfusion is greater. Consequently, ventilation-perfusion ratios $(\dot{V}/\dot{Q})$ vary throughout the lungs and the overall $\dot{V}/\dot{Q}$ is normally 0.8. Common events such as a change in position can further alter $\dot{V}/\dot{Q}$ relationships. For example, in the supine position, the gravity effect becomes anterior to posterior and the reverse in the prone position. The side-lying position distributes greater ventilation and perfusion to the dependent lung and can make an important difference to gas exchange in the person with unilateral lung disease.

NURSING ASSESSMENT

Evaluation of the client with actual or potential pulmonary compromise must include a comprehensive assessment of physiological as well as biopsychosocial aspects of the problems presented. An individualized approach based on the person's present life situation, perceptions of the problem, concurrent medical conditions, social relationships, and available support systems must be used. The nurse needs this information to identify the care, learning, and emotional needs of clients and their families.[28]

Subjective Assessment

Information obtained directly from clients is the foundation of the assessment process and allows them to identify what they perceive as problems and concerns. Subjective data should always be the first source of information in the nursing assessment. These data must be supplemented if clients have difficulty remembering or communicating. Sources of supplementation include family or friends, previous physicians, and past medical records.

Symptoms are the subjective manifestations of disease. Four respiratory symptoms frequently prompt a person to seek medical attention: (1) dyspnea, (2) cough and expectoration, (3) hemoptysis, and (4) chest pain.[49] Constitutional symptoms such as fever, weight loss, fatigue, exercise intolerance, and sleep disturbance also may be present, so a total body review of systems should be conducted. For purposes of this text, however, the four respiratory-related complaints most frequently cited are discussed.

Dyspnea

Dyspnea, the client's perception and interpretation of shortness of breath, is often a difficult symptom to evaluate, because it is so highly subjective. The person may describe breathlessness but actually mean weakness, fatigue, or chest discomfort. Breathlessness can be a reflection of the level of functioning of the total body system. It is a subjective sensation arising from a myriad of causes and is influenced by both voluntary and automatic control mechanisms. The nurse should ascertain exactly what the person means when describing symptoms. Clear, precise questions, allowing clients to describe the problem in their own terms, will allow for a better understanding of the degree of discomfort present. Tolerance for breathlessness varies among people, and the extent of dyspnea does not always correlate well with the actual physical condition. Individuals may have significant respiratory disease, but limited physical activity may be due to other medical problems. They may not consider dyspnea a problem at all but upon exertion, breathlessness becomes severe. The nurse must assess the amount of activity a person can tolerate without dyspnea.

A number of questions should be asked. For example, rather than asking only how far a person can walk, the nurse should also question pace, ability to walk on an incline, and ability to climb stairs. Does the client become breathless when performing activities of daily living? A progressive decrease in activity performance because of shortness of breath is common. The client may not be consciously aware of this change, but it can result in deconditioning to a level greater than predicted for the degree of impairment present. Early identification of the problem can prevent further disability.

Chronic dyspnea can contribute greatly to functional disability. Adequate breathing becomes a priority need. Activities that produce symptoms or decreased energy are often eliminated, despite the importance they may have had in a person's life. Life-styles and interests may change accordingly, at great cost to a person in terms of physical, social, and emotional well-being.

Contributing factors must be identified because nursing interventions for dyspnea may vary according to its cause. Questions about the onset of the symptom (acute or chronic), precipitating events, duration, associated symptoms, relieving factors, and identifiable patterns must be asked. For example, a person may complain about awakening from sleep each night with shortness of breath (paroxysmal nocturnal dyspnea). Upon questioning, the person with a primarily respiratory etiology may state that relief is found in the upright position within a short period of time after coughing and expectorating sputum. The nurse may suggest respiratory therapy maneuvers such as chest physiotherapy before bedtime, or, if the person receives bronchodilator therapy, the dosage may be scheduled to more effectively cover the nighttime interval.

Persons with cardiac decompensation may complain of the same initial symptom, that is, awakening with shortness of breath. They too may state that relief is obtained in the upright position, but the dyspnea takes a longer time to resolve. Treatment for heart failure may be required. As much information as possible should be obtained to clarify presenting complaints and place them in the proper perspective.

Cough

The presence of a cough, with or without sputum production, is another frequent finding when assessing a person with breathing dysfunction.

Coughing normally occurs to clear and protect airways. Initiating factors include inflammatory, mechanical, chemical, and temperature stimulation of cough receptors or tactile stimulation in the ear canal.[51] A cough becomes abnormal when it is persistent, irritating, painful, or productive. It can be acute or chronic, associated with other symptoms (pain, wheezing, dyspnea, syncope), productive or dry, effective or ineffective (unable to clear secretions). All data pertinent to the development of the cough must be obtained. For example, a person may note that the cough followed a recent illness or respiratory tract infection, is exacerbated by seasonal or environmental conditions, or occurs only at a certain time of day. Most persons with a chronic cough notice that it becomes worse when they lie down at night or when they arise in the morning.[33] Persons who cough during or shortly after eating may have a problem with aspiration of food or fluid into the tracheobronchial tree.

Characteristics of the cough, including quality, frequency, and alleviating factors, must be reviewed. A change in the usual characteristics of a chronic cough also should be investigated. The presence of a cough alone is nonspecific, but when associated with other signs and symptoms may suggest a diagnosis. For example, development of an acute dry cough with a respiratory tract infection is frequently attributed to a viral illness.

The production of sputum, including quantity and character, should be assessed. Generally persons with chronic bronchitis expectorate a small to moderate amount of mucoid material each day, often in the morning. A change to thick yellow or green sputum may signify respiratory tract infection and prompt early treatment. The volume of sputum is greatly increased with bronchiectasis. Anaerobic bacterial infections may produce foul-smelling sputum. Sputum production may have characteristic features that, when combined with other clinical data, contribute to the overall nursing diagnosis and management of the client.

Hemoptysis

Hemoptysis generally originates from a problem in the airways, parenchyma, or pulmonary vasculature.[49] The severity varies from blood-streaked sputum, as sometimes seen in chronic bronchitis to frank bleeding, which may accompany pulmonary infarction. Frequently, no definite diagnosis can be made. However, the symptom is always worrisome and requires further investigation.

Chest pain

Chest pain associated with respiratory disease usually occurs secondary to involvement of the parietal pleura, diaphragm, or mediastinum, all of which are extensively innervated with sensory nerve fibers. Lung tissue and visceral pleura do not have these sensory fibers and, as a result, significant disease may exist in these areas without producing any pain.

Nerve endings in the parietal pleura may be stimulated by inflammation or stretching the membrane. Involvement of the pleura may be secondary to an underlying parenchymal lesion in the same area. "Pleuritic" pain may vary in intensity but is often abrupt in onset, becomes worse with inspiration, is well localized, and is generally not relieved by splinting. Diaphragm involvement can cause pain to be referred to the neck and upper shoulder.

Disease in any of the mediastinal structures can cause pain in that area. Pain may be retrosternal or precordial with radiation to the neck or arms or through the back.[33] Causes may be of respiratory (tracheobronchitis, pulmonary emboli), cardiovascular (myocardial infarction, dissecting aneurysm), or gastrointestinal (esophageal reflux) origins, and associated symptoms will vary accordingly.

Chest wall pain also may produce considerable distress. It can originate from intercostal or pectoral muscles, ribs, and cartilage or be due to pressure or inflammation along the neural pathway. Usually chest wall pain is described as constant local aching, aggravated by movement and tender to palpation. A recent history of trauma or strain should be investigated.

Complaints of chest pain are highly subjective and may be difficult to evaluate. A detailed picture, including onset, description, frequency, duration, and precipitating and relieving factors, must be obtained. Associated factors such as dyspnea, exercise, position change, and emotional environment can help differentiate the cause.

The chronology of presenting respiratory symptoms also aids in establishing a nursing diagnosis and developing an appropriate plan of care. Previous medical data and a personal history must be obtained to correctly assess the current situation. Past or concurrent medical problems, present treatment regimens, compliance behaviors, the incidence of respiratory disease. and a complete history of smoking habits should be reviewed. Questions about smoking should include the age at which the habit began, the type and amount of tobacco used (cigarettes, cigar. pipe, snuff, chewing tobacco), current smoking habits, successful and unsuccessful attempts to quit, and reasons for continuing to smoke or for quitting. Such information can reveal the level of motivation the person may have for participating in a plan for respiratory rehabilitation.

Additional information may be elicited, depending upon the situation presented at the time of the interview. Evaluation of the psychosocial environment of the client is essential information in developing an appropriate plan of care

Objective Assessment

The physical examination is a primary source of objective data and is used initially to determine the nursing diagnosis, develop goals, and write a plan of care. Ongoing assessment and evaluation of the plan also depend upon the ability to perform a thorough and accurate physical assessment.

Respiratory dysfunction is often the result of other body system impairments, so each new client must have a complete physical examination. The focus of this discussion, however, is limited to the basic principles involved in evaluating the respiratory system.

Whenever possible, the client should be seen in a quiet, well-lit room. Examination of the chest involves the techniques of inspection, palpation, percussion, and auscultation. The underlying anatomy of the lungs and thorax must be envisioned at all times during the examination. As each area is assessed, it is always compared with the same region of the other side, so that clients actually serve as their own control.[4]

Inspection

Inspection begins during the interview. At this time, the nurse has the opportunity to observe the general appearance of the client, skin color, presence and degree of respiratory distress, character and rate of respirations, quality of voice, pattern of speech, interruptions by coughing or breathlessness, flaring nostrils, use of pursed-lip breathing, and assumed posture. These parameters give clues as to which areas to emphasize when performing the physical assessment.

Examination of the anterior thorax is best performed with the client supine with the chest exposed from the waist up. The chest cage should move symmetrically and expand equally as the person breathes. Areas of decreased movement may represent obstruction of airflow, disease of the underlying lung or pleura, or the client may be splinting part of the chest secondary to pain.

Any use of accessory muscles or abnormal retraction or bulging of the interspaces during breathing should be noted. On inspiration the abdomen should be displaced outward. Expiration normally occurs passively as the abdomen returns to the resting position. Paradoxical motion of the abdomen during quiet breathing often indicates abnormal or absent use of the diaphragm.

The shape of the chest is evaluated for pectus excavatum (depression of the lower portion of the sternum) or pectus carinatum (anterior displacement of the sternum, which increases the anteroposterior diameter).[4] The general configuration of the chest is best viewed with the client in a sitting position. The adult thorax normally has an anteroposterior diameter less than the transverse diameter. Advanced age may increase the anteroposterior diameter slightly and in the client with chronic obstructive pulmonary disease, the increase may be significant.

The thoracic spine is normally straight when viewed posteriorly and has a gentle anterior concave appearance when viewed from the side. The thoracic cage is also evaluated for deformity. Abnormalities of the thoracic cage interfere with chest expansion, causing decreased compliance and reduced lung volume. Some of the most common posterior deformities that may lead to a restrictive respiratory defect include kyphosis, scoliosis, and kyphoscoliosis. Ankylosing spondylitis causes a straight, immobile spinal column that limits expansion of the chest.

Cyanosis, a bluish discoloration of the skin and mucous membranes, also is best noted in daylight and best detected in the nail beds and buccal mucosa. Cyanosis reflects severe hypoxemia of arterial blood to a sufficient degree to desaturate Hb. Approximately 5 g/100 ml of reduced Hb must be present to change skin color from the usual pink to blue.[23] For this reason, cyanosis usually is not seen with anemia until hypoxemia is

severe, whereas clients with polycythemia may appear cyanotic with less hypoxemia present. The most common cause for cyanosis is generalized hypoxemia (central cyanosis) but hypoxemia also may occur secondary to low blood flow states (peripheral cyanosis).

Palpation

Palpation is used to evaluate the underlying structure and function of the chest, detect areas of tenderness or crepitation, and assess respiratory excursion. The anterior chest is palpated by placing the hands over the anterolateral aspect of the chest, with the thumbs extended along the costal margins. As the client inhales, the chest should expand equally and symmetrically. Posterior chest excursion is evaluated by grasping the sides of the rib cage and placing the thumbs parallel to the tenth rib.[4]

Diminished movement of the thorax can occur secondary to lung or pleural disease, neuromuscular defects, or musculoskeletal defects. Splinting also may occur to prevent pain on movement. Tenderness noted on palpation should be evaluated; it often indicates a musculoskeletal origin of chest pain. The intercostal spaces should be palpated for the presence of a tumor. Swelling or crepitation must be further investigated.

Fremitus refers to the transmission of voice-generated or vibrating sounds to the surface of the chest. By placing the palmar surface of the hands over comparative areas of the chest as the client speaks, the examiner can determine if there is normal, increased, or decreased fremitus. A variety of chest conditions can alter the transmission of sounds. Decreased transmission can be secondary to weakness of the voice, obstruction of the airway, or the collection of air, fluid, or tissue in the pleural space. Increased density of lung tissue as seen with consolidation or tumor mass increases fremitus if the airway remains patent.

Percussion

Percussion notes are produced by fingers striking the chest and creating a sound and a palpable vibration, helping to evaluate lung tissue underlying the chest wall. Percussion can be performed either directly, by tapping areas of the chest with a flexed finger, or indirectly, by tapping the distal portion of the interposed middle finger of the opposite hand. Movement of the striking finger should be from the wrist, with a quick direct blow and the lightest touch able to elicit a sound.

Symmetrical areas of the chest are percussed systematically from side to side down the chest wall. Bony structures such as the scapulae need not be percussed. Healthy, air-filled lung produces a diffeent sound from fluid-filled lung or solid tissue. The quality ranges from dull to tympanitic. Increased density is accompanied by a loss of resonance and dullness, as seen when percussing over solid organs, areas of consolidation, or fluid-filled spaces. Hyperresonance accompanies an increased accumulation of air such as hyperinflation or pneumothorax.

Diaphragm location and excursion also should be evaluated by percussion. The lower posterior lung fields are percussed down in small increments until a change in sound is heard. The distance between levels of dullness at deep inspiration and deep expiration is compared to evaluate movement of the diaphragm. Normal excursion ranges from 4 to 6 cm.[33] A low-lying diaphragm with limited excursion often accompanies hyperinflation. Diaphragm paralysis, atelectasis, or pleural effusion may be accompanied by elevation of the diaphragm and impaired movement.

Auscultation

Auscultation of the chest allows the examiner to evaluate the quality and intensity of chest sounds and added (adventitious) noises that may indicate a respiratory disorder. Every nurse should be familiar with normal breath sounds so that abnormalities can be readily noted.

Auscultation should be performed in quiet surroundings to block out extraneous environmental noise. The client should be seated in an upright, comfortable position when possible. If weakness or debilitation prohibits this position, the client should be turned from side to side to enable complete examination of all lung fields. Throughout the assessment, the underlying anatomy of the lungs must be considered in order to correctly describe the location of findings.

The diaphragm of the stethoscope is generally used because lung sounds have a high frequency. The bell may be easier to use on very thin or small clients, but it should be placed firmly so that it functions as a diaphragm. The stethoscope should always be placed directly on the chest wall because clothing produces artifact that can interfere considerably with accurate findings.

The client is instructed to breathe somewhat deeper than usual, with the mouth open in a relaxed, unforced manner. Assessment must be systematic. The examiner listens to all lobes on the anterior, posterior, and lateral chest for a complete respiratory cycle in each position and then auscultates from side to side, comparing symmetrical areas of the lungs, moving from top to bottom.[4]

Lung sounds are evaluated for location, pitch, intensity, appearance in the respiratory cycle, and distinctive characteristics. The quality of breath sounds varies from area to area, depending upon the proximity of the auscultated site to the large airways.

Vesicular breath sounds are heard over most of the pulmonary parenchyma and are considered "normal." These occur primarily during inspiration and have a soft, muffled quality likened to the rustle of trees.[33] Lung tissue is believed to serve as a filter that changes quality and intensity.

Breath sounds heard over large airways, such as the trachea and major bronchi, are described as "bronchial" and have a hollow, tubular sound. Generally the expiratory component is at least equal to or slightly longer than the inspiratory phase, often with a slight pause between the two.

Bronchovesicular sounds, those which are an intermediate sound between vesicular and bronchial sounds, can be heard around the upper half of the sternum and in the intrascapular area. Bronchovesicular sounds are more muffled than bronchial breathing, with no pause between inspiration and expiration.

Bronchial and bronchovesicular breath sounds become abnormal if heard in any areas other than the stated normal zones. If the airway remains open, lung sounds are heard much better through areas of consolidation than when transmitted through normal lung parenchyma. For this reason, auscultation over areas of lung consolidation frequently yields bronchial sounds.

Voice sounds also become transformed when listened to through a stethoscope. Normally the spoken word sounds soft, muffled, and often barely audible. In the presence of consolidation, words increase in clarity and intensity (bronchophony). Egophony refers to the transformation of the letter "E" to sound like a nasal "A" over the involved area. Whispered sound also increases in intensity and clarity (whispered pectoriloquy) and may be a useful means of identifying pulmonary consolidation.

When interpreting breath sounds, transmission depends on the patency of the airway. Increased airway resistance or obstruction from tumor, secretions, or a foreign body can cause decreased or absent breath sounds. Shallow breathing from weakness, obesity, or neuromuscular disorders may also decrease sound transmission. Decreased air entry may accompany alveolar destruction as seen with emphysema or reduced compliance states such as interstitial lung disease. Finally, transmission also may be altered by excess subcutaneous fat or air or either air or fluid in the pleural space.[33]

Adventitious sounds heard over the chest can be produced by the movement of air in the tracheobronchial tree or pulmonary tissue. There has been considerable confusion regarding the appropriate terminology to describe these sounds but a combined committee of the American College of Chest Physicians and the American Thoracic Society has established recommendations for the use of pulmonary terms.[36]

Crackles, also known as rales, is the term used to describe low- to medium-pitched, discontinuous lung sounds that have an explosive quality and are usually heard during inspiration. These range in quality and intensity from fine to coarse and represent the opening sounds in small airways or alveoli that have been collapsed secondary to fluid accumulation, poor aeration, or inflammatory exudate.[49] They may or may not clear with coughing. Crackles are commonly heard with pulmonary edema, atelectasis, pneumonia, and interstitial lung disease.[49]

High-pitched continuous sounds are referred to as *wheezes*. These can occur during inspiration, expiration, or both. Wheezes may be audible without the aid of a stethoscope, or they may be apparent only with forced expiratory effort. Wheezes are caused by airflow through obstructed airways, whether from bronchospasm, secretions, compression, mucosal swelling, or a foreign body.

The term *rhonchi* should be used only when referring to low-pitched continuous sounds that have a "snoring" quality. Rhonchi are generally associated with excess secretions in the airways and often are cleared with coughing.

Another noise that may be heard during assessment of the client with pulmonary problems is *stridor*. Stridor refers to a low-pitched, continuous, crowing sound heard over the larynx and trachea, generally during inhalation. Usually it is loud enough to hear without a stethoscope and represents upper airway obstruction. Detection of stridor should prompt quick action to evaluate the airway in an effort to prevent critical obstruction.

When pleural surfaces become inflamed or roughened, a characteristic sound, a *pleural friction rub*, can be heard. Often, a grating sound or vibration associated with breathing can be heard over the site of discomfort. Many conditions may be associated with a pleural friction rub, including pleurisy, tuberculosis, pulmonary infarction, pneumonia, and primary and metastatic carcinoma.[7]

Diagnostic Studies

Accurate medical diagnosis of a pulmonary problem usually requires additional laboratory and radiological data. Nurses must know about the indications, collection, and interpretation of these data. They play a major role in client and family education throughout the assessment and ongoing evaluation. Together with other members of the rehabilitation team, the nurse works toward establishing a complete profile of information on which client care decisions can be based.

A chest x-ray examination is performed on admission for initial assessment and baseline data and at intervals to evaluate treatment of such complications as pneumonia. Although most chest x-ray examinations are performed with the client in a semi-Fowler's or upright position, the client with a spinal cord injury should be supine initially to maintain immobilization.[52]

Establishment of nursing diagnoses often depends upon assessment of the client's functional level. Two common and helpful testing procedures that contribute to the functional assessment of the client with pulmonary problems are pulmonary function tests and arterial blood gas analysis.

Pulmonary function testing provides an objective, noninvasive means of documenting the physiological effects of disturbed pulmonary physiology. These tests may be ordered for several reasons: (1) evaluation of a pulmonary component in complaints of dyspnea, (2) determination of the type and extent of impairment of lung function, (3) early detection of small airway disease, (4) assessment of the effects of treatment on pulmonary function, and (5) preoperative evaluation of the high-risk client with pulmonary disease.

Spirometry is ordered as a means to measure lung volumes and capacities and the flow rates generated during breathing maneuvers. Primary compartments of the lung are designated as *volumes*. Combinations of lung volumes are called *capacities*. The most useful of these measurements for the nurse to know are the following[37]:

tidal volume (TV) The volume of air inhaled or exhaled with each breath during quiet breathing.

residual volume (RV) The volume of air remaining in the lungs after maximum exhalation.

vital capacity (VC) The maximum amount of air exhaled from the point of maximum inspiration.

functional residual capacity (FRC) The volume of air remaining in the lungs at the end expiratory position.

total lung capacity (TLC) The volume of air in the lungs after maximum inspiration.

Interpretation of results of pulmonary function tests depends on proper performance of the test, the client's ability to understand and perform the maneuvers, equipment, and the use of standards of measurement considering the variations attributed to age, sex, and height. There is a wide range of "normal" values, and generally at least three forced expiratory tracings should be done with each testing. The results must always be interpreted in conjunction with available clinical data. Pulmonary function testing can be repeated periodically for more dependable assessment and ongoing evaluation of change.

Measurement of arterial blood gases enables the evaluation of the effects of respiratory dysfunction on overall gas exchange. Together with available clinical data, blood gas measurement contributes vital data for assessment of respiratory, cardiac, and metabolic function.

Routine arterial blood gases are evaluated for PO_2, PCO_2, and pH. This information allows for evaluation of the adequacy of oxygenation, ventilation, and acid-base balance. Many persons with pulmonary disease have a complex, mixed picture of abnormalities that can be better understood if periodic monitoring of arterial blood gases is performed. Blood gas determinations also help determine the need for supplemental O_2, a decision that must be based on objective data.

NURSING DIAGNOSES

The subjective and objective findings, as well as the results of diagnostic tests, are used to formulate nursing diagnoses. Nursing diagnoses common to clients with impaired breathing are described in this discussion.[20]

The nursing diagnosis of *ineffective airway clearance* is made when an infection of the respiratory tract leads to an increase in tracheobronchial secretions. Constriction of the airways and an inability to effectively remove secretions by deep breathing and coughing also contribute to retained secretions.

An *ineffective breathing pattern* is frequently exhibited by individuals with physiological impairment of the respiratory tract. For example, individuals with chronic obstructive pulmonary disease often struggle to get air into and out of the lungs. Common signs and symptoms include dyspnea, tachypnea, nasal flaring, and use of accessory muscles. These clients are forced to devote most of their energy to the work of breathing, leaving little energy for other activities of daily living.

Impaired gas exchange can be caused by a number of factors. Certain disease processes such as emphysema can lead to a mismatch of ventilation and perfusion because of destruction of alveoli and pulmonary circulation. Pulmonary congestion because of retained secretions also can lead to impaired gas exchange. Other causes may include bronchospasm, such as that occurring in asthma, and diffusion impairment, which can be caused by pulmonary fibrosis. Impaired gas exchange can greatly affect the client's ability to carry out activities of daily living. Early signs and symptoms of hypoxemia and hypercapnia include headache on arising, somnolence, cardiac dysrhythmia, irritability, facial flush, diaphoresis, confusion, and tachypnea. The hypoxemia and hypercapnia can be severe enough to be life threatening.

Altered in nutrition in the client with respiratory dysfunction can be due to the lack of adequate food intake. Several factors may contribute to decreased food intake. Shortness of breath and hypoxemia are two principal causes in clients with chronic obstructive lung disease, specifically emphysema. These individuals have to work harder to breathe, leading to an increased caloric demand. At the same time, their decreased energy level makes even simple ingestion and digestion of food fatiguing and increases their need for an already depleted oxygen supply. Their decreased activity level also leads to a disinterest in food. Overall results are weight loss, muscle wasting, and decreased resistance to infection. Weight gain also can be a problem for individuals with respiratory impairment because of a decreased activity level combined with increased caloric intake. For example, individuals with bronchitis may be more likely to be overweight.

Individuals with respiratory impairment may encounter *sleep pattern disturbance* because of shortness of breath or fears of suffocation. They are afraid to sleep at night for fear of experiencing difficulty breathing or sleep apnea.

Sexual dysfunction is a common problem for individuals with respiratory impairment. Physical factors, including neurological dysfunction and psychogenic factors, can affect an individual's ability to perform sexually. Persons with chronic obstructive lung disease may fear physical exertion, because it may cause increased shortness of breath. Many of these individuals are depressed, have poor self-esteem, are hypoxic, and have reduced muscle strength.[27]

GOALS

The goals established with clients with impaired respiratory function may include all or some of the following:

1. To assist in mobilizing secretions from the respiratory tract through coughing, postural drainage, percussion, vibration, or nasotracheal or tracheal suctioning
2. To prevent respiratory tract infection
3. To establish an effective breathing pattern
4. To control or prevent development of hypoxemia or hypercapnia
5. To work with the client, dietitian, and physician in assessing the client's caloric needs, monitoring nutritional status, and maintaining adequate hydration
6. To work with the client in developing a relaxed climate conducive to sleep before retiring and implement measures to make sleeping more comfortable by improving ventilation
7. To encourage clients and partners to verbalize feelings about sexual difficulties and work with them to determine methods to improve sexual functioning

8. To prepare clients and their families for long-term mechanical ventilation if their condition so warrants.
9. To educate the client and family about:
    a. Effective coughing and skills necessary to effectively remove secretions from the respiratory tract
    b. Relaxation techniques and breathing retraining to help decrease respiratory rate
    c. Signs and symptoms of and measures to avoid development of a respiratory tract infection
    d. Early signs and symptoms of hypoxemia and hypercapnia
    e. Medications and equipment if applicable
    f. Need for increased or continued physical exercise within the bounds of clients' airflow limitations and life-style
    g. Use of oxygen therapy if appropriate
    h. Use of aids to lung expansion if indicated
    i. Nutritional management
    j. Energy conservation

REHABILITATION NURSING INTERVENTIONS

There are a number of rehabilitation nursing interventions for the client with impaired respiratory function. The interventions chosen depend upon the specific nursing diagnoses derived from the nursing assessment.

Promotion of Airway Clearance

Nursing interventions for the client with ineffective airway clearance will vary, depending on the underlying problem, the ability of the client to follow directions and perform various maneuvers, and the willingness of family to participate in the client's care. The client and family members should be involved early in goal setting and in the rehabilitation program.

Hydration

Adequate hydration is necessary for thinning tracheobronchial secretions, keeping mucous membranes moist, and facilitating the removal of these secretions from the lungs. Unless contraindicated, the client should be encouraged to drink approximately 10 glasses of liquid a day.[41] Milk should be avoided, since it tends to increase the viscosity of the secretions. Coffee and tea should not be included in the 10 glasses of liquid, since these substances tend to act as diuretics. Adequate hydration is particularly important during the winter when heating systems can cause a dry environment. Also, many individuals with shortness of breath may decrease their fluid intake, since they must hold their breath when swallowing.[44] Individuals with chronic obstructive lung disease tend to breathe through their mouths when short of breath and thereby bypass the humidification carried out by the nose.

Nebulization. Nebulization involves increasing moisture in the air by adding water droplets of varying sizes to help thin tracheobronchial secretions. Aerosol therapy is often used interchangeably with nebulization. Various types of equipment have been developed to deliver fine water particles to the respiratory tract. Medications such as bronchodilators also can be administered by nebulization.[47]

Types of equipment available for humidification and nebulization range from the simple hand-bulb nebulizer to the highly efficient ultrasonic nebulizer. It is beyond the scope of this chapter to elaborate on these devices. The nurse should instruct the client and family on the proper use and potential side effects of these devices. For example, the use of a hand-bulb nebulizer requires a coordinated breathing pattern to facilitate the deposition of water particles or medication into the lower respiratory tract.

Coughing

Coughing is an important physiological mechanism for the removal of secretions from the respiratory tract. An effective cough is performed with the client in a sitting position, preferably a chair, or in a high Fowler's position. The client's head should be flexed, with the shoulders relaxed and bent slightly forward.[41] The client is then told to breathe in slowly and deeply. Deep breathing is important. One way the nurse can assist deep breathing is to place the hands on the sides of the client's chest and tell the client to push the hands as far apart as possible with the chest.[44] After taking a deep breath, the client should be told to cough several times until it feels like there is no air left in the lungs. This coughing technique is referred to as the *cascade cough*.[44]

Individuals with obstructive lung disease may not be able to perform the cascade cough effectively because of collapse of the airways. In this case, the *end expiratory cough* may be more effective in removing secretions. To perform this cough, the individual is instructed to take a deep breath and exhale slowly through slightly parted or pursed lips to a point just below that which will cause a collapse of the airways. At this stage, the individual is told to cough. After this coughing maneuver has been carried out several times, the individual may then try the cascade cough.[44]

In persons with neuromuscular disease, the nurse may have to manually compress the abdomen during the expiratory phase of the cough. The client is instructed to take a deep breath and cough. When the client coughs, the nurse pushes abruptly in and up on the client's upper abdomen with the hand, while at the same time bending the client forward at the waist. These actions help to increase abdominal pressure and the upward movement of the diaphragm.[44]

Clients must be given privacy during the coughing procedure. They also should be provided with tissues and instructed to cover the nose and mouth. Secretions should be inspected for color, amount, and consistency. If an infection is suspected, sputum should be sent for culture and sensitivity studies.

Postural drainage

Postural drainage is a technique used to drain pulmonary secretions from the various segments of each lung by gravity. This procedure has been found to be effective in removing excessive tracheobronchial secretions from the lungs, especially in individuals with impaired mucociliary clearance.[3] Twelve positions are used in postural drainage.[44] Illustrations of these positions are found in basic respiratory texts. Most individuals do not require drainage in each position. The nurse, after checking x-ray reports, should ascertain which lobe or lobes require drainage. The client's chest should be auscultated before and after postural drainage to determine the effectiveness of the procedure. The client's physical status should be evaluated, since some of the more extreme tipping positions may not be tolerated by all individuals. The head-down position should be used cautiously and only when the uppermost lung segment is affected. Clients with increased intracranial pressure, hypoxemia, cardiovascular or hemodynamic instability, and marked bronchospasm should be treated with extreme caution and monitored carefully.[45]

Before beginning, the nurse should explain the procedure and provide the client with tissues and a sputum cup. Postural drainage should not be carried out immediately preceding or following a meal. Clients should wear loose-fitting gowns or clothes, since they will be encouraged to cough and deep breathe before positioning, between position changes, and at the end of the procedure. If they are taking bronchodilating medications, such as those given by nebulization, these should be taken approximately 15 minutes before beginning the postural drainage to facilitate the drainage of secretions through dilated airways.

The client is then placed in the appropriate positions. In the hospital, bed jacks can be used to raise the foot of the bed when more extreme tilting positions are required. Some hospital beds can be automatically put into reverse Trendelenburg's position. Extra pillows also will be needed for proper positioning. Immobilization beds, such as the Wedge Stryker turning frame also can be positioned to lower the head of the bed approximately 18 inches. Postural drainage with clients who have spinal cord injury should be carried out within the limitations of orthopedic alignment, tolerance, and type of immobilization bed in use.[52] In the home, the appropriate degree of slope can be obtained by using pillows, folded blankets, stacks of newspapers, or a tilt board.

Percussion and vibration frequently are carried out in conjunction with postural drainage to help push secretions into the upper airways, where expectoration and suctioning can be accomplished more easily. These maneuvers should not be performed when bright red hemoptysis is present or recent.[45]

Percussion

Percussion, also referred to as cupping or clapping, is carried out by cupping the hands and striking the area of the chest to be drained in an alternating, rhythmic fashion (Figure 7-6). The cupped hand creates an air pocket between the hand and chest, producing a hollow but not a slapping sound on percussion. To avoid becoming tired, the wrists should be kept loose and the elbows slightly flexed.[47] Percussion should not be done over the sternum, vertebrae, kidneys, or tender areas.[41] Individuals usually find percussion to be more comfortable when it is performed over a thin layer of clothing rather than on bare skin. This technique requires only 2 to 3 minutes and,

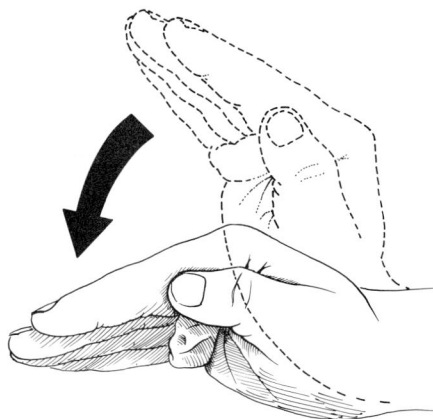

Figure 7-6
Position of hand for percussing chest.

if properly performed, should cause the client no discomfort and should assist with the removal of sputum.[47]

Vibration

Vibration usually follows percussion. In this technique, vibrations are transmitted through the chest wall at the same time the chest is compressed. Vibration is performed with arms and shoulders straight and with hands placed one on top of the other on the client's chest. The client is instructed to take a deep breath and to exhale slowly. As the client begins to exhale, the operator applies pressure over the affected area and by alternate tensing and contracting of the shoulder muscles produces fine vibratory movements that are transmitted to the client's chest wall. This maneuver continues for the duration of expiration. If a spontaneous cough is not elicited, the client should be instructed to cough following vibration. A sitting position will make it easier for the client to generate an effective cough. The vibrating procedure can be repeated several times.

Postural drainage accompanied by percussion, vibration, and coughing can be a fatiguing ordeal for the client, especially if all the lung segments require treatment. A client is usually positioned for 5 to 10 minutes to drain one segment of the lung. In the home, postural drainage with percussion and vibration is most effectively accomplished with another person assisting. Mechanical vibrators are available and are especially helpful to clients who must carry out this procedure alone.

A schedule for performing postural drainage based on the client's needs must be established. This procedure commonly is performed in the morning upon arising to remove secretions that have pooled during the night and in the evening before retiring to clear secretions from the lungs and allow optimum ventilation during sleep, when respirations tend to become more shallow. Individuals may have to perform postural drainage more frequently, for example, when there are increased secretions in the airways because of a respiratory tract infection.[41]

Suctioning

Nasotracheal suctioning. If the client is unable to effectively remove secretions from the respiratory tract by coughing, nasotracheal suctioning may be necessary. Nasotracheal suctioning is not without complications and therefore should not be instituted as a routine procedure. Complications of nasotracheal suctioning may include hypoxia, stimulation of the vagus nerve leading to cardiac dysrhythmias, irritation of the mucous membranes, and laryngospasm.[17] Suctioning is most effective when carried out in conjunction with the therapies mentioned previously. Since the lower respiratory tract is sterile, nasotracheal suctioning must be carried out as an aseptic technique. The procedure should be explained to clients even if they are unresponsive.

The head of the bed should be elevated to about 45 degrees to facilitate deep breathing and coughing. The lungs should be auscultated before and after. Necessary sterile equipment includes a glove, a catheter, a basin, and normal saline. A water-soluble lubricant and a portable or wall suction unit also are needed. Since a major complication of suctioning is hypoxemia, oxygen should be provided to the client either by mask or nasal cannula. The liter flow of oxygen should be determined by the physician. To protect the nasal mucosa from damage due to the introduction of the suction catheter, a nasopharyngeal airway can be inserted.[17]

The client should be positioned with a pillow behind the shoulder blades and the head extended backward to provide a better angle for catheter insertion. Asking the client to stick out the tongue during insertion will prevent swallowing the catheter.[17] The catheter is lubricated and inserted into the nose or through the nasopharyngeal airway without suction, gently manipulated through the turbinate bones, and advanced 6 to 8 inches, at which point it should be over the back of the tongue. The client is then instructed to inhale and the catheter is quickly advanced 1 or 2 inches into the lower airway. The suction pressure should be checked by occluding the lumen of the suction catheter and pinching it between the thumb and forefinger, putting the ungloved thumb over the suction port. The wall suction pressure should be between 80 and 120 mm Hg.[17]

As the catheter passes the epiglottis and larynx, the client will usually cough. The catheter is advanced slowly and as far as possible until resistance is met. The suction catheter is then withdrawn using intermittent suctioning. If the client has copious secretions, the suction catheter should only be withdrawn to a point between the larynx and the major carina.[44] The connecting tubing to the suction machine is then detached, and the client is instructed to deep breathe and allowed to rest for 1 or 2 minutes. Supplemental oxygen is given at this time. The tubing can then be reattached and the suctioning procedure repeated until the secretions have been removed. Leaving the catheter in place in the lower airway until the suctioning procedure has been completed avoids the trauma of repeated catheter insertions into the lower respiratory tract.

Once the procedure is completed, the client should be given oxygen and encouraged to relax and deep breathe. If a nasopharyngeal airway is used and frequent suctioning is needed, the airway can be left in place for up to but no more than 8 hours.[17] The client's tolerance of the procedure (for example, vital signs), as well as the color, consistency, and amount of secretions, should be recorded in the chart.

Tracheostomy suctioning. For individuals with ineffective airway clearance, tracheostomy tube insertion may be necessary to (1) relieve airway obstruction, (2) protect the airway from aspiration because of impaired airway reflexes, (3) facilitate the removal of respiratory tract secretions, and (4) provide for mechanical ventilation.[15, 44] Tracheostomy tubes can be made of metal or plastic (usually polyvinyl chloride or nylon). Most of the plastic tubes have a cuff to occlude or seal the trachea when mechanical ventilation or intermittent positive pressure breathing is used. Most of the metal tubes are uncuffed and are used by individuals who will have a permanent tracheostomy opening. Many tracheostomy tubes come with inner cannulas that can be removed for cleaning.[22]

An individual who has a tracheostomy requires suctioning to remove secretions from the airway. Strict aseptic technique is required to prevent infection. Sterile supplies include a suction catheter, glove, saline, and receptacle for the saline solution. As in nasotracheal suctioning, the client should receive oxygen during the treatment to prevent hypoxemia. Frequently, clients are given a high-liter flow of oxygen before, between, and at the end of suctioning using a hand-operated bag resuscitator. The risk of vagal stimulation leading to dysrhythmias also is present in tracheal suctioning. The suctioning procedure should be explained to the client and tissues provided for expectoration of any secretions from the mouth. The lungs should be auscultated before and after the procedure.[18]

The catheter is inserted without the use of suction until resistance is met at the level of the carina. This technique will usually stimulate a cough. Intermittent suction is then applied, and the catheter is slowly withdrawn while gently rotating it to remove as many secretions as possible from the airway. Suctioning should be applied for no longer than 10 seconds to prevent hypoxemia. The client is then allowed to rest and oxygen is given via a tracheotomy collar or a hand-operated bag resuscitator. If more secretions are present, the entire procedure can be repeated after 1 or 2 minutes. The catheter should be rinsed with the sterile normal saline between each insertion. It also may be necessary to suction the client's mouth at the end of the procedure, but the catheter is then considered to be contaminated and must be discarded. All equipment is discarded once the procedure is completed.

The client's response to the suctioning is then evaluated; vital signs are taken; and the color, consistency, and amount of sputum is recorded in the chart. The frequency of tracheal suctioning must be individualized for each client, depending on the amount of secretions present. Postural drainage with percussion and vibration is frequently done in conjunction with suctioning to mobilize secretions into the upper airways where they can more easily be removed.

Rehabilitation clients may be discharged from the hospital with tracheostomy tubes in place, necessitating instruction of the client or family member in suctioning techniques. Fears of causing trauma to the airways or impeding respirations may make teaching this procedure to clients and family members difficult. The client and family must be assessed both from a physical and psychological standpoint as to their willingness to learn and perform suctioning at home.

The client and caretakers should be involved in care early in the rehabilitation process. Initially the nurse should explain the procedure and answer any questions that the client or family may have. Providing the client with a mirror to visualize the procedure greatly aids the learning process.

Certain modifications in the suctioning procedure can be made once the client is discharged home. Catheters do not have to be discarded after each use but can be washed in a mild soap solution, rinsed thoroughly, and then boiled for 5 minutes. The catheters are then wrapped in a clean, ironed towel. The client does not have to purchase sterile saline, since this mixture can easily be made up by boiling water with salt added and storing the solution in a sealed container that has been boiled. A new supply of sterile water and salt should be made daily, since bacteria can form in the solution once the bottle has been opened. The client also should boil the receptacle used for the saline during suctioning.

Social service should be included in the discharge planning, since the client may require financial assistance for a portable suction machine and a visiting nurse referral. The visiting nurse will be able to assess how well the client and family are coping with tracheostomy care and suctioning.

Tracheostomy care

In addition to suctioning, a client with a tracheostomy requires cannula and stoma care, humidification, and, if present, proper management of a cuff. Disposable kits are frequently used in the hospital for tracheostomy care. Sterile equipment is needed and includes gloves, basins, hydrogen peroxide, normal saline, a brush, pipe cleaners, cotton swabs, and tracheostomy ties.

The stoma site, or area around the tracheostomy tube, should be cleaned with hydrogen peroxide to remove secretions, which provide a medium for bacterial growth. The site is then rinsed with normal saline and the area thoroughly dried. Controversy exists regarding the application of a tracheostomy or bib dressing. If a dressing is used, it should be changed whenever exudate and secretions are present to prevent irritation and infection of the stoma site.

When an inner cannula is present, it should be removed at least once a shift and cleaned with hydrogen peroxide and saline. At this time, the outer cannula can be suctioned of secretions.

Tracheostomy ties should be changed when soiled. To prevent accidental expulsion of the tracheostomy tube, it is wise to fasten the clean ties in place before removing the soiled ties.

To prevent drying of secretions, proper humidification must be provided. Humidified air or oxygen can be delivered directly to the tracheostomy by a tracheostomy collar or by a ventilator. Humidity also can be provided by means of a mechanical room humidifier.[6] The client must be instructed to avoid getting water in the tracheostomy tube while bathing or taking a shower. To prevent infection, the tubing and water in the humidifier should be changed at least every 24 hours.

If a tracheostomy tube is cuffed, proper cuff pressure must be maintained. Instructions on cuff management are provided by the manufacturers of the various tubes. The proper amount of air should be put into the cuff (at or below 15 mm Hg), since too much air can impede circulation to the tracheal mucosal lining, which leads to tissue breakdown and possible necrosis. Too little air in the cuff may allow the client to aspirate liquids or food into the lungs and, if the client requires a mechanical ventilator, can lead to ineffective ventilation. Secretions tend to pool in the oropharyngeal area above the cuff and should be removed by suctioning before deflation. This practice will prevent the aspiration of these secretions into the lungs.

Clients are usually weaned from a tracheostomy tube gradually. Initially the cuffed tube may be replaced with a noncuffed tube to make breathing around the tube easier. Even a deflated cuff can obstruct airflow. Some cuffed and cuffless tracheostomy tubes have an opening, or fenestration, in the outer cannula. These tubes enable the client to breathe through the upper respiratory tract and can be plugged when the inner cannula

is removed. When plugged, the client is able to breathe, speak, and generate a more effective cough. A cuffed tracheostomy tube should never be plugged with the inner cannula in place or with the cuff inflated, since the airway will be obstructed. If the client can tolerate a plugged tracheostomy tube and a respiratory assessment shows good tolerance, the tracheostomy tube may be removed. An occlusive dressing is placed over the site until the stoma heals.

There are instances, however, when a permanent tracheostomy is required, for example, when a client cannot be weaned from a ventilator or cannot effectively cough up secretions. Thus, in addition to correct suctioning, other aspects of tracheostomy care also must be taught. Usually inner cannula care is easier and less anxiety producing for the client and family member to learn. Again, early participation in this care facilitates learning in a relaxed and unhurried manner. In the home, equipment for cleaning the inner cannula and stoma can be washed and reused. The only purchases necessary are hydrogen peroxide, dressings, and pipe cleaners or a brush to remove secretions from inside the inner cannula. The client may need some assistance with changing the tracheostomy ties. Both the client and family member should be encouraged to repeat instructions verbally and to demonstrate proper tracheostomy care and cuff inflation and deflation if applicable.

Proper humidification of the client's air supply is an important discharge concern. A mechanical room humidifier may have to be purchased for the home or a portable source of humidified air or oxygen may have to be supplied. Sometimes, wearing a dressing dampened with sterile water over the tracheostomy tube is sufficient. However, the client should be cautioned about the danger of getting water in the tracheostomy. The client should always protect the tracheostomy opening from possible inhalation of foreign substances (for example, powder, aerosol sprays) and from dry air. The client also should maintain an adequate fluid intake. If necessary, 2 or 3 ml of saline can be instilled into the trachea to liquefy secretions before suctioning.

A duplicate sterile tracheostomy tube should be readily available in the home in case the old tracheostomy tube becomes dislodged or obstructed. Clients and family members can be taught how to insert a new tracheostomy tube.

Telephone numbers of the ambulance and physician should be posted in a visible location in the home.

The client and family members should be taught to examine the sputum for color, amount, and consistency. Any change in the normal characteristics of the sputum, as well as other signs of a respiratory tract infection (such as an elevated temperature or an increased shortness of breath) should be reported to the physician. Signs of infection around the stoma site (such as redness, pain, or purulent drainage) also should be reported. Clients should be told to avoid other individuals with respiratory tract infections, since they are particularly vulnerable to such infections. Good oral hygiene should be stressed because the oropharyngeal area contains many organisms, including anaerobes, which can be aspirated into the lower respiratory tract. Keeping the mouth clean can decrease the number of these organisms and the chance of infection.[6]

Another important concern is the client's inability to communicate verbally. Providing a magic slate or word board is one means of communication. Placing the bell of a stethoscope against the client's lips will enable whispered words to be heard. Placing a clean finger over the end of the tracheostomy tube with the cuff deflated will allow the client to produce enough air to vocalize words.[6] Speaking or talking tracheostomy tubes are available. These tubes have a line built into the cannula that, when connected to air or oxygen, allows this gas to be directed upward to the larynx so the client can talk in a low whisper.[22] Not being able to speak can be frustrating and frightening. A system should be implemented in the home to enable the client with a tracheostomy to be left alone and to contact someone if there is an emergency.

Smoking cessation

Smoking has been shown to stimulate mucus production, impair ciliary function, and increase vulnerability to respiratory tract infections. It is a definite detriment to effective airway clearance. Quitting smoking can be an involved process. The nurse should explain the hazards of smoking and work with the client to set up a regimen that will be most conducive to smoking cessation. The nurse can suggest pamphlets and organizations such as the American Lung Association to help clients stop smoking.

Environment

The client should maintain an optimum environment to decrease drying and irritation of the airways. As stated earlier, added humidity, such as that supplied by a humidifier, is required in the home during the winter because of the drying effect of heating systems. Humidity should be kept at around 40%.[41]

Individuals should avoid contact with smoke and other agents, such as cleaning substances, powders, paints, and aerosols, that can irritate the airways. Individuals with asthma should avoid allergens such as dust, fungus, molds, pollen, and animal danders.[41]

The inhalation of cold air can lead to shortness of breath and coughing. Wearing a scarf or mask over the nose and mouth can help to prevent these symptoms. Clients should be advised to avoid going outside in cold windy weather and to allow more time for walking when the weather is cold.[41]

Relaxation Techniques

Difficulty in breathing leads to anxiety and fear. Blood pressure, heart rate, and respiratory rate increase, causing increased use of oxygen and increased production of carbon dioxide.[23] The nurse should teach clients techniques that can help them relax.

The most effective techniques for decreasing oxygen consumption, carbon dioxide production, and respiratory rate are exercises leading to conscious contraction of muscles, followed by an effort to totally relax. Transcendental meditation and biofeedback also have been found to be effective relaxation methods.[23] These techniques should be carried out in a quiet environment with few distractions. The client should wear comfortable clothing and assume a comfortable posture, such as reclining in a lounge chair, to reduce muscle tension to a minimum.[41]

Breathing Retraining

Breathing retraining has been used most extensively with individuals who have chronic obstructive airway disease and cervical spinal cord injuries. Breathing exercises are taught to the client or performed by an assistant to build strength of existing muscles of respiration and to promote adequate ventilation.

The aims of breathing retraining are to reduce dyspnea and make more effective use of the diaphragm.[23] Pursed-lip breathing and abdominal-diaphragmatic breathing are the techniques most frequently taught to achieve these aims.

Pursed-lip breathing

To perform pursed-lip breathing, the client should be instructed to inhale slowly through the nose and to breathe out slowly through the mouth with lips pursed or puckered (Figure 7-7). Exhalation should take two or three times longer than inhalation to effectively empty the lungs of trapped air. Pursed-lip breathing is believed to create a back pressure within the airways, thus preventing them from collapsing prematurely and trapping air within the lungs.[41]

Abdominal-diaphragmatic breathing

Abdominal-diaphragmatic breathing and pursed-lip breathing should be used together to obtain maximum breathing efficiency. Clients can be taught these exercises while in a semisitting or supine position (Figure 7-8). They should be told that the purpose of these breathing exercises is to make use of the diaphragm rather than the accessory muscles while breathing. Unless paralyzed, clients should be instructed to place one hand on the epigastric area of the upper abdomen, about one hand breadth below the sternum, and the other hand on the apical region of the chest. They should then be instructed to breathe in slowly through the nose, while relaxing the abdominal muscles so that these protrude while inhaling. This maneuver allows the diaphragm to move downward. The upper chest should remain still. The client should then breathe out through pursed lips while tightening the abdominal muscles, if possible. This maneuver helps to move the diaphragm upward. The client should be instructed to practice this technique several times a day. Eventually, the client should be able to use abdominal-diaphragmatic breathing while walking and carrying out activities of daily living.[41] Family members also should participate in this training so that they can encourage and support the client to master this breathing technique. Although long-range beneficial effects of abdominal-diaphragmatic breathing have not been reported in the literature, individuals have indicated that this breathing pattern helps to relieve dyspnea and increases exercise tolerance, thereby enabling them to be more functional in performing activities of daily living.[23]

If the client is paralyzed, the assistant places hands on the diaphragm to help focus attention

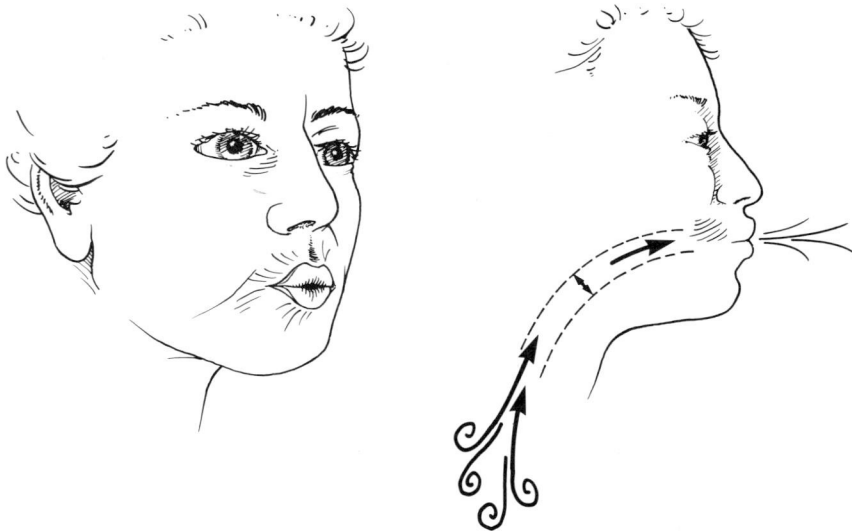

Figure 7-7
Pursed-lip breathing.

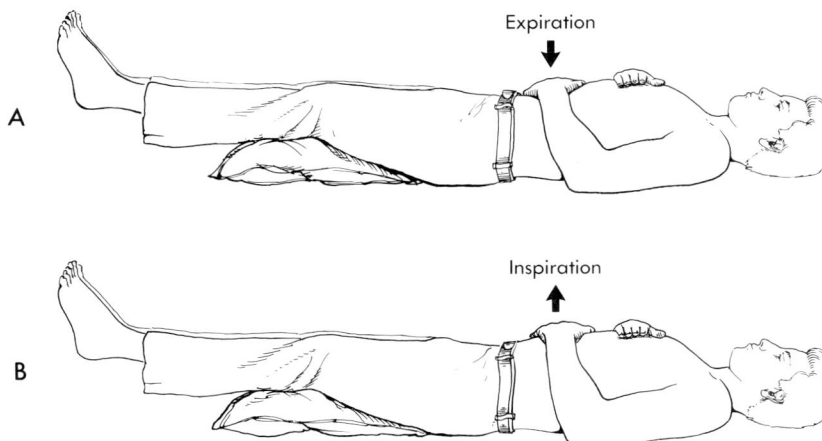

Figure 7-8
Abdominal-diaphragmatic breathing. **A,** Expiration. **B,** Inspiration.

on it, even though the client may not be able to feel the assistant's hand. The client should be instructed to take deep breaths through the nose and to exhale through the mouth at a rate of 6 to 10 breaths per minute. The person who is quadriplegic may also be instructed to rebreathe carbon dioxide to improve deep breathing and stimulate coughing. This therapy is used to prevent atelectasis. A reservoir bag is filled with a mixture of 10% carbon dioxide and 90% oxygen from a prepared tank. The client holds the mouthpiece securely in the mouth and wears a nose clip. The client is instructed to breathe in and out through the mouth until deeper breaths are taken and coughing is stimulated. If the client complains of dizziness or headache, the treatment should be discontinued.[52]

Conditioning Exercises

An ineffective breathing pattern can be a deterrent to exercise, since exercise increases the work of breathing. Thus individuals may avoid even mild exercise to prevent dyspnea from occurring or becoming worse. Curtailment of exercise has negative physiological and psychological effects, such as decreased appetite, insomnia, and depression. Exercise conditioning is considered by many to be important in the rehabilitation of the respiratory cripple. Numerous studies dealing with the physiological effects of exercise on the indi-

vidual with chronic obstructive lung disease have shown that spirometric values, lung volumes, and other measurements of pulmonary function did not improve with training.[24] Nevertheless, individuals who undergo exercise training almost always report feeling better, and their exercise tolerance increases. In effect, individuals require less energy expenditure or oxygen consumption for a given amount of work. They have greater stamina and interest in life.[24]

Many methods have been used to accomplish conditioning, including the use of a treadmill or bicycle ergometer, stair climbing, walking, swimming, and bicycling. Some experts believe it is better to condition individuals using normal walking in corridors and on stairs rather than on treadmills or bicycles.[34] Clients are taught to calculate and try to achieve their target heart rate in some types of exercise programs.[23]

One problem with exercise conditioning programs is that many individuals cannot or will not adhere to the disciplined regimen required. They need to know the importance of exercise training and its effect on the respiratory system. The client's family will need to offer support and encouragement for continuing the program in the home.

The nurse should work with the client and family to show them ways of conserving energy. For example, clients should be told to perform activities of daily living slowly, conserve energy by using proper body mechanics, and alternate periods of exercise with periods of rest. Exercise can involve the use of muscle groups used in activities of daily living. Furniture, utensils, and food should be arranged in ways to minimize energy expenditure.[24]

Promotion of Gas Exchange

Nursing interventions for the client with impaired gas exchange involve many of the interventions described in the discussion on effective airway clearance. If secretions are present, coughing and deep breathing are required, as well as suctioning. Breathing exercises also may be indicated to promote adequate alveolar ventilation.

Oxygen therapy

Individuals with significant hypoxemia (less than 55 mm Hg) are candidates for supplemental oxygen therapy.[35] Clients with chronic obstructive lung disease most frequently require long-term oxygen management. In this group oxygen therapy is primarily initiated to relieve pulmonary hypertension and cor pulmonale, to decrease secondary polycythemia, and to improve mental functioning and exercise tolerance.[23]

The oxygen is usually given at a low liter flow (1 or 2 L) to help maintain the hypoxic drive to breathe in individuals with chronic hypercapnia. The length of time that the oxygen is used each day will depend on the individual needs of the client. Results of some studies indicate that oxygen should be used at least 15 hours per day.[35] Oxygen may be ordered continuously, intermittently, at night, or only during periods of exercise. Many studies have shown that certain individuals can exercise much better with oxygen, specifically those with exercise-induced hypoxemia.[35]

Oxygen is most frequently delivered through a nasal cannula or mask. The nasal cannula is a simple, effective way to administer low to moderate oxygen concentrations. The client does not have to have oxygen flow interrupted to eat, cough, and perform other activities. One disadvantage, however, is that cannulas can cause nasal irritation, even when the oxygen is humidified. Small amounts of a water-soluble lubricant applied to the nares can reduce or prevent this discomfort.[44]

The client should consider oxygen as a medication and only use it at the liter flow and for the length of time prescribed. The client also should

know that oxygen supports combustion and therefore should not be used around flammable objects such as lighted cigarettes or gas stoves.

If the client is to be discharged home with oxygen, the proper equipment should be procured. Various oxygen systems are now available, including conventional compressed tanked oxygen and an oxygen concentrator that separates oxygen from the nitrogen in the air. The latter apparatus is electrically operated, and therefore a source of tanked oxygen must be made available in case of power failure. Advances in liquid oxygen systems now provide transfilling liquid systems for home use. These portable oxygen devices weigh approximately 11 pounds filled and give up to 9 hours of oxygen at 2 L per minute. These systems allow clients with exercise-induced hypoxemia to get out of the house for both recreational and work activities.[35]

The client and family should understand the type of oxygen system they will be using. They should also be able to perform the manual skills necessary for operation. The cost and payment for oxygen should be taken into account, since financial assistance may be needed for this therapy.

Mechanical aids to lung expansion

Mechanical aids to lung expansion have been introduced with the primary aim of preventing or treating atelectasis.

Intermittent positive-pressure breathing therapy. One of the most popular mechanical aids to intermittent lung inflation has been intermittent positive-pressure breathing (IPPB). An IPPB machine causes intermittent inflation of the lungs with air or oxygen under pressure and delivered through a mouthpiece. Aerosol medications such as bronchodilators are given through an IPPB machine.[26] The use of this form of therapy has waned since 1981. Reported complications are increased airway resistance, barotrauma, and nosocomial infections.[42] Since these machines are pressure cycled, the volume of air delivered to the lungs is smaller for the same pressure when lung compliance is decreased. Some experts state however, that IPPB should be considered for those individuals who are unable to take deep breaths spontaneously, that is, individuals with restrictive problems, severe airway obstruction, and neuromuscular disorders.[23]

Incentive spirometry. Incentive spirometry is designed to encourage and allow visual monitoring of sustained maximum inspiration.[42] The client is instructed to take a deep breath through the mouthpiece of the apparatus and hold it. Evidence as to the effectiveness of the deep breath is substantiated by how high and long the individual can suspend the ball located inside the device. Visual evidence of deep breathing may be more motivating to a client than mere instruction to take deep breaths every hour.

Mechanical ventilation

Although the care of clients receiving mechanical ventilation is primarily dealt with under acute aspects of respiratory care, some individuals may require long-term mechanical ventilation. These individuals frequently have chronic, underlying lung disease such as emphysema or neurological impairment such as cervical spinal cord injuries resulting in the inability of the individual to breathe.

The two types of ventilators most commonly used to augment respirations are pressure-cycled ventilators and volume-cycled ventilators. Pressure-cycled ventilators inflate an individual's lungs until a predetermined pressure is reached, at which point inspiration ends and expiration begins. With this type of ventilator, the volume of air delivered to the client can vary with each inspiration, depending on the compliance of the individual's airways. For example, if an individual is experiencing bronchospasm, the pressure set on the ventilator is reached quickly and only a small volume of air is delivered into the lungs. In contrast, volume-cycled ventilators deliver a fixed predetermined tidal volume of air into the lungs, and the pressure to deliver this volume of air varies, depending on airway compliance. There is a safety valve or pressure-limit setting on these ventilators above which the ventilator will no longer continue the inspiratory cycle. This mechanism prevents trauma that could occur if air was forced into the lungs under too high a pressure. Volume-cycled ventilators are preferred for both hospitalized and homebound individuals because a consistent volume of air is delivered to the lungs.

Rehabilitation of ventilator-dependent individuals requires a team approach. Clients and families must be willing to make a long-term commitment to care. Also, the physical environment of the home should facilitate effective and efficient operation of the needed equipment. The client and family should be included in establishing short- and long-range goals, participate in the se-

lection of the appropriate ventilator for home use, and become thoroughly familiar with the machine before discharge. The ventilators developed for home use are more compact than those used in a hospital. Some are mounted on motorized wheelchairs and are referred to as "mobile ventilators." These units are self-contained and self-powered. A sufficient supply of oxygen and suction equipment are included to allow for mobility up to 3 hours. Home ventilators can be driven by electrical power, batteries, or gas.

Individuals discharged with volume-cycled ventilators must understand ventilator operation and possible mechanical problems. Discharge teaching should include the use of all ventilator equipment, alarms, and backup equipment such as batteries for use in case of power failures. A self-inflating resuscitation bag also should be supplied in case there is mechanical failure of the respirator. The use of supplemental oxygen should be addressed. Instruction in general respiratory care, tracheostomy care, signs of underventilation and overventilation, and signs and symptoms of hypoxemia and hypercapnia should be given.[16]

Home support services, including visiting nurses, home health aides, and respiratory therapists may be required. Respiratory equipment is almost always maintained by the company supplying the ventilator.[31] Although third-party payment is available for home ventilator care, the financial arrangements can be confusing and frustrating, so social workers should be involved to make this aspect of care as easy as possible for the client and family.

Other types of artificial ventilation can be used in the home. Cuirass respirators are external ventilators that have replaced the iron lung and offer an alternative to the positive-pressure ventilators described previously. Individuals with chronic respiratory or neuromuscular diseases are candidates for this type of ventilator. One advantage is that no tracheal intubation is required; however, position and mobility are more limited than with the volume-cycled ventilators. Skin care is important, since this ventilator may cause tissue pressure and skin breakdown. Nutrition also may be a problem, since swallowing should be timed with the exhalation cycle of the ventilator.[11]

Rocking beds are another alternative and also offer the advantage of not requiring tracheal intubation. These beds effectively maintain adequate ventilation in clients with neuromuscular disorders.

Home care for respiratory-dependent individuals increases morbidity and mortality and the psychological burden on the family. Nevertheless, studies have shown that home care, when compared to continuous institutional care, does provide certain individuals with an improved quality of life within familiar surroundings. Home care also has been shown to be more cost-effective than hospital care.[31] Clients requiring long-term mechanical ventilation and their families require frequent assessments of how they are managing physically and psychologically.

Maintenance of Adequate Nutrition

Once the correct caloric intake has been calculated, the client identifies food preferences. A high-protein, high-caloric diet of easily digested food is indicated in most situations. High ingestion of carbohydrate calories can lead to carbon dioxide retention, an important complication to consider in respiratory disease.[10] Frequent small meals can help decrease the work of digestion and decrease abdominal distention, a situation that can further impede diaphragmatic movement and can lead to shortness of breath. Gas-forming foods also should be avoided to prevent abdominal distention. A poor food intake can be augmented by the use of supplemental foods such as high-protein caloric drinks. Some persons can tolerate puddings and milkshakes.[10]

The individual should be encouraged to eat in a relaxed and unhurried manner. Good oral hygiene before meals can help eliminate the foul odor of sputum and may help to stimulate a good appetite. Supplemental oxygen during meals may help to decrease shortness of breath when low oxygen levels exist. The client should be encouraged to rest after each meal so that needed energy will be available for the digestive process.

Clients who are unable to consume sufficient food orally to satisfy caloric needs may require the insertion of a nasogastric feeding tube or gastrostomy tube. Hyperalimentation may be implemented in severe cases of nutritional deficiency if clients cannot tolerate foods given through the gastrointestinal route.

Clients requiring long-term mechanical ventilation pose a special nutritional problem. Abdominal distention can occur because of aspiration of air into the stomach. In intubated clients, aspiration of food into the lungs also can be a problem. Cuffed tubes should be kept inflated during meals and for 1 to 2 hours after meals to prevent aspiration.

Adequate nutritional intake is important in these individuals. It has been shown that semi-starvation in clients receiving ventilation therapy can lead to a diminished hypoxic drive, especially in clients with chronic obstructive lung disease. A diminished hypoxic drive can precipitate respiratory failure, and recovery from it can be prolonged.[25]

Promotion of Optimum Sleep

The nurse should discuss sleep patterns with the client to determine if difficulties exist. The lungs should be cleared of secretions before retiring to decrease coughing and shortness of breath. Pillows should be provided or the head of the bed elevated into a position that makes breathing easier. Supplemental oxygen also may make sleeping easier. Some individuals may require mechanical ventilation at night as a safeguard against sleep apnea. Relaxation exercises or other techniques conducive to relaxation, such as listening to music or reading, should be practiced as aids to sleep.

Assistance with Sexual Problems

Sexual function should be assessed as part of the total health evaluation. The nurse should determine whether sexual difficulties exist because of the respiratory dysfunction or another problem, such as a medication side effect or feelings of decreased masculinity or femininity.

If increased shortness of breath occurs during sexual activity, the individual may be told to use supplemental oxygen or a bronchodilating medication just before this activity. The client should be instructed to use a comfortable position such as a side-by-side position that does not restrict breathing. Selecting a time for sexual activity that allows for a rest period before or afterward can be beneficial. Early morning sexual activity is frequently recommended because both partners are usually rested. Individuals with chronic obstructive lung disease should be made aware of the possible allergens in the environment. Clients should be told to postpone sexual activity for at least 3 hours after a full meal or after the ingestion of alcohol. If the environment is extremely cold or hot and humid, sexual activity should be postponed.[41]

The partner should be included in sexual counseling. Both the client and partner should realize that sexual expression can be manifested in ways other than sexual intercourse. These ways can include speaking words of endearment, embracing, handholding, and sharing feelings, all of which are important ingredients of a meaningful sexual relationship.[41]

REHABILITATION TEAM INTERVENTIONS

A primary physician, chest specialist, physiatrist, physical therapist, occupational therapist, nutritionist, respiratory therapist, social worker, vocational rehabilitation counselor, and psychologist or psychiatrist may be working with the nurse as members of the pulmonary rehabilitation team. Their roles and functions in working with the client who has impaired respiratory function are described here.[19]

Primary physicians or chest specialists: Perform history and physical examination and order extensive diagnostic tests.

Physiatrists: Evaluate clients regarding readiness to engage in vocational rehabilitation based on the results of the physical examination, record review (including radiological and bacteriological findings), complete pulmonary function studies, and electrocardiogram.

Occupational therapists: Evaluate the client's ability to perform activities of daily living and develop individualized practical, energy-saving techniques. Occupational therapists evaluate clients' upper extremity strength, sensation, range of joint motion, coordination, cognition, and performance in home activities and teach clients to properly pace activities by monitoring their pulse, coordinating breathing with activity, conserving energy in such maintenance activities as dressing, personal hygiene, and eating and with instrumental activities such as working, socializing, performing household chores, preparing meals, and washing laundry. Occupational therapists also teach relaxation techniques and explain the hazards of air pollution. Progress is measured by observing the client's use of energy conservation measures in all activities, stabilization of pulse rate with activities, and a decrease in dyspnea and fatigue.

Physical therapists: Develop an exercise program designed to diminish dyspnea, improve breathing, and increase endurance. Physical therapists teach the client ways to train the muscles of respiration and facilitate the mechanics of breathing through pursed-lip diaphragmatic breathing and segmental breathing techniques. The pulse is monitored during progressive ambulation. The client may be taught postural drainage for home use, manual and mechanical percussion and vibratory techniques for bronchial toilet, and relaxation techniques.

Nutritionists: Assess eating habits, home or other food preparation facilities, food likes and dislikes, and general nutritional status. Nutritionists teach diet modification, meal planning, principles of cooking, and ways to select food when grocery shopping. In addition, they give general instruction on proper nutrition.

Respiratory therapists: Teach clients to initiate and become competent in self-administration and care of respiratory equipment. Clients may be taught how to use oxygen, aerosol bronchodilators, and mist inhalation and perform bronchial hygiene for clearing excessive sputum. Respiratory therapists teach clients to observe the type and amount of sputum produced. They also identify previous respiratory problems and determine clients' needs for reeducation. They review pulmonary function tests and other pertinent diagnostic tests, clinical signs and symptoms, and arterial blood gases to help determine the need for equipment such as oxygen humidifiers, ventilators, compressors, and nebulizers in the home. In addition, they help determine the need for tracheostomy care and intermittent positive-pressure breathing. Respiratory therapists also assess the support given by family members and their involvement in home care.

Social workers: Obtain a social history and identify life roles of the client; reactions and perceptions of the client and family to the disability; and the client's emotional, physical, financial, intellectual, and environmental resources for coping with a disability. Social workers team up with psychologists to provide counseling for anxiety, depression, and other street responses to illness, hospitalization, and disability. In addition, they provide information and advice about community resources, such as attendant care, financial assistance, and legal and vocational aid.

Vocational rehabilitation counselors: Interview clients to establish preliminary psychosocial and vocational assessment. One of the major responsibilities of the rehabilitation program is to evaluate work tolerance and vocational potential of the client who is disabled. The type and amount of work the client can tolerate per day before experiencing discomfort is determined. Any vocational and avocational interests of the client are analyzed to ascertain proclivities. Work history is discussed in great detail and includes the client's employment history, duties and activities, job conditions, salary, ways in which jobs were obtained and reasons for leaving a job. Clients seem to fall within four groups: (1) those who can return to their previous occupation with no limitations, (2) those who have disability-related conditions that conflict with the activities and conditions of their previous occupations, (3) those who have full work tolerance, usable skills, and the ability to use public transportation but who cannot return to work under competitive employment conditions, and (4) those who cannot return to their previous occupations because the activities and conditions involved may jeopardize their health.[19]

Psychologists: Evaluate psychosocial history and reaction to illness and disability and provide counseling to assist clients and their families to adjust better to disability, cope better with illness, and adapt to the situation. Psychologists administer a battery of tests to measure anxiety, depression, somatic focus, and self-esteem. They help clients become more aware of their responses to disability and find solutions to family, economic, and other problems.

OUTCOME CRITERIA

Outcome criteria for the client with impaired respiratory function depend upon the condition of the client and the specific situation of the client and family. Generally outcome criteria include the following[43]:

1. The client maintains a patent airway, with no signs of increased secretion or airway obstruction.
2. The client remains free of respiratory tract infection.
3. The client has a regular respiratory rate and maintains acid-base balance.
4. The client uses measures to prevent or control hypoxemia.
5. The client maintains adequate nutrition, hydration, and weight for age and height.
6. The client obtains adequate rest and has a satisfactory sleeping pattern.
7. The client verbalizes feelings concerning

sexual problems and works with the partner and selected rehabilitation team member(s) to help resolve these problems.
8. The client and family manage long-term mechanical ventilation when necessary.
9. The client and family understand or can demonstrate:
   a. Effective coughing and skills necessary to remove secretions from the respiratory tract
   b. Relaxation and breathing techniques
   c. Early signs and symptoms of and measures to avoid hypoxemia and hypercapnia
   d. Signs and symptoms of and measures to avoid respiratory tract infections
   e. Administration of, indications for, and side effects of medications when prescribed
   f. Use of equipment when prescribed
   g. Continued or increased physical exercise within the bounds of airflow limitations and life-style
   h. Use of oxygen therapy if prescribed
   i. Use of aids for lung expansion if indicated
   j. Management of nutrition and hydration
   k. Energy conservation

SUMMARY

Breathing is necessary to sustain life. During the process of breathing, oxygen is delivered by the airways and the mechanical action of the chest bellows to the alveolar-capillary unit of the respiratory system. At this level oxygen is exchanged for carbon dioxide. Carbon dioxide is then delivered back to the atmosphere.

The integrity of the respiratory system depends upon proper function of the neural pathways, the chest bellows apparatus, the airways, and the alveolar-capillary unit. Neuromuscular disease, impairment of central and peripheral chemoreceptors, and impairment of pulmonary mechanoreceptors can affect both automatic and voluntary control of breathing. Failure of the chest bellows apparatus, or "ventilatory pump," may be the result of defective neural pathways, mechanical defects of the pump, or high work loads. Many conditions can narrow the lumen of the airways and increase resistance to airflow. Disturbances in gas exchange at the alveolar-capillary units are associated with diffusion defects, abnormal gas transport, and ventilation-perfusion abnormalities.

The client who has impaired respiratory function presents a complex and difficult problem to the rehabilitation team. All activities of daily living can be affected. Early diagnosis, goal setting, and intervention will help reduce the risk of secondary physical, psychosocial, and financial problems and help improve the quality of life for clients and families affected by chronic respiratory impairment.

TEST QUESTIONS

1. Which one of the following statements is true about the normal structure and function of the respiratory sysem?
   a. The medullary center in the brain establishes the basic pattern of respiration.
   b. Hypoxemia has a direct stimulating effect on the respiratory center and results in increased ventilation.
   c. The stimulant effect of Po_2 on the central respiratory centers accounts for 40% of the total chemoreceptor response to that gas.
   d. Pulmonary mechanoreceptors are sensory receptors within the carotid bodies that transmit signals to the respiratory centers through the phrenic nerves.

2. The diaphragm:
   a. Is the primary muscle of expiration.
   b. Separates the abdomen from the rib cage.
   c. May be paralyzed from the interruption of impulses through the phrenic nerve.
   d. Accounts for greater than one third of the volume entering the lungs during tidal breathing.

3. In caring for a client with C6 quadriplegia, the nurse is aware that:
   a. Diaphragmatic function is impaired.
   b. Marked expiratory muscle weakness is present.
   c. The ability to cough effectively is maintained.
   d. Diaphragmatic fatigue and atelectasis are not significant problems.

4. Which statement is true about the lower airway?
   a. The right lung has eight bronchopulmonary segments as opposed to ten in the left lung.
   b. Mucous glands are most numerous at the level of the bronchioles.
   c. The alveoli are the basic units of gas exchange with a normal volume of approximately 3,000 ml.
   d. Secretions from the tracheobronchial tree are estimated to range from 100 to 1,000 ml per day in a normal adult.

5. When performing a nursing assessment for the client with impaired respiratory function, the nurse is aware that:
   a. Objective data are always gathered first during the assessment.
   b. Dyspnea is easy to evaluate because it is a highly objective symptom.
   c. A cough becomes abnormal when it is irritating, persistent, painful, and productive.
   d. Clients with chronic bronchitis expectorate large amounts of mucoid material, often in the morning.

6. When performing an objective assessment of the client with impaired breathing, the nurse knows that:
   a. Paradoxical motion of the abdomen during quiet breathing often indicates abnormal or absent use of the diaphragm.
   b. Approximately 1 g/100 ml of reduced hemoglobin must be present to change the skin color from pink to blue.
   c. Examination of the anterior chest is best performed with the client seated and the chest exposed from the neck down.
   d. Percussion is used to detect areas of tenderness or crepitation, and to assess respiratory excursion.

7. The term crackles describes:
   a. Discontinuous lung sounds, low to medium pitched, that have an explosive quality and are usually heard during inspiration.
   b. High-pitched, continuous sounds occurring during inspiration, expiration, or both.
   c. Low-pitched, continuous sounds that have a snoring quality.
   d. Low-pitched, continuous crowing sounds heard over the larynx and trachea generally during inspiration.

8. Tidal volume refers to:
   a. The maximum amount of air exhaled from the point of maximum inspiration.
   b. The volume of air remaining in the lungs after maximum exhalation.

c. The volume of air inhaled or exhaled with each breath during quiet breathing.

d. The volume of air in the lungs after maximum inspiration.

9. To promote airway clearance in a client with ineffective lung clearance, the nurse teaches the client to:
a. Limit fluid intake to five glasses daily.
b. Increase coffee and tea intake to promote diuresis.
c. Increase moisture in the air through use of humidification equipment.
d. Increase milk intake to decrease secretion viscosity.

10. To promote effective coughing, the nurse instructs the client to:
a. Hold the head in an extended position with the shoulders bent slightly backward.
b. Breathe rapidly for several seconds while lying in a supine position.
c. Take a deep breath and cough several times until there is no air left in the lungs.
d. Inhale deeply while the nurse's hands are on the client's anterior and posterior chest wall.

11. A nursing intervention for the client with compromised respiratory function is postural drainage. Postural drainage is performed:
a. Immediately before or after a meal.
b. To drain pulmonary secretions from the lungs by gravity.
c. Whenever bright red hemoptysis is present or recent.
d. Approximately 1 hour before administration of bronchodilating drugs.

12. When caring for the client requiring tracheostomy suctioning, the nurse:
a. Applies suction for no longer than 40 seconds to prevent hypoxemia.
b. Rotates the catheter upon withdrawal for more adequate secretion removal.
c. Rinses the catheter with tap water between each suctioning.
d. Suctions the oral cavity first to remove any loose secretions.

13. Which of the following statements is true concerning lung sounds?
a. Vesicular breath sounds are heard over the large airways and are considered abnormal.
b. Increased sound transmission may result from airway obstruction, secretions, or neuromuscular disorders.

c. Rhonchi refers to high-pitched, continuous sounds that have a snoring quality.
d. Bronchovesicular sounds can be heard over the upper half of the sternum and in the intrascapular area.

14. When auscultating the chest, the nurse:
a. Uses the bell of the stethoscope because lung sounds generally have a low frequency.
b. Instructs the client to breathe deeper than usual with the mouth open.
c. Places the client comfortably in a lying, supine position.
d. Taps areas of the chest with a flexed finger to evaluate lung tissue underneath the chest wall.

15. All of the following statements regarding the care of the client with impaired gas exchange are true except:
a. Clients with hypoxemia (less than 55 mm Hg) are candidates for supplemental oxygen therapy.
b. Incentive spirometry allows visual monitoring of intermittent maximum expiration.
c. Volume-cycled ventilators deliver a consistent predetermined tidal volume of air into the lungs.
d. Pressure-cycled ventilators inflate the client's lungs until a predetermined pressure is reached.

16. In providing health education for the client with impaired respiratory function and family, the nurse teaches:
a. A self-inflating hand operated resuscitator bag should be supplied for the client receiving home mechanical ventilation.
b. Suctioning and chest physical therapy are not performed to promote sleep and relaxation before the client goes to bed.
c. A high-carbohydrate, high-fat diet is usually ordered for the client to aid digestion.
d. Cuffed tracheostomy tubes should be deflated during eating to prevent aspiration.

17. All of the following statements about health teaching for the client discharged with a permanent tracheostomy are true except:
a. The equipment for cleaning the client's inner cannula and stoma may be washed and reused.
b. The client's air supply should be adequately humidified.

c. Good oral hygiene must be provided, since the client's oropharynx contains many organisms.

d. A finger may be placed over a cuffed tracheostomy tube to allow for client vocalization.

Answers: 1. a, 2. c, 3. b, 4. c, 5. c, 6. a, 7. a, 8. c, 9. c, 10. c, 11. b, 12. b, 13. d, 14. b, 15. b, 16. a, 17. d.

LEARNING ACTIVITIES

In the classroom:

1. Invite a respiratory therapist to discuss and demonstrate postural drainage, percussion, and vibration techniques.

2. Demonstrate chest assessment. Divide students or staff members into pairs and ask each person to perform a chest assessment on his or her partner. Document findings.

3. Invite a primary physician from a rehabilitation team to discuss the history and physical examination plus diagnostic test findings for clients with various respiratory impairments.

4. Demonstrate nasotracheal suctioning, tracheostomy suctioning, and tracheostomy care. Ask each class participant to provide a repeat demonstration.

5. Invite a physical therapist to discuss exercise programs, breathing techniques, and relaxation techniques for the client with impaired breathing.

In the clinical unit:

6. Assign each student or staff member to design and implement a rehabilitation education plan for the client with compromised respiratory function.

7. Assign clients with selected respiratory impairments to students or staff members and ask them to discuss the pathophysiological process responsible for the respiratory impairments of their clients.

8. Assign clients with ineffective airway clearance and ask each student or staff member to establish mutually determined goals with the client that would assist in removing secretions from the lower respiratory tract.

9. Invite a social worker to a postcare conference to discuss the social history, environmental resources, and community resources available to clients coping with a respiratory disability.

10. Invite a respiratory therapist to discuss and demonstrate the use of IPPB equipment, incentive spirometry, and mechanical ventilators. Allow time for students and staff members to become familiar with the equipment.

11. Assign each student or staff member to perform a chest assessment on clients with selected respiratory impairments and present findings at a postcare conference.

12. Assign each student or staff member to design and implement an educational plan to convey information and skills necessary for the client and family to maintain respiratory therapy at home.

REFERENCES

1. Altose MD: Assessment and management of breathlessness, Chest 88(2):77S, Aug 1985.

2. Altose MD: Pulmonary mechanics. In Fishman A, editor: Assessment of pulmonary function, New York, 1982, McGraw-Hill Book Co.

3. Bateman JRM and others: Is cough as effective as chest physiotherapy in the removal of excessive tracheobronchial secretions, Thorax 36:683, 1981.

4. Bates B: A guide to physical examination, ed 4, Philadelphia, 1987, JB Lippincott Co.

5. Bogrand B: Impairment of respiratory function. In Snyder M: A guide to neurological and neurosurgical nursing, New York, 1983, John Wiley & Sons, Inc.

6. Brown I: Trach care? Take care—infections on the prowl, Nurs '82 12:44, May, 1982.

7. Burton GC and Hodgkin JE, editors: Respiratory care, Philadelphia, 1984, JB Lippincott Co.

8. Cherniak NS: The regulation of ventilation. In Fishman A, editor: Assessment of pulmonary function, New York, 1982, McGraw-Hill Book Co.

9. Crofton J and Douglas A: Respiratory diseases, Oxford, 1975, Blackwell Scientific Publications, Ltd.

10. Curgian L and Pagano K: Nutrition in chronic respiratory disease, Rehabil Nurs 10:22, July/Aug 1985.

11. Curgian L and Sparapani M: The chest cuirass and related nursing management, Rehabil Nurs 11:17, July/Aug 1986.

12. Dantzker DR, editor: Cardiopulmonary critical care, Orlando, Fla, 1986, Grune & Stratton, Inc.

13. DeTroyer A and Deisser P: The effects of intermittent positive pressure breathing on patients with respiratory muscle weakness, Am Rev Respir Dis 124:132, Aug 1981.

14. Fanta C and Ingram R: Airway responsiveness and chronic airway obstruction, Med Clin North Am 65:473, 1981.

15. Feldman J: Chronic obstructive pulmonary disease. In Traver G, editor: Chronic care in respiratory nursing: the science and the art, New York, 1982, John Wiley & Sons, Inc.

16. Fischer DA and Prentice W: Feasibility of home care for certain respiratory-dependent restrictive or obstructive lung disease patients, Chest 82:739, 1982.

17. Fuchs P: Streamlining your suctioning techniques. I. Nasotracheal suctioning, Nurs '84 14:55, May 1984.

18. Fuchs P: Streamlining your suctioning techniques. III. Tracheostomy suctioning, Nurs '84 14:39, July 1984.

19. Glaser EM, editor: Pulmonary rehabilitation programs, Los Angeles, 1980, Human Interaction Institute.

20. Gordon M: Nursing diagnosis: process and application, ed 2, New York, 1987, McGraw-Hill Inc.

21. Guyton A: Basic human physiology: normal function and mechanisms of disease, ed 5, Philadelphia 1981, WB Saunders Co.

22. Harper R: A guide to respiratory care: physiology and clinical applications, Philadelphia, 1981, JB Lippincott Co.

23. Hodgkin J: Pulmonary rehabilitation. In Simmons P, editor: Current pulmonology, New York, 1981, John Wiley & Sons, Inc.

24. Hudson L and Pierson D: Comprehensive respiratory care for patients with chronic obstructive pulmonary disease, Med Clin North Am 65:629, 1981.

25. Irwin M and Openbrier D: Feeding ventilated patients safely, Am J Nurs 85:274, May 85.

26. Keller C, Solomon J, and Reyes V: Respiratory nursing care, Englewood Cliffs, NJ, 1984, Prentice-Hall, Inc.

27. Kieran J: No end to love, Bull Am Lung Assoc 67:10, Dec, 1981.

28. Krider SJ: Interviewing and the respiratory history. In Wilkins RL, Shelton RL, and Krider SJ, editors: Clinical assessment in respiratory care, St. Louis, 1985, The CV Mosby Co.

29. Luce JM and Culver BH: Respiratory muscle function in health and disease, Chest 81:82, 1982.

30. Macklem PT: Respiratory muscles: the vital pump, Chest 78:753, 1980.

31. Make B and others: Rehabilitation of ventilator-dependent subjects with lung diseases: the concept and initial experience, Chest 86:358, 1984.

32. Murray JF: The normal lung, ed 2, Philadelphia, 1986, WB Saunders Co.

33. Pare JAP and Fraser RG: Synopsis of diseases of the chest, Philadelphia, 1983, WB Saunders Co.

34. Petty TL: Intensive and rehabilitative respiratory care, ed 3, Philadelphia, 1982, Lea & Febiger.

35. Petty TL: Ambulatory oxygen, New York, 1983, Thieme-Stratton, Inc.

36. Report of the ATS: ACCP ad hoc subcommittee on pulmonary nomenclature, ATS News 2:8, Winter 1981.

37. Report of the ATS: ACCP ad hoc subcommittee on pulmonary nomenclature, Chest 67:583, 1975.

38. Rochester DF: Respiratory muscle function in health, Heart Lung 13:345, 1984.

39. Rochester DF: Fatigue of the diaphragm. In Fishman A, editor: Update: pulmonary disease and disorders, New York, 1982, McGraw-Hill Book Co.

40. Roussos C and others: Voluntary factors affecting the distribution of inspired gas, Am Rev Respir Dis 116:457, 1977.

41. Sexton D: Chronic obstructive pulmonary disease: care of the child and adult, St. Louis, 1981, The CV Mosby Co.

42. Shapiro B, Peterson J, and Cane R: Complications of mechanical aids to intermittent lung inflation, Resp Care 27:467, April 1982.

43. Standards of nursing care of patients with COPD, ATS News, p 31 Summer 1981.

44. Traver G: Respiratory nursing: the science and the art, New York, 1982, John Wiley & Sons.

45. Tyler M: Complications of positioning and chest physiotherapy, Respir Care 27:458, 1982.

46. Wachter-Shikora N: Chemoreceptors of respiration: physiology and nursing implications, J Neurosurg Nurs 10(2):68, 1978.

47. Wade J: Comprehensive respiratory care: physiology and technique, St. Louis, 1982, The CV Mosby Co.

48. Weibel ER: Design and structure of the human lung. In Fishman A, editor: Assessment of pulmonary function, New York, 1982, McGraw-Hill Book Co

49. Weinberger SE: Principles of pulmonary medicine, Philadelphia, 1986, WB Saunders Co.

50. West JB: Pulmonary pathophysiology, ed 2, Baltimore, 1982, The Williams & Wilkins Co.

51. Wilkins R: Techniques of physical examination. In Wilkins RL, Sheldon RL, and Krider SJ: Clinical assessment in respiratory care, St. Louis, 1985, The CV Mosby Co.

52. Zejdlik CM: Management of spinal cord injury, Monterey, Calif, 1983, Wadsworth Health Sciences Division.

ADDITIONAL READINGS

Belman MJ and Sieck GC: The ventilatory muscles, Chest 82:761, 1982.

Braun N: Respiratory muscle dysfunction, Heart Lung 13:327, 1984.

Brown H and Wasserman K: Exercise performance in chronic obstructive pulmonary disease, Med Clin North Am 65:525, 1981.

Devito A: Rehabilitation of patients with chronic obstructive pulmonary disease, Rehabil Nurs 10:12, March/April 1985.

Dudley DL and others: Psychosocial concomitants to rehabilitation in chronic obstructive pulmonary disease, Special Report, Chest 77:413, 1980.

Frasca C and Weimer M: Establishing a respiratory therapy program in the home: the South Hills Program, Home Health Care Nurse 3(2):8, 1985.

Howell JBL and Campbell EJM, editors: Breathlessness, Philadelphia, 1966, FA Davis Co.

Johnson DL, Giovannoni RM, and Driscoll SA: Ventilator-assisted patient care: planning for hospital discharge and home care, Rockville, Md, 1986, Aspen Publishers, Inc.

CHAPTER 8

Controlling Body Temperature

Mary Sue Niederpruem

Objectives

After completing Chapter 8, the reader will be able to:

1. Discuss the physiological basis of body temperature control.

2. Identify the alterations in body temperature that occur with specific diseases and conditions.

3. Conduct a nursing assessment specific to the client with altered body temperature.

4. Formulate nursing diagnoses associated with elevated body temperature, hyperthermia, and hypothermia.

5. Develop goals to assist the client in controlling altered body temperature.

6. Determine the nursing interventions for elevated body temperature, hyperthermia, and hypothermia.

7. Explain the interventions of other rehabilitation team members in assisting a client with altered body temperature.

8. List outcome criteria used as a basis for evaluation of the client's response to interventions for altered body temperature.

The maintenance of normal body temperature is vital to life. Normally, body temperatures range from 96.4° to 100° F (35.8° to 37.8° C), but can vary from person to person. For every degree of elevation of body temperature, the body's demands for oxygen and nutrients increase; when body temperature decreases, body demands decrease.

Under normal circumstances, the internal body temperature remains relatively constant. Even in abnormal circumstances, a constant body temperature is maintained by use of defense mechanisms, when the naked body is exposed to temperatures ranging from as low as 55° to 140° F (12.7° to 60° C).[5]

The nurse working in a rehabilitation setting is responsible for monitoring alterations in body temperature. Therefore, this chapter includes the physiology of altered body temperature, factors that affect control of body temperature, and the problem of extremes in body temperature. The focus of nursing interventions is on management of rehabilitation clients with spinal cord injury, cerebrovascular accidents, multiple sclerosis, head trauma, and the special needs of elderly clients. Responsibilities of other rehabilitation team members in relation to maintenance of body temperature are discussed.

MECHANISMS OF BODY TEMPERATURE CONTROL

The hypothalamus, located in the brain beneath the thalamus, is the center for control of body temperature. It consists of several structures and forms the wall of the third ventricle (Figure 8-1). The hypothalamus also controls metabolic activities such as maintenance of water balance, glucose levels, and fat metabolism.

The temperature control function of the hypothalamus is regulated by neural feedback. Sensitive receptors located in the preoptic area of the anterior hypothalamus maintain body heat equilibrium. Heat-sensitive receptors increase their output as the environmental temperature decreases; cold-sensitive receptors decrease their output when the environmental temperature increases. Heat and cold receptors in the skin transmit impulses via the spinal cord to the hypothalamus to help control body temperature.

Figure 8-2 depicts the precision with which the hypothalamic thermostat can control heat loss

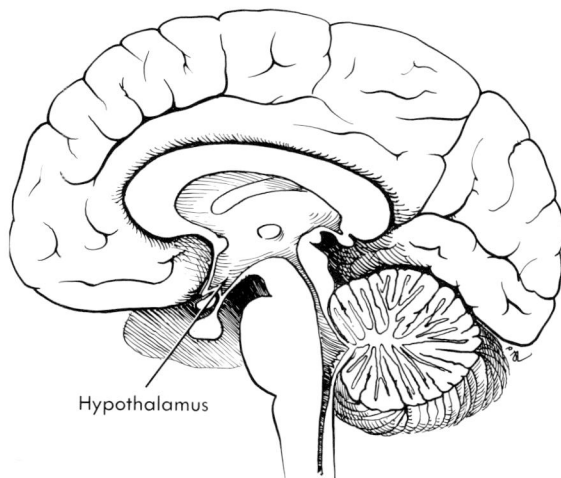

Figure 8-1
Location of hypothalamus.

and heat production. Sweating begins at precisely 37° C and increases rapidly as the temperature rises. Conversely, sweating ceases when the temperature falls below this level. This point, referred to as the *set point* of the body, can be compared to a standard household thermostat and appears to change under the influence of all types of stimuli. Roe[14] reports changes in the set point from the diurnal variation in body temperature (low body temperature in the morning, high body temperature in the evening), during the menstrual cycle, and when the body is invaded by pyrogens. When the temperature falls below 37° C, shivering and other heat-producing mechanisms are activated.

Heat is lost from the body by conduction, convection, radiation, and evaporation.[3,5] The amount of heat lost by each of these mechanisms varies with atmospheric conditions. Only small amounts of heat are lost by conduction from the body surface to other objects, although loss of heat by conduction to air represents a considerable proportion of body heat loss. Conduction of body heat is self-limiting unless the heated air moves away from the skin, so that new, unheated air is brought into contact with the skin.[5]

Convection is the movement of air. A small amount of convection always occurs around the body because air tends to rise as it is heated.[5] Heat loss by radiation refers to loss of heat in the form of infrared heat rays. If body temperature is greater than the temperature of the surroundings, a greater amount of heat is radiated from the body than is radiated to the body. On hot days, the surroundings become hotter than the body temperature; therefore more heat is radiated to the body.[3]

Evaporation is the removal of moisture on the body surface by vaporization. Moisture is brought to the surface by the sweat glands. The vaporization of moisture enables the body to maintain a stable temperature on hot summer days without the symptoms of heatstroke. Heat also is lost from the body through the lungs, urine, and stool.[3]

Shivering

The dorsomedial portion of the posterior hypothalamus is the primary motor center for shivering. This area is inhibited by the preoptic thermostatic area. When the preoptic area is cooled, the normal inhibition of the primary motor area

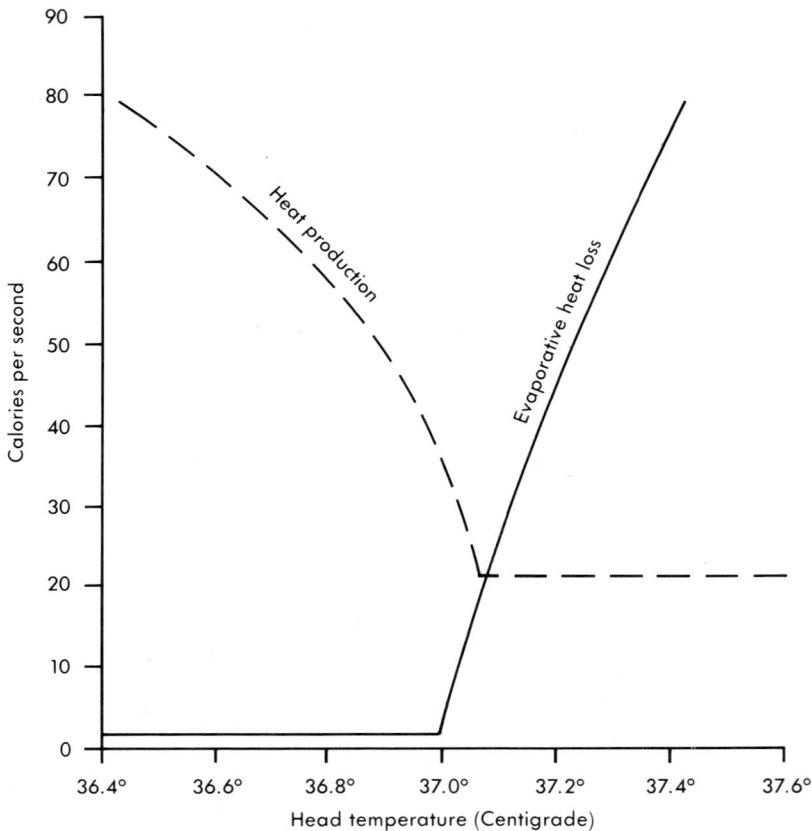

Figure 8-2
Effect of hypothalamic temperature on evaporative heat loss and heat production caused primarily by muscular activity and shivering. Note extremely critical temperature level at which increased heat loss begins and increased heat production stops. *(From Guyton, AC: Textbook of medical physiology, ed 5, Philadelphia, 1976, WB Saunders Co. Based on data from Benzinger, Kitzinger, and Pratt. In Hardy, JD, editor: Temperature, part 3, New York, 1963, Reinhold Publishing Corp).*

is denervated. The self-excitation mechanism of this area causes it to transmit impulses through the bilateral tracts of the brain to the brainstem and the lateral columns of the spinal cord, increasing tone of the skeletal muscles throughout the body. When the tone increases to a certain level, shivering begins. During shivering, body heat production rises as high as 100% to 200% above normal.[5] The intensity of the shivering response depends on the activity of the anterior hypothalamus and cerebellum. The cerebellum controls the rhythm of the shivering, and tracts in the spinal cord control the frequency.

Sweating

Overstimulation of the preoptic thermostatic area of the hypothalamus results in sweating. Sweat glands, located in the subcutaneous layer of the skin, can be stimulated, thus causing heat loss by evaporation. Most of these glands are controlled by the sympathetic postganglionic cholinergic division of the autonomic nervous system. Vasodilation of blood vessels occurs when the sympathetic centers of the posterior hypothalamus are inhibited.[5] Figure 8-3 shows the temperature-regulating mechanism of the hypothalamus.

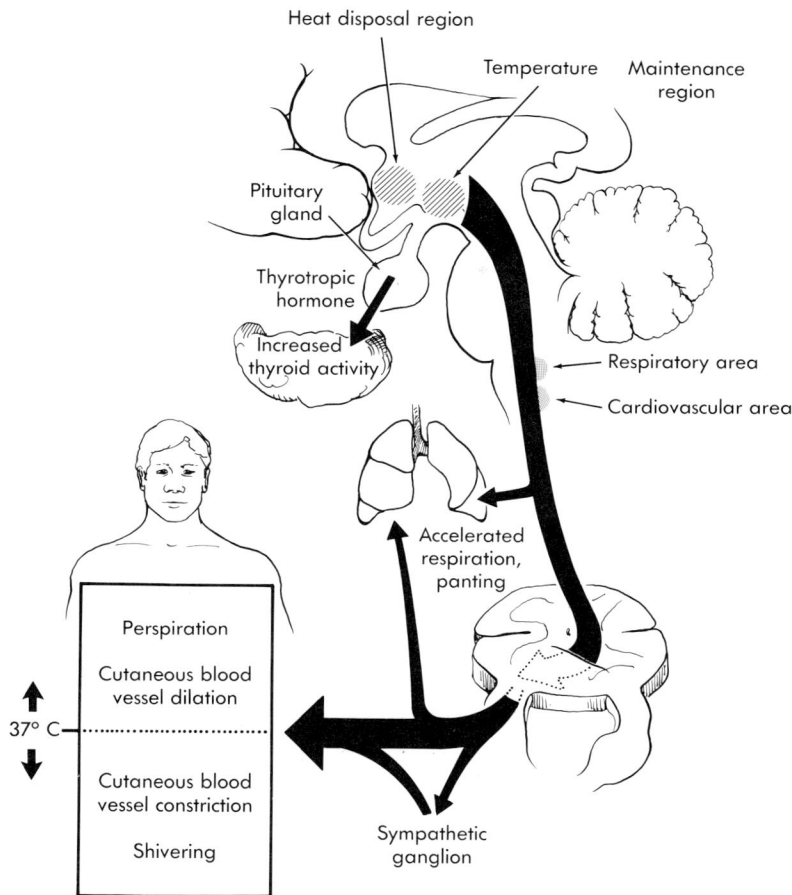

Figure 8-3
Temperature-regulating mechanism of hypothalamus.

When internal body temperature falls below 98.6° F (37° C), sympathetic areas located in the posterior hypothalamus send impulses to constrict blood vessels over the entire skin surface.[7] In response to these skin receptors, the preoptic thermostatic area is inhibited and causes sweating to cease. The body's evaporative cooling mechanism is then halted.

ALTERATIONS IN BODY TEMPERATURE

The hypothalamus plays a key role in maintaining body heat within the narrow range necessary for proper functioning of the central nervous system. Regulation of body temperature is of prime im-

portance and is used as an indicator of health. Elevated body temperature, hyperthermia, and hypothermia are common problems in the rehabilitation of clients with specific neurological conditions. Temperature elevations can exceed 106° F (41.1° C) in a very short time in the client with neurological problems.[8] Clients treated with steroids may have infections without exhibiting an elevated temperature, because steroids tend to mask the classical symptoms of infections.

Elevated Body Temperature

Elevated body temperature is not a disease entity in itself; rather, it is part of the body's response to injury. When injury occurs, the hypothalamus is set at a higher level in an attempt to maintain normal body temperature. The resulting fever may have a known or unknown etiology. For instance, clients with spinal cord injury often demonstrate a fever that may be caused by interruption of autonomic nervous system communication with the hypothalamus during the acute phase. When local reflex activity resumes, the severity of this problem subsides.[17] Some known causes of fever are infections, deep vein thrombosis, pulmonary embolus, drug hypersensitivities, and heatstroke.

Fever results from the effects of pyrogenic substance secretion by injured cells. The exudate formed contains substances that, when injected into healthy animals, produce a fever.[14] Pyrogens cause the set point of the hypothalamic thermostat to rise, and within hours of the rise the body temperature becomes elevated.

Pyrogens can be endogenous or exogenous. Endogenous pyrogens originate from within the body when such situations as graft rejection, hypersensitivity reaction, tumor, and tissue damage occur. Exogenous pyrogens, such as bacteria, fungi, yeast, and viruses, are substances introduced into the body.

Endogenous pyrogens are probably activated by an exogenous pyrogen. Kluger[10] points out that the areas most sensitive to endogenous pyrogens are the preoptic and anterior portions of the hypothalamus. It has been postulated that these endogenous pyrogens cross the blood-brain barrier in the region of the preoptic area, in the anterior portion of the hypothalamus or brainstem, or in both areas.[7]

When fever occurs as part of a disease state, the controlling mechanisms of the hypothalamus fail, and temperature continues to rise unless measures are taken to increase heat loss. Neurogenic fever, caused by injury to the anterior hypothalamus, results when the ability to increase heat loss is impaired. This sign is observed in some clients with severe closed head injuries and basilar skull fractures.[7]

It is not always possible to determine the cause of a fever. Jacoby and Swartz[9] identify criteria for diagnosis of fever of unknown origin as (1) an illness of at least 3 weeks' duration, (2) temperatures exceeding 101° F (38.3° C) on several occasions, and (3) no established diagnosis after 1 week of hospital investigation. The majority of these fevers are found to be caused by (1) infections (40%), (2) neoplasms (20%), and (3) collagen-vascular diseases (15%).[9] Regardless of the cause, these clients must be protected from thermal injury to cells.

Hyperthermia

Hyperthermia, a body temperature of 106° F (41.1° C) or above, is caused by elevated body and environmental temperatures. Manifestations include heat cramps, heat exhaustion, and heatstroke. Elderly persons are at particular risk for this condition because of their slowed circulation and because of structural and functional changes in the skin. Clients with diabetes mellitus, cardiovascular disease, obesity, and alcohol ingestion also are vulnerable to the effects of excessive high or low environmental temperatures. Certain medications, such as phenothiazides, anticholinergics, diuretics, and some antihypertensives can interfere with heat loss.

Heat cramps, painful muscle spasms triggered by inadequate serum sodium levels, occur in muscles that are used during strenuous activity, usually the leg muscles. Increased sodium intake usually alleviates the problem. Figure 8-4 illustrates the body's physiological responses to heat stress.

Heat exhaustion is the most common heat-related illness. Signs and symptoms include weakness, nausea, and lightheadedness caused by excessive sodium and water loss from heavy sweating. If left untreated, heat exhaustion can lead to heatstroke.

Heatstroke is characterized by a body temperature at least 40% above normal and a failure of all body cooling mechanisms. The absence of sweating is caused by a failure or exhaustion of the sweat glands. Signs and symptoms include faintness, dizziness, headache, nausea, rapid pulse, and flushed skin. The affected person may be agitated, confused, stuporous, or comatose. Cerebral and motor dysfunctions, such as ataxia and hemiparesis, may be caused by cerebral edema.

Hypothermia

Hypothermia, body temperature below 96.4° F (35.8° C), occurs when cold persists and heat loss exceeds heat production. The body attempts to

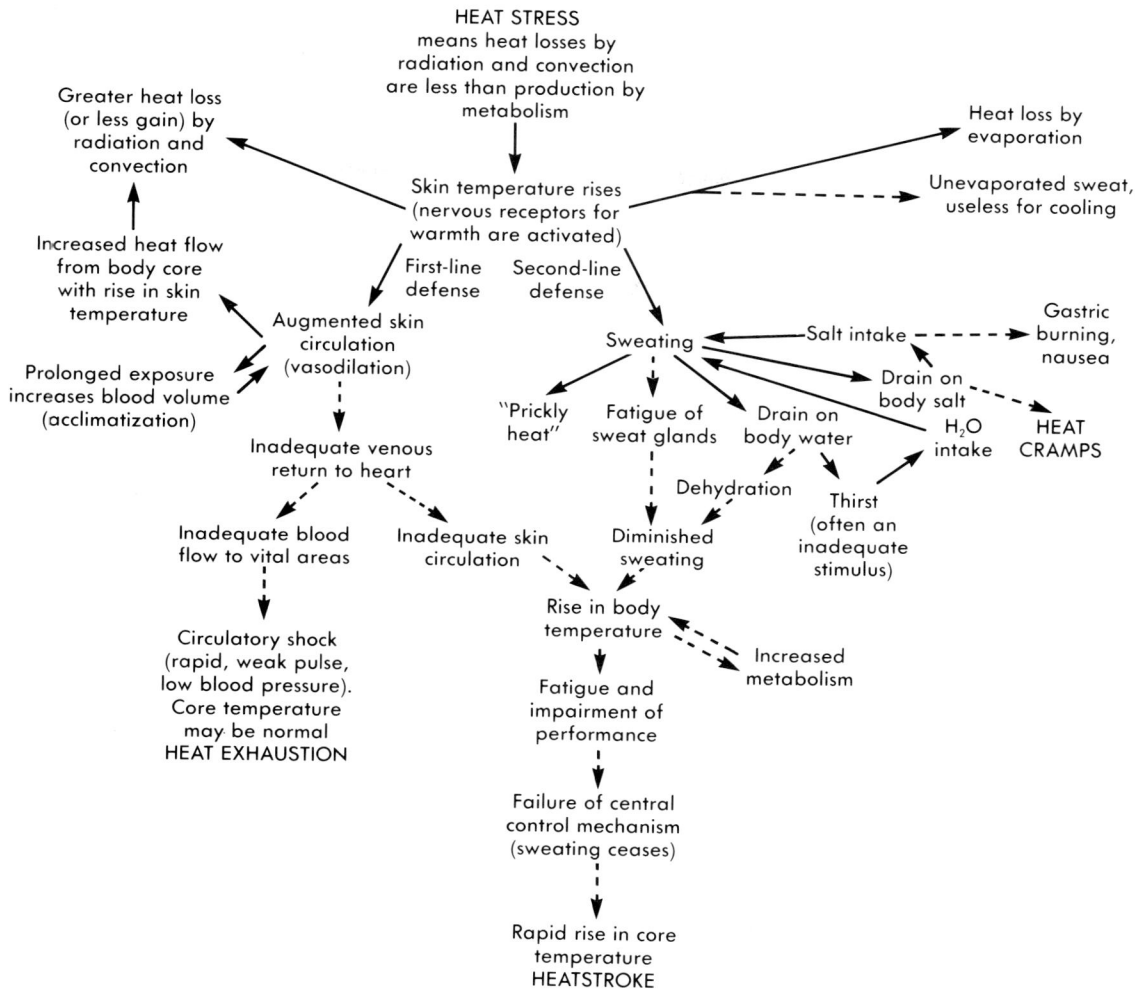

HEAT STRESS
means heat losses by
radiation and convection
are less than production by
metabolism

Greater heat loss
(or less gain) by
radiation and
convection

Heat loss by
evaporation

Skin temperature rises
(nervous receptors for
warmth are activated)

Unevaporated sweat,
useless for cooling

Increased heat flow
from body core
with rise in skin
temperature

First-line
defense

Second-line
defense

Gastric
burning,
nausea

Augmented skin
circulation
(vasodilation)

Sweating

Salt intake

Prolonged exposure
increases blood volume
(acclimatization)

Drain on
body salt

"Prickly
heat"

Fatigue of
sweat glands

Drain on
body water

H_2O
intake

HEAT
CRAMPS

Inadequate venous
return to heart

Dehydration

Thirst
(often an
inadequate
stimulus)

Inadequate blood
flow to vital areas

Inadequate skin
circulation

Diminished
sweating

Rise in body
temperature

Increased
metabolism

Circulatory shock
(rapid, weak pulse,
low blood pressure).
Core temperature
may be normal
HEAT EXHAUSTION

Fatigue and
impairment of
performance

Failure of central
control mechanism
(sweating ceases)

Rapid rise in core
temperature
HEATSTROKE

Figure 8-4
Physiological responses to heat stress. Solid lines indicate usual response; directions of arrows
show cause-and-effect relationships. Broken lines denote events leading to injury. (*From Beland
IL and Passos JY: Clinical nursing: pathophysiological and psychosocial approaches, ed 4, New York,
1981, Macmillan Publishing Co., Inc.)*

compensate for heat loss by shivering. This mechanism of maintaining body temperature is usually
adequate when the environmental temperature is
adequate (59° to 80.6° F; 15° to 27° C). Warm
clothing and adipose tissue also help prevent heat
loss.

Body core temperature (temperature of the internal organs such as the heart and liver) must

remain constant to prevent adverse physiological
changes. However, extremities can withstand environmental temperature changes ranging from
86° to 104° F (30° to 40° C).

Causes of hypothermia include prolonged
periods of outdoor exposure to subzero temperatures without adequate clothing or with wet
clothing; consumption of alcohol combined with

exposure to cold temperatures, resulting in vasodilation and consequent heat loss; and depression of the central nervous system by morphine and barbiturates. A low metabolic rate accompanied by a slow pulse, hypotension, oliguria, and atrial arrhythmias can contribute to hypothermia.

Hypothermia also can be artificially induced by external or surface cooling, internal or body cavity cooling, or extracorporeal cooling.[7] These procedures are used to decrease oxygen needs of the brain when open heart surgery and neurosurgery are performed.

Specific Conditions Accompanied by Altered Body Temperature

Specific diseases or conditions often accompanied by altered body temperature are spinal cord injury, heat trauma, cerebrovascular accidents, multiple sclerosis, malignancies, burns, and infections.

Spinal cord injury

Spinal cord injury is one of the most devastating survivable catastrophies known to humans and affects primarily young men age 15 to 35 years old. After a spinal cord injury, every body system may be involved in attempts to maintain homeostasis.

Fever is common in clients who sustain cervical spinal cord injuries. It is thought that disturbed thermoregulatory control in clients with spinal cord injury is caused by loss of autonomic control over vasomotor activity and the sweating mechanism. This problem is particularly prominent in clients with quadriplegia who are unable to maintain a desirable central temperature when not protected from changes in environmental temperatures.[17] After injury, individuals with damage to the spinal cord above the thoracolumbar outflow of the sympathetic nervous system lose function in the hypothalamic thermoregulatory mechanisms. They are unable to internally control temperature below the level of the lesion, mainly because of absence of vasoconstriction, loss of ability to shiver to conserve body heat, and loss of thermoregulatory sweating to dissipate heat. With chronic loss of vasomotor tone and passive vasodilation, body heat tends to be continually lost.

Clients with complete spinal cord lesions sweat only above the level of the lesion. However, those with incomplete lesions can sweat both above and below the level of the lesion. When sweating becomes excessive in persons with lesions above the T6 spinal cord level, autonomic dysreflexia should be suspected, and measures should be instituted to treat the problem. (See Chapter 10.)

Infection, deep vein thrombosis, and emboli are common causes of fever in clients with spinal cord injuries. Because controlling body temperature is difficult in clients with high cervical injuries and possible damage to the hypothalamus and brainstem, these individuals must be closely monitored for alterations in body temperature that might be signs of brainstem or medullary dysfunction.

Head trauma

Head trauma, a result of catastrophic, debilitating, survivable injury, occurs most often in males between 14 and 30 years of age. Major causes of head trauma are falls, gunshot wounds, and motorcycle accidents. The prognosis for these individuals depends upon the severity of the injury, the area of the brain involved, and the duration of coma.

Hyperthermia during the acute phase of head trauma is an indicator of damage to the hypothalamus or brainstem. Other causes of elevated body temperature are dehydration and infection. When the temperature becomes elevated, the metabolic demands increase, producing an increase in the elimination of carbon dioxide to the cells. Carbon dioxide acts as a vasodilator and causes an increase in intracranial pressure. If the client already has increased intracranial pressure, hyperthermia will lead to further damage. When oxygen supply to the cerebral tissue is insufficient, cerebral ischemia develops. Therefore it is necessary to treat hyperthermia in the client with head injury rapidly and effectively.[8]

Cerebrovascular accidents

A cerebrovascular accident is caused by interruption of blood flow to an area of the brain, resulting in ischemia, necrosis, and often permanent damage to neurons and neural pathways. Among the contributing factors are hypertension, diabetes, obesity, heavy smoking, high cholesterol levels, and sedentary life-styles. Arteriosclerosis, hardening of the arteries, and atherosclerosis, narrowing of the arteries caused by the accumulation of fatty deposits, are commonly found in clients who have suffered a cerebrovascular accident.

Hyperthermia in the acute phase of a cerebrovascular accident can result from damage to the brainstem or hypothalamus. Substantial temperature elevations seen in clients with hemorrhagic stroke or subarachnoid hemorrhage can be caused by blood in the cerebrospinal fluid contributing to hypothalamic dysfunction or the development of aseptic meningitis.[7] Elevated temperatures also can be caused by dehydration and infection.

Multiple sclerosis

Multiple sclerosis, a disease of the central nervous system, is characterized by plaques forming in the spinal cord, cerebellum, cerebrum, brainstem, and optic nerve. These plaques cause demyelination of the myelin sheaths, subsequently causing destruction of the nerves traveling to the lower limbs, eyes, and, to a lesser extent, the upper limbs.

Although the reason is unknown, there is increased thermosensitivity in clients with demyelinating disease. This is a critical problem, because increased core body temperature exacerbates neurological symptoms. Thus the use of the "hot bath test" as a diagnostic tool for multiple sclerosis is discouraged.

Infections

Elevated body temperatures are the most evident sign of infection. Infections have numerous causes, ranging from gram-negative and gram-positive bacteria to viruses, and can be found in every area of the body. The fever of infections must be treated effectively to prevent complications that could lead to death. The fever of infections can be caused by deep vein thrombosis, pulmonary embolism, heterotopic ossification, osteomyelitis, urinary tract infection, respiratory tract infection, infected pressure sores, brain abscess, wound infection, and generalized sepsis.

Burns

Burns are a result of excessive external body temperature. Second- and third-degree burns alter clients' metabolic state, increasing their susceptibility to infection along with other cardiovascular, renal, respiratory, and musculoskeletal complications.

Malignancies

Elevation of body temperature also occurs with various types of malignancies. Kluger[10] associated an elevated temperature with production of a toxin by a tumor that releases pyrogenic substances. Bacterial or viral infections in the client with malignancies also causes elevation of body temperature. Often, however, no cause is found.

Anesthesia

General anesthesia renders the temperature-regulating mechanism inactive. Spinal anesthesia causes the core body temperature to fall quickly.[14] This rapid reduction is associated with the pharmacological inactivation of the temperature-regulating mechanism in the hypothalamus.

The Elderly

The elderly are especially prone to changes in body temperature. Thermoreceptors in the hypothalamus may be impaired because of disease, injury, or degenerative changes. Thus heat exhaustion and heatstroke are both major threats. Elderly clients with cardiovascular disease and diabetes are particularly at high risk. High temperatures can interfere with the absorption of certain medications taken by elderly clients. Additionally, anesthesia is potentially hazardous for these persons when they are undergoing lengthy surgery, because it is difficult for them to use the heat-producing and heat-conserving mechanisms of the body.

NURSING ASSESSMENT

An accurate nursing assessment of changes in body temperature begins with taking a client's temperature. Other vital signs, along with laboratory values, must be incorporated into a comprehensive nursing assessment. Subjective and objective data must be collected.

Temperature Measurement

Accurate body temperature determination is based on three major factors: accuracy of the instrument used, accurate placement of the instrument in the body cavity for a precise amount of time, and accurate reading of the instrument.

A wide range of thermometers is currently in

use. These include traditional oral and rectal glass thermometers, disposable thermometers, and electronic thermometers. Oral and rectal glass thermometers require safety measures because glass can break and cause injury. The mercury in these thermometers also can be toxic if fumes are inhaled. Although disposable thermometers are safe and convenient, these are not as accurate as the glass or electronic type. Electronic thermometers are fast, accurate, safe, convenient, and cost-effective.

Three types of body temperatures are routinely taken: oral, rectal, and axillary. It is generally accepted that the rectal route is the most accurate. Normal rectal temperatures are 1° F above oral recordings of body temperature or 99.6° F (37.6° C). Rectal temperatures are taken for confused, disoriented, or comatose clients to obtain the most accurate recording and minimize the chance of accidents. Two to five minutes are needed to obtain an accurate reading. Nichols[12] found that an average of 2 minutes was required for accurate temperature measurement in both men and women. A room temperature of 65° to 79° F (18.3° to 26.1° C) required 3 minutes of placement, and a room temperature of 80° to 95° F (26.7° to 35° C) required 2 minutes of placement to obtain an accurate body temperature measurement.

The normal oral temperature is 98.6° F (37° C). Although the oral route is the most accessible, factors such as smoking and drinking cold or hot beverages can alter the reading. Most nursing texts recommend 3- to 5-minute placement for an accurate oral temperature measurement. Nichols and Kucha,[13] in a study of 390 subjects, found that 1 to 12 minutes was required to obtain an accurate measurement. The majority of subjects reached an accurate temperature after 8 minutes. Clients above the age of 40 required 7 minutes, and 8 minutes was required for clients ages 18 to 39 years. Men required 7 minutes and women 8 minutes. When the temperature of the room ranged from 65° to 75° F (18.3° to 23.9° C), Nichols and Kucha[13] found it necessary to place the thermometer for 8 minutes. When the room temperature ranged from 76° to 86° F (24.4° to 30° C), it was necessary to place the thermometer for 7 minutes to achieve an accurate reading.

Numerous studies have been conducted to investigate the relationship between oxygen use via nasal cannula and the accuracy of oral temperature measurement.[6,11,16] Results of these studies have shown that there are no significant differences between clients who receive oxygen via nasal cannulas and those who do not in relation to the accuracy of their body temperature measurements.

Axillary temperatures are usually 1° F below the oral reading, or 97.6° F (36.4° C). This method is often recommended for infants under 1 year of age but also can be used for confused or comatose clients. The axillary method is safe and easily accessible. Furthermore, it does not stimulate defecation and avoids the danger of rectal or colon perforation. The length of time required for accurate measurement is 10 minutes, with the arm placed so that it is hugging the body.[15]

A client's temperature can be altered according to circadian rhythm. Usually an early morning reading is lower than normal, whereas a temperature taken around 7 PM is usually higher. Thus it is important for the nurse to take temperatures around the clock and determine the clinical significance of an elevated temperature according to the time of day or other factors. Low and high temperatures are reversed for people who sleep during the day and work at night. Other factors that influence temperature are age, sex, menstrual cycle, pregnancy, type of clothing, and chemicals such as phenothiazines, barbiturates, and alcohol. Regardless of how, when, or where a temperature is taken, it is vital to record it accurately. Prompt documentation of the temperature measurement in the proper place in a client's chart helps to ensure accuracy. All vital signs should be recorded on the same sheet. This documentation provides nursing and medical personnel a chance to see temperature fluctuations in relation to changes in other vital signs.

Other Objective Data

Certain laboratory values should be monitored. Arterial blood gases are assessed for signs of metabolic or respiratory acidosis or alkalosis. Decreased Pao_2 values can be a sign of increased oxygen consumption, temperature, and metabolism. Electrolytes are monitored for signs of dehydration. However, the cornerstone of laboratory values as a sign of possible infection is the white blood cell count.

The electrocardiogram should be monitored

for changes in the conduction system of the heart. Lower levels of consciousness, particularly in postoperative clients or those with head trauma, could be a sign of a nonfunctioning hypothalamus. Cultures should be taken from possible sources of infection, namely wounds, urine, blood, sputum, and stool. Any type of unusual drainage from the body also should be cultured.

The integument should be monitored. Observations should be made of the skin color and turgor, shivering, or sweating. Sensation should be checked.

The external temperature should be considered when hyperthermia or hypothermia occur. The amount and type of clothing should be judged as to appropriateness. Dietary intake should be assessed for its value in meeting the client's metabolic needs.

Age, sex, time of ovulation, pregnancy, absent or deficient sweat glands, and emotions also should be considered when assessing the client for altered body temperature. Infants and younger persons have a higher metabolic rate, thus resulting in a higher body temperature. Men have a metabolic rate that is 10% to 15% higher than women. Women who are ovulating have a body temperature that often falls and rises, but during the time following ovulation, the temperature remains elevated. It then falls before the onset of menstruation. When sweat glands are absent or deficient, the body cannot decrease heat by sweating. Emotional states lead to increased metabolic rates, probably caused by interactions of nervous system stimulation, hormone secretion, and muscle contraction.[1]

Subjective Data

Subjective data are difficult to obtain when there is decreased sensation, altered neurological or mental status, and possible unconsciousness. However, the nurse should be able to obtain some basic data, including whether the client is hot or cold, sweating, shivering, nauseous, confused or lethargic, and experiencing pain in any area of the body where sensation is not altered.

NURSING DIAGNOSES

Nursing diagnoses are based on nursing assessment. Because normal body temperature is vital to life, there are a wide variety of nursing diagnoses that can be made. The primary nursing diagnoses are *ineffective thermoregulation* secondary to the medically diagnosed cause of the altered body temperature, *hypothermia or hyperthermia*. Other nursing diagnoses that might be made, depending upon the individual and the specific body system involved, include the following[4]:

• Ineffective breathing pattern
• Alterations in cardiac output
• Fluid volume deficit or excess
• Impaired physical mobility
• Altered nutrition
• Altered tissue perfusion
• Potential or impaired skin integrity

An ineffective breathing pattern affects body temperature because the lungs help control body temperature by increasing or decreasing respirations. If respiration is impaired by spinal cord injury, heat trauma, or cerebrovascular accident, nursing interventions must be instituted to maintain body temperature.

Altered cardiac output also affects body temperature because vasoconstriction or vasodilation can lower or raise body temperature. Thus in clients suffering from hypothermia, hyperthermia, or head trauma, cardiac output can become impaired.

Altered body temperature can be caused by alterations in fluid volume that occur with blood loss from trauma or overhydration in clients who have burns. Excessive diaphoresis from fever or hyperthermia can cause decreased body fluid volume.

Impaired physical mobility is a problem for many clients involved in the rehabilitation process. One of the many problems resulting from altered mobility is altered body temperature, manifested as sepsis, fever, and hyperthermia or hypothermia.

Decreased nutritional intake can cause body temperature to fall. Increased sodium intake also causes an alteration in body temperature because of dehydration. The elderly are especially at risk.

Altered tissue perfusion as a result of hypothermia, burns, or tissue ischemia causing pressure sores, affects body temperature. The elderly also are at high risk for hypothermia. The individual immobilized because of spinal cord injury or cerebrovascular accident is prone to tissue ischemia and pressure sores.

Impaired skin integrity can affect body temperature. For example, a pressure sore can be a source of infection, causing an elevated body temperature. Burns, heatstroke, frostbite, and fevers from infected pressure sores require constant nursing intervention. These problems are frequently seen in the client involved in the rehabilitation process.

GOALS

The goals when the body temperature is altered are to teach the client and family ways to prevent elevated body temperature, hypothermia, and hyperthermia; teach the client and family how to treat elevated body temperature, hypothermia, and hyperthermia; and teach the use of appropriate institutional and community resources to assist in prevention and treatment of altered body temperature.

REHABILITATION NURSING INTERVENTIONS

Since the most common alteration in body temperature is fever, interventions for fever are discussed first. The controversy over the advantages and disadvantages of treating a fever has raged for decades. Both arguments for and against treatment are valid. The principal argument against treatment is that an elevated body temperature is a normal body defense mechanism. Leukocytes are produced more rapidly in the febrile client to fight the infection. Treatment of a fever masks the cause, however, often making it more difficult to treat.[1]

Proponents for treatment argue that lowering a client's temperature produces a sense of comfort and well-being. Most clients feel uncomfortable when they have a fever. This discomfort is related to feelings of heat, thirst, anorexia, and malaise and is demonstrated by shivering and diaphoresis. Whether the body temperature is decreased by physical or pharmacological means, the client usually feels better. The reduction in body temperature also decreases the body's demand for oxygen, thus lowering metabolic rate and decreasing the demands placed on the cardiopulmonary system.

When the physician orders treatment of the fever, the nurse incorporates the physician's or-

ders into the nursing care plan. The body temperature is taken at least every 4 hours using the method specified or judged most appropriate. Medications often ordered for treatment are acetylsalicylic acid (aspirin) or acetaminophen (Tylenol) suppositories.

If a cooling blanket is ordered, rectal temperatures usually should be taken. To prevent preventricular contractions, the individual placed on a cooling blanket should have body temperature decreased at no more than 1° C every 15 minutes. If a nondisposable or rubber blanket is ordered, a sheet between the client and the blanket assures comfort. If the client is immobile, such as the person with spinal cord injury, cerebrovascular accident, heat trauma, or coma, turning at least every 2 hours is essential to prevent skin breakdown. Shivering, the body's mechanism for increasing body temperature, can be controlled by administering chlorpromazine as ordered. A cooling blanket is often chosen over ice bags and alcohol sponges because these methods tend to be very uncomfortable. With a cooling blanket, the desired body temperature can be maintained at a constant level.

Fluid and electrolyte balance must be maintained. Laboratory values must be monitored continually and appropriate electrolyte and fluid replacement given via mouth or intravenous routes.

Since increased temperature can lead to dehydration, fluids must be replaced. If the client is unable to take fluids orally, intravenous or nasogastric routes may be chosen to maintain fluid balance. If antibiotics are ordered, these should be administered promptly, and the client should be monitored for harmful side effects or anaphylactic reaction. The exudate of any infection should be cultured and the appropriate antibiotic administered to the client. Regardless of the route of administration, therapeutic levels of the antibiotic must be maintained to ensure eradication of the pyrogen.

Prompt and accurate administration of antipyretics also is important. Antipyretics cross the blood-brain barrier and enter the hypothalamus to alter its response to pyrogens. These medications lower the set point, thereby lowering body temperature.

Comfort measures to be taken include application of a cool cloth to the forehead, a darkened room if the client also has a headache, a backrub or position change, and administration of adequate fluids if there is no fluid restriction imposed by the physician because of other medical diagnoses. Informing the client and family of what is to occur helps to lessen anxiety.

Nursing intervention in heat disorder is determined by the signs and symptoms attributed to excessive heat. Ingestion of salt and water usually alleviates heat cramps. Heat exhaustion requires additional interventions, including replacement of fluids and electrolytes. Heatstroke is considered a medical emergency, and immediate measures must be instituted to prevent circulatory collapse. Boyd, Shurett, and Coburn[2] identified four components to the treatment of heatstroke: (1) monitoring vital body functions, (2) cooling the body, (3) preventing or treating complications, and (4) supporting the client. Temperature is monitored constantly to guard against hypothermia, and blood pressure and pulse are monitored to assess the cardiopulmonary status. A cooling blanket or immersion in an ice bath are used to decrease the client's temperature rapidly. Electrocardiograms are monitored for signs of myocardial infarction caused by heat and ventricular arrhythmias caused by hypothermia.

Level of consciousness also must be closely monitored. The hyperthermic client can be severely confused or even comatose. The conscious client should be assessed for irritability and restlessness or any other signs indicative of a changing level of consciousness.

Client and Family Education

A major goal in the rehabilitation of all clients is the prevention of complications and maintenance of functions by client and family. Formal and informal education programs can be used to teach the client about the prevention and treatment of complications occurring with alteration in body temperature. Information about changes in body temperature should be incorporated into educational programs for all clients with cerebrovascular accidents, spinal cord injuries, head trauma, and multiple sclerosis. Community-based educational programs for elderly persons can help them prevent hyperthermia and hypothermia.

Inpatient programs should stress prevention of infections and fever. For example, the majority of clients with spinal cord injury readmitted to hospitals are admitted because of infected pressure sores, urinary tract infections, respiratory tract infections, and generalized septicemia. With proper education, a client and family can learn to prevent these complications and decrease the length and cost of hospitalization.

Since clients with altered neurological sensation have difficulty differentiating hot and cold, they must always be conscious of extremes in temperature. Clients with cerebrovascular accidents and spinal cord injuries must beware of hot stoves, hot water in bathtubs, and overexposure to the sun. These clients can be severely burned in short exposures to the sun. Excessive heat in the form of hot baths also can exacerbate symptoms in clients with multiple sclerosis.

Prevention of hyperthermia can be accomplished in several ways. The elderly are particularly susceptible to the effects of heat, especially if they are hypertensive, diabetic, obese, consume large quantities of alcohol, or have poor dietary habits. Risk factors can be reduced by teaching the client to stay inside or in the shade during the heat of the day and to wear light, loose-fitting clothing and a hat when going outside. The family also should be informed about these precautions. The home can be made cooler by the use of shades and drapes to block the sun, the use of fans or air conditioners if the client can afford them (tax deductible if medically prescribed), and by cooking only during the coolest part of the day. Clients should drink plenty of fluids and limit exercise to cool times of the day.

Hypothermia is also preventable. To reiterate, the ingestion of alcohol is contraindicated during prolonged exposure to the cold. Clients susceptible to cold, especially the elderly, should pay attention to weather reports, especially wind chill factors. Clothing should be worn in layers, preferably natural fibers that conserve body heat. Any layers that become wet should be removed promptly to prevent heat loss. The home should be adequately heated. With the high cost of home heating fuel, this can be difficult, but community agencies can aid clients in defraying costs. Clients should be cautioned against the use of kerosene, space heaters, and wood-burning stoves, or when there is no other choice they should be warned of precautions to take. These items can be possible fire hazards and have the potential to emit toxic fumes.

Referrals

Since rehabilitation is an ongoing process, it is necessary to make referrals for clients once they are discharged from the acute care or rehabilitation setting. Clients may be referred to many different medical specialists such as neurologists, neurosurgeons, orthopedic surgeons, urologists, internists, radiologists, endocrinologists, and psychiatrists.

Psychologists can be helpful in assisting the client with adjustment to disability. Many rehabilitation centers offer peer-group counseling to discharged clients. These centers also offer counseling and discussion groups for significant others and parents of clients.

Once the client is discharged from the acute care or rehabilitation setting, various community agencies can become involved. Referrals are often made to a community health nurse so progress can be monitored, problems can be resolved, and complications can be prevented. Complications that affect body temperature, such as fevers from infections of the urinary tract, respiratory tract, pressure ulcers, hyperthermia, or hypothermia can be prevented. If more therapy is required for the client to adapt to the environment, referrals can be made for speech, occupational, and physical therapy in the home. Various community agencies funded by state and federal governments aid the elderly and disabled. Financial help is available to those who qualify for assistance in payment of heating bills and food purchase. If medically necessary, funds can be allocated to provide air conditioning in the home and automobile.

If a client cannot be discharged to home, referrals can be made to apartments for the elderly, skilled nursing facilities, extended care facilities, and domiciliaries. These residential arrangements provide safe, supervised environments for elderly and disabled persons. If relocation is chosen, agencies may provide assistance in locating suitable housing and assist with

moving expenses for those who qualify. By providing an optimum temperature environment, the complications of excessive heat or cold can be avoided.

Further prevention and treatment of problems associated with altered body temperature can be accomplished by close follow-up of the client. Clients return to the acute care setting or rehabilitation center for physician appointments and reevaluation of function. Hospital-based home care programs from within the rehabilitation center can provide the client with a smooth transition from the hospital environment.

REHABILITATION TEAM INTERVENTIONS

All members of the rehabilitation team play a part in assessment and intervention aimed at controlling body temperature. The physiatrist orders diagnostic tests and establishes the medical regimen for the client. It is the responsibility of the other rehabilitation team members to incorporate these orders into their specific treatment plans and into the team plan for rehabilitation.

Physical therapists help the client improve mobility, thus preventing the hazards of immobility that can cause fever. Occupational therapists play a part in teaching the client to avoid hot stoves and baths and extreme cold. Speech/language pathologists help the client in making needs known by improving speech/language function or using alternatives, such as communication boards or electronic vocal cords.

Social workers assist clients in obtaining financial help for climate controls in the automobile and home. Social workers also investigate community resources to obtain assistance with transportation to hospitals and physicians and counsel the client and family.

The registered nurse assesses the client's function; plans, implements, and evaluates nursing interventions; reinforces the educational programs of all disciplines; and provides emotional support.

OUTCOME CRITERIA

Outcome criteria for the client and family affected by ineffective thermoregulation, hypothermia, or hyperthermia are as follows:

1. The client and family will understand ways to prevent elevated body temperature, hypothermia, and hyperthermia.
2. The client and family will take appropriate actions for the treatment of elevated body temperature, hypothermia, and hyperthermia.
3. The client and family will seek institutional and community resources to assist in the prevention and treatment of elevated body temperature, hypothermia, and hyperthermia.

SUMMARY

This chapter provides information about clients with altered body temperature. Body temperature is characterized as a balance between heat produced by the body and heat lost from the body. Alterations in body temperature are discussed in the context of specific diseases related to altered body temperature. The rehabilitation nurse is responsible for applying the nursing process and functioning as a client and family educator, a role that is vital to maintaining a healthy life-style. The client is the focus of the rehabilitation team, and prevention and treatment of complications related to altered body temperature are paramount to maintaining and restoring function.

TEST QUESTIONS

1. Temperature control receptors are located in the:
   a. Anterior hypothalamus
   b. Skin
   c. Posterior hypothalamus
   d. All of the above
2. Heat is lost from the body by means of all of the following *except:*
   a. Shivering
   b. Sweating
   c. Conduction
   d. Convection
3. Elevated body temperature:
   a. Is a response to a specific disease
   b. Occurs when the hypothalamus is set at a lower level to maintain body temperature
   c. Requires measures to decrease heat loss
   d. Is part of the body's general response to injury
4. Hyperthermia results when:
   a. Body temperature exceeds 106° F (41.1° C)
   b. Persons who have diabetes, ingest alcohol, and are obese are exposed to high environmental temperatures
   c. Body cooling mechanisms fail
   d. All of the above
5. Hypothermia results when:
   a. Body temperature falls below 96.4° F (35.8° C)
   b. Heat loss exceeds heat production
   c. Cold persists
   d. All of the above
6. The accurate objective measurement of body temperature depends upon:
   a. Accuracy of the instrument
   b. Accurate placement of instrument in body cavity for a precise amount of time
   c. Accurate reading of the instrument
   d. All of the above
7. The most accurate route(s) for measurement of body temperature is:
   a. Oral
   b. Rectal
   c. Axillary
   d. All of the above
8. A client's body temperature can be altered by:
   a. Circadian rhythm
   b. Menstrual cycle
   c. Age
   d. All of the above
9. Reduction in body temperature:
   a. Is always desirable
   b. Helps the client feel more comfortable
   c. Increases the body's metabolic work
   d. Increases the demands on the cardiovascular system
10. Antipyretic medications:
    a. Enter the thalamus to alter its response to pyrogens
    b. Increase the set point, thereby lowering body temperature
    c. Lower the set point, thereby increasing body temperature
    d. Lower the set point, thereby lowering body temperature
11. Comfort measures to help the client with elevated body temperature become more comfortable include:

a. Application of a cool cloth to the forehead
b. Back rub
c. Administration of fluids if there is no fluid restriction
d. All of the above
12. To prevent hyperthermia, clients and their families should be taught to:
    a. Keep all doors and windows open
    b. Wear dark-colored clothing
    c. Cook only during cool parts of the day
    d. Drink fluids high in sodium
13. To prevent hypothermia, clients and their families should be taught to:
    a. Wear clothing in layers during prolonged exposure to the cold
    b. Drink alcohol to keep warm
    c. Listen only to temperature reports and ignore the wind chill factor
    d. Keep the temperature down in the home
14. The rehabilitation team can help the client prevent complications of altered body temperature by:
    a. Allowing a fever to run its course no matter how high the temperature
    b. Giving the client acetaminophen (Tylenol) every 4 hours
    c. Keeping the client in a climate-controlled environment at all times
    d. Teaching the client about body temperature control and providing follow-up care

Answers: 1. d, 2. a, 3. d, 4. d, 5. d, 6. d, 7. b, 8. d, 9. b, 10. d, 11. d, 12. c, 13. a, 14. d.

LEARNING ACTIVITIES

1. Visit a senior citizens' center and make arrangements to teach elderly persons about the hazards of hypothermia and hyperthermia and measures that can be taken to avoid these conditions.
2. Monitor a graphic sheet of a febrile client and assess temperature fluctuations with time of day. Determine how the client's body temperature responds to the prescribed treatment plan.

3. Teach the client and family the effects of alterations in body temperature, ways to prevent complications, and actions to take should complications occur.

REFERENCES

1. Beland IL and Passos JY: Clinical nursing: pathophysiological and psychosocial approaches, ed 4, New York, 1981, Macmillan Publishing Co, Inc.
2. Boyd LT, Shurett PH, and Coburn C: Heat and heat-related illnesses, Am J Nurs 81:1298, July 198_.
3. Feely EM, Shine MS, and Sloboda SB: Fundamentals of nursing care, New York, 1980, D Van Nostrand Co.
4. Gordon M: Nursing diagnosis: process and application, ed 2, New York, 1987, McGraw-Hill Book Co.
5. Guyton AC: Basic human physiology: normal function and mechanisms of disease, ed 2, Philadelphia, 1977, WB Saunders Co.
6. Hasler ME and Cohen JA: The effect of oxygen administration on oral temperature assessment, Nurs Res 31:265, Sept/Oct 1982.
7. Heideman CA: Alterations in body temperature. In Snyder M, editor: A guide to neurological and neurosurgical nursing, New York, 1983, John Wiley & Sons, Inc.
8. Hickey JV: The clinical practice of neurological and neurosurgical nursing, ed 2, Philadelphia, 1986, JB Lippincott Co.
9. Jacoby GA and Swartz MN: Fever of undetermined origin, New Engl J Med 289: 1407, Dec 27, 1973.
10. Kluger MJ: The evolution and adaptive value of fever, Am Scientist 66:38, Jan/Feb 1978.
11. Lim-Levy F: The effect of oxygen inhalation on oral temperature, Nurs Res 31:150, May/June 1982.
12. Nichols GA: Rectal measurements, Am J Nurs 72:1092, June 1972.
13. Nichols GA and Kucha DH: Oral measurements, Am J Nurs 72:1091, June 1972.
14. Roe CF: Temperature regulation and energy metabolism in surgical patients, Progr Surg 12:96, 1973.
15. Saxton DF and others: The Addison-Wesley manual of nursing practice, Menlo Park, Calif, 1983, Addison-Wesley Publishing Co, Inc.
16. Yonkman CA: Cool and heated aerosol and the measurement of oral temperature, Nurs Res 31:354, Nov/Dec 1982.
17. Zejdlik CM: Management of spinal cord injury, Monterey, Calif, 1983, Wadsworth Health Sciences Division.

ADDITIONAL READINGS

Berger JR and Sheremata WA: Persistent neurological deficit precipitated by hot bath test in multiple sclerosis, JAMA 249:1751, April 1983.

Durham ML, Swanson B, and Paulford N: Effect of tachypnea on oral temperature regulation: a replication, Nurs Res 4:211, July/Aug 1986.

Hayter J: Hypothermia, hyperthermia in older persons, J Gerontol Nurs 6:65, Feb 1980.

Price SA and Wilson LM: Pathophysiology: clinical concepts of disease processes, ed 3, New York, 1986, McGraw-Hill Book Co.

Sugarman B: Fever in recently injured quadriplegic persons, Arch Phys Med Rehabil 63:639, Dec 1982.

Sugarman B, Brown D, and Musker D: Fever and infection in spinal cord injury patients, JAMA 248:66, July 2, 1982.

Sullivan-Bolyia JZ and others: Hyperpyrexia due to air conditioning failure in a nursing home, Public Health Rep 94:466, Oct 1979.

CHAPTER 9

Eating and Swallowing

Elizabeth C. Phelps

OBJECTIVES

After completing Chapter 9, the reader will be able to:

1. Identify the anatomical structures involved in eating and swallowing.
2. Describe the physiological process of eating.
3. List the cranial nerves used in deglutition.
4. Identify neuromuscular and anatomical impairments that alter deglutition.
5. Conduct a nursing assessment for an individual who has difficulty with eating and swallowing.
6. Formulate nursing diagnoses associated with eating and swallowing.
7. Establish goals with the client who has difficulty eating and swallowing.
8. Determine possible nursing interventions used in eating and swallowing difficulties.
9. Explain the contributions of other rehabilitation team members in assisting the client who has difficulty eating and swallowing.
10. List outcome criteria for the client and family affected by eating and swallowing difficulties.

The process of swallowing (deglutition) begins during the second trimester of fetal life, and by the time the individual is an adult, securing and ingesting food is usually accomplished without difficulty.[5] An individual must ingest proper nutrients to maintain health and function. Eating meals usually occurs in social situations associated with feelings of sharing, belonging, and friendship. When an individual can no longer secure or ingest nutrients in an efficient or normal manner, a biological, social, or psychological crisis may occur. This chapter includes a review of normal patterns of eating and swallowing, factors that can alter normal deglutition, nursing assessment of persons with eating difficulties, and interventions used to assist individuals in the process of eating and swallowing.

MECHANICS OF EATING

The ability to eat and swallow food and drink depends upon the appropriate position and function of intact structures within the alimentary tract. The primary structures involved with eating and swallowing and the stages in these processes are discussed.

Anatomical Structures

The primary structures involved in eating and swallowing include the oral cavity, pharynx, larynx, and esophagus. Ingestion of food begins in the oral cavity, which is composed of the lips, cheeks, gums, hard and soft palate, uvula, palatoglossal arch, palatopharyngeal arch, palatine tonsils, salivary glands, teeth, mandible, and tongue (Figure 9-1).

The oral cavity communicates with the pharynx via the oropharyngeal isthmus. The pharynx is a 12 to 14 cm musculomembranous tube extending from the soft palate to the cricoid cartilage where it connects to the esophagus. The pharynx is composed of three constrictor muscles: the superior, medial, and inferior. These muscles propel food along the pharynx during deglutition. The cricopharyngeal muscle, the most inferior structure of the pharynx, acts as a valve at the top of the

esophagus, preventing air from entering the esophagus during respiration and allowing the bolus of food to enter the esophagus during deglutition.[10]

The esophagus is a hollow muscular tube approximately 23 to 25 cm long with a sphincter at each end. The bolus of food enters the esophagus from the pharynx and is transported to the stomach by the muscular peristaltic action of the esophagus.

The larynx, which begins with the epiglottis found at the base of the tongue, includes the false and true vocal cords (Figure 9-2). The epiglottis prevents food from entering the airway during swallowing.

The larynx, esophagus, pharynx, and oral cavity are the primary structures associated with eating and swallowing. The secondary structures include the eyes, brain, arms, and legs. To remain functionally independent, a person must not only swallow food, but must locate, prepare, and deliver the food to the oral cavity. Although sight can be compensated for, it is essential for finding food either in the home or at the store. Securing and preparing food involves use of the arms and

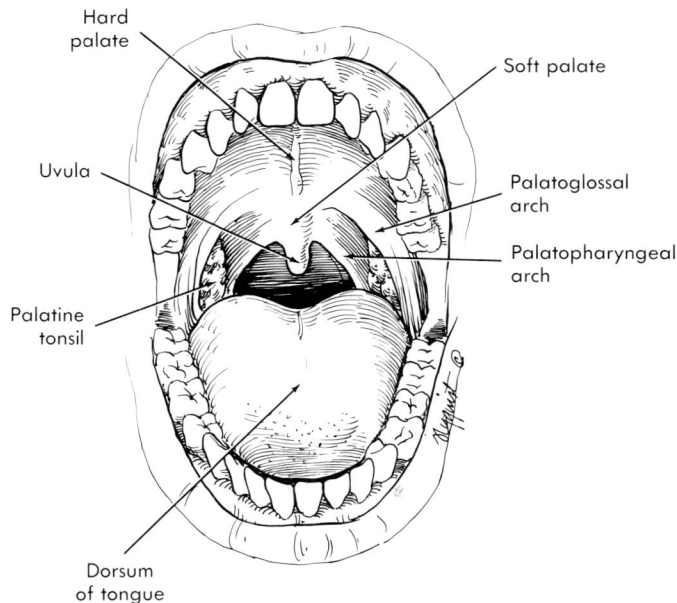

Figure 9-1
Anatomy of oral cavity.

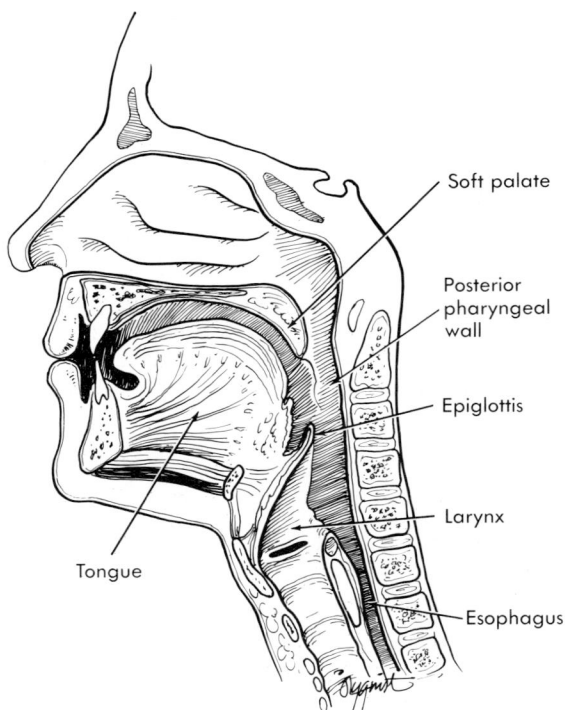

Figure 9-2
Anatomy of larynx.

legs. Today food preparation is simpler if pre-packaged meals are used, but these are sometimes expensive, making them less desirable.

The brain has an impact upon adequate nutrition in several ways. The brain retains knowledge of likes and dislikes, and it records the social significance of foods. Certain diseases that affect the nervous system can alter the rate and quantity of food consumed or can alter the concepts of appropriate foods.[9,13] In addition, an intact nervous system is essential for selecting, planning, and securing food.

Physiological Basis

The process of eating and swallowing can be divided into seven stages: (1) selecting and securing food; (2) preparing food; (3) anticipatory motor stage, when food is placed in the mouth; (4) oral preparatory phase, when food is manipulated within the mouth; (5) lingual stage, when the food bolus is centrally located and pushed posteriorly toward the oropharynx; (6) pharyngeal stage, when the bolus is carried by the swallowing reflex through the pharynx; and (7) esophageal phase when peristalsis carries the bolus to the stomach.

As noted earlier, the body parts involved in the first three stages of eating and swallowing are the eyes, brain, arms, and legs. Vision is important because it allows an individual to locate and choose foods. A meal that appeals to an individual can visually stimulate the appetite as well. To have a clear visualization of food, a clear image must be transmitted to the retina and then be transferred to the brain via the optic tract. Anything that prevents or alters the light as it passes through the cornea, anterior chamber, pupil, and lens to the retina may affect the ultimate visual acuity. In addition, the retina may be affected by systemic diseases such as hypertension, arteriosclerosis, and diabetes. Poor visual acuity can, in some instances, be corrected with lenses.

The arms and hands perform essential tasks in securing and preparing foods. Motions of the wrist that are particularly necessary include flexion and extension. Necessary motions of the thumb include flexion, extension, and opposition. Good range of motion, including rotation, abduction, adduction, extension, and flexion of the shoulder and extension and flexion of the elbow, permit easy lifting and reaching for objects. The ability to locate and secure materials easily depends upon mobility. The least restrictive mobility is independent ambulation that requires adequate function of hips, knees, ankles, and feet.

Adequate functioning of the brain means adequate integration of all systems. The cerebrum stores knowledge and controls sensory and motor functions. The brainstem controls reflex activity and acts as a passageway for many of the afferent and efferent tracts.

The first three stages of eating and drinking may be accomplished by a caregiver without serious physiological consequences to the individual. The social and psychological consequences of loss of independent function, however, are significant.

The final stage of the eating process is called deglutition, or the act of swallowing. The inability or difficulty of the individual in completing this process effectively has serious consequences for physiological status. Once the food enters the oral cavity, deglutition begins. Swallowing is a complex body reflex requiring little thought or difficulty and is normally accomplished within 5 to 10 seconds.[5]

During the oral preparatory stage, food is manipulated within the oral cavity. The type of manipulation performed depends upon the consistency of the material ingested. Any material requiring mastication involves the rotary lateral movement of the tongue and mandible, using the upper and lower teeth to crush the material. The material is then collected medially on the tongue before the swallow is begun. If the food ingested is soft, it may be held on the tongue or between the tongue and hard palate. Liquids are generally pulled together and held between the tongue and anterior palate until the lingual stage begins.

The lingual or oral stage begins as the tongue moves posteriorly toward the oropharynx, squeezing the bolus of food centrally. This stage ends when the root of the tongue is forced against the posterior pharyngeal wall and the pharynx elevates to receive the bolus. This phase of the swallowing process is considered voluntary and is under the control of the fifth, seventh, and twelfth cranial nerves (Table 9-1).

The pharyngeal stage, the most complex part of swallowing, consists of moving the bolus along the pharynx while maintaining airway integrity. This process is considered reflexive; however, the reflex must be initiated voluntarily during the oral stage and does not automatically occur any time something is placed in the oral cavity.[12] When the oral stage of deglutition begins, the swallowing reflex can be triggered as the bolus touches the sensory receptors of the tongue, epiglottis, or palatoglossal arch. The impulses travel to the swallowing center in the brainstem via the glossopharyngeal nerve. The fifth, seventh, tenth, and twelfth cranial nerves carry the motor impulses that produce the swallowing reflex (Table 9-1). Once the swallowing reflex has been initiated, the following events occur: (1) closure of the pharyngeal port to prevent material from entering the nasal cavity, (2) beginning of pharyngeal peristalsis by constriction of the pharyngeal constrictors to carry the bolus past the pharynx, (3) elevation and closure of the larynx, and (4) relaxation of the cricopharyngeal sphincter to permit the bolus to enter the esophagus.

The last stage of deglutition, the esophageal phase, begins as the bolus enters the esophagus at the cricopharyngeal junction. Gravity and peri-

TABLE 9-1

Cranial nerves used for deglutition

Cranial nerve	Motor (M)/ sensory (S)	Function
V, Trigeminal	S	Maxillary, mandibular
	M	Mandibular muscles
VII, Facial	S	Taste—anterior two thirds of tongue
	M	Submandibular and sublingual salivary glands
		Facial expression
IX, Glossopharyngeal	S	Taste—posterior third of tongue Sensation of palate and uvula
	M	Stylopharyngeus muscle
X, Vagus	S	Membrane of larynx and pharynx
	M	Pharynx and larynx
XI, Spinal branch	M	Muscles: sternocleidomastoid
XII, Hypoglossal	M	Intrinsic tongue

staltic waves along the esophagus help to transport the bolus to the stomach where the esophageal phase ends.

ASSOCIATED FACTORS

Since swallowing is such a complex neuromuscular process, many factors can impair its efficiency. The factors of age and neuromuscular impairment are reviewed, and structural deficiencies that alter swallowing are outlined.

Age

Swallowing for infants begins with the sucking reflex, which is present at birth and remains throughout the first 7 months. The tongue is elevated during sucking and then thrusts the liquid to the posterior oral cavity. This movement makes the intake of solids difficult, because they are forced against the hard palate and then forced out of the mouth. By the third to fourth month, however, most infants can begin to swallow soft solid foods.

Few studies are concerned with swallowing in aged individuals. The available data suggest that changes in deglutition do not occur until the eighth decade.[2] Then reduced pharyngeal peristalsis occurs along with increased esophageal transit time.

Neuromuscular Impairment

Neuromuscular impairments usually affect multiple systems and frequently involve several stages of deglutition. The major neuromuscular impairments that can affect deglutition are summarized in Table 9-2.

Impairments in the oral preparatory stage frequently result from poor perception about the quantity and location of the food when it is in the mouth. There may be poor mastication and tongue control, resulting in inadequate chewing of food, or food may pocket in the side cavities of the mouth formed by the palatoglossal and palatopharyngeal arches.

The child with cerebral palsy may be multiply handicapped by poor deglutition, poor head and trunk control, and a lack of sitting balance. Re-

flexes that normally disappear in infancy may be present, affecting the process of eating. The risk of aspiration in these children during feeding is extremely high.[8]

The impairment most frequently seen in the lingual stage of deglutition is a delayed swallowing reflex that results in frequent aspiration as the bolus of food or liquid invades the larynx. Those persons who have had a cerebrovascular accident may exhibit lingual hemiparesis, which interferes with tongue control and preparation for swallowing. It has been shown that even the most experienced bedside observers do not identify 40% of the individuals who aspirate.[10]

Impaired pharyngeal motility results in a poorly coordinated swallowing reflex. Food then becomes lodged within the valleculae or pyriform sinuses and drains into the trachea, causing aspiration.

Frequently, neuromuscular impairments involve more than one stage of deglutition. Robbins, Logemann, and Kirshner[11] found that all of their subjects with Parkinson's disease "exhibited

TABLE 9-2
Neuromuscular diseases associated with poor deglutition

Stages of deglutition	Disease	Characteristics
Oral preparatory	Cerebral palsy	Poor suck reflex
		Inappropriate reflexive behaviors
	Parkinson's disease	Poor mastication
	Multiple sclerosis (when cranial nerve XII is involved)	Foods inadequately chewed
	Amyotrophic lateral sclerosis	Poor tongue control or mobility
	Cerebrovascular accident	
	Head trauma	
Lingual	Cerebrovascular accident	Delay in swallow reflex
	Head trauma	Choking or coughing
	Cerebral palsy	
	Parkinson's disease	
	Multiple sclerosis (when cranial nerve IX is involved)	
	Cerebrovascular accident	Lingual hemiparesis
Pharyngeal	Parkinson's disease	Impaired pharyngeal motility and peristalsis
	Poliomyelitis	
	Cerebrovascular accident	Residue remains in valleculae and pyriform sinuses
	Myasthenia gravis	
	Myotonic dystrophy	Aspiration
	Head trauma	
	Amyotrophic lateral sclerosis	

abnormal oropharyngeal movement patterns and timing during the volitional oral and pharyngeal stages of swallowing."

Difficulty with swallowing is common after a stroke.[1] Persons affected by cerebrovascular accidents and head trauma may find their difficulty with deglutition will be reversed. However those individuals with cerebral palsy, Parkinson's disease, multiple sclerosis, and amyotrophic lateral sclerosis find that swallowing and eating problems are chronic.

Anatomical Impairments

Cleft lips and cleft palates, anatomical impairments found in children, require surgical correction. A cleft lip may be only a small notch, or it may extend to the floor of the nose. Cleft palates occur alone or in conjunction with cleft lips. These abnormalities sometimes involve only the uvula or may extend through the hard and soft palate, exposing one or both nasal cavities. Until surgical repair is completed, sucking and swallowing liquids is complicated by nasal regurgitation. Inadequate nutritional intake at this rapid stage of growth and development has serious consequences and must be avoided.

The first sign of carcinoma of the esophagus is often a difficulty in swallowing. This type of cancer tends to develop quickly, and only half of those diagnosed can be considered for surgical repair.[7]

Zenker's diverticulum, an abnormal pouch arising in the pharyngeal area, results in severe dysphagia and repeated regurgitation of undigested food. The formation of the diverticulum appears to be secondary to latent relaxation of the cricopharyngeal muscle and is referred to as *achalasia*.[4] Food collects abnormally at the base of the pharynx. Surgery is usually required to correct this dysfunction.

Persons who have had radical head and neck surgery often experience poor deglutition. The severity of the eating problem depends upon the extent of the surgery.

NURSING ASSESSMENT

The nursing assessment is central in reviewing an individual's eating process and identifying specific deficits. A complete assessment, including a history of difficulties in eating, an actual review of food and fluid intake, and a physical assessment, are necessary.

Nursing History

The purpose of the nursing history is to establish the present eating patterns of the client, to describe the present difficulties, to determine areas of evaluation for the physical assessment, and to evaluate the client's need for education. The history should focus on three broad areas: (1) ability of the client to obtain and prepare food, (2) adequacy of the diet, and (3) difficulties in eating the food.

Caregivers who obtain and prepare food should be included in the history taking regarding adequacy of the diet. If the client shops for and prepares food, the following questions should be asked in the history: How do you get to the store? How frequently do you shop? What storage and preparation facilities are available to you at home? The types of foods selected by the client are frequently determined by the above variables.

Answers given to the following questions help determine the adequacy of the diet:

- How much money is available for food on a weekly basis?
- Do you eat alone regularly?
- Are meals eaten out?
- Are any meals provided and brought to the home by someone else?
- Do you take medications that may alter nutritional status?
- Has a special diet ever been recommended by your physician?
- Is there a particular type of food used (such as canned, frozen, or fresh)?
- Who prepares your food? If you prepare your own food, do you have any difficulty?
- Are there adequate utensils, safety features, and space in your home?
- Do you feed yourself? If so, do you have any difficulties or are foods modified to help you with eating or drinking?
- What is your actual food intake based on a 3-day diet history?

Economics can play an important role in the types of foods available to the client. Convenience or prepared foods may be easier, but are frequently more expensive. Fresh foods may have more nutrient value, but are more difficult to prepare and also may be more expensive. It is well established that those individuals who eat alone are more prone to poor nutrition. The nurse should be aware of what medications the client is taking and what alterations in diet need to be made. If the client has difficulty with arm and hand range of motion or coordination, dietary alterations may be made so foods can be more easily eaten. A description of the difficulty the individual has with feeding is helpful information to use when performing the physical assessment.

The next phase of the history elicits the client's ability to swallow food effectively. Factors to be considered include the following:

- Is there pain with swallowing?
- Do foods get stuck in your throat?
- Is there difficulty with swallowing solid foods?
- Do foods regurgitate nasally?
- Do you choke and cough when eating?
- Is there difficulty with swallowing liquids?
- Can you sit upright during meals without difficulty?

Obstruction of the pharynx is usually associated with pain and difficulty in swallowing solid foods, whereas a neuromuscular difficulty is associated with more difficulty in swallowing liquids and the presence of nasal regurgitation. The upright sitting position is the most efficient for eating and drinking and allows a more adequate swallow to be performed.

By the end of the history the nurse, through conversations with the client, should be able to assess the following:

- The degree to which loneliness or depression is contributing to a poor nutritional intake
- The amount of fear the person has regarding eating
- The degree to which lifelong eating habits are contributing to a poor nutritional intake
- The degree of willingness and motivation the client has to work in a rehabilitation program

It is difficult to change lifelong eating habits, and these can hamper the client's rehabilitation. However, highly motivated clients can frequently overcome these habits and conquer their fear.

Physical Assessment

The physical assessment focuses on the client's ability to obtain and prepare food, place food in the oral cavity, and swallow food. Weight is a key indicator of the degree of difficulty with eating and should be monitored closely. The physical assessment begins with examination of the head and neck and should include the following:

- Inspect the lips for color, symmetry, and moisture. Malignant lesions of the oral cavity may occur on the lip.
- Ask the client to close the lips tightly. Observe ability to perform this activity.
- Inspect the mucosa of the oral cavity. In dehydration, it will appear dry.
- Inspect the teeth for number and state of repair. Two opposing incisors and two opposing molars are needed to adequately chew.
- If there are dentures, inspect for proper fit. Remove them and inspect the gums.
- Test cranial nerve XII (hypoglossal) by inspecting the tongue for irregular movement or asymmetry, both while the tongue is in the mouth and when it is protruded.
- Test cranial nerves IX (glossopharyngeal) and X (vagus) by asking the client to say "ah." The uvula and soft palate should rise. Deviation of the uvula is found when there is paralysis. If the uvula is touched with a tongue depressor, a gag reflex should occur, indicating that motor function of the vagus nerve is intact. Although the gag reflex is closely associated with the swallowing reflex, it does not have to be present for the normal swallow to occur.[12]
- Inspect the pharynx for color, edema, and ulcerations. This observation includes the palatoglossal arch, palatopharyngeal arch, and palatine tonsils.
- Test cranial nerve V (trigeminal) for strength and symmetry by asking the client to clench the teeth. The examiner palpates the temporomandibular area to determine muscle strength during contraction. The sensory component of the nerve is tested by asking the client to identify sharp and dull sensations on the sides of the face, forehead and cheeks.
- Test cranial nerve VII (facial) by observing throughout the examination for the presence of tics and unusual movements or asymmetry of the face. Motor function is tested by the ability to clench the teeth and smile. The

sensory component of this cranial nerve is used to identify sweet (sugar), salt, sour (lemon), and bitter (aspirin) tastes.
- Test cranial nerve XI (spinal accessory) by applying pressure to the sternocleidomastoid muscle as the person shrugs the shoulders.
- If indicated, test the client for the presence of primitive reflexive behaviors. These behaviors are usually seen in infants, and when present in later life indicate a disturbance of the upper motor neuron system. These reflexes include the rooting reflex, stimulated by stroking the lips or corners of the mouth and having the client's head reflexively turn toward the stimulus; and the tonic neck reflex, sometimes called the fencing position. The tonic neck reflex is a total body pattern that occurs by turning the head to one side, resulting in extension of the extremities on the face side when the extremities on the skull side are flexed.
- Throughout the examination, evaluate the client's voice. Oral and palatal dysfunction are highlighted by dysarthria or hypernasality.[4]
- Finally, ask the client to swallow water. Can the client form a seal with the lips? How long does it take to complete the swallow? and Is a cough reflex present?

The remainder of the physical examination should focus on the client's ability to eat independently. The following areas should be assessed:
- Does the client have sufficient mobility, muscle strength, and control to lift eating utensils from plate to mouth?
- Are grip and strength sufficient to hold eating utensils?
- Does a tremor or involuntary movement interfere with coordination?
- Can the client cut food?
- Is the client limited to the use of one hand?
- What is the client's visual acuity? Is vision limited (such as hemianopsia, half visual fields)?

If the client prepares meals, include the following questions in the history:
- How is balance when standing?
- Is there any difficulty with mobility?
- Is there sufficient strength and dexterity in the arms and hands to manipulate, open, and prepare foods?
- Is there sufficient muscle strength and head control to remain upright for meals?

The nursing history and physical assessment should provide data to describe adequately the client's disability and to form the basis for the nursing diagnoses.

NURSING DIAGNOSES

Nursing diagnoses that may be used for eating and swallowing problems are (1) impaired gas exchange, (2) fluid volume deficit, (3) potential fluid volume deficit, (4) altered nutrition: less than body requirements, (5) altered nutrition: more than body requirements, and (6) knowledge deficit in proper nutrition, adaptive equipment, or availability of community resources.[6]

Nutritional status is influenced not only by physical ability to consume food, but by psychological and sociocultural factors as well. In American society, many ethnic groups define food choices differently and attach different emotional significance to food. It is important in the assessment to identify these characteristics and to realize that cultural choices may affect the client's nutritional choices. Additionally, food is frequently associated with social events and therefore has significant psychological meaning. Traditional foods for holidays are a good example. As one ages or becomes ill, the lack of significant interactions at meals or lack of other significant social interactions can significantly reduce nutritional intake.

Physical impairments that reduce the ability to swallow effectively can result in aspiration of food or fluids. The client frequently becomes frustrated and disappointed and reduces nutritional intake further. Clients with a neuromuscular disorder are particularly susceptible to aspiration.

In those clients with other physical disabilities contributing to reduced activity, a potential increase in nutritional intake above requirements may result in obesity. When other physical activity is reduced, eating frequently becomes an important daily activity. Unfortunately, a significant increase in calories leads to obesity and hampers an active rehabilitation program.

Finally, clients may have an inadequate nutritional intake because of a knowledge deficit. They may be unaware of what nutrients compose an adequate diet, what adaptive equipment is available for use, or what community resources are available.

GOALS

Goals established by the nurse and client should relate to the specific diagnoses and be based on information obtained from the client during the nursing assessment. Impaired gas exchange may result because of a poor swallowing reflex, in which case the nurse should decrease the episodes of aspiration and choking by improving the swallowing process. A potential or actual deficiency of fluid volume means increasing liquid intake either through alternate forms or by more frequent feedings. Liquids are usually the most difficult food for someone with an inadequate swallowing process. As a result, the client may have a great deal of fear when taking liquids. It is important to ensure that everything is done to maximize the swallowing process and to provide encouragement when the client is taking liquids. An inadequate caloric intake, particularly of solid foods, necessitates alternate and more frequent feedings. If the poor intake is a result of depression, the underlying problem must be addressed. A complete diet history that includes food preferences and the significance of food to the client should be completed to find foods the client might eat. If the client is consuming too many calories, the goal is to reduce caloric intake by substituting reduced-calorie foods. Frequently it is necessary to look for meaningful activities that the client can use to substitute for time previously spent in eating.

The goals then for the client experiencing difficulty with eating and swallowing may include all or some of the following:

1. To improve or maintain gas exchange
2. To improve or maintain fluid volume
3. To maintain adequate nutrition
4. To teach the client and family:
   a. Measures to prevent and alleviate choking
   b. Proper nutrition
   c. Use of adaptive equipment
   d. Availability of community resources to assist in promoting adequate nutrition

REHABILITATION NURSING INTERVENTIONS

Once an assessment is completed, nursing diagnoses formulated, and goals established, specific nursing interventions must be considered. If the primary difficulty is a neuromuscular swallowing disorder, interventions are directed to improving the swallowing process. Steps to improve the swallowing process are as follows:

- Begin by placing the client in an upright sitting position with the head bent slightly forward. The forward tilt of the head is important to prevent food from hitting the posterior pharyngeal wall before the swallow reflex begins.
- If the client has poor head control and the head falls forward, hold the head up by using the palm of your hand against the client's forehead.
- Sit down when assisting the client with eating. This action communicates time and willingness to help.
- Initially use small amounts of soft food that are easy to swallow (applesauce, purees).
- Place half a teaspoonful on the middle to back part of the tongue. However, if the client has tongue or facial paralysis or has had a partial laryngectomy, the correct placement is on the strong intact side, not midline.
- With the spoon, push on the tongue as you remove the food from the spoon.
- If swallowing does not occur, remove the spoon from the client's mouth.
- Instruct the client to move the food around and toward the rear of the mouth.
- If the swallow comes slowly, press on the tip of the client's head with the palm of your hand. This action will decrease laryngeal tension and facilitate swallowing.[3]
- Check to see that the client's lips are sealed or the swallowing reflex will not begin. Manually seal the lips together or use a jaw-control maneuver to pull the jaws together (Figure 9-3).
- If swallowing does not occur, try placing your thumb on the client's chin, moving the chin downward toward the sternum to facilitate the swallow.[3]

The client with a neuromuscular disorder has more difficulty with liquids than soft foods. The

Jaw control from front
  Thumb on chin
  Index finger on jaw bone
  Middle finger under chin

Jaw control from side
  Thumb on jaw bone
  Index finger on chin
  Middle finger under chin

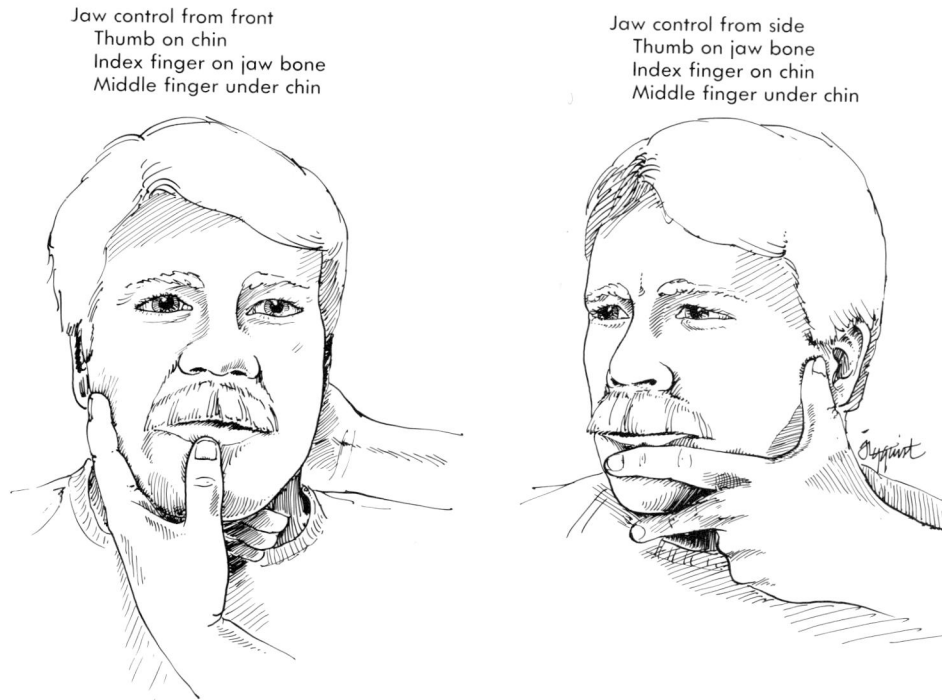

Figure 9-3
Jaw control from front (**A**) and side (**B**).

difficulty appears to be a lack of tongue control and coordination to form the liquids into a bolus. In these cases, liquids may first be placed on a spoon and put posteriorly on the tongue. If this procedure does not give the client any difficulty, try using a syringe and placing small amounts of liquids posteriorly. A straw usually requires the complex functioning of the oral musculature and as a result is less useful for these clients. If the client can drink from a cup, remember that when the glass is less than half full, it becomes necessary to tilt the head back to drink. This position increases the risk of aspiration and should be avoided. Specially designed cups should be used (Figure 9-4).

Choking, a protective device for the airway, is expected to occur in individuals with swallowing difficulties and is frightening to the client. If the coughing and choking can be minimized, fear and anxiety associated with feeding will be decreased. When coughing or choking begins, the nurse

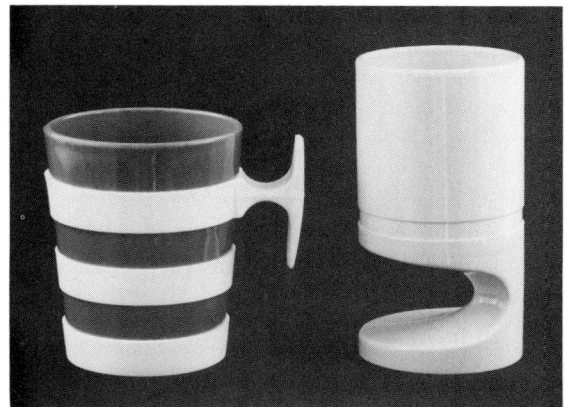

Figure 9-4
Specially designed cups.

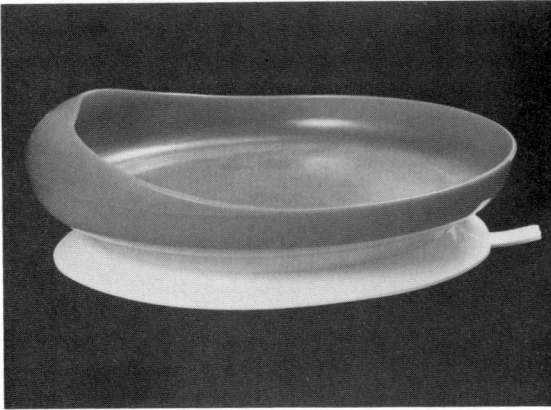

Figure 9-5
Scoop dishes.

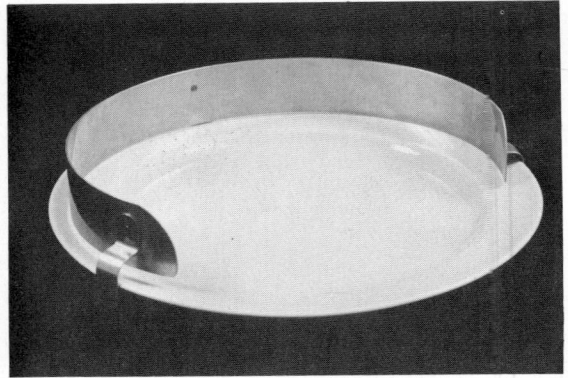

Figure 9-6
Plate guards.

should instruct the client to flex at the waist or neck if possible. Waist or neck flexion assists in more efficient airway clearance. If food becomes lodged in the larynx and compromises breathing, sharp blows between the shoulders are administered. If this action is ineffective, the Heimlich maneuver should be used.

Milk and milk products should be avoided, since these tend to form tenacious secretions that are poorly handled. If the client can chew, a textured food may be more desirable. Above all, the nurse should encourage the client and family to keep the diet flexible and reevaluate it often to avoid monotony.

For the client who has difficulty eating independently, the nurse should work closely with occupational and physical therapists in muscle strengthening, coordination, and use of adaptive equipment. The nurse's role is to understand the use of the equipment and to encourage the client to use the equipment properly and participate in therapy. Examples of adaptive equipment include scoop dishes (Figure 9-5) and plate guards (Figure 9-6). Silverware can be modified so that it is held more effectively (Figure 9-7).

In addition to understanding the exact nature of the eating problem, the client and family need to be involved in establishing goals and planning care. Without total cooperation, rehabilitation will be ineffective. The nurse is essential in pro-

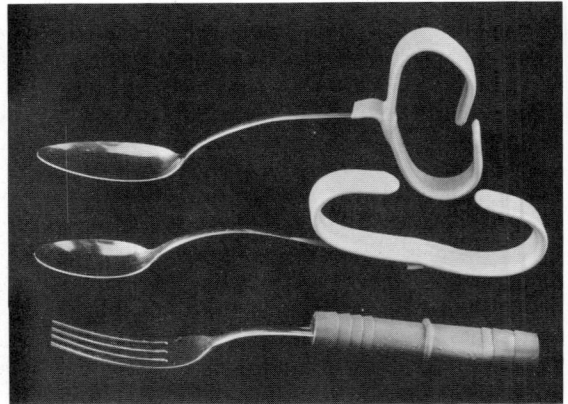

Figure 9-7
Adapted silverware.

moting good communication with the family. In between care plan meetings, the nurse acts as advocate for the family, explains new treatment approaches, and reports progress. The client and family should demonstrate knowledge of dietary modifications, use of adaptive equipment if needed, the process for feeding, and use of emergency measures in case of coughing and choking.

In the case of excessive caloric intake, it is particularly necessary to work with the family and client. For this client, food is frequently substituted for other activities or reinforcements. Family may bring food to the client because it brings pleasure. The nurse should work with the client and family to develop long-term goals for rehabilitation and help the client to see the result of overeating.

REHABILITATION TEAM INTERVENTIONS

Because of the complex nature of eating difficulties, the nurse should use other rehabilitation team professionals in the treatment. As noted earlier, physical therapy helps improve muscle tone, strength, and coordination. Treatment is directed at improving muscle tone for the primary eating muscles, as well as secondary muscles of arms, legs, head, and neck. The occupational therapist should take an active role in the use of adaptive equipment, exercises to improve hand control and coordination, and assistance in food preparation. The therapist also helps find meaningful activity for the client to engage in during the day as a substitute for eating. A planned program for exercise of the oropharyngeal musculature can be carried out through the speech therapist. The dietitian can help develop a menu plan that is adequate and teach proper diet to the client and family. It is the nurse's responsibility to be aware of each therapist's expertise and refer clients appropriately after consulting with other members of the team.

OUTCOME CRITERIA

For the client with a progressive neuromuscular disorder, maintaining the maximum level of independence in eating and maintaining adequate nutritional intake are realistic goals. Clients with neuromuscular insults, such as cerebrovascular accident or head trauma, may anticipate a return to normal function after an active rehabilitative period, but this depends on the extent of the injury. Three months appears to be the critical period in which maximum return of function can be anticipated.[10]

Measurable outcome criteria that can be used to evaluate treatment results follow:

1. Client maintains adequate gas exchange.
2. Client manipulates utensils for independent eating.
3. Client cuts and prepares foods to be eaten.
4. Client chews without difficulty.
5. Client swallows soft foods without difficulty.
6. Client drinks liquids without difficulty.
7. Client maintains adequate body weight.
8. Client and family describe emergency measures for choking.
9. Client and family describe nutritional requirements.
10. Client and family use adaptive equipment as appropriate.
11. Client and family know of community resources to assist in the provision of adequate nutrition.

For the client who has caloric intake above requirements, the major goal of the treatment program is to reduce caloric intake. Measurable outcome criteria used to evaluate treatment results follow:

1. The client and family describe nutritional requirements.
2. The client and family describe the emotional significance of food to the client.
3. The client consumes the appropriate amount of calories for the physical condition.

SUMMARY

Eating and swallowing are essential to an individual's survival physiologically. Psychologically, food and eating are important to feelings of self-worth and community. When one can no longer eat without difficulty, fear is frequently an over-riding emotional reaction. It includes not only fear for one's survival and ability to function, but fear or actual loss of significant social interactions. For persons with significant physical disability, excessive food consumption is an emotional response to the loss of function and the decreased need of the body for calories. The nurse is crucial in assisting these individuals and their families, and may be the first health care professional to realize that there is an eating problem. The nurse has the ability to draw in other rehabilitation team members. Patience, understanding, and ability to teach the client and family about this aspect of rehabilitation have many positive rewards and outcomes for the client, family, and nurse.

TEST QUESTIONS

1. All of the following are primary anatomical structures involved in the eating process *except* the:
   a. Pharynx
   b. Oral cavity
   c. Trachea
   d. Larynx

2. Which of the seven stages for normal eating and swallowing occurs when the bolus of food is centrally located and pushed posteriorly toward the oropharynx?
   a. Lingual stage
   b. Pharyngeal stage
   c. Oral preparatory phase
   d. Esophageal phase

3. Which of the following groups contains the cranial nerves used in deglutition?
   a. III, V, VII, X, XI, XII
   b. V, VII, IX, X, XI, XII
   c. I, III, V, VI, VII, X
   d. I, III, VII, IX, X, XII

4. Which one of the following neuromuscular disorders is *not* associated with difficulty in pharyngeal deglutition?
   a. Parkinson's disease
   b. Cerebrovascular accident
   c. Cerebral palsy
   d. Head trauma

5. Mr. C is a 69-year-old man who had a cerebrovascular accident. He ambulates infrequently and spends most of his time watching television. In the 6 months since the cerebrovascular accident, he has gained 20 pounds. Of the following nursing diagnoses for clients with eating and swallowing problems, which *one* would be *most* appropriate?
   a. Nutrition, alteration in, less than body requirements
   b. Nutrition, alteration in, more than body requirements
   c. Fluid volume deficit, actual
   d. Fluid volume deficit, potential

6. Which *one* of the following rehabilitation nursing interventions is appropriate for improving the swallowing process in the client with a neuromuscular swallowing disorder?
   a. Place client in upright sitting position with head bent slightly backward.
   b. Stand up when assisting the client to eat.
   c. Initially use large amounts of food that are easy to swallow.
   d. Instruct the client to move food around and toward the rear of the mouth.

7. Outcome criteria that can be used to evaluate treatment for the client and family affected by an eating and swallowing disorder include all of the following *except:*
   a. The client drinks liquids without difficulty.
   b. The client ambulates the distance of the hallway twice daily.
   c. The client and family describe nutritional requirements.
   d. The client manipulates utensils for independent eating.

Answers: 1. c, 2. a, 3. b, 4. c, 5. b, 6. d, 7. b.

LEARNING ACTIVITIES

1. Prepare and eat a meal with one arm immobilized. Have a friend feed you your dinner.
2. Try to complete your food shopping from a wheelchair.
3. As you eat, pay particular attention to how you chew your food and how you swallow.

REFERENCES

1. Axelsson K, Norberg A, and Asplund K: Relearning to eat late after a stroke by systematic nursing intervention: a case report, J Adv Nurs 11:553, 1986.
2. Blonsky E and others: Comparison of speech and swallowing function in patients with tremor disorders and in normal geriatric patients: a cinefluorographic study, J Gerontol 30(3):299, 1975.
3. Buckley J, Addicks C, and Maniglia J: Feeding patients with dysphagia, Nurs Forum 15(1):69, 1975.
4. Dobie R: Rehabilitation of swallowing disorders, Am Fam Phys 17:84, May 1978.
5. Fisher S, Painter M, and Melmoe G: Swallowing disorders in infancy, Ped Clin North Am 28(4):845, 1981.
6. Gordon M: Nursing diagnosis: process and application, New York, 1987, McGraw-Hill Book Co.
7. Griffin J and Tollison J: Dysphagia, Am Fam Phys 22:154, Nov 1980.
8. Helfrich-Miller KRK, Rector KL, and Straka JA: Dysphagia: its treatment in the profoundly retarded patient with cerebral palsy, Arch Phys Med Rehabil 67:520, Aug 1986.
9. Leopold N and Kage M: Swallowing, ingestion, and dysphagia: a reappraisal, Arch Phys Med Rehabil 64:372, Aug 1983.

10. Logemann J: Evaluation and treatment of swallowing disorders, San Diego, 1983, College Hill Press, Inc.
11. Robbins JA, Logemann JA, and Kirshner HS: Swallowing and speech production in Parkinson's disease, Ann Neurol 19:283, March 1986.
12. Roueche J: Dysphagia: an assessment and management program for the adult, Minneapolis, 1980, Sister Kenny Institute.
13. Wolanin M and Phillips L: Confusion: prevention and care, St Louis, 1983, The CV Mosby Co.

ADDITIONAL READINGS

Griffin CW and Lockhart JS: Learning to swallow again, Am J Nurs 87:314, March 1987.
Linden P and Siebens A: Dysphagia: predicting laryngeal penetration, Arch Phys Med Rehabil 64:281, June 1983.
Zimmerman JE and others: Swallowing dysfunction in acutely ill patients, Phys Ther 61:1755, Dec 1981.

CHAPTER 10

Bladder Elimination

Sharon S. Dittmar

OBJECTIVES

After completing Chapter 10, the reader will be able to:

1. Explain the anatomy and physiology of normal bladder function.

2. Identify the location and causes of lesions that interrupt the neural pathways to the bladder.

3. Describe the complications associated with neurogenic bladder dysfunction.

4. Conduct a nursing assessment specific to a client with impaired bladder function, including collection of subjective and objective data.

5. Identify the diagnostic studies commonly used for clients with impaired bladder function.

6. Formulate nursing diagnoses for the client with impaired bladder function.

7. Develop rehabilitation goals with the client with impaired bladder function.

8. Determine the possible nursing interventions for the client with difficulty emptying urine from the bladder.

9. Determine the possible nursing interventions for the client with difficulty storing urine in the bladder.

10. Specify the nursing interventions for the prevention and treatment of autonomic hyperreflexia.

11. Give the category, dosage, action, therapeutic use, and nursing implications of pharmacological agents ordered to manage clients with lower urinary tract dysfunction.

12. Determine the possible nursing interventions for the client who has a urinary diversion procedure performed.

13. Identify the indications for transurethral procedures, implantation of artificial sphincters, and implantation of electrodes.

14. List the information and skills needed by the client and family to assume responsibility for the bladder rehabilitation program.

15. Relate the discharge planning process to rehabilitation of the client with impaired bladder function.

16. Explain the contributions of rehabilitation team members in rehabilitation of the client with impaired bladder function.

17. List the outcome criteria used as a basis for evaluation of the client's response to a bladder rehabilitation program.

The person with impaired bladder function faces many physical, social, and psychological impediments to performing activities of everyday living. Impairment of bladder function resulting in involuntary control interferes with a person's physical, mental, and social well-being. The bladder performs a basic physiological function by storing and emptying urine from the body. Disease and trauma can seriously affect the bladder's ability to perform this function. The inability to eliminate or store urine can ultimately threaten a person's life if the kidneys become damaged.

Involuntary urination is expected and tolerated in infants and small children. The adult, however, is expected to maintain control over this body function. In addition to the destructive effect on self-esteem and restrictive effect on performance of social roles, the person with impaired bladder function must face and deal with many physical and social inconveniences in daily living. Skin irritation, the constant need to change clothing or carry additional clothing, restriction in social activities and a decrease in leisure activities involving others, interrupted sleep, interruption of the sleep of others involved in care, difficulties in competitive employment, and difficulties with intimate relationships are just some of the problems faced.[6] Moreover, the physical and mental energy required to anticipate and "clean up" after incontinence episodes consumes time needed for other more productive pursuits. Additional time and money are required for laundry and become another source of frustration for the affected individual or primary caretaker. As a result, the individual's total life-style may revolve around the bladder and bladder management.

Fortunately, within the last decade, major advances have been made in the diagnosis and treatment of impaired bladder function. In the rehabilitation practice setting, the major problems seen are the result of interruption of nerve supply to this organ and anatomical changes that impede urine flow.

NORMAL BLADDER FUNCTION

The complex function of the physiologically normal bladder depends upon neuroanatomical integrity and coordination. Structures responsible for the transport and elimination of urine from the kidneys include the ureters, bladder, and urethra. Muscles lining and supporting the urinary tract facilitate and inhibit urine flow. Urinary elimination is controlled by neural pathways in the brain, spinal cord, and spinal reflex arc.

Anatomy

The bladder serves as a reservoir. This hollow, muscular organ can store 350 to 450 ml of urine. When empty, it lies behind the pubic symphysis. Smooth muscle (detrusor) lines the bladder. This muscle is continuous with and lines the urethra, allowing the bladder and urethra to function as one unit. Contraction of the detrusor forces urine from the bladder; relaxation of the detrusor permits storage of urine within the bladder.

The two ureters drain urine from the kidneys to the bladder. These tubes lie retroperitoneally and enter the posterior surface of the bladder through an oblique tunnel that functions as a valve to prevent backflow of urine when the detrusor contracts.[2]

The urethra is a small tube located behind the symphysis pubis. It is anterior to the vagina in females and extends through the prostate gland, fibrous sheet, and penis in males. The female urethra serves only the urinary tract, whereas the male urethra serves both the urinary and reproductive tract, also functioning to eliminate semen from the body.[2]

Muscles used to assist in urination include the internal sphincter, the external sphincter, and the pelvic diaphragm. The internal sphincter, or bladder neck, is not a true sphincter but a thickening formed by interlaced and converging muscle fibers of the detrusor as they pass distally to become the smooth musculature of the urethra.[40] The external sphincter is composed of striated skeletal muscle and can be voluntarily relaxed and contracted. Pelvic floor muscles support the bladder and relax and descend as urine is expelled from the body.

The bladder and sphincters are under the control of the autonomic nervous system. Both parasympathetic and sympathetic fibers flow to and from major integrating systems in the spinal cord.[11] Suprasacral centers inhibit and facilitate micturition by permitting voluntary contraction and relaxation of the external sphincter and pelvic musculature (Figure 10-1).[18]

Sacral innervation

Sympathetic afferent fibers are believed to travel from the detrusor muscle of the bladder to the T9 to L2 segments of the spinal cord. Pain and proprioceptive sensation are believed to be transmitted along this pathway. Sympathetic efferent fibers proceed via the anterior nerve roots T11 to L2 of the spinal cord and through the sympathetic ganglia to the hypogastric plexus to innervate the detrusor muscle and internal sphincter.

Parasympathetic afferent fibers travel via the pudendal nerve to the S2 to S4 spinal nerve roots to convey pain, touch, temperature, and muscle stretch sensation from the bladder and internal sphincter. Parasympathetic efferent fibers travel from S2 to S4 spinal nerve roots to innervate the

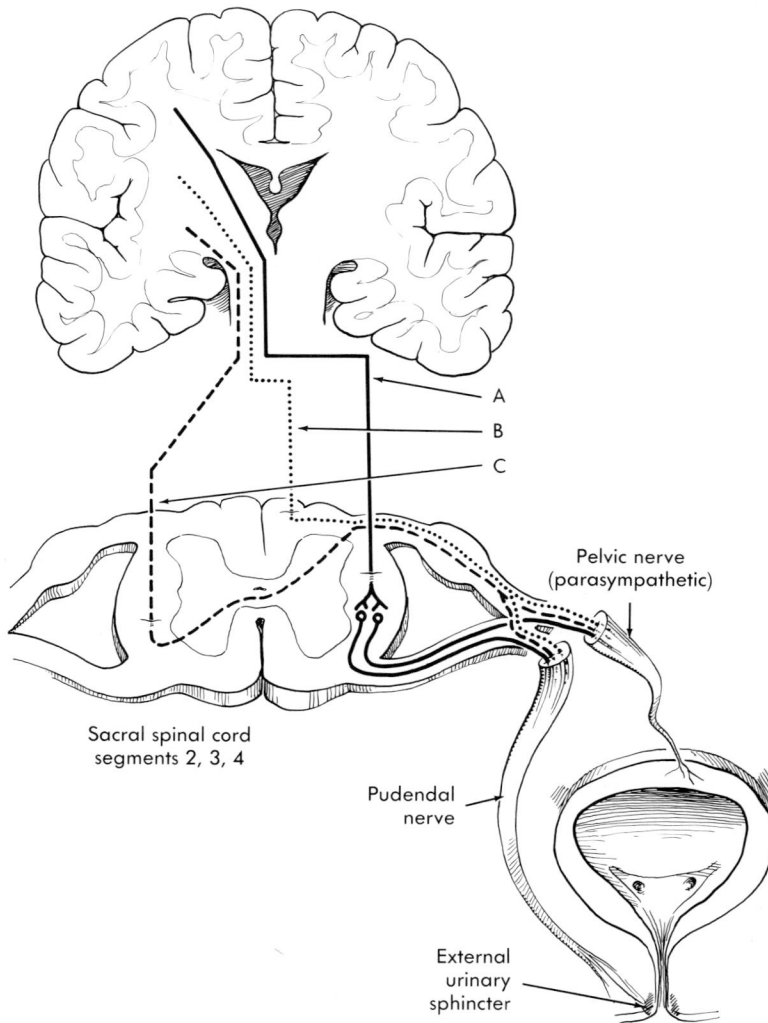

Figure 10-1
Neural pathways involved in control of bladder function. *A*, Cortical regulatory tract (voluntary control); *B*, Dorsal column tract (filling and distention); *C*, Lateral spinothalamic tract (pain and temperature). *(From Johnson JH: Nurs Clin North Am 15:295, 1980.)*

detrusor muscle and internal sphincter. The action of these fibers is mainly upon the detrusor muscle, permitting contraction.[9] This spinal reflex arc is referred to as the *micturition reflex* and operates without higher control in infancy, unconsciousness, and certain lesions of the central nervous system.[18]

The external sphincter and perineal musculature are innervated by pudendal nerve fibers that pass from S2 to S4 segments of the spinal cord. Afferent fibers within the pudendal nerve transmit sensation from the external sphincter and the posterior urethra.[11]

Suprasacral innervation

Suprasacral pathways allow for voluntary control of urination. Afferent impulses are sent from the spinal cord via the spinothalamic tracts and posterior columns to centers in the midbrain. Efferent impulses travel from these centers via the corticoregulatory tract to contract the external sphincter and directly inhibit the parasympathetic reflex, thus preventing micturition. When voiding occurs, centers in the brain send impulses via the corticoregulatory tract to allow for complete relaxation of the external sphincter and pelvic floor musculature.[18]

Physiology of Micturition

Voluntary relaxation of the external sphincter and pelvic floor musculature is necessary to initiate voiding. The normal tone of the pelvic diaphragm, including the levator and sphincter urethrae and the bulbocavernosus muscle (in the male), facilitates urinary continence. When a person begins to void, the posterior diaphragm progressively descends and the posterior urethra fills. When the diaphragm reaches its lowest level, a wavelike contraction of the detrusor muscle occurs and continues until the bladder is emptied. If a person voluntarily contracts the external sphincter, the urethral stream ceases and the pelvic diaphragm rapidly returns to a higher position, elevating the bladder. In the female, the distal urethra empties immediately; in the male, the bulbourethral muscle contracts to immediately empty the distal urethra.

A relatively constant intravesical pressure is maintained by the detrusor muscle through variation in muscle tone, despite varying urine volumes. The first sensation of bladder filling is usually felt when the bladder contains approximately 100 ml of urine. When the bladder contains 300 to 400 ml of urine, the desire to void is felt. When intravesical pressure reaches a very high level, the suprasacral inhibition may be involuntarily overcome. After voiding occurs, voluntary contraction of the ischiocavernosus and bulbocavernosus muscles closes off the bladder. Strong voluntary contractions of these muscles must occur to interrupt the urinary stream.[11]

IMPAIRED BLADDER FUNCTION

Interference with the neuroanatomical integrity of any part of the lower urinary tract can seriously affect the ability of the bladder to store and eliminate urine. Neurogenic bladder dysfunction is the most common form of bladder impairment seen in rehabilitation practice. Depending upon the level and extent of the neurological lesion, clients may experience difficulty with voluntary retention or expulsion. Immediately following damage to the spinal cord, the person affected experiences *spinal shock*, a temporary condition of flaccid paralysis and loss of all reflex activity below the level of the lesion.

Spinal Shock

The signs of spinal shock resemble the signs of autonomous neurogenic bladder. Complete anesthesia and flaccid paralysis are present below the level of the lesion, regardless of the site of damage. The bladder, innervated at the lower level of the spinal cord, demonstrates similar characteristics. Reflexes are absent; perception of fullness, pain, and temperature is absent; and the bladder fills to overflowing.[40] The cystometrogram shows a very large bladder capacity, absence of detrusor contractions, and low intravesical pressure. Spinal shock may last from a period of a few weeks to 6 months or more but usually resolves in 2 to 3 months. Signs of resolution vary according to the level of the lesion and the type of neurogenic bladder.

The variations in recovery time from spinal shock make it particularly difficult for the client and the rehabilitation nurse to establish specific goals and interventions for bladder retraining. The client should be aware that symptoms, prob-

Classification of Neurogenic Bladders

Neurological	Sensory, motor, sensory-motor
	Complete, incomplete
	Sacral, suprasacral (cord, brainstem, cerebrum)
Clinical	Asymptomatic, symptomatic
	Balanced, unbalanced (significant residual)
Radiological	Normal, abnormal upper tracts
	Normal, abnormal cystourethogram
Urodynamic	Bladder dysfunction (normal, hyperreflexic, areflexic)
	Urethral dysfunction (normal, hyperactive, inactive)

From Raz S and Bradley W: Neuromuscular dysfunction of the lower urinary tract. In Harrison JH and others, editors: Campbell's urology, ed 4, vol 2, Philadelphia, 1978, WB Saunders Co.

lems, and interventions will change as the specific neurological bladder dysfunction is determined.

Classification of Neurogenic Bladders

Despite numerous attempts at classification of neurogenic bladder dysfunction,[4,23] a categorical system that fully describes the problems encountered by the client and provides a blueprint for treatment strategies has been elusive. Attempts have been made to describe bladder status in terms of a neurological, clinical, radiological, and urodynamic view of neurogenic bladder dysfunction. (See box.) This classification system includes a reference to urethral dysfunction that many earlier systems did not. In addition, it emphasizes the need for a thorough diagnostic evaluation.[36]

Lapides and Diokno[23] classified neurogenic bladders into five groups to help pinpoint the underlying pathological process: (1) reflex, (2) autonomous, (3) uninhibited, (4) sensory paralytic, and (5) motor paralytic neurogenic bladders. Most neurogenic bladders represent a combined motor and sensory impairment. For ease of description, the types of neurogenic bladder are described here according to the schema proposed by Lapides and Diokno.

Reflex neurogenic bladder

The *reflex neurogenic bladder* also is referred to as an upper motor neuron, suprasacral, spastic, and central neurogenic bladder. This dysfunction occurs when both the sensory and motor tracts (posterior columns, spinothalamic tracts, and corticoregulatory tracts) of the spinal cord that send messages between the bladder and the supraspinal center are disrupted. Figure 10-2 demonstrates where damage may occur and lists the causes of this dysfunction.[23]

Voiding is involuntary because of the lack of cerebral control and also is incomplete because of bladder spasticity. The reflex arc remains intact and can be stimulated by various facilitory techniques in bladder retraining programs to trigger spontaneous voiding. The bulbocavernosus reflex is present and increased. A cystometrogram shows uninhibited contractions with decreased bladder capacity. The detrusor muscle frequently hypertrophies, leading to vesicoureteral reflux, hydronephrosis, and permanent renal damage because of obstruction of the valvelike ureteral mechanism. In addition, the external sphincter and perineal muscles become spastic, resulting in increased resistance to urine outflow and a large residual urine volume.[27]

The client is unable to sense fullness, pain, or temperature and is unable to void volitionally. Therefore micturition cannot be started or stopped in the normal manner. If the urethral sphincter and external urinary sphincter are coordinated, spontaneous voiding will occur when the micturition reflex arc is stimulated. If the two events are uncoordinated, however, pressure within the bladder wall will increase as the detrusor attempts to contract against the contracted external urinary sphincter. The resulting dysfunction is termed *detrusor sphincter dyssynergia*. The force and size of the urinary stream will decrease, and large amounts of residual urine will remain in the bladder.[35]

Autonomous neurogenic bladder

The *autonomous neurogenic bladder* also is referred to as a lower motor neuron, flaccid, atonic, sacral, and peripheral bladder. It is difficult to determine when spinal shock subsides when the client has an autonomous neurogenic bladder, because the characteristics are similar. Damage occurs to the cauda equina (lesions involving the reflex arc), disrupting pathways that carry sensory impulses from the bladder to the cord, motor impulses from the spinal cord to the detrusor muscle, and motor impulses from the spinal cord to the external sphincter. Figure 10-3 illustrates areas where damage may occur and lists the causes of this dysfunction.[23]

Voiding is involuntary and occurs when the bladder overflows. Peripheral reflexes and the

bulbocavernosus reflex are absent or hypoactive. Sensation and motor control also are absent. The cystometrogram demonstrates the absence of uninhibited contractions, a bladder capacity above normal (600 to 1,000 ml), and decreased intravesical pressure. Residual urine is present.[18]

The client cannot sense fullness, pain, or temperature; cannot void volitionally; and therefore cannot start or stop voiding in a normal manner.

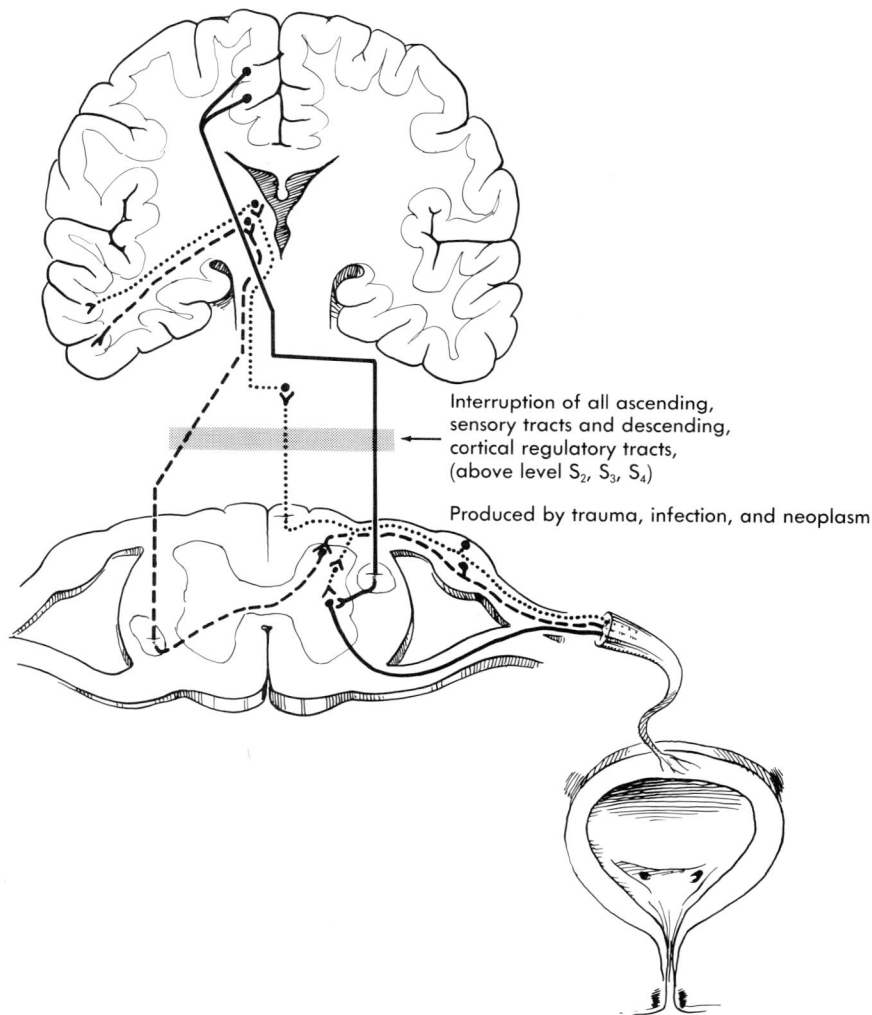

Interruption of all ascending, sensory tracts and descending, cortical regulatory tracts, (above level S_2, S_3, S_4)

Produced by trauma, infection, and neoplasm

Figure 10-2
Reflex neurogenic bladder can be produced by complete transection of spinal cord above sacral level. *(From Lapides J and Diokno AC: Urine transport, storage, and micturition. In Lapides J, editor: Fundamentals of urology, Philadelphia, 1976, WB Saunders Co.)*

The bladder can be partially emptied with manual pressure and straining. Two patterns of external sphincter activity may occur: (1) no motor activity and (2) some uncontrollable activity. In the former pattern, the client can void while maintaining low intravesical pressure. In both patterns, the amount of residual urine depends upon how well the individual can expel urine by applying pressure, the tone of smooth muscle and elasticity of the bladder wall, and the amount of muscle re-sistance offered by the internal and external urinary sphincters.[35]

Uninhibited neurogenic bladder

The *uninhibited neurogenic bladder* results from a disruption of the corticoregulatory tract or a malfunction of the supraspinal center that regulates voiding. Figure 10-4 shows areas of the nervous system where damage may occur and lists the causes of this dysfunction.[23]

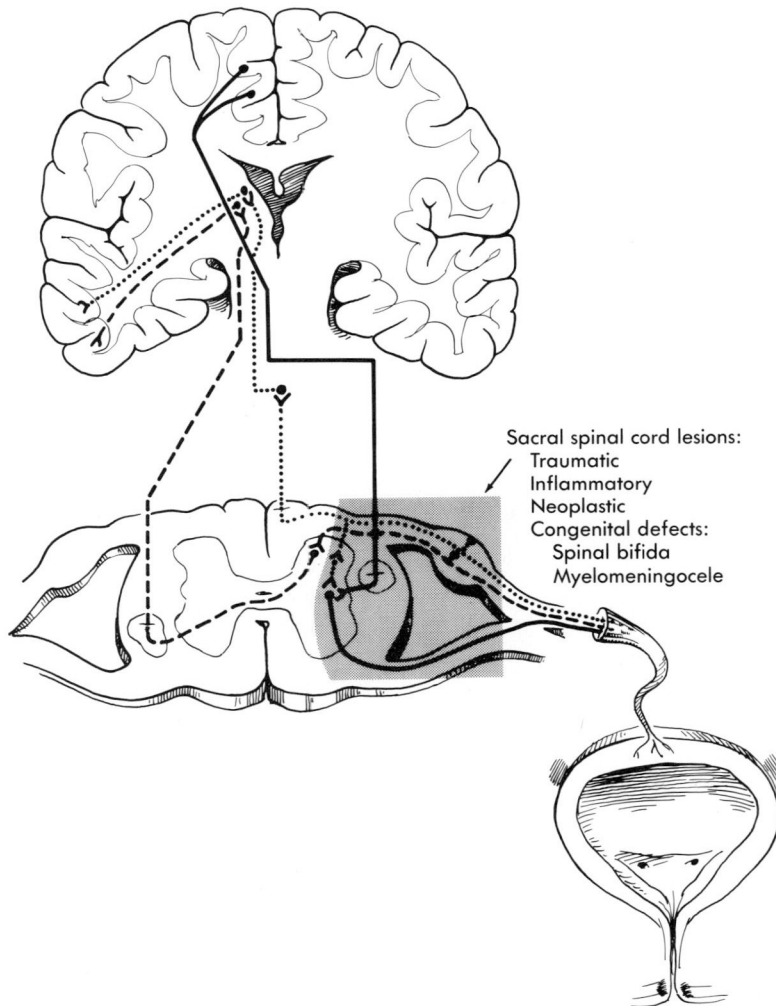

Sacral spinal cord lesions:
Traumatic
Inflammatory
Neoplastic
Congenital defects:
Spinal bifida
Myelomeningocele

Figure 10-3
Autonomous neurogenic bladder is produced by lesion involving both limbs of reflex arc.
(From Lapides J and Diokno AC: Urine transport, storage, and micturition. In Lapides J, editor: Fundamentals of urology, Philadelphia, 1976, WB Saunders Co.)

Frequent uninhibited contractions occur, but the bladder usually empties completely, resulting in no residual urine. The micturition reflex remains intact. Sensation is present as is the bulbocavernosus reflex. A cystometrogram will demonstrate strong, uninhibited contractions as the bladder is filled. The capacity of the bladder is decreased and involuntary voiding will take place long before "normal" capacity is reached.[40]

Clients with uninhibited neurogenic bladder frequently complain about the urgency and frequency of urination and nocturia. They can initiate micturition but cannot inhibit flow. When the external sphincter is voluntarily contracted, partial control of urination, even with strong voiding contractions, is possible. The intravesical pressure, however, remains high because of the force of detrusor contractions.[35] Perkash[33] indi-

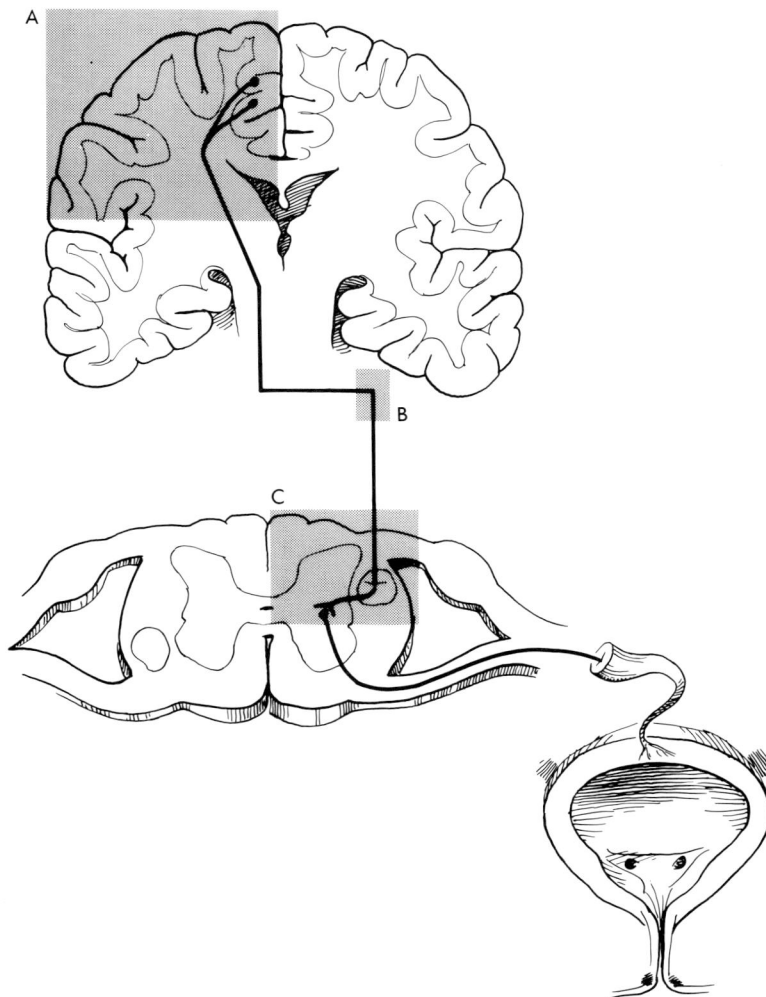

Figure 10-4
Uninhibited neurogenic bladder can be produced by lesion anywhere along corticoregulatory tract. *A*, Cerebrovascular accidents, cerebral palsy, luetic palsy, enuresis. *B*, Multiple sclerosis, complication of cordotomy. *C*, Spina bifida (occasionally), myelomeningocele. *(From Lapides J and Diokno AC: Urine transport, storage, and micturition. In Lapides J, editor: Fundamentals of urology, Philadelphia, 1976, WB Saunders Co.)*

cates these clients may be able to avoid incontinence by voiding before the bladder is full enough to trigger the micturition reflex. Therefore an important part of nursing intervention is scheduled voiding and attention to fluid intake.

Sensory paralytic bladder

The *sensory paralytic bladder* occurs when the afferent or sensory side of the micturition reflex arc is damaged. Figure 10-5 shows where dam-

age occurs and lists the causes of this dysfunction.[23]

The client can volitionally void, but the sensation of bladder fullness is absent. The cystometrogram demonstrates the absence of uninhibited contractions with an increased bladder capacity. The presence of residual urine is variable as is the presence of the bulbocavernosus reflex and perineal sensation.[18]

The client senses no fullness, pain, or tem-

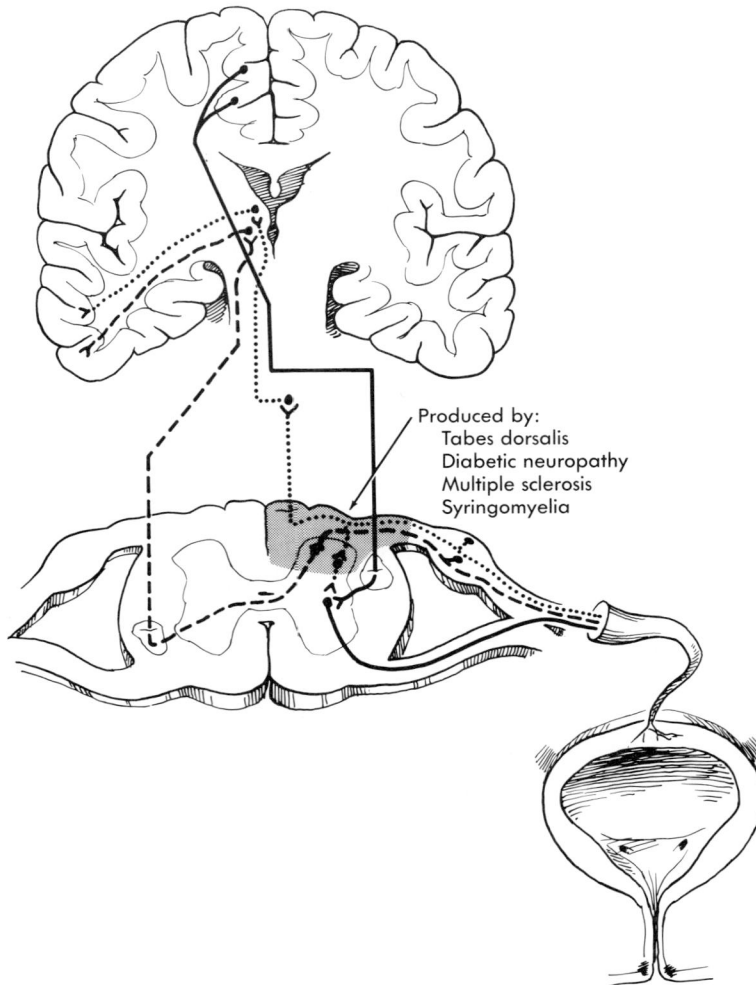

Produced by:
Tabes dorsalis
Diabetic neuropathy
Multiple sclerosis
Syringomyelia

Figure 10-5
Any process that interrupts sensory limb of lower reflex arc or long afferent tracts to brain may give rise to sensory paralytic bladder. *(From Lapides J and Diokno AC: Urine transport, storage, and micturition. In Lapides J, editor: Fundamentals of urology, Philadelphia, 1976, WB Saunders Co.)*

perature but is able to initiate voiding unless the bladder has become markedly atonic because of prolonged periods of overdistention. A loss of bladder wall tone may develop because of the large volumes of urine that collect in the bladder between voids.

Motor paralytic bladder

The *motor paralytic bladder* occurs when the efferent or motor side of the micturition reflex arc

is damaged. Figure 10-6 demonstrates areas where damage may occur and lists the causes of this dysfunction.[23]

Voluntary control of urination is variable and sensation is normal. The bulbocavernosus reflex is absent. The cystometrogram demonstrates no uninhibited contractions with increased bladder capacity. Residual urine is markedly increased.[18]

Since sensory nerves are still intact, the client will sense fullness, pain, and temperature. Motor

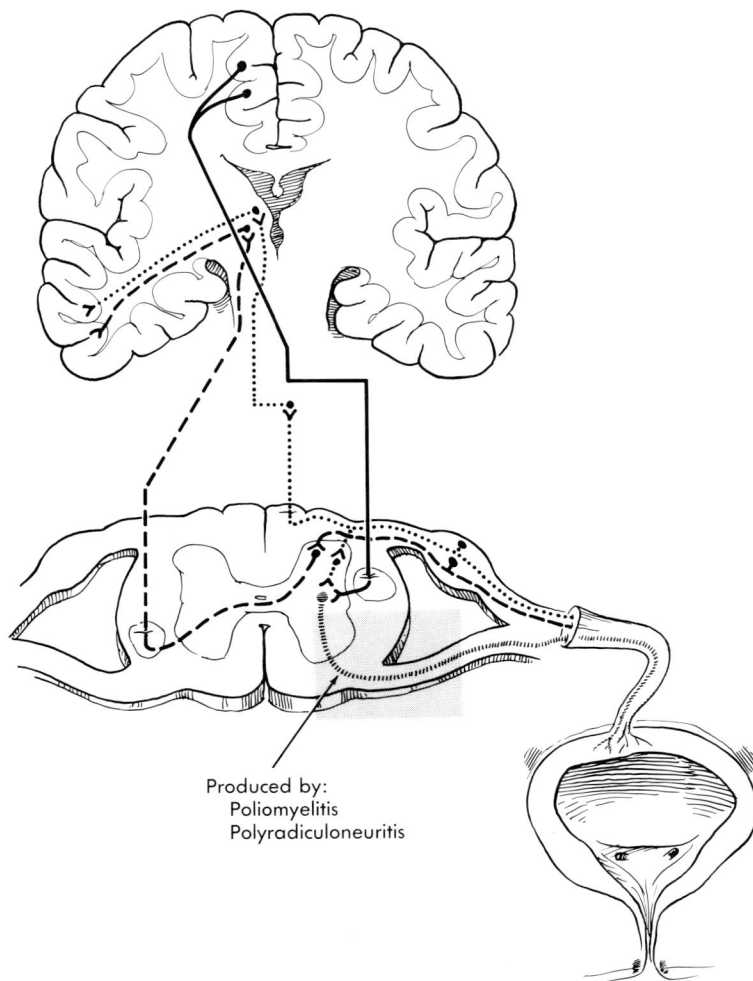

Produced by:
Poliomyelitis
Polyradiculoneuritis

Figure 10-6
Motor paralytic bladder is frequently associated with poliomyelitis and polyradiculoneuritis as result of involvement of lower motor neurons or motor fibers. *(From Lapides J and Diokno AC: Urine transport, storage, and micturition. In Lapides J, editor: Fundamentals of urology, Philadelphia, 1976, WB Saunders Co.)*

loss, however, will be partial or complete. When the onset of a motor paralytic bladder is slow and left untreated, the detrusor muscle will stretch and lose tone, resulting in large residual urine volumes. The client will complain of difficulties in initiating voiding, decreased force of the urinary stream, and a need to strain to void. These signs and symptoms are from loss of motor function and a decrease in muscle tone.[35]

Complications Associated with Neurogenic Bladder

The rehabilitation nurse should recognize the complications that commonly occur with neurogenic bladder dysfunction and exercise vigilance in their prevention. Complications include autonomic hyperreflexia, detrusor sphincter dyssynergia, hydronephrosis, vesicoureteral reflux, urinary tract infections, and urinary calculi. Other complications that may contribute to the person's problems are urethral stricture and a preexisting or coexisting prostate hyperplasia.

Autonomic hyperreflexia

Almost every activity in the autonomic nervous system has sympathetic stimulation with an opposing parasympathetic response aimed at restoring balance. Sympathetic neurons arise between T5 and L2 spinal cord segments, whereas parasympathetic outflow occurs from the brainstem and from the second to fourth sacral spinal cord segments.

Autonomic hyperreflexia, also known as autonomic dysreflexia, paroxysmal hyperactive reflex, and distention syndrome, results from unchecked reflex sympathetic activity in response to an afferent stimulus arising from the skin or viscera below the level of the lesion.[3] It is a serious medical emergency that occurs in 80% of neurologically impaired individuals with lesions above the T6 spinal cord segment.[3] Stimulation of the sympathetic nervous system produces a mass response leading to vasoconstriction of the blood vessels to the skin and viscera and vasodilation of blood vessels to the brain, skeletal muscles, and heart. With no interruption in neural circuits, stimulation of sensory receptors leading to sympathetic reflex activity normally would be inhibited by an outflow from supraspinal centers. With a complete or incomplete transection of the cord, these inhibitory reflexes fail to reach below the

level of the lesion. Thus the reflexes continue to build, resulting in autonomic hyperreflexia. The return of bladder tone, the return of the bulbocavernosus reflex, and the beginning of spasticity signal the potential for autonomic hyperreflexia to occur. Without proper recognition and treatment, the affected person may experience convulsions, intracranial hemorrhage, and even death.

Sudden hypertension results from the sympathetic vasoconstriction. To counteract the hypertension, baroreceptors in the aortic arch, carotid sinus, and cerebral vessels send afferent impulses along the ninth and tenth cranial nerves to the vasomotor center in the medulla. The vasomotor center sends vasodilator and bradycardic impulses to the blood vessels and heart, causing bradycardia and flushing, warmth, and perspiration above the level of the lesion. The vasodilation results in temporal and neck vessel engorgement, nasopharyngeal congestion, and blurred vision. Because the vasodilation cannot occur below the level of the lesion, hypertension persists, causing severe bitemporal, bifrontal, or occipital headaches. The rise in systolic pressure is frequently more dramatic than the rise in diastolic pressure. Other symptoms include anxiety before the onset of obvious symptoms, nausea, piloerection, difficulty in breathing, and chest pain. The resulting symptoms are not always present in the same sequence or severity in each person or in each episode.

A diagnosis of autonomic hyperreflexia should be anticipated in persons with spinal cord lesions above T4 to T6 spinal cord segments. Clients should be observed for signs and symptoms of this condition. When nursing interventions discussed later in this chapter fail to alleviate the hypertension, the physician is notified. Parenteral therapy and nonsurgical interventions may be ordered.

Parenteral therapy. Parenteral therapy includes (1) drugs that have a fast action and a direct vasodilator effect, such as hydralazine (Apresoline), nitroprusside (Nipride), or diazoxide (Hyperstat); and (2) drugs that can immediately counteract the massive sympathetic outflow, such as ganglionic blockage with trimethaphan (Arfonad) or spinal anesthetics. Pharmacological agents given for long-term prevention include methantheline (Banthine), oxybutynin (Ditropan), phenoxybenzamine (Dibenzyline), propantheline (Pro-Banthine), and mecamylamine (Inversine).[10]

Nonsurgical procedures. Nonsurgical procedures for long-term management include subarachnoid or phenol blocks. The client should be informed that nerve blocks may affect bladder training and the ability to have an erection. Surgical procedures such as sympathectomy, sacral neurectomy, rhizotomy, and cordectomy are permanent and also result in the loss of erection. These procedures do not prevent hyperreflexia from stimuli below the surgical site.[30]

Detrusor sphincter dyssynergia

Detrusor sphincter dyssynergia occurs when smooth muscle of the bladder wall contracts and effects a reflex contraction of the external urinary sphincter. The asynchrony of the internal and external sphincters results in poor urinary stream, residual volumes of more than 150 ml, and persistent urinary tract infections. Although detrusor muscle contraction can overcome some functional obstruction at the bladder outlet, eventually it will be unable to compensate fully.[39]

Drugs such as diazepam (Valium), dantrolene sodium (Dantrium), and baclofen (Lioresal) may be valuable in decreasing the spasticity of skeletal muscle, including that of the external sphincter. The dosage required for good sphincteric relaxation, however, may produce severe weakness and diffuse muscle relaxation. This generalized relaxation becomes a major problem for persons who take advantage of extensor spasms to walk or perform other activities.[27]

When a pharmacological approach is unsuccessful, an external sphincterotomy may be considered. This procedure decreases the tension caused by the increased activity of the periurethral striated muscle. It is believed that an external sphincterotomy prevents bladder neck hypertrophy. Since this procedure renders the person incontinent, an external collection device must be worn. This procedure is performed in persons with a high spinal cord injury. In persons with low lesions, a transurethral resection may be performed. The individual should be informed that removing tissue from the bladder neck may result in retrograde ejaculation.[39]

A procedure whereby the spastic bladder and extremities are made flaccid may be performed when the person has a small bladder capacity and severe involuntary spasms of the extremities when voiding. Another reason for performing this procedure is the occurrence of upper renal tract damage despite other treatments or continuous catheter drainage. By performing a subarachnoid block, anterior or posterior sacral rhizotomy, or selective sacral nerve section, the upper motor neuron lesion is "converted" to a lower motor neuron type.[27]

Hydronephrosis

Hydronephrosis can occur at any time after a neurological injury and refers to dilation of the kidneys secondary to reflux, infection, or obstruction. With reflux, urine regurgitates from the bladder and travels back up to the kidneys because of a faulty ureterovesical valve or a lower tract obstruction. The greater the length of time or seriousness of the obstruction, the greater the renal damage. Monitoring urine output is vital to detection and management.

The excretory urogram indicates the severity of the dilation. Depending upon the outcome of the test, the hydronephrosis may be classified as severe (grades III and IV) or less critical (grades I and II). Treatment is aimed at decreasing the resistance to urine outflow and restoring free urinary drainage. For severe hydronephrosis the urologist may order the insertion of an indwelling catheter for 1 to 3 months followed by intermittent catheterization. For less critical hydronephrosis intermittent catheterization may resolve the problem. Transurethral resection of the bladder neck and an external sphincterotomy may be necessary to relieve obstruction in a male.[40]

Vesicoureteral reflux

Vesicoureteral reflux is a common complication resulting from congenitally short intramural ureters, bladder inflammation, neurogenic bladder disease, bladder outlet obstruction, or vesical neck surgery. Ureterovesical valvelike action is impaired, producing a regurgitation and backflow to the kidneys. This condition is an important contributing cause to pyelonephritis.

When the bladder decompensates with chronic distention and increased intravesical pressure, an outpouching of mucosa from the detrusor muscle bands *(trabeculation)* may change the oblique angle at which the ureters transverse the muscle or may mechanically obstruct the ureteral opening.[39] Consequently, urine backs up into the kidneys.

Surgical intervention is necessary with any of the following conditions: (1) urine remains infected and reflux persists, despite a strict medical regimen and long-term suppressive antimicrobial therapy; (2) increased renal damage is demonstrated on serial excretory urograms; and (3) reflux continues for 1 year after institution of therapy. Temporary or permanent urinary diversion may be required when kidney function is impaired to allow renal function to improve and dilated ureters to regain tone. Later, definitive relief of obstruction by surgical intervention can be performed at the optimum time.[40]

Urinary tract infections

Urinary tract infections account for approximately 40% of all nosocomial infections. High-risk clients are pregnant women, the elderly, persons with diabetes, and persons with structural or neurological abnormalities of the urinary tract. These infections are, for the most part, preventable by careful attention to need for invasion of the urinary tract, proper procedures during insertion of instruments, and meticulous care of urinary drainage systems.[21]

The insertion of catheters is a major cause of urinary tract infections. According to Kunin,[21] 3% to 10% of hospitalized persons who have indwelling catheters will incur significant bacteriuria. Even otherwise healthy young adults have a 1% to 2% chance of infection with a single catheterization.

The concept of significant bacteriuria is defined as 100,000 (10^5) or more organisms demonstrated in a clean-catch specimen. Because contaminants can be introduced in collection containers from periurethral tissues, the urethra, the anus, and the vagina, nonsignificant organisms are found normally in clean-catch specimens. On the other hand, organisms of any number found in a catheterized specimen would be significant.[27]

There are a number of reasons for the high incidence of urinary tract infections in rehabilitation settings. Frequent catheterization and instrumentation provide a portal of entry for resistant nosocomial organisms. High residual urine volumes in persons with neurogenic bladders offer an ideal reservoir for the growth and multiplication of bacteria. Bladder overdistention and increased intravesical pressure decrease blood circulation, interfere with the antibacterial defenses, and disrupt the structural integrity of urinary tract tissues.[21]

Introduction of a urethral catheter creates a convenient pathway for organisms to ascend the urinary tract and interferes with the normal voiding mechanism, which washes out offending organisms that colonize the distal urethra and perineum. Lower urinary tract infections frequently result in renal complications. Despite the advances made in urinary tract care, urinary tract infections remain a major cause of death in spinal cord–injured persons.[1]

Anderson and Hsieh-ma[1] found that persons undergoing intermittent catheterization often suffer asymptomatic bacteriuria. They found that gram-positive *Staphylococcus epidermidis* and *Streptococcus faecalis* produced a minimum white cell response even in high colony counts. Conversely, gram-negative and fungal organisms elicited significant pyuria. They recommend that analysis of pyuria in conjunction with urine cultures serve as a clinical guide to treatment of significant bacteriuria.[1]

Urinary calculi

Urinary calculi can develop in almost any part of the urinary tract but are most commonly found within the kidney (*nephrolithiasis*). The composition of urinary stones varies. Approximately three fourths are composed of calcium oxalate or calcium phosphate; other stones are composed of magnesium ammonium phosphate (struvite), uric acid, or cystine.

Calcium oxalate stones are small, rough, hard, and dark in color with sharp spicules. Formation of horns (staghorns) is rare. These stones are opaque and can be seen on x-ray examination.[20]

Calcium phosphate stones are yellow-brown. These may be soft or hard, often form staghorn masses, are opaque, and can be readily seen on x-ray examination. These stones are soluble in acidic urine.

Struvite stones, also known as stones of infection, are yellowish, moderately opaque, and somewhat friable. Staghorn formation is common. Often the organism responsible for infection is *Proteus mirabilis*.

Uric acid stones form only in acid urine. These small, hard, and yellowish-brown stones may be multiple and usually are nonopaque on plain films. These stones may appear as filling defects on the excretory urogram.

Cystine stones are a light yellow or yellow-brown and resemble maple sugar. The stones may coalesce to form staghorn masses. Because cystine stones are the result of an inherited disorder of amino acid metabolism and are characterized by an early age of onset, they are not seen as a secondary complication in rehabilitation practice.[29]

Predisposing factors to stone formation. A number of theories have been postulated regarding the formation of urinary tract stones. Since calcium and struvite stones are commonly seen in rehabilitation practice, the possible causes of these stones are discussed. The following three theories currently account for the formation of calcium stones[27]:

1. Excessive excretion of calcium in the urine, hypercalciuria, is the first step in stone formation.
2. A relative excess of urinary oxalate excretion exceeds certain critical values of oxalate in the urine, which results in a relative hyperoxaluria.
3. The calcium oxalate or phosphate crystals grow over other crystals in the urine.

Magnesium ammonium phosphate stones are associated almost exclusively with persistently alkaline urine and with urea-splitting bacteria such as *Proteus*. The basic abnormality is the maintenance of alkaline urine. Two other associated conditions that contribute to infection and thus the tendency to form struvite stones are the presence of foreign bodies within the bladder and neurogenic bladder. Infection increases the amount of organic matter around which minerals can precipitate and increases the alkalinity of the urine by production of ammonia. The presence of residual urine in the bladder also precipitates organic matter and minerals. Urinary tract infections, rather than immobility and its associated urinary calcium and magnesium imbalance, are now believed to be the cause of struvite stones. Constantly alkaline urine leads to supersaturation with magnesium ammonium phosphate and when its formation product is exceeded, a spontaneous nucleus of stones can form.[27]

Clinical signs and symptoms. The clinical signs and symptoms of urinary tract stones vary with the size, location, and movement of the stone and the integrity of neural sensory pathways.

The person with intact neural sensory pathways generally will feel pain only when the stone becomes trapped in a calyx, the ureteropelvic junction, the pelvic brim, the posterior pelvis, or the ureterovesicular junction. Pain of renal colic is extreme. Stones that obstruct the calyx or ureterovesicular junction result in dull flank pain because of parenchymal and capsular obstruction. As the stone moves to the middle of the ureter, pain radiates to the lateral flank and abdominal area. If the stone ceases to move, inflammation may occur in the area of impaction and pain becomes localized to that area. Usually the client with urinary stones has "moving irritation" and is constantly trying to find a comfortable position to remove the discomfort. Costovertebral tenderness may be present. With prolonged ureteral obstruction, a mass in the flank may be observed, palpated, or percussed. Pain and irritation may cause the pulse and blood pressure to rise. Rebound tenderness may be elicited, particularly in the presence of infection.[27] Nausea and vomiting may accompany renal colic.

The person with damage to the neural sensory pathways may not feel pain but will exhibit other symptoms when the stone becomes trapped. Movement of the stone may trigger profuse sweating. An increase in bladder and lower extremity spasms also may occur.[39]

Diagnosis. Stones can be identified by blood, urine, and x-ray evaluation. Frequently used laboratory studies include serum calcium, phosphorus, magnesium, uric acid, and creatinine; protein electrophoresis; urine analysis and culture; 24-hour creatinine clearance; cystine, oxalate, and uric acid excretion; and fasting urinary pH.[29]

Roentgenographic studies include x-ray examination of the kidneys, ureters, and bladder and an upright film; excretory urography; and retrograde pyelography. Calcium and struvite stones and at least 90% of all stones are radiopaque. A renal scan will be done if excretory urograms indicate poor renal function. Ultrasound scanning also may be performed. These diagnostic tests, in conjunction with data from the history and physical examination, determine the definitive treatment.

Treatment. Treatment depends upon the cause of stone formation; composition, size, and location of the stones; and persistence of signs and symptoms. About 90% of stones are passed spontaneously. The urine should be strained by placing two 4×8-inch gauze strips over a funnel. Fluids, preferably 4 L/24 hours, unless otherwise contraindicated, promote passage of stones and prevent infection in the normally functioning bladder. Morphine sulfate and meperidine hydrochloride (Demerol) are given for pain. Antispasmodics also may be prescribed to relax smooth muscle of the ureters and lessen pain from spasm.[7]

Treatment of the client who is immobilized, has a neurogenic bladder, urinary tract infection, or an acid or alkaline pH that is conducive to a specific type of stone formation is directed toward the cause. The "best" treatment for calcium calculi remains controversial. Oral thiazides and oral neutral phosphates may be ordered. Decreased urinary calcium excretion is the therapeutic response of clients receiving thiazide therapy. The client may be instructed to test the pH of the urine and try to keep it below 6.0 because calcium phosphate stones form more rapidly in neutral or alkaline urine. Cranberry juice (200 ml) five times daily, ascorbic acid (1 g) four times daily, or potassium acid phosphate may be given to acidify the urine.[27] Restriction of calcium intake for those who drink more than a quart of milk per day has been recommended to establish a baseline should hypercalciuria occur. Persons who drink excessive amounts of milk and absorbable alkali usually can avoid hypercalciuria by reducing milk and alkali intake to normal dietary levels.[39]

Because it is impossible to cure a urinary tract infection in the presence of stones, infected urinary calculi must be removed surgically. Recurrence of struvite stones postoperatively is usually caused by small fragments that were left behind. After removal of the stone, the client's urine must be kept sterile. Two other therapies that may be suggested are restriction of exogenous phosphate using a low-phosphate diet and lowering the intestinal absorption of phosphate through the administration of aluminum. A low-phosphate diet (the Shorr regimen) modified from Drach* follows:

1. The daily dietary intake of phosphorus is restricted to less than 300 mg/day; calcium is restricted to less than 700 mg/day.
2. The patient takes 40 ml of basic aluminum carbonate gel four times daily.
3. A fluid intake of at least 3,000 ml/day and more as needed is prescribed to keep urinary output at 2,000 ml/day.
4. Analysis of urinary phosphorus excretion, which should be less than 250 mg/day, is done at intervals.

---

*From Harrison JH, et al: Campbell's urology, vol 1, ed 4, Philadelphia, 1978, WB Saunders Co; modified from Marshall VF, Lavenwood RW Jr, and Kelly JS: Ann Surg 162:366, 1965.

Phosphatic calculi develop in alkaline urine; therefore prevention depends upon keeping the urine acid and preventing urinary tract infection. Medications such as ascorbic acid or ammonium chloride may be given for a time to increase urine acidity.

A new technique, lithotripsy, removes calculi that are too large to pass spontaneously. To perform this procedure, the client is supported and suspended in a large tank of water, and a lithotripter sends shock waves through the water to the calculus. The calculus is shattered and excreted within several days. Another method used to break down kidney stones is ultrasound vibration. This procedure requires an incision about 0.33 inch (0.84 cm) long. The kidney stone is flushed out with water after the ultrasound treatment. Both of these procedures, if successful, allow the client to avoid major surgery.[7]

Urethral strictures

Urethral strictures can be congenital or acquired through trauma to the urethra. Introduction of a catheter, cystoscopy that produces bleeding, placement of an indwelling catheter, introduction of a foreign body, or a periurethral abscess that heals with subsequent fibrosis can produce trauma and a potential urethral stricture. Meatal stenosis and urethral papillomas also can cause urethral strictures. According to Shields,[39] "urethral strictures can be noted by resistance when a catheter is introduced." The extent of the stricture is determined by urethral calibration or retrograde urethrography.

Treatment consists of periodic urethral dilation with steel sounds. A large number of these strictures resist dilation and therefore require reconstructive surgery.[27]

Prostate hyperplasia

As men age, the periurethral glands that surround the prostate begin to multiply abnormally or the number of normal cells increases (hyperplasia). Although the normal adult prostate cannot be truly divided into lobes, lobulation occurs as prostatic hypertrophy progresses.

Physiological problems are not caused by enlargement of the prostate in and of itself. Over a period of time, however, urine outflow is hindered and may become totally blocked. Hypertrophy of the detrusor muscle, trabeculation of the bladder wall, reflux, hydroureter, hydronephrosis, and ultimately renal insufficiency may result.[27] Bladder diverticula, which retain urine and become sites for infection and calculi, also may develop.

Benign prostatic hypertrophy is diagnosed by a general physical examination, including a rectal examination, laboratory studies, x-ray examinations, cystography, and cystoscopy. Medical approaches are conservative and include avoidance of excessive fluid intake in a short period of time, avoidance of alcohol because of its diuretic effect, and voiding as soon as the urge is felt to avoid overdistention of the bladder. When conservative measures fail and acute urinary problems exist, surgery becomes necessary. A number of surgical procedures are available. The surgical approach depends upon the size and configuration of the prostate and the client's health.[27]

NURSING ASSESSMENT

The nursing assessment of the person with altered bladder function depends upon the collection of subjective and objective data. Data obtained from client and family interviews help determine the abilities and disabilities of the client in relation to the bladder dysfunction. Data collected from the family contribute to an understanding of support available in continuation of the rehabilitation process in the community. Information from the history, physical assessment, and diagnostic tests determine the actual physical, social, psychological, spiritual, and vocational problems. Nursing interventions are guided by the identified problems in each area. When the client cannot furnish information, the family may be the only source of the history.

Subjective Data

Several questions elicit information about the client's past and present health status, the nature and history of impaired bladder function, socioeconomic status, management of bladder function, and goals for rehabilitation of bladder function (Figure 10-7). With this information, the nurse identifies the client's self-care abilities, disabilities, desired health state, and feasible health state.[5]

While conducting the client interview, the nurse also assesses hand function and intellectual ability. The client's potential for managing the various treatment modalities available is assessed with a recognition that abilities will change during the rehabilitation process and require recurrent evaluation.

Family members frequently give the nurse additional information about the client's bladder impairment and ability to perform a bladder management routine with or without help. The nurse validates information given by the client and also assesses the intellectual abilities and capacities of those called upon to assist in the individualized plan for bladder management.

Objective Data

Objective data are collected by means of a physical assessment, performance of diagnostic studies, and review of results obtained from diagnostic studies.

Physical assessment

The rehabilitation nurse inspects, palpates, and percusses to physically assess the client's bladder status. The lower abdomen is observed for fullness. In addition, the urine is observed for color, amount, precipitates, cloudiness, and blood. The lower abdomen is palpated for the presence of a distended bladder. The bladder, normally not palpable, can be identified as a smooth and round tense mass when distended. A rectal examination is performed in the male to palpate the prostate gland. The nurse should be able to identify two lobes of the prostate gland separated by a medial sulcus when palpating anteriorly. The gland should feel smooth and rubbery with no irregularities or nodules. The gland will vary in size but when markedly enlarged, symptoms of urinary problems usually will be present. Percussion of the abdomen is performed to elicit any change to dullness in the suprapubic area that might indicate bladder distention.[37] Vital signs are taken and clinical signs such as fever, malaise, nausea, and vomiting are considered in relation to a possible lower urinary tract problem.

Nurses may be the first rehabilitation team members to notice the clinical signs and symptoms of urinary tract infection. They daily observe the urine for color, appearance, composition, and

Text continued on p. 169.

GENERAL HISTORY RELATED TO ALTERED BLADDER FUNCTION

Do you have any health problems other than the problem with your bladder (e.g., nervous system disease, diabetes mellitus, cerebrovascular or spinal vascular disease, hypertension, collagen disease)?

Have you had any operations (e.g., spine, rectum, uterus) or injuries (e.g., head, spine)?

Have you had any major infections (e.g., encephalitis, Guillain-Barré syndrome)?

Do you have any other symptoms (e.g., numbness in your extremities, visual change, weakness, dizziness, bowel problem, sexual problem, rigidity and stiffness of your extremities)?

Are you taking any medications for your bladder (e.g., bethanechol chloride, propantheline bromide, oxybutynin chloride, baclofen, phenoxybenzamine) or other medications (e.g., antihypertensives)?

Does any member of your family have a chronic illness (e.g., spinal cord tumor, diabetes mellitus, vascular disease, multiple sclerosis)?

Are you allergic to any medicines, foods, insects?

Have you been hospitalized before? If yes, for what, when, and where?

HISTORY AND NATURE OF ALTERED BLADDER FUNCTION

When did you begin to have problems with your bladder?

What symptoms did you notice then?

What did you do about those symptoms?

Did that relieve your symptoms?

What happened afterwards?

Figure 10-7
Interview guide for obtaining history from client with altered bladder function. *(Modified from Cantanzaro M: Impairment of bladder function. In Snyder, M editor: A guide to neurological and neurosurgical nursing, Philadelphia, 1983, John Wiley & Sons, Inc.)*

HISTORY AND NATURE OF ALTERED BLADDER FUNCTION—cont'd

Have you had any tests done previously to determine the reason for your bladder impairment (e.g., excretory urogram, cystometrogram)? If yes, where?

What were you told about the tests?

Have you ever experienced other problems associated with your bladder impairment (e.g., autonomic hyper-reflexia, urinary tract infection, detrusor sphincter dyssynergia, stones, skin irritations)?

What other symptoms did you experience when you first had a problem with your bladder?

What is your urine usually like (e.g., color, smell, particles, amount daily)?

PRESENT BLADDER STATUS

Tell me about your bladder problem now (e.g., frequency, urgency, incontinence, hesitancy, force of stream, burning, pain)?

Does anything make these symptoms worse (e.g., position, stress, coughing, bending, cold)?

Have these symptoms changed since you first noticed them?

What is your urine like now (e.g., color, smell, particles, amount daily)?

How much do you drink each day and when?

Is your sleep interrupted by your bladder symptoms?

Do you do anything to help you urinate?

What equipment/appliances do you use to assist with urination (if applicable)?

Figure 10-7, cont'd
Interview guide for obtaining history from client with altered bladder function.   *Continued.*

PSYCHOSOCIAL/ECONOMIC STATUS
What are your toileting facilities like at home? At school or work?

What is your occupation?

Has your bladder impairment interfered with your work, social, or sexual activities? If yes, in what way?

Do you have any financial assistance for purchase of medications/supplies/equipment (e.g., Medicaid, Medicare, insurance)?

Do you need help from others to manage (e.g., toileting, changing clothes, searching for bathroom facilities ?

Does anyone help you with your bladder management (e.g., family member, friend, personal care attendant ?

Does your bladder routine interfere with the activities of others?

Who is available to learn about your bladder problem and its management?

GOALS
What changes would you like to see occur in your bladder function?

What do you think might contribute to this desired change?

What do you think your family expects regarding your bladder problem and its management?

Figure 10-7, cont'd
Interview guide for obtaining history from client with altered bladder function.

odor. Daily observation of the client for mental status, intake and output, and vital signs allows the nurse to identify subtle signs of infection and possible septic shock. Successful treatment of septicemia depends on early recognition and immediate therapy.

Diagnostic tests

The rehabilitation nurse should have knowledge of normal and abnormal results of diagnostic tests used to determine the underlying pathophysiological process of altered bladder function. Diagnostic tests performed include laboratory examination of blood and urine and urine cultures, urodynamic studies, roentgenographic studies, radioisotopic studies, and ultrasound examination. Additional tests may be ordered, depending upon the suspected etiology.

Blood and urine tests. Blood tests are routinely ordered to rule out kidney damage when there is a history of lower urinary tract complications. Diagnostic tests ordered include blood urea nitrogen (BUN) level, serum creatinine level, and creatinine clearance, which is a combination of blood and urine examination.

Urea is formed in the liver. It is the most important nonprotein nitrogenous compound of blood and is the chief end product of protein metabolism. Normally it is excreted entirely by the kidneys. The normal BUN value varies widely from 5 to 20 mg/100 ml because the ingestion of dietary protein varies widely. Elevations may indicate dehydration, prerenal failure, or renal failure. Excessive breakdown of protein also may occur with sepsis, fever, or gastrointestinal bleeding. Once a client is hydrated, the BUN level should return to normal; if it does not, renal insufficiency should be suspected. Kidney diseases that result in an elevated BUN level include glomerulonephritis, extensive pyogenic infections, and posttraumatic renal insufficiency. In older persons the BUN level may be higher because of a decrease in the number of nephrons. In addition, some drugs such as antibiotics, diuretics, and antihypertensives raise the BUN level. Elevation of the BUN level does not occur until at least two thirds of the nephrons have stopped functioning.[19,27] The nurse should assess the client's dietary intake because a low protein intake and a high carbohydrate intake can decrease the BUN level, whereas a high-protein diet will increase the BUN level unless adequate fluids are given. Hydration status should be assessed routinely. Overhydration can tax the cardiovascular system, especially in the aged and in cardiac patients, resulting in hypervolemia and a decreased serum BUN level. Clients with a slightly elevated BUN level should be taught to increase fluid intake unless medically contraindicated.

A serum creatinine test also is done to determine levels in the blood. The nurse should explain the purpose of the test and instruct the client that there is no food or water restriction before the test. Except for antibiotics, medications should be held for 24 hours before the test with the physician's permission. Medications not withheld should be listed on the client's chart. Creatinine is a byproduct of muscle catabolism and is derived from the breakdown of muscle creatine phosphate. The daily production of creatinine is proportional to the muscle mass and ranges from 0.6 to 1.5 mg/100 ml in adults. This value remains constant, because it is not affected by diet or fluid intake or other factors that affect BUN values. It is considered a more sensitive and specific indicator of renal disease than the BUN value. Elevation of serum creatinine occurs in all kidney diseases in which 50% or more of the nephrons are destroyed. Nonrenal causes of creatinine elevation are extremely limited.[19,27] The nurse should be able to relate the creatinine levels to clinical problems. Since the kidneys excrete creatinine normally, a high serum creatinine level indicates renal disease. If both the BUN and creatinine levels are elevated, the client's problem is most likely kidney disease. The nurse should instruct the client whose creatinine level is extremely elevated to eat less beef, poultry, and fish. Normally food intake does not effect the serum creatinine level.

The creatinine clearance test is the most accurate measure of renal function in routine usage. Since creatinine is excreted by glomerular filtration and is not reabsorbed or secreted by the tubule cells, the serum creatinine level rises when the glomerular filtration rate falls. The nurse instructs the client to omit meats, poultry, fish, tea, and coffee for 6 hours before the test and during the test. The procedure for blood and urine collection follows: Blood is drawn in the morning, the client voids and the urine is discarded, and then all urine is saved for 12 or 24 hours in a urine container. About 100 ml of water per hour should be taken throughout the test. When the creatinine clearance rate is determined on a 24-hour basis, it also should be low. The creatinine clearance rate is calculated by the following formula:

$$\frac{\text{Urine creatinine} \times \text{Urine volume}}{\text{Serum creatinine}}$$

A decreased creatinine clearance corresponds to decreased renal function.

Urine creatinine is reported as the number of grams of creatinine excreted in the 24-hour urine specimen. Volume refers to the amount of urine excreted in that period, and the serum creatinine value is the creatinine concentration in the serum recorded in milligrams per 100 ml. The serum is collected the morning of the test. The result of the glomerular filtration rate is expressed in milliliters per minute, and the average normal rate is 120 ml/minute. In older persons, the creatinine level may be as low as 60 ml/minute. This value varies with an individual's age and muscle mass and is corrected to an average standard body size of 1.73 square meters.[19,27]

Urinalysis. Gross general examination of the urine is not a reliable method of detecting bacteria. Although a urinalysis can be one of the most important tests in diagnosing urological problems, all too often specimens are collected improperly, the analysis is delayed, or analysis of the urinary sediment is incomplete. Information obtained from a urinalysis includes pH, specific gravity, glucose, protein, appearance, color, odor, and the presence of cells.

The normal pH of urine ranges from 4.5 to 7.5. Urine pH is a reflection of the hydrogen ion concentration and of the plasma pH. An alkaline urine may be found when urea-splitting bacteria are present, after administration of alkalizing medications such as sodium bicarbonate or acetazolamide or after ingestion of low-protein diets high in vegetables and citrus fruits. Since most diets are high in protein foods that are metabolized into acid end products, the urine is usually acidic. Although the serum pH is low in renal tubular acidosis associated with renal disease, the urine pH remains between 6.0 and 7.0. In other conditions, such as hypercalciuria and nephrocalcinosis, the urine pH is high.[27]

Specific gravity, measured by a urinometer, normally ranges from 1.005 to 1.030. The urinometer measures the concentration of dissolved solids in the urine and is used to estimate general hydration. When a client's fluid level is depleted, the specific gravity is high because the kidneys "conserve fluid," causing the urine to be concentrated. When kidneys lose their ability to concentrate and dilute urine, the specific gravity becomes fixed at a level about equal to that of plasma (1.010). The specific gravity can be elevated in persons with diabetes mellitus, vomiting, diarrhea, hepatic diseases, adrenal insufficiency, and heart failure. Other reasons for elevation of the specific gravity include decreased fluid intake, fever, administration of intravenous dextran or albumin, and injection of x-ray contrast media.

All urinalyses include examination for glucose, primarily to screen for diabetes mellitus. Normally no glucose should be found in the urine and its presence indicates the need for further testing. The absence of glucose does not necessarily rule out diabetes mellitus because some older clients with arteriosclerosis have high renal thresholds for glucose and may have diabetes without glucosuria. Glucose also may be present in the urine of clients who have a cerebrovascular accident, meningitis, Cushing's syndrome, severe stress, infections, or take drugs such as ascorbic acid, cephalothin sodium (Keflin), streptomycin sulfate, epinephrine, or aspirin.[19,27]

Very small amounts (100 mg/day) of protein may be found in normal urine. Larger amounts are characteristically found in disorders involving the glomeruli. The size of the protein molecule determines the ease with which it passes through the damaged membrane. Since albumin has the smallest molecule, it is the protein most often found in the urine.

The color, appearance, and odor of urine are routinely examined. The normal color of urine is a relatively clear, golden yellow. Colorless or very pale urine is found in clients with a large fluid intake, diabetes insipidus, chronic kidney disease, alcohol ingestion, and nervousness. A pale color usually indicates diluted urine whereas a dark yellow or amber color indicates concentrated urine. Many drugs and foods can change the color of the urine. The urine may appear hazy or cloudy in the presence of bacteria, pus, tissue, red blood cells, white blood cells, phosphates, prostatic fluid, spermatozoa, urates, or uric acid. The urine may be milky in the presence of fat or pus. Persons may initially contact a physician because of the change in color and smell of urine. Foul odors may be present when there is a urinary tract infection. *Escherichia coli* infections may smell like feces or sulfur. In the presence of urea-splitting organisms such as *Proteus*, the urine frequently smells like ammonia. Methylmercaptan, found in asparagus, gives a pungent odor to the urine.[19,27]

The urinary sediment is examined microscopically for the presence of red blood cells, white blood cells, and hyaline casts. Red blood cells greater than two per low power field are found in trauma to the kidney, renal disease, renal calculi, cystitis, lupus nephritis, and when drugs such as anticoagulants, sulfonamides, and aspirins in excess are taken. Menstrual discharge also may contaminate the urine. White blood cells greater than four per low power field are found in urinary tract infection, fever, strenuous exercise, lupus nephritis, and renal diseases. If white blood cells are found, a culture and sensitivity should be done. Hyaline casts are found in renal diseases and heart failure.[19,27] Clients who are bringing a specimen for urinalysis to the clinic should be instructed to place the fresh morning urine specimen in the refrigerator immediately after obtaining it and to bring it to the laboratory within the hour, because bacterial growth begins within ½ hour after collection. Refrigeration may retard this growth. The nurse also should know the diet and medications the client takes in order to evaluate the urinalysis report.

Urine cultures. Urine cultures are required to identify infecting organisms. With few exceptions (for example, the woman who has bacteriuria, very frequent voiding, and bladder irritation), clean-voided, midstream urine samples should be obtained. Significant bacteriuria, that is, bacteriuria above that which might occur with contamination, exists when the colony count from a single culture is over 100,00 organisms/ml (10^5) with bacteria and pus cells visible microscopically in a clean-catch specimen.[39] The presence of any amount of bacteria is considered significant when aseptic methods of collection are used to obtain urine from the renal pelves, ureters, or bladder.[27]

Roentgenographic studies. A flat plate of the abdomen usually precedes any other x-ray films of the urinary tract. Views of the kidney, ureters, and bladder (KUB) are taken to determine the size, shape, and placement of the kidneys and to note any stones in the kidneys, pelves, or ureters. KUB views are usually used in conjunction with a more definitive examination, such as the excretory urogram.[27]

The excretory urogram is the most commonly ordered diagnostic test when renal impairment is suspected. By means of a series of x-ray films, the absence, presence, location, and size of each kidney, as well as the filling of the renal calyces, pelves, and outlines of the ureters are determined. Irregularities, opacities, and other noted defects are compared in various x-ray views, which are usually taken at 2-, 5-, 10-, and 15-minute intervals after injection of contrast media. The last film also is a postvoid film. Before the test is performed, the client's sensitivity to the contrast medium should be determined.[27]

Roentgenograms of the kidney are called *nephrotomograms* and are taken with a rotating x-ray tube moved in the direction of an arc. These films are taken to further define abnormalities detected on excretory urograms. They are also used to evaluate renal lacerations and nonperfused areas after trauma, as well as localizing adrenal tumors. A radiopaque dye is injected or infused before the films are taken. A circulation time also is recorded before the procedure to assist in the timing of the x-ray series.[27] The nephrotomogram gives pictures of sections of the kidney and delineates tissues at the level at which the x-ray tube radiates.

Computed tomography (CT scan) also may be used for examining sections of the kidneys for a pathological condition. Through a series of complex manipulations, the computer "reconstructs" the cross-sectional image as an array or grid of picture elements and displays the image as an integrated, recognizable picture on a screen. One of the many advantages of this procedure is the elimination of contrast material, which has been known to cause allergic reactions. This procedure is completely noninvasive.[27]

Cystoscopy is a method of direct visualization of the bladder. A metallic instrument with illumination provides remarkable magnification and clarity. Both the bladder and urethra are inspected. Encouraging the client to take deep breaths promotes relaxation and facilitates the passage of the cystoscope. The bladder is distended with sterile saline to make visualization more effective. During bladder filling, the client may feel the urge to void. This feeling should be tolerable, however, if the nurse continues to encourage relaxation.[27] This procedure usually is performed under local anesthesia. Cystoscopy is indicated for the evaluation of hematuria, chronic or recurrent urinary tract infection, unexplained urological symptoms, evaluation of congenital anomalies, or in any clinical situation in which excretory urograms have suggested pathological changes but have not furnished enough information for definitive diagnosis and treatment. Cystoscopy is contraindicated in acute urinary tract infection, since trauma may exacerbate the infection and when severe symptoms of prostatic obstruction are present because trauma may produce just enough edema of the bladder neck to cause complete urinary retention.[40]

Other x-ray examinations of the bladder and urethra include retrograde cystography, delayed cystography, voiding cystourethrography, and retrograde urethrography. These x-ray examinations demonstrate a clear outline of the bladder, show any diverticula, and may demonstrate vesicoureteral reflux.

Urodynamic studies. Urodynamic studies are designed to measure pressure from within the bladder, urethra, and abdomen; urinary flow; and striated muscle activity. In a broad sense, urodynamic studies include *urine flow rate, cystometrography, urethral pressure profile, voiding cystourethrography,* and *sphincter electromyography.* These studies have been developed specifically to evaluate bladder and voiding problems.

The urine flow rate is measured by asking the client to void into an instrument that simultaneously records the peak urine flow and graphically records the characteristics of voiding. The total volume divided by the time taken to void will give the urine flow rate per second. Modern equipment allows the client to be left alone and instructed to push a button on the machine when voiding is initiated. Normal values for the client who voids 200 to 400 ml are as follows: a peak flow rate should be greater than 15 ml/second; a normal flow pattern should be a smooth, bell-shaped curve without any interruptions or sharp peaks and sustained over a period of 20 seconds. Variations from normal can result from decompensation of the detrusor muscle or outflow obstruction, obstructing effects of prostatic hypertrophy or an overdistended areflexic bladder.[27,33]

A cystometrogram helps assess bladder function by providing a volume-pressure relationship when the bladder is gradually filled with water or carbon dioxide. The bladder pressure during filling and voiding is continuously recorded. Information is obtained about the presence or absence of residual urine, contractility of the detrusor muscle, capacity for stretch, sensation of fullness, desire to void, and pain.[27,33] Normally uninhibited contractions are absent, the capacity of the bladder is 450 ml, the voiding stream is normal, and there is no residual urine. The first desire to void is present when the bladder is filled with 150 ml and the perception of fullness occurs when the bladder is filled with 400 ml.[40]

A urethral pressure profile is intended to provide an index of urethral resistance to bladder output, assist in the assessment of urinary incontinence, provide a distinction between a distensible and fibrotic urethral segment, and contribute information regarding coordination of the detrusor muscle and the external urinary sphincter.[33] Any weakness or hyperactivity in either the smooth or voluntary muscle can be detected.[40]

The voiding cystourethrogram may reveal ureteral reflux. Cystourethrograms combine simple cystography with urethrography to visualize abnormalities of the bladder and urethra such as stenosis of the urethra, enlargement of the prostate, diverticula, fistulas, or other conditions of the urethra. Radiopaque dye is instilled in the bladder through a catheter. With the catheter clamped off, an x-ray film is taken to determine if there is reflux. The catheter is then removed and the client is asked to void. When voiding occurs, an x-ray film is taken to outline the urethra.

Sphincter electromyography can be compared to electrocardiography in that electrodes are used to pick up electrical activity in the muscles. Used for some time in studying the muscles of the extremities, it is only within the last few years that it has become possible to study the activity of the striated (voluntary) muscles within the perineal area. This test is almost never performed alone because the major objective is to evaluate the relationship of perineal muscle activity to detrusor contractions.[27]

Radioisotopic studies. These studies are becoming increasingly important because of the major advantages they have over traditional techniques. All are noninvasive, result in less radiation exposure than with traditional x-ray studies, and require no client preparation. The currently available radioisotopes provide a means of evaluating the internal organs without disturbing normal physiological processes. They are used to measure overall renal function, evaluate regional renal function and structure, and evaluate the condition of the ureters and bladder.[27]

Ultrasound examination. Ultrasound techniques are used to visualize deep structures within the body by recording the reflection of ultrasound or high-frequency waves directed into the tissues. These techniques also have major advantages over traditional techniques, but have been used as a complement in the investigation of many urinary tract disorders. In addition to diagnosing renal conditions, ultrasound examination can be used to evaluate bladder lesions and diverticula and in estimating residual urine. More recently these techniques have been used to delineate the prostate and seminal vesicles. The ultimate clinical utility is unknown at this time.[35]

NURSING DIAGNOSES

The person with altered bladder function presents a nursing diagnosis of an *altered pattern of urinary elimination*.[15] The problems in daily living resulting from this nursing diagnosis have been explained in the introduction to this chapter. The nurse may diagnose several other client problems as a direct result of the altered pattern of urinary elimination.

The client may experience difficulty coping with a problem in urinary elimination and have a diagnosis of *ineffective individual coping*.[15] Living with additional appliances and adjusting time and fluid schedules to need for elimination is a change with which some individuals cannot cope. Some individuals may have to have an indwelling catheter inserted because they cannot or will not follow an intermittent catheterization program. Clients who are totally dependent on a family member to manage a bladder program may find that family members either refuse to learn or cannot adjust their schedule to assist the individual. The bladder program may be disruptive to the overall family life-style. In this instance, the nursing diagnosis might be *ineffective family coping*.[15] The nurse should consider the family from the beginning of the rehabilitation process and include them in planning the client's rehabilitation program.

Potential or impaired skin integrity occurs in clients with bladder impairment.[15] The use of external collection devices and stoma bags can result in skin irritation if not properly managed. Episodes of incontinence are irritating to the skin. The client and nurse must routinely inspect the skin several times a day when potential or actual interruption of skin integrity exists. Nursing interventions are designed to prevent this occurrence or restore skin integrity should irritation be present.

A diversional activity deficit also may occur if the client continues to be embarrassed about the bladder problem and the requirements to maintain bladder elimination. Matter-of-fact approaches to the problem, the opportunity to socialize in the rehabilitation setting, wearing and managing regular clothes, visits with friends and family, passes to the community, and the chance to be catheter free encourage the client to continue activities and promote social adjustment to the demands of the bladder program.

Home management of urinary elimination can be a problem if toileting facilities are not accessible, appliances are not available, and medications are difficult to obtain. Several members of a family residing in a small house can make it difficult to obtain privacy and may further inhibit progress in the bladder program. The nurse may diagnose *impaired home maintenance management*[15] after a home assessment is made and prescribe appropriate nursing intervention.

A knowledge deficit about the bladder management program should be identified while the client remains in the tertiary care facility. The nurse documents these knowledge deficits and devises teaching plans and programs to educate the client and family members regarding the specific knowledge deficit.

Initially the client may totally depend on others for assistance with expelling or retaining urine. As clients progress in the total rehabilitation program, they should become progressively independent and assume increasing responsibility for toileting. In some clients a diagnosis of *toileting self-care deficit*[15] may be identified. The bladder management program is either adjusted accordingly or additional emphasis is given to other aspects of the rehabilitation program to help improve independence and responsibility.

Impairment in bladder function also can disturb a person's *self-concept in relation to body image, self-esteem, role performance, and personal identity*. If this nursing diagnosis is identified, the plan and intervention must indicate nursing actions to maximize the person's growth potential despite the bladder impairment.

Sexual dysfunction may be identified as a result of bladder impairment. Clients may be hesitant to discuss this aspect of daily living and may be more open if given permission by the nurse. A good time to inquire about this area is during the initial assessment, opening the door for future discussion.[15]

A nursing diagnosis of *altered patterns of urinary elimination* can affect many aspects of a person's life. The above additional nursing diagnoses must be considered in developing a comprehensive plan of rehabilitation for the person with altered bladder function.

GOALS

The goals for the client with altered bladder function are developed so that the client will achieve optimum physiological bladder status with minimum interference in social role performance. The rehabilitation goals are individualized for each client. Generally the goals are as follows:

1. To achieve a low amount or no residual urine with adequate emptying of the bladder at predictable intervals
2. To prevent complications and preserve renal function
3. To maintain skin integrity
4. To promote a catheter-free state involving the least amount of time, money, and assistance of other persons
5. To establish a bladder program that can be maintained with little interference in social role performance after discharge
6. To maintain the client's self-esteem and dignity
7. To educate the client and family about:
   a. Medications and equipment prescribed when applicable
   b. Prevention and recognition of complications
   c. Performance of the bladder management program
8. To assist the client in making any necessary modifications in the home to assure appropriate toileting facilities

9. To obtain maximum client and family participation in and responsibility for the bladder management program

REHABILITATION NURSING INTERVENTIONS

No single nursing intervention is appropriate for clients with altered bladder function. The goals and nursing interventions will vary from client to client. In planning the nursing interventions, the underlying pathological condition, the ability of clients to perform specified maneuvers with their hands, the ability to move around and reach equipment and facilities, and the reliability, intelligence, and cooperation of clients and their families in the planning and implementation of the bladder elimination program are paramount to success. Changes in the client's status from the occurrence of the initial problem to functional stability affect the goals and interventions.

Bladder Retraining Programs

Bladder retraining programs have become safer, more successful, and more widespread since the introduction of intermittent catheterization.[28] Bladder retraining takes place during the recovery from spinal shock in the person with spinal cord disease or injury. Regardless of the underlying problem, bladder retraining is a dynamic process that changes as the neurological/urological status changes.

General considerations

The goals during the acute phase after a neurological insult are to prevent overdistention of the bladder with resultant interruption of blood flow, lowered resistance to bacteria, infection, and possible damage to the upper urinary tract. The preferred nursing intervention during this period is intermittent catheterization with careful attention to fluid intake and output.[36] In some rehabilitation settings an indwelling catheter may be inserted for 2 to 3 days after the neurological insult until fluid and electrolyte balance is reestablished.

When the acute phase of spinal shock is subsiding and there is progressive reappearance of bladder and extremity function, bladder training is initiated while observations of neurological/urological status continue. Maneuvers to empty the bladder and intermittent catheterization are performed. Drugs to assist in bladder contraction and relaxation may be given.[1,12,16,36]

In the final stage of neurological recovery, usually after complete recovery of the lesion, the nurse continues with procedures used during the transitional phase but establishes the definitive interventions and bladder management program with the client and family. The ultimate goal is to assist the client in achieving a "balanced" or "rehabilitated bladder." A *balanced bladder* is one in which the client can pass adequate urine on reflex or easily with the Credé maneuver and abdominal strain, the residual urine volume is approximately 150 ml or less, and there are no pathological changes in the genitourinary tract.[33]

Psychosocial responses of the client. A successful bladder retraining program depends upon the participation of the client and those persons who will be assisting in the bladder program. The response to procedures that invade the intimate personal space of the individual can be tempered through the nurse's attention to the client's dignity, self-esteem, and need for privacy; complete explanation of diagnostic tests and nursing procedures; and validation of goals with the client and persons assisting.

Psychological response to self-insertion of catheters is influenced by the individual's age, sex, culture, and beliefs. Older individuals grew up in a time when handling of the genitals was thought to cause psychiatric problems. Women frequently have more familiarity with handling the genitals through tampon insertion and thus may be more comfortable with self-care. Different cultures have different norms and practices regarding the genital area. In Western cultures, the practice of elimination is performed in private. Rituals surround the bathroom and the activities carried out in this area of the home. People incorporate their beliefs regarding this area of the body into their value system. The nurse must assess the client's value system in planning the bladder program.

Motor skills. Performance of voiding facilitory techniques and self-catheterization require hand dexterity. The client must be able to transfer to a commode or toilet, place equipment within easy reach, exert enough pressure to either push urine manually from the bladder or stimulate the micturition reflex, and care for equipment. Clients who lack finger flexion may pick up, hold, and manipulate equipment by using tenodesis, the

normal flexion caused by extension of the wrist. Some finger contraction is necessary to make the grip functional. The use of flexor-hinge hand splints assists some clients in applying external collection systems.[14]

Clothing. In a general hospital setting, the majority of clients are issued hospital clothing that comes in "one size fits all." In rehabilitation settings, clients should be encouraged to dress in their own clothes as soon as the acute phase of their illness has passed.

Certain clothing choices and adaptations facilitate life for the client involved in a bladder retraining program. For men, trousers a size larger than usually worn provide extra room for collection devices and tubing. Boxer shorts rather than briefs also provide extra room. For women, dresses and skirts are preferred because they are easier to manipulate than slacks. The use of Velcro closures instead of snaps, buttons, or zippers makes it easier for both men and women to remove clothing to accommodate evacuation needs.

Privacy. As mentioned previously, in Western society, elimination is performed in private. There are closed doors in public bathrooms, at work, and at school. At home it is unusual for persons to void without closing the bathroom door. Yet in hospitals and specialized rehabilitation settings, clients frequently begin their bladder retraining program in bed, often in wards with other clients and with nursing staff members of recent acquaintance. The nurse should make every effort to work with the client in a private room, private area, or bathroom. When it is impossible to provide a private area, drapes should be drawn around the bed or commode before any discussion of the bladder program and before bringing equipment to the individual's unit.

Equipment. Many types of catheters, catheter insertion sets, external collection devices, tubes, leg straps, collection bags, and skin protection ointments are available. The equipment available in rehabilitation settings depends on the cost and evaluation by clients and rehabilitation team members. Problems with any kind of equipment should be brought to the attention of administration. The choice for equipment needs in the home depends on cost, third-party reimbursement, client satisfaction, availability, and convenience of replenishing supplies.

Fluids. Fluid intake is closely monitored for the individual involved in a bladder retraining program. Intermittent catheterization programs require scheduled and restricted fluid intake until a pattern is established or until the client learns to adjust fluid intake according to urine output. According to Perkash,[33] "prolonged intermittent catheterization with limitation on fluid intake is frustrating for spinal cord–injured patients with complete lesions and is even a hindrance to their rehabilitation." He suggests that we recognize early those clients in whom intermittent catheterization may not be successful and recommends careful urological intervention to establish a catheter-free state.

For clients with uninhibited bladders and those with urinary tract infections, fluids at regular intervals of up to 4,000 ml/day should be encouraged unless otherwise contraindicated. Scheduled voiding should be strictly followed.

External collection devices

External collection devices are used to guard against episodes of incontinence between scheduled voids in males. Unfortunately, women usually rely on absorbent padding because external devices have not been that successful with them. A variety of male external collection devices are available. All consist of a condom, drainage tubing, and adhesives or stretchable tape to attach the condom to the penis.

Tape that stretches should be used and wrapped in a spiral fashion to secure the condom to the penis. To maintain circulation, the tape should be wrapped downward without overlaps. The condom should be checked frequently to ensure free urine outflow without twisting and changed daily to prevent buildup of bacteria and odor.

The penile shaft should be washed, gently dried, and exposed to air between condom applications. The penis can be placed in a urinal while airing to collect spontaneous voids. Removing the external condom at night allows for longer periods of airing.[39] The penis should be checked regularly during the day and night for redness, allergic reaction, and swelling. If these conditions occur, the condom should be removed to permit healing. When swelling occurs, the penis should be elevated on a folded pad or linen roll. Cold applications, when ordered, should be covered before placement and should never be left on longer than 20 minutes.[39]

Concerns of nursing are to maintain skin integrity, circulation to the penis, and free flow of urine without pooling. The client or person assisting should be able to apply the collection device without difficulty and be able to purchase the chosen device at a minimum cost in a convenient location.

The Client with Difficulty Emptying the Bladder

The client with urine retention may have suprasacral or sacral lesions, with or without asynchrony of the voluntary external urinary sphincter muscle and the involuntary smooth muscle of the urethra and detrusor muscle. Voiding maneuvers, intermittent catheterization, administration of medications, electrical stimulation, urinary diversion, and other surgical interventions are used to assist this individual in emptying the bladder. The method chosen depends upon the underlying pathological problem, as indicated by neurological/urological diagnostic testing, and the person's psychosocial, intellectual, and motor status.

Voiding maneuvers

Voiding maneuvers differ according to the type of neurogenic bladder dysfunction. The nurse should know why specific voiding maneuvers are used and assist the client and family in adhering to the timing.

Upper motor neuron bladders: suprapubic triggering. Persons with suprasacral lesions void by stimulation of the micturition reflex arc. Stimulation of the sacral-lumbar dermatomes by manually tapping the suprapubic area, pulling pubic hairs, stroking or squeezing the genitalia, or stimulating the anus digitally are effective in stimulating bladder contraction and external sphincter relaxation.

These techniques are used in conjunction with intermittent catheterization. Once the client voids, the client or nurse immediately performs a straight catheterization to determine the amount of residual urine in the bladder. The amount of urine expelled spontaneously and the amount of urine obtained on catheterization are recorded.

At the beginning of the bladder retraining program, suprapubic triggering and catheterization are performed at 2- to 4-hour intervals. When 3 successive days pass without the residual urine exceeding 150 ml at each catheterization, one catheterization period is eliminated while the client or nurse maintains the schedule of suprapubic triggering. Urine pH is documented after each catheterization, with pH values above 7.0 invariably indicating infection with urea-splitting organisms. Also, residual amounts less than 50 ml are invariably associated with bladder infection.[33] Eventually all catheterizations are eliminated, and the client is maintained indefinitely with micturition reflex arc stimulation and periodic monitoring of residual urine volume. Men can wear an external collection device to minimize problems of incontinence between scheduled voids. As noted previously, women have had limited success with external devices.[27]

Lower motor neuron bladders: Credé method and abdominal strain. Persons with sacral lesions manually express urine from the bladder by applying external suprapubic pressure from above the abdomen toward the pubic area or exerting internal pressure if capable by use of abdominal strain (Valsalva maneuver). These techniques are contraindicated in persons with suprasacral lesions because reflex contraction of pelvic musculature increases the obstruction and inhibits the flow of urine.[36]

These techniques also are used in conjunction with intermittent catheterization. Clients use their fists or palms to press down over the bladder area while straining with the abdominal muscles. They are instructed to bear down as if having a bowel movement, wait 30 seconds to 1 minute before repeating the procedure, and continue to repeat the procedure until no more urine is expressed. Initially this procedure is performed every 4 hours, followed by intermittent catheterization. The amount of urine expressed manually and the amount of residual urine are measured and recorded. When the amount of residual urine is within a "safe" range, usually 50 to 150 ml at a certain time of day, the catheterization is stopped at that time and the client continues with only the voiding technique. As the residual urine decreases at the scheduled catheterization times, the catheterizations are gradually eliminated while the voiding techniques are continued at the scheduled times.

If the client does not have the manual dexterity to perform this maneuver or intermittent catheterization, then intermittent catheterization procedures alone may be performed by a helper.[27] Men are usually more successful in minimizing the problems of incontinence between scheduled

voids because of the availability of an external collection device.

Asynchrony of sphincters: anorectal stimulation. Persons who have asynchrony of the smooth muscle of the detrusor and the skeletal muscle of the external sphincter may be able to expel urine when anorectal stimulation is used. Although the response of the bladder and sphincters to anal stimulation is in dispute, it is mentioned as another technique helpful to some clients. Wu, Nanninga, and Hamilton[42] found that anal stretch inhibited the bulbocavernosus reflex and was a useful alternative technique for bladder emptying when clients with paraplegia had normal hand function and detrusor-sphincter dyssynergia. O'Shaughnessy, Clowers, and Brooks[32] found that in some clients, the detrusor reflex and the external sphincter contraction are inhibited. The simultaneous inhibition results in a detrusor-sphincter unit that assumes a lower motor neuron pattern. They suggest this occurrence as a rationale for the incorporation of the Credé and abdominal strain maneuvers in the anal stretch technique to allow clients with asynchrony to void. Other commonly accepted uses for anal sphincter stretch are to stimulate bowel evacuation and to allow easier catheter passage in those persons with external urethral spasm.

Intermittent catheterization

Intermittent catheterization was introduced in Great Britain by Guttmann[17] as the preferred method of treatment for World War II soldiers with neurogenic bladder dysfunction. He advocated a nontouch sterile technique performed in the operating room. It was not until the late 1960s that this treatment gained widespread acceptance in the United States. Now intermittent catheterization is the preferred treatment for persons with neurogenic bladder dysfunction resulting from trauma and a number of neurological diseases.

Intermittent catheterization has several advantages over indwelling catheterization and suprapubic cystostomy. The latter procedures invariably lead to bladder infection. Intermittent catheterization has the advantage of allowing the bladder mucosa, which has a decreased tone and tolerance to pressure immediately after an insult, to become gradually accustomed to a foreign body. Intermittent catheterization encourages the physiological stimulus to micturition, namely, some bladder distention while preventing overdistention, by setting up the appropriate impulses to the micturition reflex center in the spinal cord and promoting early return of detrusor activity. Thus physiological stretching of the bladder is maintained even during the period of spinal shock.[17]

Lapides and associates[25] postulated that bladder overdistention interrupted blood flow to the bladder, resulting in ischemia and lowered resistance to gram-negative bacteria found in the person's own intestinal tract. Thus they believed clients could learn to catheterize themselves because the key to prevention of infection was the prevention of overdistention rather than the sterility of the technique. Other studies have supported their findings.[9,24,26]

Goals. The goals of this procedure are to retrain the bladder, simulating a nearly normal voiding schedule; to assist the client in achieving a catheter-free state with use of external collection devices for males and pads for females for occasional incontinence; to eliminate the risks of infection, bladder calculi, penoscrotal abscess, and urethral diverticula associated with indwelling catheters; and to reduce the odor, appliances, lack of freedom, and inconvenience of indwelling catheters.

Procedure in institutions. Although the specifics of intermittent catheterization vary among institutions, the procedure is uniformly carried out under aseptic technique. The client and family should participate in the bladder retraining program from its inception.

In a typical intermittent catheterization program, catheterization is started at 2- to 4-hour intervals. Intake is restricted to 1,500 to 2,000 ml/24 hours. Careful attention is given to monitoring and recording intake and output. During the period of spinal shock, spontaneous voiding does not occur. As detrusor activity, bulbocavernosus reflex, and anal sphincter tone return, triggering of the micturition reflex or manual expression, depending upon the type of bladder, is performed before each catheterization. Catheter intervals are decreased if more than 400 to 500 ml of residual urine is obtained in order to prevent overdistention of the bladder. As residual urine decreases and spontaneous voiding increases in amount, the intervals between catheterizations are increased to 6, 8, 12, 24, 48, 72 hours, weekly, and finally monthly.[33] Stimulation

of the micturition reflex or Credé and abdominal strain maneuver is continued every 4 hours except when the client is sleeping. Intermittent catheterization is stopped when a balanced bladder is achieved. A bladder is considered balanced when the client can (1) pass adequate urine on reflex or easily with the Credé-Valsalva maneuver, (2) achieve a residual urine volume of 150 ml or less, and (3) remain free of pathological changes in the genitourinary tract.[33]

Self-catheterization in the home. Based on the findings of Lapides and associates,[25] intermittent self-catheterization using the clean technique was introduced. Although the clean technique is not used in institutional settings because of the number and variety of organisms present, the client and family are taught the sterile and clean procedure in the institutional setting. Compliance is improved if the procedure is simplified and performed in as nearly normal a position and location as possible. If the associated disability permits, women should sit on the toilet and men should stand in front of the toilet.[27] No lubricant is needed for females. A water-soluble lubricant is necessary for males to avoid traumatic urethritis.[22]

Techniques for cleaning and storing the catheters also should be kept simple. The catheter can be washed with ordinary soap and water or a detergicide if preferred. The catheters can be stored in a plastic sandwich bag in a pocket, purse, or bathroom.[27] Separate bags are kept for dirty catheters.

Clients should be taught to keep a daily record of times and amount of intake, amount of spontaneous void, and amount of residual urine on catheterization. They should be taught to observe the urine for color, odor, and particles. Any changes in output or the character of urine should be reported to the nurse or physician immediately. Clients should be advised to adhere strictly to the fluid restriction and catheterization schedule.

Special nursing considerations. The length of time during which intermittent catheterization must be continued varies according to the type of neurological bladder dysfunction and the condition of the client. The time required for persons with spinal cord injury to become catheter free varies from a few days to several weeks. Clients who have additional neurogenic bladder complications, such as an areflexic sphincter or detrusor sphincter dyssynergia may continue intermittent catheterization for months.

Problems and possible complications must be carefully monitored by the nurse. Persistent urinary calculi, frequent infection, and atrophic bladder requiring very frequent catheterizations interfere with attempts to become catheter free. The inability to adjust to the routine can become a problem for the client and for those who may be assisting with the bladder retraining program. When the client has an acute infection and is unable to take fluids, intravenous therapy may be required for short periods of time. An indwelling catheter may be inserted until oral fluid intake can be resumed.[39]

Not all clients are good candidates for intermittent catheterization. Many who have functioned with indwelling catheters for years are reluctant to comply with an intermittent catheterization program. Others may have harmful effects to the genitourinary tract after a long catheter-free period. Some clients have progressive disabilities, and decreasing hand function becomes a problem in maintaining the regimen. Early recognition of those who may not be candidates for an intermittent catheterization program prevents frustration for the client, family, and nursing staff.[39]

Administration of medications

The rehabilitation nurse is responsible for administering medications that assist the client in emptying the bladder. Many of these medications can be used singly or in combination to effect bladder function. The nurse must understand the category of drug, dosage, action, use, and nursing implications for each of the drugs prescribed (Table 10-1).

The Client with Difficulty Storing Urine

Clients with difficulty storing urine include those with uninhibited neurogenic bladders, those with surgical interruption of the sphincters, women with abnormally short urethras and resultant stress incontinence, and women with scar tissue and decreased tonicity of muscle and elastic tissues in the wall of the urethra. Urinary fistulas in women also may result from operative trauma, neoplasms, auto accidents, and gunshot wounds. Consequently, urine drains through a tract from the ureter, bladder, or urethra into

the vagina. In the male, a constant dripping incontinence may be associated with prostatectomy.[23]

Mild stress incontinence in women may be treated with perineal exercises involving isometric contractions of the periurethral muscles and the use of drugs producing sustained tonic contracture of urethral adrenergic smooth muscle. Those clients with severe stress incontinence frequently require surgery.[23]

Incontinence in the male after a prostatectomy is extremely difficult to treat, and the client may have to rely on an external collection device. The implantation of an artificial urinary sphincter has met with success in some males.

Scheduled voiding at regular intervals and attention to timing of fluid intake is helpful to persons with uninhibited neurogenic bladders. The prognosis for return of normal bladder function is excellent, because the reflex arc may remain intact, partial sensation of bladder filling may remain, and there may be partial voluntary control over voiding. Bladder training should start immediately. Accurate recording of intake and output, frequency of voids, the force of the urinary stream, and subjective sensations of the client should be closely observed and recorded. Treatment of any existing urinary tract infection may alleviate urgency and incontinence.

Drugs to decrease bladder contractility and increase bladder outlet resistance may be prescribed, depending upon the underlying pathological process (Table 10-1). Side effects of other drugs should be reviewed if the cause of incontinence cannot be determined.

The Client with Autonomic Hyperreflexia

As with any complication of neurogenic bladder, an ounce of prevention is worth a pound of cure. Excellent bowel, bladder, and skin care assist in preventing autonomic hyperreflexia. Elevating the head of the bed before any diagnostic procedure reduces intracranial pressure and blood flow. The urethra and bladder should be anesthetized before any diagnostic procedure, particularly if there is a history of autonomic hyperreflexia. Urinary tract infections should be treated appropriately to avoid bladder spasm.[10] The client and family should be made aware of the signs and symptoms of this condition. In many spinal cord

Text continued on p. 185.

TABLE 10-1 _____
Pharmacological agents commonly used to manage lower urinary tract dysfunction

Agent	Category	Oral dosage	Mode of action	Therapeutic use	Nursing implications
Bethanecol chloride (Urecholine)	Cholinergic	50-400 mg/day, divided doses; most effective when given subcutaneously 2.5-5 mg three or four times a day	Releases acetylcholine in terminals of postganglionic parasympathetic fibers; acts directly on smooth muscle of detrusor, increasing detrusor tone and decreasing bladder capacity	Hypotonic bladder dysfunction with high residual volumes	Hypotension usually occurs on rising; caution client to change positions slowly in stages, particularly from recumbent to sitting position; to avoid standing still; to avoid hot baths or showers; to lie down at first sign of faintness or lightheadedness Taking drug with meals minimizes hyperacidity, hypersalivation Contraindicated in mechanical outlet obstruction, peptic ulcer, asthma, hyperthyroidism, coronary artery disease, Parkinson's disease, pregnancy
Oxybutynin hydrochloride (Ditropan)	Antispasmodic activity with anticholinergic properties	5-20 mg/day, divided doses	Inhibits muscarinic action of acetylcholine on smooth muscle; directly depresses smooth muscle, produces local anesthesia	Detrusor hyperreflexia with urgency incontinence, no residual urine	May cause dizziness, drowsiness, blurred vision; warn client to avoid driving and other hazardous activities until reaction to drug is known Instruct client to avoid hot temperature because drug suppresses sweating See propantheline bromide

Modified from Cantanzaro M: Impairment of bladder function. In Snyder M, editor: A guide to neurological and neurosurgical nursing. New York, 1983, John Wiley & Sons, Inc.

TABLE 10-1 _____

Pharmacological agents commonly used to manage lower urinary tract dysfunction—cont'd

Agent	Category	Oral dosage	Mode of action	Therapeutic use	Nursing implications
Flavoxate hydro-chloride (Urispas)	Urinary anti-spasmodic, smooth muscle re-laxant	100-800 mg/day, divided doses	Exerts papaverine-like spasmolytic action on smooth muscle; reported to increase bladder capacity in clients with spastic bladder, possibly by direct action on detrusor muscle	Detrusor hyperreflexia, symptomatic relief of dysuria, frequency, urgency, nocturia, incontinence, suprapubic pain associated with various urological disorders	May cause drowsiness, confusion, blurred vision; caution clients to avoid driving or other hazardous activities that require alertness and physical coordination until reaction to drug is known Advise clients to report adverse reactions and lack of favorable response to nurse or physician See propantheline bromide
Pro-panthe-line bro-mide (Pro-Ban-thine)	Anticholin-ergic	7.5-240 mg/day, divided doses	Inhibits muscarinic effect of acetylcholine at receptor level; has ganglionic blocking effect; competes with acetylcholine for cholinergic receptors	Detrusor hyperreflexia; decreases bladder activity	Potentiated by antihistamines and other anticholinergic agents, including over-counter cold, allergy, and sleep medications Instruct client to notify nurse or physician about inability to void Manage constipation preventively with increased fluids, bulk, fruit Manage dry mouth by having client chew gum, suck hard candy Instruct client to avoid tricyclic antidepressants unless taken under medical supervision Contraindicated in glaucoma

Continued.

TABLE 10-1 _____

Pharmacological agents commonly used to manage lower urinary tract dysfunction—cont'd

Agent	Category	Oral dosage	Mode of action	Therapeutic use	Nursing implications
Pro-pantheline bro-mide (Pro-Ban-thine) —cont'd					Use with caution in clients with prostatic hypertrophy, gastrointestinal obstruction, coronary artery disease, megacolon, myasthenia gravis, obstructive uropathy of lower tract, pregnancy
Imipramine hydrochloride (Tofranil)	Adrenergic	10-40 mg/day, divided doses	Inhibits reuptake of norepinephrine at postganglionic sympathetic nerve endings; increases adrenergic effect, tonicity in bladder neck area; has relaxing effect on bladder dome	Hyperreflexic but inefficient detrusor contraction	May take up to 4 weeks to improve clinical symptoms; over-the-counter drugs for colds and allergies may potentiate effects; Large doses may have depressive effect in nonclinically depressed clients; Few side effects with low doses used for neurogenic bladder; usually dry mouth, constipation, blurred vision; Potentiates vasopressors in many over-the-counter drugs; Blocks action of guanethidine (Ismelin), clonidine (Catapres); Do not give concurrently or within 14 days of monoamine oxidase inhibitor
Phenyl-propanolamine hydrochloride (Ornade)	Alpha-adrenergic	1 capsule twice a day	Stimulates activity of beta-receptors of urethra and bladder	Sometimes effective in true stress incontinence	May cause insomnia, epigastric distress, palpitations, cardiac arrhythmias

TABLE 10-1 _____

Pharmacological agents commonly used to manage lower urinary tract dysfunction—cont'd

Agent	Category	Oral dosage	Mode of action	Therapeutic use	Nursing implications
Phenoxy-benza-mine (Diben-zyline)	Alpha-adren-ergic blocking agent	10-40 mg/ day in sin-gle or di-vided doses	Decreases bladder outlet resistance; occasionally com-bined with betha-necol to increase bladder pressure; blocks alpha-recep-tors in urethra and bladder neck	Functional outflow obstruction	Use cautiously in clients with car-diovascular dis-ease, hyperten-sion, hyperthy-roidism, prostatic enlargement, glaucoma Instruct client to contact nurse or physician if light-headed, espe-cially on rising, and if heart rate increases Contraindicated if client is receiving tranquilizers or sedatives or when sudden fall in blood pressure might be danger-ous
Dantro-lene so-dium (Dan-trium)	Skeletal mus-cle relax-ant	25-200 mg/ daily; highly in-dividual-ized	Directly relaxes spas-tic muscle by inter-fering with calcium (contraction activa-tor) release from sarcoplasmic reticu-lum; clinical doses produce about 50% decrease in con-tractility of skeletal muscles but no ef-fect on smooth or cardiac muscles	Relaxation of skel-etal muscle, in-cluding external urinary sphincter	Most common side effects are drows-iness, dizziness, fatigue, muscular weakness, general malaise, head-ache, diarrhea Risk of hepatotoxic-ity; perform base-line and regularly scheduled hepatic function tests (alkaline phospha-tase, serum glu-tamic-oxaloacetic transaminase, se-rum glutamic-pyruvic transami-nase, total biliru-bin), blood cell counts, and renal function Persistent diarrhea may necessitate drug withdrawal

Continued.

TABLE 10-1 _____

Pharmacological agents commonly used to manage lower urinary tract dysfunction—cont'd

Agent	Category	Oral dosage	Mode of action	Therapeutic use	Nursing implications
Dantrolene sodium (Dantrium) —cont'd					Warn client of possibility of dizziness and drowsiness; advise client to avoid driving and other potentially hazardous activities until reaction to drug is known Good tonicity in extremities is required by some clients to walk or carry out activities; this is major impediment to use of drug
Diazepam (Valium)	Anxiolytic	8-40 mg/day, divided doses	Appears to act at both limbic and subcortical levels of central nervous system to inhibit skeletal spasms	Detrusor sphincter dyssynergia	Most adverse reactions are dose related: drowsiness, ataxia, confusion, paradoxic rage Addiction-prone individuals, such as drug addicts or alcoholics, predisposed to dependency on this drug
Baclofen (Lioresal)	Skeletal muscle relaxant	5 mg three times a day, increased by 5 mg every 3 days until optimum response obtained; total daily dosage not to exceed 80 mg	Centrally acting skeletal muscle relaxant; precise mechanism of action unclear; decreases frequency and amplitude of muscle spasms by inhibiting transmission of monosynaptic (extensor) and polysynaptic (flexor) afferent reflexes at spinal cord level; may also act at supraspinal level, since it produces generalized central nervous system depression when given in large doses	External urinary sphincter spasticity; detrusor sphincter dyssynergia	May affect client's ability to stand or walk because of decrease in extensor spasms Instruct client to avoid alcohol and other central nervous system depressants because effects of these drugs are addictive Instruct client to avoid driving and other potentially hazardous activities Advise client to report adverse reactions

injury units, clients and family members are given printed instructions that help them recognize signs and symptoms and specify actions to take should these occur. These instructions can be shown to other health care providers, many of whom are unaware of this condition.

When signs and symptoms of autonomic hyperreflexia appear, the nurse should raise the head of the bed immediately to take advantage of orthostatic hypotension.[3] The blood pressure should be monitored at 3- to 5-minute intervals. If an indwelling catheter is in place, it should be checked for patency and replaced if plugged. If the client does not have an indwelling catheter, the tip of a catheter should be lubricated with an anesthetic agent and the client catheterized.

When a distended bladder is not the cause of an episode, the anal area should be anesthetized with Nupercainal ointment and the bowel checked for impaction. If an impaction is present, it should be removed with care and gentleness. Appropriate measures should be taken to produce near-normal body temperatures.

Hypertension usually subsides with the previously mentioned nursing interventions. If, however, neither the bladder nor bowel is responsible and other possible stimuli have been removed, the physician should be notified at once. Persistent diastolic hypertension in excess of 130 to 140 mm Hg may be treated with antihypertensive agents or nonsurgical interventions.

The Client with a Urinary Diversion

Urinary diversion procedures are performed when the person with a neurogenic bladder has progressive and severe ureteral renal damage because of vesicoureteral reflux or chronic infection. Several methods can divert the urinary stream so that it passes through the urethra or a new opening. Common urinary diversion procedures include indwelling catheterization, ileal conduit, ureterosigmoidostomy, and cystostomy (vesicostomy) with or without tubes.

Indwelling catheterization

Indwelling catheterization is probably the easiest and least aggressive form of urinary diversion. It is not without problems, however, and should be performed only when administration of medications, intermittent catheterization, neural blocks,

and various surgical procedures have failed.[36] An indwelling catheter left in the bladder and urethra for any length of time acts as a foreign body and irritates the mucosal walls of the urinary tract. To reiterate, the presence of the catheter predisposes the client to the development of penoscrotal abscesses, urethral diverticula, and urethral abscess.

Only nursing staff members familiar with aseptic insertion techniques and catheter care should handle catheters. Clients and staff members should be taught to wash their hands before and after handling any part of the catheter. The following sterile equipment is required: sterile gloves, a fenestrated drape, sterile sponges and an iodophor solution for periurethral cleansing, a basin, lubricant jelly, waste receptacle, and the appropriate size indwelling catheter. After insertion, the catheter should be anchored to the abdomen in males to prevent penoscrotal abscess. The catheter is attached to the thigh in females to prevent pull on the urethra.

The nurse should maintain a closed system of drainage and carry out the following practices:

1. The junction of the catheter with the drainage tube should never be broken except when obstruction is suspected and irrigation is required. Obtain specimens from the port with a syringe and introduce a small-gauge needle at an angle after cleaning with an alcohol sponge.
2. When the client ambulates, the drainage bag should remain attached to the catheter. Empty the drainage bag before suspending it from a belt around the client's waist. When the client is being bladder trained, the tubing may be clamped at prescribed intervals but never disconnected from the catheter.
3. Empty collection bags at least every 8 hours and take care to avoid contaminating the mouth of the spigot.
4. Collection bags may be suspended from the sides of beds, chairs, and stretchers, but should never be tipped upside down or raised above the level of the client's bladder.
5. Care of the perineum consists of washing with soap and water two times a day. This recommendation is simply to keep the periurethral area clean. Conflicting results have

been found regarding the use of povidine ointment.

6. Catheters should not be irrigated unless an obstruction is suspected. When it is necessary to irrigate, maintain sterile technique.[22]

7. Any time a catheter system is contaminated by inappropriate technique, accidental disconnections, leaks, or other means, it should be immediately replaced.

8. Catheterized clients should be separated from one another whenever possible. Separation of clients with infections from clients who do not have infections is particularly important.[41]

Certain rules guide the maintenance of good flow. The collection bag must *always* be kept below the level of the bladder and *never* be held upside down while emptying in order to prevent urine backflow. The bag must *never* touch the floor because of the possibility of ascending organisms. Careful attention should be given to the tubing and bag whenever the client moves in bed, sits up in a chair, or ambulates. Urine should always flow well from the drainage tube. If the entire tube is filled with urine, an obstruction should be suspected.[22]

Three liters of fluids per day should be encouraged, unless otherwise contraindicated, to reduce stasis and decrease the concentration of minerals in the urine. Renal and ureteral drainage can be improved by raising the head of the bed and encouraging the client to move about in a wheelchair.

When encrustation is observed around a catheter or when the drainage tube feels gritty as it is rubbed between the fingers, the catheter and tubing should be changed. If urine is draining well and there are no encrustations, there is no need to change the catheter.

The catheter is easily removed by aspirating fluid or air from the balloon with a syringe and a small-gauge needle at the filling port. When the balloon fails to deflate, the urologist should be contacted. One ml of lightweight mineral oil injected into the inflating lumen of the catheter may be prescribed. The bag will usually break within 5 minutes to an hour. Mineral oil should be washed out by irrigating the catheter before removal.[22] Intake and output should be monitored closely for 24 hours after removal of a catheter.

Failure to void may require intermittent catheterization or the reintroduction of the indwelling catheter.

Even when all necessary precautions have been taken, urine usually does not remain sterile beyond 7 days after catheter insertion. Most catheterized clients will remain asymptomatic despite the presence of organisms in the urine. It is impossible, however, to achieve sterile urine when a catheter is in place. Since the eventual outcome of antibiotic therapy used on a long-term basis is recolonization with bacteria resistant to most chemotherapeutic agents, the current thinking is that antibiotics should not be prescribed as a routine prophylactic measure.[27]

Ileal conduit

The most frequently performed urinary diversion procedure in which a new opening is created is the *ileal loop,* or *conduit.* This procedure also is referred to as ureteroileal urinary conduit, ileal bladder, ileal loop, Bricker's procedure, or ureteroileostomy.[8] In this procedure a short segment of the terminal ileum is isolated with its intact mesentery. Intestinal continuity is reestablished by anastomosis. The proximal end of the isolated segment of ileum is closed, the ureters are implanted in this segment of ileum; and the distal end is brought through the abdominal wall and secured to the skin. The client must wear an ileostomy appliance on the skin stoma to collect urine. Peristalsis in the ileal loop prevents stasis of urine, and there is no cross-contamination with feces.

Postoperatively the collecting device should be changed every 4 to 5 days or whenever it is leaking. A skin barrier or protectant should be applied if needed. Gentle pressure is applied around the appliance to remove air bubbles and to secure the adhesive or cement and the appliance to the skin. Tape around the appliance will give the client added security.

The time the nurse spends with the client before and after the surgery influences the retention of information regarding care of the stoma. Age, intelligence, dexterity, and visual acuity influence the rehabilitation process. The cost and availability of equipment and the client's economic resources must be considered in choosing urinary appliances on a short- and long-term basis. The client must be taught about accessories and skin care. Problems can occur with odor, stoma, skin, and diet.

Foods such as tomatoes and asparagus give the urine a strong odor and should be avoided. Also, wearing an appliance too long without cleaning it will result in an unpleasant odor. The ingestion of ascorbic acid and cleaning the pouch with white vinegar will help alleviate odors. The bag should be rinsed in warm water and then soaked in a vinegar and water solution for 30 to 60 minutes. It can then be rinsed, dried (avoiding sunlight), and powdered with cornstarch for storage until its next use.[8]

Adjusting to an external stoma is frequently very difficult. Clients must deal with a change in body image and potential alterations in self-concept, self-esteem, and sexual identity. Some recreational pursuits such as exercising at health clubs may be avoided because of the lack of privacy. The nurse should take time to assist the client in learning self-care and adjusting to these changes.[8]

Ureterosigmoidostomy

Ureterosigmoidostomy procedures are appealing because external appliances do not have to be worn. The flow of urine is directed into the rectum. In this surgical procedure the ureters are implanted into the colon as low as possible. The spread of bacteria and reflux of urine back to the kidneys is minimized because the ureters are attached to a section of the ileum rather than directly to the sigmoid colon.

Any fecal incontinence or the expulsion of flatus will result in urinary incontinence. The skin around the perianal area may become excoriated because of contact with feces and urine if diarrhea or incontinence develops. Because of the potential for reabsorption of electrolytes and fluid, leading to hyperchloremia, metabolic acidosis, and hypokalemia; magnesium deficit; hypercalcemia predisposing the client to calculi; pyelonephritis from urinary reflux; increased absorption of urinary ammonia, which may raise serum ammonia blood levels, and other complications, this procedure usually is not considered for young persons who have a normal life expectancy.[8]

Life-styles of these clients are changed because of altered body image and the need to adjust the diet to prevent complications. A diet high in potassium, low in chloride, and low in calcium will help prevent some of the complications just mentioned. Additionally, males need to adjust to the sitting position to urinate. Embarrassment results for both sexes with incontinence.[8]

Cystostomy (suprapubic procedure)

A cystostomy (*vesicostomy*) involves opening the bladder and draining urine through an abdominal wound either with or without a catheter. In some rehabilitation centers, this method is preferred to intermittent catheterization because of easier maintenance, the greater sexual freedom afforded the client, and the lack of availability of personnel and supplies to continue an intermittent catheterization program.[39]

A temporary cystostomy may be performed to treat a penoscrotal abscess with fistula or diverticula formation and epididymitis. Permanent cystostomies provide an entry portal for bacteria. The rehabilitation nurse takes the precautions suggested for indwelling urethral catheters to minimize the incidence of infection.

Namiki, Ito, and Yasuda[31] emphasize the difficulty in actually managing the nontouch intermittent catheterization technique during the acute phase of spinal cord injury in terms of proper staff and time. They believe that the results obtained with a closed, aseptic cystostomy in the acute stage of spinal cord injury are nearly as good as those obtained by the nontouch intermittent method. They do, however, point out the lower rate of urine sterility in those clients who can void without a catheter. Most of their paraplegic and quadriplegic clients acquired the ability to void without a catheter.

The Client with Selected Surgical Procedures

Other selected surgical procedures to assist the client in emptying the bladder are transurethral operations, implantation of artificial sphincters, and implantation of electrodes. Transurethral operations are performed for a number of reasons listed below. The success of implantation of artificial sphincters and electrodes is under evaluation.

Transurethral operations

The aim of transurethral operations is to decrease bladder outlet resistance in persons who have upper tract changes with high intravesical pressure and spastic external sphincters, areflexic bladders with inability to open the bladder neck, repeated urinary tract infections with high residual urine volumes, autonomic hyperreflexia with high residual urine volumes, or prolonged intermittent catheterization.[34] Commonly performed transurethral operations are transurethral resection of the bladder neck and external sphincterotomy. Neither operation should be performed until neurological stability is established (at least 3 to 4 months after the injury).

There are two types of external sphincterotomy. The first type involves both internal and external sphincterotomy and results in complete incontinence that requires constant use of an external collection device. This procedure is performed mainly in males who have outlet obstruction at both the bladder neck and at the external sphincter. The second type is performed when there is obstruction related solely to the external sphincter. Following this procedure, continence can be maintained and complete bladder emptying accomplished by use of Credé and abdominal strain maneuvers.[27]

Nursing interventions are directed toward support, information giving, and observation postoperatively for hemorrhage, extravasation, and infection. After removal of the indwelling catheter, intermittent catheterization may be performed for weeks to months until an acceptable residual urine volume is established. The nurse should be aware that males may be particularly troubled if rendered incontinent by a sphincterotomy because they experience dribbling during sexual intercourse and have difficulty changing clothes without becoming wet. The advantages of these procedures are that they do not interfere with erection as do phenol blocks and pudendal neurectomies. Bladder retraining programs should be reestablished with consideration of changes needed as a result of operative procedures.[39]

Implantation of artificial sphincter

The surgical implantation of prosthetic artificial sphincters in humans was first accomplished by Scott, Bradley, and Timm[38] in 1972. Their goals were to (1) render clients with neurological bladder dysfunction continent, (2) determine the safety of this procedure in humans, (3) establish the reliability of an internal device with external control, (4) demonstrate maintenance of normal lower tract function, and (5) show unobstructed flow during voiding.[38] The device also has been used in persons with stress incontinence, incontinence after a prostatectomy, and epispadias.

The principle is relatively simple. The silicone rubber prosthetic sphincter consists of four parts: (1) a reservoir, (2) an inflatable occlusive cuff, (3) an inflating pumping mechanism, and (4) a deflating pumping mechanism. The purpose of the cuff is to occlude the urethra, thus preventing urinary incontinence. The cuff surrounds the urethra and occludes urine flow when it is inflated. When the cuff is deflated, urine flows freely.

The reservoir is attached behind the rectus muscle where it is unlikely to be punctured accidentally. The inflatable occlusive cuff is placed at the bladder neck, membranous urethra, or around the bulbous urethra. The inflating bulb mechanism is implanted on the right side of the labium or scrotum; the deflating bulb on the left side of the labium or scrotum. The sphincter, reservoir, and bulbs are connected by a series of silicone tubes with one-way valves. Pressing on one bulb forces fluid from the bulb to the reservoir. When pressure on the bulb is released, the sphincter cuff is deflated and urine flows freely. Pressing the bulb on the opposite side inflates the sphincter cuff and occludes urine flow. When pressure on the second bulb is released, fluid flows from the reservoir to again fill the first bulb. These sphincters have been effective in controlling incontinence in a number of clients.

The nurse must understand the purpose and operation of the artificial urinary sphincter in order to observe for possible malfunction. She must be aware that this is an expensive mechanical device that could be damaged by urethral catheterization. This procedure has potential for controlling incontinence and promoting self-esteem.

Implantation of electrodes

Another surgical approach still being researched is the implantation of electrodes. Stimulation of the spinal cord, pelvic innervation of the detrusor muscle, one or more of the sacral ventral roots that innervate the detrusor, and direct application of electrodes to the detrusor muscle have been tried. The principle of synchronicity of anal and urinary sphincters has been used in the stimulation of the anus by means of an anal plug connected to an electrical unit. Drawbacks of current spread and spasticity of striated muscles have occurred with electrical stimulation. These procedures do not have widespread use and are under further investigation.[36]

Client and Family Education

The aims of client and family education are the prevention and recognition of urinary tract complications; prevention of lost time from work, school, or leisure activities because of urinary tract problems; and the return to social roles with some adaptations to accommodate the bladder retraining program.

Involvement of the client in the bladder program should begin as soon as possible after admission to a rehabilitation setting. Client goals for bladder management should be established either verbally or in a written contract. Clients should know from the beginning that the program may change as neurological/urological status changes. The family, with agreement on the part of the client, should be taught all aspects of bladder care.

Assessment of the learner before offering information is essential for learning to occur. The nurse must determine the client's physical ability, mental and intellectual ability, emotional response to altered bladder function, hand dexterity, and functional potential. Teaching a client who has no grip, no strength, and a low activity tolerance despite high motivation to perform self-catheterization can be extremely frustrating for the client and the nurse.

Knowledge is needed in the following areas: anatomy and physiology of the urinary tract; prevention of infection; recognition of symptomatic urinary tract infection, autonomic hyperreflexia when applicable, urinary retention, and urinary tract stones; actions to take when complications occur; and cleaning and care of urinary equipment. The client should be able to perform voiding facilitation maneuvers and intermittent catheterization, insert and change indwelling catheters, and apply external collection devices according to the prescribed bladder retraining program. The name, dose, reason for taking, and side effects of any urinary tract medications should be known. The client should know when the drugs are to be taken, where to obtain them, and when to obtain refill prescriptions. Those clients who continue intermittent catheterization at home should know how to measure residual urine volume after spontaneous voids and be taught to keep an accurate record of date, time, and amount of fluid intake and urine output. The importance of keeping follow-up appointments should be stressed.

Clients who are unable or unwilling to participate in the bladder retraining program should be consulted regarding preferences for a family member to assume the responsibility. Family members may be placed in awkward positions if the participation in this intimate area of rehabilitation affects their relationship with the client. For example, a mother may agree to catheterize her 20-year-old quadriplegic son, but performance of this procedure may be detrimental to their preinjury relationship. In such instances, the son may be able to identify a willing person whom he would prefer to perform the procedure. When the client and family member are unwilling or unable to participate in the bladder retraining program, referral is made to a public health or visiting nurse.

Correct performance of procedures requires demonstration by the nurse and redemonstration by the client or family. Guidance and supervision is needed initially. Aseptic technique is taught in the rehabilitation setting but instructions for use of clean technique at home are given. Printed instructions supplement verbal instructions and are used for reference and reinforcement when the client returns to the community.

Documentation of what was taught, when, by whom, and the client's response should be recorded on a continuing basis in the chart. Consistency in instruction among team members is promoted when the chart reflects the teaching-learning process. Close communication between the client and family or community nurse helps determine further learning needs regarding the bladder program after discharge.

DISCHARGE PLANNING AND FOLLOW-UP

Discharge planning begins immediately after the acute phase of illness has passed. Conferences planned between the client, family, and rehabilitation team members as soon as possible after admission to the rehabilitation facility assist in clarifying perceptions of the disability and in establishing goals during the rehabilitation process.

The goals in effect at admission will change as the client's functional level improves. Likewise, the goals in effect at discharge may not be relevant

3 months later. The client and family should know that the neurological/urological status of the bladder may change. They should know what the client may or may not do to remain free of complications, and what assistance is needed in bladder management activities.

Home assessments before discharge ascertain the availability of bathroom facilities. These assessments may be made by asking the family to bring measurements and information about the home to the rehabilitation team or by visits of team members to the home. Recommendations are made for modification when the client, family, and team members deem them necessary for maintenance of the home bladder management routine.

Before discharge, all aspects of bladder management should be reviewed and any additional questions answered. The telephone number of the primary nurse, physiatrist, primary physician, or urologist should be given to the client so that any questions that arise at a later time can be answered. The availability of team members establishes a supportive connection in the transition from institution to community. Additional anxiety can be decreased by assuring that all supplies are available for the first day at home.

The client should be reminded to call the nurse or physician any time danger signs occur. Danger signs to be reported include urine retention, high temperature, severe headache with sweating or chills, abdominal pain, just feeling sick, bloody urine, and swelling or abscess of the scrotum.[39]

Referral to a community nursing agency is necessary when the client and family are unwilling or unable to carry out the bladder management program. Even when they can assume responsibility, a brief period of supervision after discharge can help the client adjust to equipment, adapt to home problems, and continue the bladder management program.

Despite strict adherence to the bladder management program, the potential exists for bladder complications to occur throughout the person's life. The client with no clinical evidence of complications should have an annual x-ray examination of the abdomen to rule out calculous disease. In addition, blood studies, including a complete blood cell count, BUN level, and creatinine clearance should be done annually.[33] Clients with recurrent complications should be monitored more frequently for urine culture and sensitivity and other tests deemed appropriate. The frequency of follow-up visits will depend upon the specific problems of the client.

REHABILITATION TEAM INTERVENTIONS

The coordination, communication, and cooperation of all rehabilitation members is necessary for successful bladder rehabilitation. Short- and long-term goals are established for the bladder program. The client and family members are the most important members of the team and should be involved from the beginning of rehabilitation in establishing these goals. All team members must be aware of the bladder program and consider the timing of the specifics of the client's bladder program as the individual participates in other aspects of the total rehabilitation process. The physiatrist, neurologist, and urologist are responsible for the medical and surgical management of the neurogenic bladder dysfunction. Other team members may participate directly in bladder rehabilitation by helping the client to work independently with assistive devices to insert catheters and apply external collection devices. The social worker may work indirectly by arranging financial resources for purchase of medications and supplies, securing homemaking or nursing assistance from community agencies, and suggesting resources for adaptations to the home. In many rehabilitation units, the nurse, occupational therapist, and physical therapist will assess the home situation and make recommendations for adaptation of bathroom facilities.

A system of recording and communicating among team members should include potential problems or activities that may interfere with the client's bladder management routine, the effect of specific activities on the client's ability to control urine flow, and reinforcement of the bladder management program when the client is away from the nursing unit. Other team members should understand the effect of medications received by the client for bladder management. In addition, all rehabilitation team members should have knowledge of the signs and symptoms of autonomic hyperreflexia and know the actions to take when these occur. Information should be provided on a daily basis among team members regarding the client's discussion of the bladder elimination routine, the frequency of visits to the toilet, adaptations in current activities, and proposed adaptations that might help the client maximize independence. Information given about the bladder management routine to family members should be documented in the record to maintain consistency in the rehabilitation process.

OUTCOME CRITERIA

The success of bladder rehabilitation can be measured in terms of outcome. Outcome criteria are based on goals and provide a blueprint for evaluation. It is easier to measure objective criteria, in other words, criteria that can be quantified. Some criteria will necessarily relate to the client's perceived feeling of well-being and self-esteem in relation to control of bladder elimination, and measurement depends upon self-reports.

Objective outcome criteria that can be quantified are as follows:

1. The client and family can demonstrate cleansing technique related to bladder elimination.
2. The client and family can demonstrate, as applicable, care of an indwelling catheter, straight catheter, external urinary device, or stoma collection bag and the equipment associated with these appliances.
3. The client and family can arrange clothing for bladder elimination.
4. The client and family can name the drugs prescribed, dose, action, reason for use, possible side effects, and actions to take should these occur.
5. The client and family can describe the signs and symptoms of urinary tract infection and actions to take should these occur.
6. The client and family can describe the signs and symptoms of autonomic hyperreflexia and actions to take should these occur (when applicable).
7. The client and family can describe how, where, and when to obtain medications and supplies.
8. The client maintains a residual urine volume below 150 ml.
9. The client remains free of significant bacteria.
10. The client remains free of complications.
11. The client keeps follow-up appointments.

Subjective outcome criteria depend upon self-reports of clients and family and include the following:

1. The client and family follow a bladder management program consistent with and useful in their daily pattern of living.
2. The client maintains self-esteem and performs social roles.

SUMMARY

The client with neurogenic bladder dysfunction poses a challenge for rehabilitation nurses. The rehabilitation nurse must understand normal bladder function and alterations that may cause problems in storing urine and expelling urine from the bladder. A comprehensive assessment of bladder function is necessary to identify the specific bladder problem and to establish goals with the client and family. Nursing interventions are designed to maximize bladder elimination. Integral to the success of bladder rehabilitation is the participation of the client and family from the time of admission to the rehabilitation setting and communication and collaboration among rehabilitation team members in relation to the bladder management program designed for each client.

TEST QUESTIONS

Circle the most appropriate response.
1. The normal bladder can store _____ ml of urine.
   a. 150-250
   b. 250-350
   c. 350-450
   d. 450-550
2. The bladder and sphincters are under the control of the _____ nervous system.
   a. Autonomic
   b. Somatic
   c. Peripheral
   d. Central
3. Lesions that interrupt the neural pathways to the bladder may occur in the:
   a. Spinothalamic tract
   b. Cauda equina
   c. Cortex
   d. All of the above
4. Complications of a neurogenic bladder include:

   a. Autonomic hyperreflexia
   b. Detrusor sphincter dyssynergia
   c. Hydronephrosis
   d. All of the above
5. While eliciting a history from the client related to bladder impairment, the nurse assesses the client's:
   a. Hand function
   b. Intellectual function
   c. Self-care abilities
   d. All of the above
6. Significant bacteriuria exists when the colony count obtained from a single culture is:
   a. 10^2
   b. 10^3
   c. 10^4
   d. 10^5
7. A diagnostic test used to determine glomerular filtration rate is:
   a. BUN level
   b. Creatinine clearance
   c. Urinalysis
   d. Urine culture and sensitivity
8. Assessment of a client with an autonomous neurogenic bladder indicates:
   a. Absent or hypoactive peripheral reflexes
   b. Spastic paralysis
   c. Presence of a bulbocavernosus reflex
   d. Presence of sphincter tone
9. Assessment of a client experiencing autonomic hyperreflexia indicates:
   a. Tachycardia, hypotension, and perspiration below the level of the lesion
   b. Bradycardia, hypertension, and perspiration above the level of the lesion
   c. Flushing and warmth below the level of the lesion
   d. Dramatic rise in the diastolic blood pressure
10. General considerations when planning interventions for a bladder retraining program are:
    a. Psychosocial responses of the client to various interventions
    b. Hand dexterity
    c. Type of clothing and equipment needed
    d. All of the above
11. A nursing intervention used to assist the client with an autonomous neurogenic bladder to void is:
    a. Pulling pubic hairs
    b. Digital stimulation of the anus
    c. Tapping the suprapubic area

   d. Applying pressure over the bladder by use of the Credé maneuver and abdominal strain
12. A nursing intervention(s) used to assist the client with a reflex neurogenic bladder to void is (are):
    a. Tapping the suprapubic area
    b. Pulling pubic hairs
    c. Stroking the genitalia
    d. All of the above
13. A nursing intervention(s) used to assist the client with uninhibited neurogenic bladder to void is (are):
    a. Scheduled voiding
    b. Pulling pubic hairs
    c. Applying pressure over the bladder by use of the Credé maneuver and abdominal strain
    d. All of the above
14. A nursing intervention that should be carried out immediately for the client experiencing autonomic hyperreflexia is to:
    a. Lower the bed and place the client in a supine position
    b. Raise the head of the bed and put the client in an upright sitting position
    c. Monitor the blood pressure every hour
    d. All of the above
15. The nurse teaches that intermittent catheterization
    a. Allows physiological stretching of the detrusor muscle
    b. Invariably leads to bladder infection
    c. Requires proper placement of the urinary collection bag
    d. Is a foreign body that remains in the bladder
16. A drug administered by the nurse to relax skeletal muscle of the external sphincter is:
    a. Bethanechol chloride (Urecholine)
    b. Oxybutynin hydrochloride (Ditropan)
    c. Baclofen (Lioresal)
    d. Phenylpropanolamine (Ornade)
17. Nursing interventions when the client has an indwelling Foley catheter include all of the following *except:*
    a. Maintain a closed system of drainage.
    b. Obtain specimens from the port of the catheter tube with a small-gauge needle introduced at an angle after cleaning with an alcohol sponge.
    c. Raise the collection bag above the level of

the bladder when the client is transported for therapy.

d. Empty the drainage bag at least every 8 hours, taking care to avoid contaminating the mouth of the spigot.

18. Nursing interventions postoperatively for the client who has had a transurethral operation include:
    a. Support and information giving
    b. Observation for hemorrhage, extravasation, and infection
    c. Reestablishment of the bladder retraining program with consideration of changes needed as a result of the operative procedures
    d. All of the above
19. Information needed by the client and family to assume responsibility for the bladder rehabilitation program includes:
    a. Signs and symptoms of urinary tract infection
    b. Name, dose, reason for taking, and side effects of urinary tract medications prescribed for the client
    c. Cleaning and care of urinary equipment
    d. All of the above
20. All rehabilitation team members should understand:
    a. The timing of the bladder training program
    b. Signs, symptoms, and actions to take when autonomic hyperreflexia occurs
    c. The effect of specific activities on the client's ability to control urine flow
    d. All of the above

Answers: 1. c, 2. a, 3. d, 4. d, 5. d, 6. d, 7. b, 8. a, 9. b, 10. d, 11. d, 12. d, 13. a, 14. b, 15. a, 16. c, 17. c, 18. d, 19. d, 20. d.

LEARNING ACTIVITIES

1. Using the interview guide for obtaining a history from a client with altered bladder function, perform a nursing assessment by talking to and observing the client, talking to the family, and reviewing the results of diagnostic tests. State your nursing diagnoses.
2. With the client and family assessed as described in the preceding activity, establish realistic goals for the bladder rehabilitation program. Share these goals with other rehabilitation team members at a team conference.

3. Visit a local medical supply store. Examine the various types of catheters, external collection devices, and urine collection bags available. Obtain the cost of each appliance. Report the pros and cons of each appliance to your classmates or staff members.
4. Prepare to teach one of your clients to perform self-catheterization. In writing your lesson plan, consider the client's mental status and intellectual ability, hand dexterity, and fatigue tolerance. State your objective, teaching method, audiovisual resources, content, and client activities, as well as your method of evaluation. Use the lesson plan to teach one of your clients to perform self-catheterization.

REFERENCES

1. Anderson RU and Hsieh-ma ST: Association of bacteriuria and pyuria during intermittent catheterization after spinal cord injury, J Urol 130:299, 1983.
2. Anthony CP and Thibodeau GA: Textbook of anatomy and physiology, ed 11, St Louis, 1983, The CV Mosby Co.
3. Bell J and Hannon J: Pathophysiology involved in autonomic hyperreflexia, J Neurosci Nurs 18:86, April 1986.
4. Bors E and Comarr AE: Neurological urology, Baltimore, 1971, University Park Press.
5. Cantanzaro M: Impairment of bladder function. In Snyder M, editor: A guide to neurological and neurosurgical nursing, New York, 1983, John Wiley & Sons, Inc.
6. Cantanzaro M and others: Urinary bladder dysfunction as a remedial disability in multiple sclerosis: a sociologic perspective, Arch Phys Med Rehabil 63:472, 1982.
7. Chambers JK and Hawks JH: Specific disorders of the kidneys and urinary system. In Kneisl CR and Ames SW, editors: Adult health nursing: a biopsychosocial approach, Reading, Mass, 1986, Addison-Wesley Publishing Co, Inc.
8. Chambers JK and Hawks JH: Surgical approaches to kidney and urinary system dysfunction. In Kneisl CR and Ames SW, editors: Adult health nursing: a biopsychosocial approach, Reading, Mass, 1986, Addison-Wesley Publishing Co, Inc.
9. Champion V: Clean technique for intermittent self-catheterization, Nurs Res 25:13, Jan/Feb 1976.
10. Chui L and Bhatt K: Autonomic dysreflexia, Rehabil Nurs 8:16, March/April, 1983.
11. Chusid JG: Correlative neuroanatomy and functional neurology, ed 19, Los Altos, Calif, 1985, Lange Medical Publications.
12. Cotterell M and Miller M: Nursing implications of drug therapy, Geriatr Nurs 1:271, 1980.

13. Drach GW: Urinary lithiasis. In Harrison, JH and others, editors: Campbell's urology, ed 4, vol 1, Philadelphia, 1978, WB Saunders Co.
14. Ford JR and Duckworth B: Physical management for the quadriplegic patient, ed 2, Philadelphia, 1987, FA Davis Co.
15. Gordon M: Nursing diagnosis: process and application, ed 2, New York, 1987, McGraw-Hill Book Co.
16. Govoni LE and Hayes JE: Drugs and nursing implications, ed 5, Norwalk, Conn, 1985, Appleton-Century-Crofts.
17. Guttmann L: Spinal cord injuries: comprehensive management and research, ed 2, Oxford, 1976, Blackwell Scientific Publications, Ltd.
18. Johnson JH: Rehabilitative aspects of neurogenic bladder dysfunction, Nurs Clin North Am 15:293, 1980.
19. Kee JL: Laboratory and diagnostic tests with nursing implications, Norwalk, Conn, 1983, Appleton-Century-Crofts.
20. Kracht H and Buscher HK: Formation of staghorn calculi and their surgical implications in paraplegics and tetraplegics, Paraplegia 12:101, 1974.
21. Kunin CM: Urinary tract infections, Surg Clin North Am 60:223, 1980.
22. Kunin CM: Detection, prevention and management of urinary tract infections, ed 3, Philadelphia, 1979, Lea & Febiger.
23. Lapides J and Diokno AC: Urine transport, storage, and micturition. In Lapides J, editor: Fundamentals or urology, Philadelphia, 1976, WB Saunders Co.
24. Lapides J and others: Further observations on self-catheterization, J Urol 116:169, 1976.
25. Lapides J and others: Clean intermittent self-catheterization in the treatment of urinary tract disease, J Urol 107:458, 1972.
26. Maynard FM and Glass J: Management of the neuropathic bladder by clean intermittent catheterization: 5-year outcomes, Paraplegia 25(2):106, 1987.
27. McConnell EA and Zimmerman MF: Care of patients with urologic problems, Philadelphia, 1983, JB Lippincott Co.
28. Merritt JL: Residual urine volume: correlate of urinary tract infection in patients with spinal cord injury, Arch Phys Med Rehabil 62:558, 1981.
29. Metheny N: Renal stones and urinary pH, Am J Nurs 82:1372, 1982.
30. Monson R: Autonomic dysreflexia: a nursing challenge, Rehabil Nurs 6:18, Nov/Dec 1981.
31. Namiki T, Ito H, and Yasuda K: Management of the urinary tract by suprapubic cystostomy kept under a closed and aseptic state in the acute stage of the patient with a spinal cord lesion, J Urol 119:359, 1978.
32. O'Shaughnessy EJ, Clowers DW, and Brooks G: Detrusor reflex contraction inhibited by anal stretch, Arch Phys Med Rehabil 62:128, 1981.
33. Perkash I: Management of neurogenic dysfunction of the bladder and bowel. In Kottke FJ, Stillwell GK, and Lehmann JF, editors: Krusen's handbook of physical medicine and rehabilitation, ed 3, Philadelphia, 1982, WB Saunders Co.
34. Perkash I: An attempt to understand and to treat voiding dysfunctions during rehabilitation of the bladder in spinal cord injury patients, J Urol 115:36, 1976.
35. Piotrowski MM: Functioning of the normal and neurogenic bladder, ARNJ 5:13, March/April 1980.
36. Raz S and Bradley W: Neuromuscular dysfunction of the lower urinary tract. In Harrison JH and others, editors: Campbell's urology, ed 4, vol 2, Philadelphia, 1978, WB Saunders Co.
37. Saxton DF and others: The Addison-Wesley manual of nursing practice, Menlo Park, Calif, 1983, Addison-Wesley Publishing Co, Inc.
38. Scott FB, Bradley WE, and Timm GW: Treatment of urinary incontinence by an implantable prosthetic urinary sphincter, J Urol 112:75, 1974.
39. Shields L: Urinary function. In Martin N, Hot NB, and Hicks D, editors: Comprehensive rehabilitation nursing, New York, 1981, McGraw-Hill Book Co.
40. Smith DR: General urology, ed 10, Los Altos, Calif, 1981, Lange Medical Publications.
41. Stamm WE: Guidelines for prevention of catheter-associated urinary tract infections, Ann Intern Med 82:386, 1975.
42. Wu Y, Nanninga JB, and Hamilton BB: Inhibition of the external urethral sphincter and sacral reflex by anal stretch in spinal cord–injured patients, Arch Phys Med Rehabil 67:135, 1986.

ADDITIONAL READINGS

Abramson AA: Neurogenic bladder: a guide to evaluation and management, Arch Phys Med Rehabil 64:6, 1983.
Anderson TP and others: Urinary tract care: improvement through patient education, Arch Phys Med Rehabil 64:314, 1983.
Bataille P and others: Effect of calcium restriction on renal excretion of oxalate and the probability of stones in the various pathophysiological groups with calcium stones, J Urol 130:218, 1983.
Brink C: Assessing the problem, Geriatr Nurs 1:241 Dec 1980.
Brunner L and Suddarth D: The Lippincott manual of nursing practice, ed 3, Philadelphia, 1982, JB Lippincott Co.
Conti MT and Eutropius L: Preventing UTIs: what works? Am J Nurs 87:307, 1987.
DeVivo MJ and Fine PR: Predicting renal calculus occurrence in spinal cord injury patients, Arch Phys Med Rehabil 67:722, 1986.
Erickson RP and others: Bacteriuria during follow-up in patients with spinal cord injury. I. Rates of bacteriuria in various bladder-emptying methods, Arch Phys Med Rehabil 63:409, 1982.
Finkbeiner A: Helpful drugs, Geriatr Nurs 1:270, 1980.

Fleming WC: Recurrent bacteriuria in complete spinal cord injury patients on external condom drainage, Arch Phys Med Rehabil 61:178, 1980.

Gonzalez R and DeWolf WC: The artificial sphincter AS-721 for the treatment of incontinence in patients with neurogenic bladder, J Urol 121:71, 1979.

Halstead LS and others: Neurologically active drugs in spinal cord injury: a clinical coding system, Arch Phys Med Rehabil 59:358, 1978.

Hanak M and Scott A: Spinal cord injury: an illustrated guide for health care professionals, New York, 1983, Springer Publishing Co, Inc.

Implementing urologic procedures, Horsham, Pa, 1981, Nursing '81 Books.

Killian A: Reducing the risk of infection from indwelling urethral catheters, Nurs '82 12:84, May, 1982.

Kinney AB and Blount M: Effect of cranberry juice on urinary pH, Nurs Res 28:287, 1979.

Kuroiwa Y and others: Frequency and urgency of micturition in hemiplegic patients: relationship to hemisphere laterality of lesions, J Neurol 234(2):100, 1987.

Lapides J: Mechanisms of urinary tract infection, Urology 24:217, Sept 1979.

Lindner A, Kaufman JJ, and Shlomo R: Further experience with the artificial urinary sphincter, J Urol 129:962, 1983.

Martin N, Holt NB, and Hicks D: Comprehensive rehabilitation nursing, New York, 1981, McGraw-Hill Book Co.

Merritt JL, Erickson RP, and Opitz JL: Bacteriuria during follow-up in patients with spinal cord injury. II. Efficacy of antimicrobial suppressants, Arch Phys Med Rehabil 63:413, 1982.

Merritt JL, Lie M, and Opitz JL: Bladder retraining of paraplegic women, Arch Phys Med Rehabil 63:416, 1982.

Mohler JL, Cowen DL, and Flanigan RC: Suppression and treatment of urinary tract infection in patients with an intermittently catheterized neurogenic bladder, J Urol 138:336, 1987.

Nelson AL and Kelley B: Patient and family workshops: a new teaching approach in spinal cord injury, Rehabil Nurs 8:13, Nov/Dec 1983.

Newman E and Price M: Bacteriuria in patients with spinal cord lesions: its relationship to urinary drainage appliances, Arch Phys Med Rehabil 58:427, 1977.

Niederpruem MS: Autonomic dysreflexia, Rehabil Nurs 9:29, Jan/Feb 1984.

Patterson BM: A new approach to an old problem, Rehabil Nurs 12:257, 1987.

Ramphal M: Urinary incontinence among nursing home patients: issues in research, Geriatr Nurs 8:249, Sept/Oct 1987.

Ruge CA: Shock (wave) treatment for kidney stones, Am J Nurs 86:400, 1986.

Snyder M, editor: A guide to neurological and neurosurgical nursing, New York, 1983, John Wiley & Sons, Inc.

Sperling KB: Intermittent catheterization to obtain catheter-free bladder function in spinal cord injury, Arch Phys Med Rehabil 59:4, Jan 1978.

Steinberg R and others: Construction of a low pressure reservoir and achievement of continence after "diversion" in end stage vesical dysfunction, J Urol 138:39, 1987.

Voith AM: A conceptual framework for nursing diagnoses: alterations in urinary elimination, Rehabil Nurs 11:18, Jan/Feb 1986.

Wells T and Brink C: Helpful equipment, Geriatr Nurs 1:264, 1980.

CHAPTER 11

Bowel Elimination

Elizabeth L. Sharkey
Denise Hanlon

OBJECTIVES

After completing Chapter 11, the reader will be able to:

1. Explain the anatomy and physiology of bowel elimination.

2. Describe impairments in bowel elimination as these relate to the rehabilitation client.

3. Assess a client's bowel function and ability to manage bowel elimination.

4. Formulate nursing diagnoses associated with impaired bowel elimination.

5. Develop goals with the client and family that foster maximum independence in bowel elimination.

6. Determine nursing interventions to assist the client in maintaining and restoring bowel elimination.

7. Identify the interventions of other rehabilitation team members in assisting the client to maintain and restore bowel elimination.

8. List outcome criteria used to evaluate the effectiveness of planned intervention for impaired bowel elimination.

Control of bowel function is a basic human need that is the subject of varying levels of concern throughout a person's life. Children learn early that successful control of bowel function gains them praise and signifies that they are maturing. Thus, bowel function is an area of intense concern for the young child. As children mature into teenagers and then adults, other developmental tasks become the primary focus and normal bowel function is given little thought. Bowel function then reemerges as an area of concern to the older population whose main focus tends to be on regularity rather than control. However, when bowel function is compromised by any of various disorders, it may become an area of intense concern at any age.

Although not discussed openly, bowel function is an area of concern to most individuals, and down through the ages the subject has been embellished by myths and old wives' tales, advertising, and even medical fads. At one time "autointoxication from the colon" was regarded as a causative factor in a number of diseases of unknown etiology. It was taken so seriously that some surgeons performed colectomies for this reason. Today's elderly were brought up during this era and were led to believe that taking laxatives regularly was necessary for good health. Today we continue to hear advertisements promoting products that prevent constipation and imply that a daily bowel movement is necessary. Despite this heightened awareness of bowel function and habits, most people seldom think or talk about the subject unless they are faced with a problem in controlling or regulating function.

The ability to control bowel function may be compromised by a variety of neuromuscular disorders, including multiple sclerosis, stroke, traumatic head injury, tumor, syringomyelia, spina bifida, transverse myelitis, diabetes, intervertebral disk disease, and traumatic injury to the spinal cord. Altered bowel function may occur whenever the central nervous system (CNS) has been impaired. When disease or disability results in loss of control of the bowels, the incontinence may become as devastating a problem as the disability itself.

Disorders of regularity also cause considerable difficulties for some individuals. Constipation is a problem faced by most persons at one time or another and is especially persistent among the elderly. Much remains unknown or poorly understood about chronic constipation, but among the many known causes, the two most common are improper diet and inactivity. Constipation not only causes discomfort, but if neglected, it may lead to impaction and possibly bowel obstruction. Diarrhea is the opposite problem from constipation. Causes of diarrhea range from psychosomatic (irritable bowel) origins to infectious (bacterial, viral, or protozoal) agents with hosts of other causes in between, such as enzyme deficiency, gastrointestinal surgery, and drug side effects.

Management of impaired bowel function is primarily under the guidance of the rehabilitation nurse. Planning nursing care requires an in-depth knowledge of normal function. Normal bowel functioning is altered in many of the injuries or disorders in which rehabilitation nurses become involved, such as the young person with paraplegia or the elderly individual who suffers a stroke. The rehabilitation nurse also assists otherwise healthy individuals experiencing altered bowel function.

NORMAL BOWEL FUNCTION

The primary function of the alimentary tract is to provide the body with a continual supply of water, electrolytes, and nutrients via digestion and absorption. Figure 11-1 illustrates the entire alimentary canal, showing major anatomical differences among its parts. The portion of the tract from the stomach to the anus is the gastrointestinal (GI) tract. Most digestive activity takes place here, but the term GI tract often is loosely applied to the entire alimentary tract.

A myriad of autoregulatory processes keeps food moving along the GI tract at an appropriate pace—slow enough for digestion and absorption to occur and fast enough to provide the body with nutrients. Food that is neither digested nor absorbed while passing through the GI tract is excreted as feces (defecation). Defecation is a function requiring a complex integration of voluntary and involuntary mechanisms, and any interruption of these mechanisms may result in impaired bowel function.

In this section, normal function of the GI tract is discussed in relation to those functions that affect bowel elimination: secretion, innervation, functional movements, and defecation.

Secretion

Secretory glands located throughout the entire GI tract serve two primary functions. First, digestive enzymes are produced from the mouth to the end of the ileum. These secretions are composed of enzymes and electrolytes formed in response to food in the alimentary tract, and the quantity secreted in each segment is the amount necessary for proper digestion. Second, mucous glands from the mouth to the anus produce mucus to protect and lubricate the walls of the tract and to ease the passage of food and partially digested products.

Innervation

The GI tract is composed of several layers of smooth muscle fibers. Figure 11-2 illustrates a

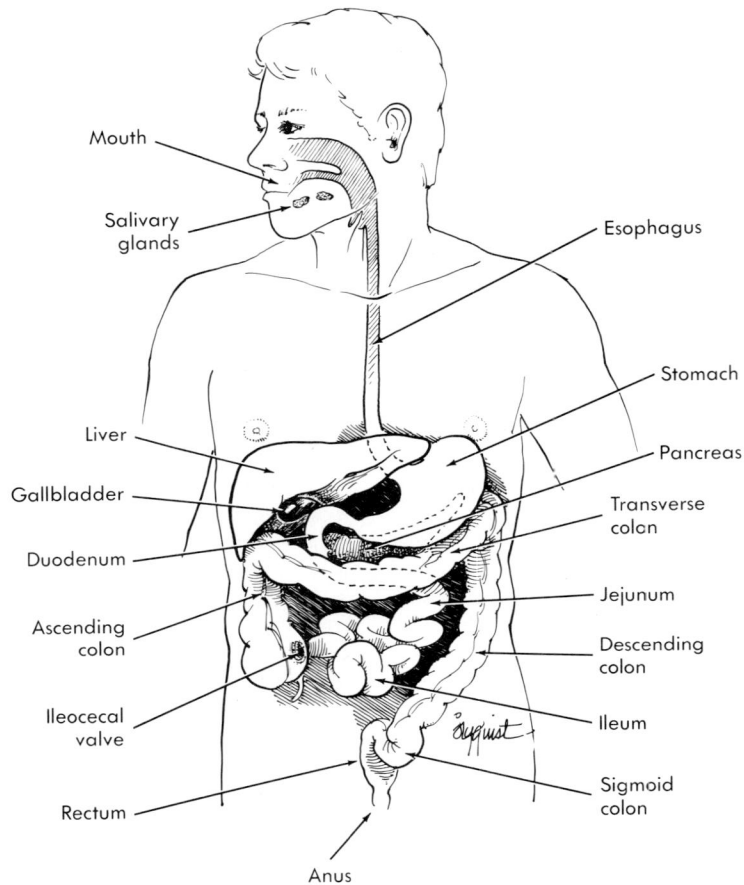

Figure 11-1
Alimentary tract.

typical section of the intestinal wall. Individual cells lie in extremely close contact. Therefore intracellular electrical impulses can travel easily from one smooth muscle fiber to another. The smooth muscle of the GI tract exhibits "pacemaker" activity similar to heart muscle in that electrical signals originating in one smooth muscle fiber are generally propagated from fiber to fiber.

Electromyographic studies have shown that this smooth muscle exhibits tonic contractions that maintain a steady pressure on the contents of the GI tract. The internal anal sphincter, composed of circular smooth muscle, also is in a state of tonic contraction and thus acts as a safeguard

against loss of small amounts of fecal material into the anal canal. In addition to tonic contractions, different parts of the GI tract also exhibit rhythmic contractions. These contractions are responsible for phasic functions, such as mixing of food and peristalsis.

Intrinsic innervation

In addition to the tonic and rhythmic contractions of the smooth muscle itself, the GI tract functions through its own intrinsic (originating entirely within the gut) nerve supply. The intramural nerve plexus begins in the esophagus and extends all the way to the anus. It is composed of two layers: (1) the outer or myenteric plexus located

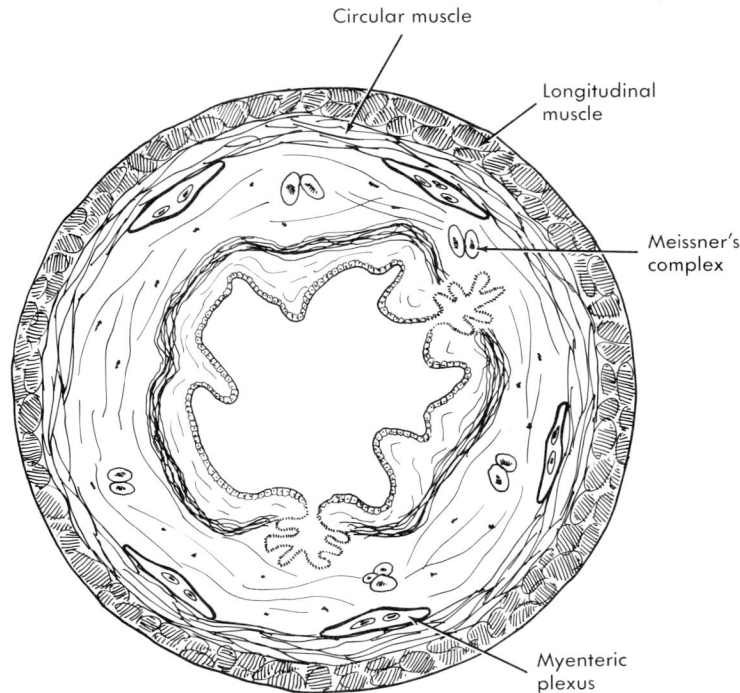

Figure 11-2
Cross section of gut. *(From Guyton AC: Basic human physiology, Philadelphia, 1977, WB Saunders Co.)*

between the longitudinal and circular muscle layers and (2) the inner layer or submucosal plexus in the submucosa (Figure 11-2). The myenteric plexus is far more extensive than the submucosal plexus and controls mainly the GI movements. The submucosal plexus controls secretion and also receives signals from the gut epithelium and stretch receptors in the gut wall, facilitating many sensory functions.

The entire intramural plexus is responsible for neurogenic reflexes occurring locally in the gut, such as a localized secretion of digestive juices by the submucosal glands. In addition, the plexus is responsible for coordinating the functional motor movements of the gut (segmentation and peristalsis). This intrinsic nervous system allows the gut to continue to function in isolation from its extrinsic nerve supply. However, signals from the brain via the autonomic nervous system can alter the degree of activity of the intrinsic nervous system.

Extrinsic innervation

The autonomic nervous system extensively innervates the entire GI tract. Sympathetic and parasympathetic activity may alter the overall activity of the gut or specific parts.

The parasympathetic supply is divided into cranial and sacral divisions. The cranial supply is transmitted almost entirely by the vagus nerve and provides extensive innervation to the esophagus, stomach, and to a lesser extent the small bowel, gallbladder, and first half of the large bowel. The sacral fibers originate in S2, S3, and S4 segments of the spinal cord and pass through the nervi erigentes to the distal half of the large bowel (Figure 11-3). The sigmoid, rectal, and anal regions of the large intestine are abundantly supplied with parasympathetic fibers that function to facilitate the defecation reflexes.

The postganglionic neurons of the parasympathetic system are part of the myenteric plexus.

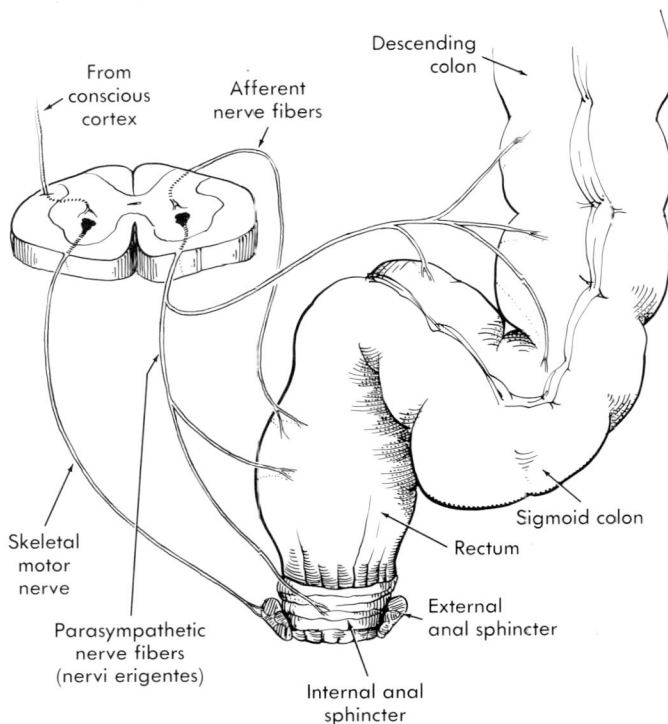

Figure 11-3
Afferent and efferent pathways of parasympathetic mechanism for defecation reflex. *(From Guyton AC: Basic human physiology, Philadelphia, 1977, WB Saunders Co.)*

Stimulation of the parasympathetic nervus results in increased activity of the plexus and therefore excites the gut wall, which in turn facilitates the intrinsic excitatory nerve reflexes of the GI tract.

The sympathetic fibers originate in the spinal cord between spinal cord segments T8 and L2 and innervate essentially all of the GI tract. After leaving the cord, the preganglionic fibers enter the sympathetic chains and pass through the chains to the outlying ganglia, that is, celiac ganglia and mesenteric ganglia. The postganglionic neuronal cell bodies are located here, and the postganglionic fibers spread from them along with blood vessels to all parts of the gut.

Stimulation of the sympathetic nervous system generally results in decreased activity of the GI tract, causing effects opposite to parasympathetic stimulation. Strong stimulation of the sympathetic system can totally halt movement of food through the GI tract.

Functional Movements of the GI Tract

The two basic types of movement in the GI tract are *mixing* and *propulsive*. The basic propulsive movement is referred to as *peristalsis*. Mixing keeps the intestinal contents blended thoroughly at all times during transit, and peristalsis keeps the food moving along the GI tract at an appropriate rate for digestion and absorption. To a great extent, however, some mixing and propulsion occur simultaneously. These actions are discussed according to occurrence in the small intestine and large intestine.

The small intestine

The mixing contractions of the small intestine occur when a portion becomes distended with

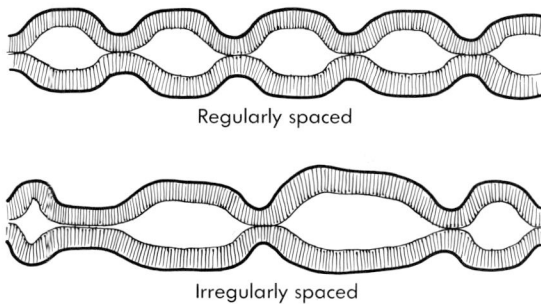

Regularly spaced

Irregularly spaced

Figure 11-4
Segmentation movements of small intestine.

chyme, a gruel-like material produced by the action of gastric juice on food. Localized, concentric ring–like contractions are elicited and spaced at intervals along the intestine. These areas of segmentation give the intestine the appearance of a chain of sausage (Figure 11-4). As one set of contractions subsides, another occurs at a different point along the intestine, thus promoting chopping and progressive mixing of the intestinal contents with the secretions of the small intestine.

Peristalsis is a series of waves. These waves are caused by distention and excitation of the stretch receptors in the gut wall, which in turn elicit a local myenteric reflex. The longitudinal muscles contract over a distance followed by a contraction of the circular muscle. The contractile process of peristalsis spreads toward the anus.

The myenteric plexus controls the movement of the peristaltic contraction down the GI tract. Passage of chyme from the pylorus to the ileocecal valve normally requires 3 to 10 hours. After meals this peristaltic activity is greatly increased, partly because of distention from entry of chyme and partly because of the gastrocolic reflex. This reflex occurs when food enters the stomach and stimulates the myenteric plexus to increase peristalsis and secretions in the small intestine. The small intestine also can increase peristalsis significantly when irritation or overdistention occurs. This mechanism is known as *peristaltic rush*. The waves travel the entire length of the small intestine in a very short time and can sweep the contents of the small bowel into the colon in a few minutes, thus relieving the small intestine of its irritation or distention.

The ileocecal valve located at the terminal ileum has the principal function of preventing backflow of fecal contents from the colon into the small intestine. The wall of the ileum is thickened near the end immediately preceding the ileocecal valve. This thickened area, known as the *ileocecal sphincter*, remains mildly constricted at all times and slows the emptying of small intestine contents into the cecum except after meals when the gastrocolic reflex intensifies peristalsis. This resistance to emptying at the ileocecal valve prolongs the stay of intestinal contents and therefore facilitates digestion and absorption. Approximately 450 ml of chyme empties from the ileum into the cecum every day.

The large intestine

The two main functions of the colon are to absorb water and electrolytes from the intestinal contents and to store fecal material until it can be expelled. Very little movement is required for these functions, so movement of the colon is normally sluggish.

Mixing and segmentation movements occur in the colon but differ somewhat from those of the small intestine. The colon bulges outward into baglike sacs called *haustral contractions*. These contractions occur at a very slow rate, thereby allowing the fecal material to be gradually exposed to the entire surface of the colon. Fluids are progressively absorbed until only 80 ml of the 450 ml load of chyme is lost in the feces.

Propulsion in the colon occurs in mass peristaltic movements. Mass movements propel the feces toward the anus. These movements occur only a few times each day, most frequently immediately after breakfast. The mass movement occurs when a distended or irritated portion of the colon, most often the transverse or descending colon, constricts, forcing the fecal material en masse down the colon. When the fecal mass has been forced into the rectum, the desire to defecate is felt.

Mass movements are caused in part by stimulation of the gastrocolic and duodenocolic reflexes when the stomach and duodenum are distended, and these movements are transmitted via the myenteric plexus. However, irritation in the colon also can initiate mass movements. For example, a person with ulcerative colitis has mass movements almost all of the time. Temperature changes with ingestion of hot and cold liquids also stimulate mass movements.

Defecation

The rectum is empty of feces most of the time. When mass movement forces feces into the rectum, the process of defecation is initiated and includes a reflex contraction of the rectum and a relaxation of the internal and external anal sphincters. These sphincters are normally in a state of tonic contraction to prevent constant dribbling. The internal anal sphincter is composed of smooth muscle, and the external sphincter is composed of striated voluntary muscle controlled by the somatic nervous system. Both autonomic and somatic systems are involved in the act of defecation.

The defecation reflex begins when sensory nerve fibers in the rectum are stimulated by the presence of fecal material. Signals are transmitted into the sacral portion of the spinal cord (S2-4) and then reflexly back to the descending colon, sigmoid, rectum, and anus by the parasympathetic nerve fibers (Figure 11-3). These signals initiate strong peristaltic waves to evacuate the rectum and at times the descending colon.

The afferent signals entering the spinal cord initiate other concurrent activities associated with defecation, such as taking a deep breath, closing the glottis, contracting the abdominal muscles (*Valsalva maneuver*), and raising the levator muscles around the rectum to aid in expulsion of the feces. However, voluntary straining may be eliminated without impeding defecation.

Along with the reflex mechanism, somatic control also is necessary for voluntary defecation to take place. The conscious mind controls the external sphincter and either inhibits its action to allow defecation or further contracts it if it is not convenient to defecate. When contraction of the sphincter is maintained, the defecation reflex dies out, not to return until additional feces enter the rectum. Voluntary inhibition can thus disrupt the normal defecation mechanism. New defecation reflexes may be initiated at a later, more convenient time by taking a deep breath, moving the diaphragm down, and contracting the abdominal muscles to increase abdominal pressure, forcing fecal contents into the rectum and eliciting new reflexes. These reflexes, however, are not as effective as those that arise naturally. People who inhibit their natural defecation reflexes too often become constipated.

IMPAIRED BOWEL ELIMINATION

Impaired bowel elimination is manifested by constipation, diarrhea, and incontinence. Discussion of each of these conditions follows.

Constipation

Constipation is a condition experienced by most persons at some time during life. The term constipation has different subjective meanings to different persons. Some define it as frequency of bowel movements less than it used to be or less than the person *thinks* it should be; others define it as movements that are difficult and require undue straining. Often both factors are present together. Other characteristics of constipation may include a feeling of incomplete emptying of the rectum and production of very small stools. Few studies have been done to evaluate the bowel habits of a healthy population eating a standard diet. Connell and others[4] studied frequency of bowel movements and found that 98% of the population moved their bowels between three times a day and three times a week.

Transit time through the colon can be measured clinically by the radiopaque colonic transit time study. This procedure is carried out by giving the client radiopaque markers in small capsules that are swallowed and then following with either direct x-ray examination of the abdomen or radiographs of the feces on successive days. A person with normal bowel motility passes 80% of the swallowed markers within 5 days, whereas constipated individuals experience delayed transit time of the markers through the colon.

Many clinicians now agree that there is more than one type of constipation. Carnevali and Patrick[3] describe three types of constipation hypotonic, hypertonic, and "habit."

Hypotonic constipation is noted when the rectum reveals soft, puttylike stool on digital examination. The colon is full of stool, and impaction is a common problem. This type of constipation is caused by lack of motility both in the segmental contractions and in those that cause mass movements.

Hypertonic constipation is characterized by hard, dry stools and in some cases, lower abdominal pain. In this type of constipation, there is an increase in activity of the segmental contractions but not of the propulsive type. This activity results in decreased transit time but increased reabsorption of water.

Habit constipation is primarily the result of poor eating habits—a diet lacking fiber. It also may be caused by consciously or unconsciously ignoring or preventing the urge to defecate.

Etiology

A variety of factors contribute to constipation. The most frequent cause of constipation in the adult population is irregular bowel habits developed through a lifetime of inhibition of the normal defecation reflexes. Failure to allow defecation to take place when the defecation reflexes are excited or overuse of laxatives to take the place of normal bowel function results in progressively weaker reflexes over a period of time. Consequently, the colon becomes *atonic*.

Immobility also seems to be a crucial factor predisposing to constipation, especially in the older population. It should be noted that the ingestion of food *alone* does not produce mass movement of the colon in the *resting* client— physical movement also is important.

The gastrocolic reflex combines with morning physical activity to cause mass propulsive movements, forcing the feces into the rectum. Distention of the rectum then produces the urge to defecate. If the urge is ignored or deliberately inhibited, it passes, and feces may move back from the rectum into the sigmoid colon.

Therefore the immobile person may have two reasons for becoming constipated. First, physical activity to stimulate the mass propulsive movement is lacking, and second, dependence on a nurse to allow the person to respond to the urge to defecate is necessary. If not given the opportunity to respond to that urge at the appropriate time, the urge may pass, and later it may not be possible for the person to defecate.

Constipation also has been linked to dietary habits, specifically a low-residue diet. Several studies have concluded that the addition of fiber to the diet provides faster passage of digested substances, reduces long transit time, and increases the water content of the stool.[6,19] Mechanisms of this process remain unknown, but shorter transit time in the colon decreases the chance of becoming constipated.

Constipation may be the first symptom of many diseases, such as hypothyroidism, hypercalcemia, and depression, or it can be a side effect of various drugs such as codeine. In determining the cause of constipation, a differential diagnosis is necessary.

Psychosomatic factors are known to affect bowel function. Emotional disturbances, expressed as either depression or enhancement of activity, frequently are accompanied by altered functioning of the colon. A direct correlation has not been found between certain emotional states and resulting colonic activity, but a strong association has been demonstrated. "In general, reactions to pain, fear, and anxiety produce pallor of the mucosa, reduced secretion of mucus, and inhibition of motility."[5]

Complications associated with constipation

A fecal impaction occurs when a hard compacted mass of fecal material that cannot be expelled accumulates in the rectum. Impaction usually is seen when the person has been constipated for several days. However, there may be some leakage of liquid stool and fecal incontinence. The diagnosis of impaction is validated by the presence of hard stool upon rectal examination.

Fecal incontinence is often a complication of untreated or improperly treated constipation. Unfortunately, fecal incontinence is all too prevalent among nursing home residents and those in extended care facilities. Fecal incontinence is frequently accepted by nursing staff members and family when it could be prevented through proper treatment of constipation. There are many other causes of incontinence, and if the individual is not constipated or continues to be incontinent after adequate treatment of constipation, other causes must be considered. Among other causes are carcinoma of the rectum or colon, diverticular disease, ischemic colitis, Crohn's disease, ulcerative colitis, or rectal prolapse. Persons with cerebrovascular disease and Alzheimer's disease also may have a form of fecal incontinence.

Diarrhea

Diarrhea results from rapid movement of fecal matter through the large intestine. Diarrhea is a too frequent emptying of the bowel with passage of stool in a liquid or very loose form. Normally the colon absorbs water from solid wastes received from the small intestine. When something interferes with that absorption or causes the bowel to secrete rather than absorb liquid, or when something speeds the passage of wastes through the bowel so that there is insufficient time to absorb fluid, diarrhea results.

The greatest hazard of diarrhea is the loss of water and electrolytes needed for normal cell function. Severe dehydration and electrolyte imbalance can cause cardiac arrhythmias, severe hypotension, renal failure, and death, especially in infants and very young children, elderly persons, and persons debilitated by extreme illness. Most of the time, however, diarrhea is not that severe or life threatening. It may be chronic and recurring or most frequently, an acute symptom lasting for only a day or so. In any case, diarrhea is a signal that something has disrupted normal function of the GI tract.

Etiology

The major cause of diarrhea is an infection called *enteritis*, which is caused by bacteria, protozoa, or a virus in the GI tract. The usual sites of this infection are the terminal ileum and the large intestine. Wherever the infection is present, the mucosa of that area of the bowel becomes irritated and increases its rate of secretion. Additionally, the motility of the bowel greatly increases. As a result, large amounts of fluid are available to wash the infectious agent away, and the strong propulsive movements move the fluid toward expulsion by the anus. Diarrhea, then, is an important mechanism for ridding the intestinal tract of debilitating infections.

Psychosomatic factors also have been linked to diarrhea. Everyone has experienced the cramps and urgency associated with fear, anxiety, or intense excitement just before an important occasion. In general, anger, resentment, embarrassment, and overt or subconscious hostility are associated with hyperemia, engorgement, increased secretion of mucus, and increased motility of the colon. Extreme responses to emotional states may lead to irritable bowel syndrome, characterized by uncoordinated and abnormal motor function, abdominal pain, flatulence, and constipation usually alternating with diarrhea. This syndrome affects some 22 million Americans, with signs and symptoms generally starting between the ages of 20 and 40 years and affecting twice as many women as men.

Irritable bowel syndrome is frequently caused or aggravated by stress, but recent studies have linked it to an intolerance of certain foods, such as wheat, corn, dairy products, coffee, tea, and citrus fruits.[13] Persons with irritable bowel syndrome also are unusually prone to migraine headaches and severe menstrual pain, suggesting that they may have a generalized, underlying disorder of the smooth muscles. Lack of fiber in the diet also has been linked to this condition. Signs and symptoms almost always improve when foods high in fiber are added to the diet.

A common but frequently overlooked cause of diarrhea and excessive flatulence may be an insufficiency of the enzyme lactose, which digests milk sugar. Eliminating such foods as milk, cottage cheese, ice cream, and yogurt from the diet for about a week determines if lactose insufficiency is the cause. Lactose insufficiency can often be overcome by pretreating milk with the enzyme or by taking mild digestant tablets just before consuming milk products.

Food allergies, although rare, also may cause diarrhea. In this case, severe cramps and other allergic reactions such as hives may accompany severe diarrhea. Some persons develop diarrhea by eating too many bowel-stimulating foods such as prunes, bran, or figs or by drinking too much coffee. Once identified, the diarrhea can be controlled by simply avoiding the offending food.

Diarrhea also may be caused by various drugs. Excessive consumption of certain sugar substitutes such as sorbitol and mannitol found in dietetic foods may cause the problem. Antibiotics often cause diarrhea by killing many bacteria that normally reside in the colon and are responsible for digesting unabsorbed foods passed along from the small bowel. This type of diarrhea ends when the antibiotic therapy is stopped.

Incontinence

To reiterate, the process of voluntary defecation is controlled by the autonomic nervous system (involuntary) and the somatic nervous system (voluntary). When any of these motor and sensory pathways are compromised, voluntary bowel control is altered. Impairment of cerebral control (the awareness of urge and ability to inhibit defecation), anal sphincter control, or anal sphincter sensation results in fecal incontinence.

When damage has occurred to the CNS, bowel function is initiated and regulated without mediation by the cerebral cortex. This condition is referred to as *neurogenic bowel*. There are five categories of neurogenic bowel dysfunction, but only three types are commonly seen in rehabilitation practice. These types are uninhibited, reflex, and autonomous neurogenic bowel. Motor paralytic and sensory paralytic neurogenic bowel are rarely seen. It is important to determine the classification of bowel dysfunction in order to plan an appropriate bowel program for each affected individual.

In differentiating the types of neurogenic bowel dysfunction, certain motor and sensory tests can be used. To plan successful bowel programs to cope with these dysfunctions, it is necessary to understand the significance of such tests and their use.

Saddle sensation is a perianal sensation elicited in response to a pinprick or light touch. The presence of sensation indicates intact sensory function at the sacral spinal cord level. An awareness of the urge to defecate helps establish bowel control.

The *bulbocavernosus reflex* may be elicited by gently squeezing the clitoris or glans penis and observing for a visible contraction of the external anal sphincter and a palpable contraction of the bulbocavernosus and ischiocavernosus muscles. A positive response indicates that reflex bowel function may be expected to return after spinal shock subsides. *Spinal shock* (spinal areflexia) is a transient condition occurring after complete disruption of the spinal cord. There is decreased synaptic excitability of neurons manifested by absence of somatic reflex activity and flaccid paralysis below the level of damage. Hypotension, bladder paralysis, and interference with defecation may occur because of autonomic nervous system involvement, especially in higher level lesions. Spinal shock may last anywhere from hours to weeks. A return of reflex activity in a shorter period of time may be expected in persons with incomplete lesions.

The *anal reflex* (anal wink) may be elicited by a pinprick to the skin adjacent to the external anal sphincter. A visible contraction (or wink) of the sphincter indicates a positive response and signifies that reflex bowel function will return following the period of spinal shock.

Uninhibited neurogenic bowel

In cortical and subcortical lesions above the C1 vertebral level, as seen in cerebrovascular accident, multiple sclerosis, and certain types of brain trauma and tumors, bowel function is classified

as *uninhibited*. There is damage to the upper motor neurons located in the cerebral cortex, internal capsule, brainstem, or spinal cord, with sparing of lower motor neurons located in the anterior gray matter throughout the entire length of the spinal cord. Bowel sensation is intact, as is saddle sensation, and the bulbocavernosus reflex is intact or increased.

Sensory impulses travel through the sacral reflex arc to the brain, but the brain is unable to interpret the impulses to defecate. As a result of decreased cerebral awareness of the urge to defecate, there is decreased voluntary control of the anal sphincter. Involuntary elimination occurs when the sacral reflex is activated. Because sensation is not impaired, the incontinence is accompanied by a sense of urgency.

Reflex neurogenic bowel

Reflex neurogenic bowel function (also referred to as automatic) occurs with spinal cord lesions above the T12 to L1 vertebral level. Lesions in this area involve the upper motor neurons and sensory tracts but spare the lower motor neurons. Quadriplegia, high thoracic paraplegia, and multiple sclerosis are associated with this dysfunction. Other possible etiologies include tumor, vascular disease, syringomyelia, and pernicious anemia. In most cases, bowel sensation and saddle sensation are diminished or absent, and the bulbocavernosus reflex is increased.

Nerve pathways between the brain and spinal cord are interrupted. This interruption may be complete or incomplete. In either type of lesion, there is no voluntary control of defecation or of the anal sphincter. Fecal incontinence occurs suddenly without warning as part of a mass reflex. The sacral nerve segments of S2-4 are intact, and it is therefore possible to develop a stimulus-response type of bowel control using the mass reflex. The intact spinal reflex arc functions when feces accumulate in the rectum and create distention, causing the bowel to empty by reflex. The parasympathetic innervation via the sacral segments of the spinal cord maintains anal sphincter tone so that fecal incontinence between mass reflex emptyings is not a problem.

Autonomous neurogenic bowel

Autonomous (flaccid) bowel function occurs with spinal cord lesions at or below the T12 to L1 vertebral level. Lesions in this area affect the lower motor neurons and are usually associated with paraplegia, spina bifida, tumor, and intervertebral disk disease. Sensation is diminished to absent, and the bulbocavernosus reflex is absent.

Nerve pathways between the brain and spinal cord are interrupted, but the extent of neural compromise depends on whether the injury is complete or incomplete. As in reflex bowel function, there is neither cerebral control of defecation nor voluntary control of the anal sphincter. Unlike reflex bowel function, however, the lesion directly involves the S2-4 segments, and the activity of the spinal reflex arc is destroyed. Therefore, no reflex emptying of the bowel occurs. Additionally, both the internal and external anal sphincters lack tone. Since there is little or no resistance to stool in the rectum, fecal incontinence is frequent.

Other factors contributing to incontinence

Diseases of peripheral nerves supplying the external anal sphincter may result in fecal incontinence. Bowel problems also may be the result of disease of the anal sphincter or weakness of the diaphragm, the abdominal muscles, or muscles of the pelvic floor.

NURSING ASSESSMENT

Before any bowel program can be implemented, the nurse must perform a comprehensive assessment of the client. When combined with a knowledge of normal and impaired bowel function, this assessment becomes the foundation for successful management.

To develop a safe, effective bowel program for the particular needs of the individual, there are many factors to be considered:

- Physical status
- Past bowel routine
- Dietary habits
- Functional status
- Medications
- Potential for cooperation
- Future life-style

Physical Status

The overall physical condition of the client must be assessed with special notation made of the cause of the disability, the neurological status, and any other factors that might affect bowel function and ability to participate in a bowel program. The

three commonly seen neurogenic bowel dysfunctions discussed previously have specific interventions that are discussed in detail later in this chapter. The level of neural dysfunction of the bowel can be assessed using the motor and sensory tests described previously in the discussion on incontinence.

The client's ability to recognize and communicate should be evaluated. Does the client understand the staff when questioned about the need to toilet? Speech and language, visual, or auditory impairments may prevent the client from locating or being able to use the call button and thus from participating fully in a bowel program.

Past Bowel Routine (Bowel History)

The admission history elicits a detailed description of the present illness, as well as the perceived bowel problem. From observation and interview, the nurse should note the consistency of the stool; episodes of incontinence, diarrhea, or constipation; and the presence of fecal impaction. Impaction may be suspected if there is abdominal distention along with diarrhea-like movements, but manual examination is more definitive. Any past history of sphincter disturbances, ulcerative colitis, diverticulitis, or hemorrhoids requires a more detailed history. Chronic overuse of laxatives or enemas should be determined. Former bowel habits, including time of evacuation frequency, and personal habits to stimulate defecation should be reviewed. Neurological disease or disability significantly alters life-style, and it may not be easy to reestablish former patterns. The nurse must attempt to determine former habits and anticipate future life-style to plan an effective, client-centered bowel plan with the client, family, and other team members.

Dietary Habits

The client's diet and appetite should receive careful attention. Assessment of preonset habits should include food preferences, cultural practices, and nutritional adequacy. The sufficiency of the diet for facilitating elimination should then be reviewed. Diets poor in fiber and fluid and high in gas-forming foods, as well as inconsistent diets, must be evaluated and changed because these create problems in regulating routine and consistency of stool. For instance, foods that caused diarrhea, excessive flatus, or constipation before the onset of disability are likely to cause the same response now.

Certain aspects of the disability may impact negatively on the client's dietary needs. For example, the person with a stroke may suffer from dysphagia, making chewing and swallowing difficult. Individuals who have lost a great deal of weight following their disability may now have ill-fitting dentures that affect their ability to chew food properly. Those who must use adaptive equipment to feed themselves often select only foods that are managed easily. Disability-related data should be thoroughly assessed when planning food intake to facilitate regular bowel function.

The client's endurance level should be considered when assessing dietary habits. Does the client tire easily and consequently have difficulty completing a large meal? Should small frequent feedings be considered? Is the energy level sufficient to prepare balanced meals while at home, or will "fast foods" dominate the diet? Is there a support system in place at home to assist with food preparation if necessary?

Functional Status

The client's ability to manage a bowel routine independently affects planning for the bowel program. For example, it is necessary to teach family members or attendants to help a person with high quadriplegia, whereas a person with paraplegia may require only assistive devices and equipment. The elderly client may suffer from degenerative joint disease that makes getting to the toilet difficult. Ability to transfer from bed to toilet or commode should be assessed and, if necessary, adaptations made to allow the client to perform the bowel program with the greatest degree of independence possible. Ambulation and the ability to perform personal hygiene activities should be assessed as these relate to bowel habits.

Medications

Following disease or disability, the client may be taking many medications. For purposes of establishing a bowel program, the nurse should be aware that those medications fall into two broad categories—those that assist in the bowel program and those that are prescribed for other medical reasons.

To assist with the bowel program, stool softeners and bulk formers are often prescribed. These medications are discussed more specifically later in this chapter. The nurse should determine the effect of the currently prescribed medications in order to plan the bowel program appropriately. For instance, if the client is reporting continuous soft stools throughout the day, the nurse may want to consider increasing the bulk formers within the prescribed range.

Medications prescribed for other medical conditions also must be evaluated, since they may have undesirable side effects (e.g., antibiotics can destroy normal bowel flora and result in diarrhea). Propantheline (Pro-Banthine) and oxybutynin chloride (Ditropan), used in the management of urinary incontinence, can cause constipation.

Potential for Cooperation

For any bowel program to be successful, full cooperation of the client on a day-to-day basis is essential. The client's suggestions and preferences should be incorporated into the plan. The nurse should know the individual's mental and physical capabilities when planning a program, so that realistic goals can be established mutually by the nurse and client.

Future Life-Style

Plans for discharge should be considered from the time of initial assessment. Will the client be attending school or returning to work? An evening program of bowel evacuation may be preferable for someone with morning deadlines. Will assistance be necessary for the client to fully participate in the program? If so, it may be necessary to plan the program for a time when assistance is available. If the plan initiated in the rehabilitation setting cannot be followed at home, it is of little use. A practical plan, easily carried out on a long-term basis by the client or primary care giver, requires active client and family participation. The successful plan allows the individual to integrate bowel control conveniently into everyday life.

NURSING DIAGNOSES

The nursing diagnoses for the client with impaired bowel function are constipation, diarrhea, and bowel incontinence.[8]

GOALS

Goals are established with the client and may vary according to disability, type of bowel dysfunction, and life-style. Goals that may be established are as follows:

1. To achieve control on a regular basis (a bowel movement every 1 to 3 days) without the need for laxatives or enemas
2. To eliminate or minimize accidents caused by incontinence
3. To avoid complications of diarrhea, constipation, and impaction
4. To help the client with an uninhibited neurogenic bowel to plan and regulate bowel elimination at a time when there is likely to be a response
5. To help the client with a reflex neurogenic bowel stimulate reflex activity that moves feces into the rectum for predictable elimination
6. To assist the client with an autonomous neurogenic bowel in maintaining firm stool consistency and keeping the distal colon empty

REHABILITATION NURSING INTERVENTIONS

The nurse should be aware that certain factors influence the efficiency of and are common to all bowel programs. In addition, there are specific nursing interventions for bowel management in diarrhea, constipation, and incontinence. The type of neurogenic bowel also influences the development of a bowel management plan.

Basic Components of a Bowel Program

Certain factors are common to all bowel programs. These include a "clean" bowel to start, timing, proper diet and fluid intake, physical exercise, privacy, and positioning.

A "clean" bowel

The bowel must be free from impaction before starting any new bowel program. Manual disimpaction, cleansing saline, or tap water enemas may be used to free the bowel from impaction. If cleansing enemas do not relieve the problem, oil retention enemas can be tried. According to Brandt[1] and Goldberg,[7] soapsuds enemas should

not be used because they cause excessive irritation. Enemas are not used routinely in bowel programs because of stretch to the colon walls and resultant loss of elasticity. With continued use of enemas, the bowel responds poorly to reflex stimulation, possibly leading to dependence on enemas and laxatives.

Timing

Scheduling a bowel program to accommodate the client's preonset routine and to fit in with anticipated discharge plans and future life-style is important. For example, defecation may be attempted every morning. However, this schedule may have to be evaluated and modified according to the client's physical condition and response. Some individuals find an every-other-day routine satisfactory; others have good evacuation with a 3-day routine.

A key element is establishing a *consistent* habit time for elimination. Clinical experience has demonstrated that for prompt bowel response to stimulation (a bowel movement within 30 minutes), the stimulation method must take place at the same hour every time. The gastrocolic reflex also should be used in the bowel routine. After breakfast or the evening meal is an ideal time, but a hot cup of coffee or tea or an evening snack also assists in producing the gastrocolic reflex at a more convenient time.

Diet and fluid intake

The client's preonset dietary habits are evaluated before implementing a bowel program. Physical condition is considered, and personal preferences are incorporated as much as possible into the diet. The diet should be high in nutrient value and well balanced, containing a variety of foods from the four basic food groups.

For a successful bowel program, the diet must be high in fiber. Dietary fiber is that part of plant food that traverses the small intestine and is not digested by the endogenous secretions within. The most important function of fiber is to bind water in the intestine in the form of a gel to prevent overabsorption from the large bowel. This action ensures that the fecal content is both bulky and soft and also that its passage through the intestine is not delayed. Delayed transit time of the fecal contents generally results in constipation. Dietary fiber is beneficial in the management of both constipation and diarrhea. Its bulking action helps alleviate diarrhea, and its softening action helps alleviate constipation.

The chief sources of dietary fiber are whole-grain cereals and breads, leafy vegetables, legumes, nuts, and fruits with skins. By simply replacing white bread with whole-grain bread, the fiber content of the diet can be greatly increased. At least three daily servings of vegetables and fruits, two of which should be raw, are recommended. Granola, bran, and wheat germ are excellent sources of fiber and may be easily added to soups, cereals, meatloaf, baked goods, and other foods. Fiber should be introduced into the diet gradually to allow the GI tract time to adapt. Too rapid an increase in the amount of fiber may lead to distressing side effects such as flatulence, distention, or diarrhea.

Unless fluid intake is restricted for medical reasons, clients should drink 2 to 3 quarts of liquid daily to maintain soft stool consistency. Drinking hot coffee, hot water, or prune juice every morning for breakfast is helpful to some persons in initiating a bowel movement. Prunes and prune juice stimulate intestinal motility and therefore act as natural laxatives. Large quantities of prune or other fruit juices, however, may result in loose stools. If loose stools are the result of antibiotic therapy, some clinicians advise eating one-half cup of yogurt two to three times per week to maintain the natural flora of the bowel.[18]

Preventing constipation and obtaining soft, bulky stools are goals of the bowel program better achieved through dietary measures than with laxatives and stool softeners. Medications should not be introduced until dietary means have been attempted to achieve effective bowel response. In the long run, a healthy diet is more beneficial and much less costly than dependence on medication.

Exercise

Physical activity is vital to a successful bowel program. Prolonged bed rest has an adverse effect on bowel motility and tends to cause fecal retention. The client who can be out of bed and involved in physical activities increases muscle tone and has return of bowel function more quickly. Physical status and type of disability determine exercise capabilities. Encouraging the client to perform activities of daily living with minimum assistance from others helps compensate for the decreased activity level as a result of physical disability. When subjected to extended periods of bed rest for medical reasons, the client must be urged to continue to carry out as many activities as possible. Turning in bed, lifting the hips, bathing, performing range–of–joint motion exercises, and carrying out other self-care activities aid in preventing decreased bowel motility and constipation.

Privacy

The act of elimination, in most cultures, is performed in private. Privacy facilitates relaxation, which in turn facilitates the act of defecation. Privacy also ensures that embarrassing sounds or odors will not be detected by others. The disabled person in an institution has little privacy. The more dependent the client, the less privacy there is. The individual benefits psychologically when privacy is incorporated into the bowel program. Whenever possible, the nurse should assist the client out of bed and onto a toilet where the bathroom door may be closed. If a portable commode must be used, privacy can be achieved by rolling it into a bathroom or other secluded area.

Positioning

Whenever possible, the client should assume an upright sitting position to defecate. This normal physiological position allows gravity to assist in peristalsis and stool expulsion. Unless absolutely necessary, bedpans should not be used. If unavoidable, care should be taken when positioning the client to limit sacral pressure exerted by the bedpan. To limit sacral pressure, the nurse should elevate the head of the bed, support the back and legs with pillows, and bridge the hips and legs as necessary. To avoid excessive pressure and potential skin breakdown, the client should not remain on the bedpan or sit on a toilet or commode for longer than 30 minutes. Persons with spinal lesions should not use a bedpan. An incontinence pad is a safe and satisfactory alternative. As soon as the client receives medical approval to get out of bed, bedpans should be abandoned.

A squat position with the knees slightly higher than the hips helps to increase abdominal pressure and thus facilitate stool passage. For those persons with weak abdominal muscles, an abdominal binder can be used to increase abdominal pressure. Abdominal massage also may stimulate and hasten the defecation process. Persons with all types of disabilities find it helpful to massage the abdomen in the direction of the bowel from right groin upward, across, and down to the left groin.

Medications and Digital Stimulation

Suppositories and medications must be ordered by a physician. However, protocols may be developed in collaboration with the physician that specify ranges and guidelines so that the nurse can make adjustments according to the individual client's response.

Digital stimulation is a technique used to induce reflex contraction of the colon, resulting in elimination.

Suppositories and medications

Suppositories are used to initiate reflex emptying of the bowel. To have an optimum effect, the suppository must come in contact with the bowel wall. Before inserting a suppository, the rectum should be checked for stool. If stool is present, enough should be removed to ensure proper placement of the suppository against the bowel wall. The suppository should be stored at room temperature before insertion, because refrigeration delays action and temperatures over 90° F (32.2° C) cause the suppository to melt. Table 11-1 summarizes the three types of suppositories commonly used in rehabilitation settings.

Stool softeners and bulk formers are often prescribed to aid in the establishment of a bowel program. For example, dioctyl sodium sulfosuccinate (Colace), 100 mg, two to three times per day, is used initially and the dosage adjusted according to the consistency of the stool. When hard stools accompanied by constipation or frequent soft, pasty stools are a problem, bulk-forming laxatives can be given to alter the consistency by making stools soft and bulky. Laxatives should not be routinely prescribed in any bowel routine because of the potential for developing atonic colon. Whenever a mild laxative is needed, senna tablets and granules assist in moving the stool to the lower bowel so that a suppository or digital stimulation can completely empty the bowel. Fecal impaction may require a stronger laxative. Some clinicians argue that laxatives aggravate the problem of impaction and prefer to use only enemas to clean the colon of impacted feces. The nurse should remember that the terminal goal of any bowel program is continence and control without the need for medication.

Digital stimulation

To perform digital stimulation, the index finger is gloved, lubricated, and gently inserted into the rectum. To stimulate the inner sphincter to relax, the finger is rotated against the anal sphincter wall. It may take from 30 seconds to 2 minutes for relaxation of the sphincter to occur; then the finger is removed. Reflex peristaltic activity then produces evacuation. If after a reasonable time no evacuation occurs, the procedure may be repeated.

In successful bowel programs, digital stimulation may replace the suppository once a reflex-response defecation pattern is established. However, digital stimulation also may be used to trigger a bowel movement if a suppository has been less than successful. Additionally, it may be used to ensure complete emptying of the colon following a bowel movement.

The Client with Constipation

To assist the client with constipation in achieving elimination of soft bulky stool on a regular basis, a bowel program based upon a comprehensive assessment and data base, as previously described, should be developed. Laxatives and enemas should be avoided because the client can develop a dependency on these methods and treatment may be complicated. These measures may be necessary after all other avenues have been fully explored.

If the client's constipation is not related to a pathological process, then the rehabilitation nurse should proceed to develop the bowel program. Based upon the individual's bowel history and assessment, a nursing care plan is developed incorporating diet, fluid intake, exercise, and timing. The following medications should be reviewed carefully as potentially causative factors:

1. Analgesics
2. Anticholinergics
3. Anticonvulsants
4. Antidepressants
5. Antiparkinsonism agents
6. Diuretics
7. Opiates
8. Psychotherapeutic agents

TABLE 11-1
Suppositories

Suppository (strength)	Action	Time when results expected	Disadvantages
Glycerin (mild/moderate)	Softens stool by irritating bowel, which responds by secreting fluid; irritation stimulates reflex peristalsis	Approximately 30 min	Irritant property may cause injury to mucous membrane with prolonged use
Vacuetts (mild/moderate)	Activated in water before insertion; suppository releases carbon dioxide, which distends bowel and initiates reflex peristalsis	Varies	Use of petroleum lubricants negates effectiveness of suppository
Bisacodyl (Dulcolax) (strong)	Contact suppository that stimulates sensory nerve endings in colon and results in reflex peristalsis	15-20 min	Abdominal cramping possible

Diet and fluid intake

The most important dietary factor when considering constipation is the amount of fiber ingested. The normal American diet has little dietary fiber. A high-fiber diet includes increasing the intake of foods containing fiber (Table 11-2). Authorities disagree about the amount of dietary fiber that constitutes a high-fiber diet. Hull and others[11] recommend 5 to 15 g of dietary fiber per day and in their research were successful in managing constipation in the majority of subjects, even though many had been laxative users. In an unpublished study by Hanlon and colleagues,[10] it was determined that 4 to 8 g of dietary fiber, in the form of unprocessed bran, was sufficient to manage constipation in a group of elderly clients with multiple functional and physical problems.

In adding fiber to the diet, the rehabilitation nurse must be cognizant of the person's likes and dislikes and especially of ability to chew, since many high-fiber foods require adequate mastication. This consideration is extremely important with persons whose residual deficits affect either the innervation or muscle function of the face, mouth, and throat. If the person is unable to handle high-fiber foods adequately, then supplementing the diet with unprocessed bran should

be considered. Cann and others[2] demonstrated the efficacy of using bran in the management of constipation.

The action of fiber on the GI tract to alleviate constipation is explained by its osmotic properties, stimulating effect, and water-retaining properties. A U.S. Food and Drug Administration study indicates "that increased dietary fiber provides bulk, gentle laxation, and ease of elimination."[20] Fiber should be introduced gradually into the diet to avoid untoward effects such as abdominal discomfort, flatulence, and diarrhea. These symptoms might occur in mild forms during the first 2 weeks of treatment but are only transient.[1] Bran is considered the most practical source of dietary fiber.[13] Its use in the treatment of constipation is outlined in the box on p. 215. Additionally, bran is considered superior to other bulk laxatives, since it is most effective in increasing fecal weight.[9,12] Bran should not be taken concurrently with digitalis, nitrofurantoin, oral anticoagulants, or salicylates because it binds orally with these medications.[14] Excessive use of fiber can cause the loss of certain nutrients such as calcium, iron, and zinc.[11]

Prune juice is used in conjunction with bran as a stimulant, since bran acts primarily as a bulk-

Text continued on p. 215.

TABLE 11-2

Fiber content of common foods

Food	Common measure	Weight (g)	Fiber (g)
Vegetables			
Peas, dried whole, raw	½ C	100	16.7
Beans, baked in tomato sauce	½ C	128	9.3
Parsley, raw, leaves	3½ oz	100	9.1
Plantain, ripe, fried in oil	1 small 5 in	100	5.8
Peas, split, cooked	3½ oz	100	5.1
Beans, butter, boiled	½ C	90	4.6
Peas, canned, drained solids	½ C	66	4.2
Peas, fresh boiled whole, no pods	½ C	75	3.9
Turnip greens, boiled	½ C	100	3.9
Yam, boiled, flesh only	½ C	100	3.9
Lentils, boiled	½ C	100	3.7
Mustard greens, raw, leaves and stems	½ C	100	3.7
Broccoli top, raw	Scant cup	100	3.6
Beans, summer, boiled	½ C	100	3.4
Beans, boiled, French style	½ C	100	3.2
Broccoli top, boiled	½ C	78	3.2
Eggplant, raw, diced	½ C	100	2.5
Beets, boiled	2.2-in diameter	100	2.5
Mushrooms, raw, small	10	100	2.5
Parsnips, boiled, flesh only	½ C	100	2.5
Potatoes, white, baked, flesh only	2½-in diameter	100	2.5
Cabbage, boiled	½ C	85	2.4
Carrots, boiled	½ C	78	2.4
Brussels sprouts, boiled	½ C	78	2.3
Carrots, raw	1 (⅛ × 7½ in)	81	2.3
Sweet potatoes, boiled, flesh only	1 small	100	2.3
Cabbage, white, raw shredded	1 C	80	2.2
Tomatoes, raw, flesh, skin and seeds	1 medium	150	2.2
Turnips, white, boiled, flesh only	⅔ C (diced)	160	2.2
Bean sprouts, canned	½ C	63	1.9
Cauliflower, raw	1 C	85	1.8
Celery, boiled	½ C	75	1.7
Onions, boiled, flesh only	½ C	100	1.3
Onions, raw, flesh only	2¼-in diameter	100	1.1
Cauliflower, boiled	½ C	63	1.1
Celery, raw, chopped	½ C	60	1.1
Potatoes, white boiled, flesh only	2¼-in diameter	100	1.0
Peppers, green raw, flesh only	1 large	100	0.9
Potatoes, white, flesh only, mashed with margarine and milk	½ C	100	0.9
Tomatoes, canned, drained	½ C	100	0.9
Asparagus, boiled	4 spears	100	0.8
Lettuce, raw		50	0.7
Cucumber, raw (sliced)	1 C	105	0.4
Watercress, raw, leaves and stem	10 sprigs	10	0.3

From Walser M, and others: Nutritional management, Philadelphia, 1984, W.B. Saunders Co.

TABLE 11-2 _____

Fiber content of common foods—cont'd

Food	Common measure	Weight (g)	Fiber (g)
Fruits			
Prunes, stewed without sugar, fruit and juice, no stones	½ C	125	10.1
Peaches, dried uncooked	¼ C	40	5.7
Blackberries, raw	¼ C	72	5.3
Lemons, whole fruit, with skin, no seeds	1	100	5.2
Grapes, white, raw, flesh and skin; no seeds or stalks	12	50	5.0
Raspberries, raw, whole fruit	½ C	67	5.0
Cranberries, raw, whole	1 C	95	4.0
Apricots, dried, raw	2 whole	16	3.8
Prunes, dried raw, flesh and skin, no stones	2 large	20	3.2
Figs, dried	1 small	15	2.8
Banana (8 × ½ in)	½	70	2.4
Damson plums, raw, weighed with stones	6, 1-in diameter	66	2.4
Apples, eating	2½-in diameter	115	2.3
Pears, eating, flesh only, no skin or core (3 × 2½ in)	½ pear	100	2.3
Rhubarb, stewed with sugar, stems, and juice	⅜ C	100	2.2
Strawberries, raw, whole fruit	10 large	100	2.2
Plums, Victoria dessert, raw, flesh and skin, no stones	2 medium	100	2.1
Oranges, raw, flesh only, no peel or seeds	1 small	100	2.0
Tangerines, raw, flesh only, no peel or seeds	1 large	100	1.9
Pears, canned, fruit halves and 2 tbs syrup	2 small	100	1.7
Apricots, raw, with skin, no stone	2	76	1.6
Apricots, canned, halves, no stones	4	112	1.5
Mango, raw, flesh only	½ medium	100	1.5
Cherries, raw, large	10	83	1.4
Dates, dried, no stones	2	16	1.4
Peaches, fresh, raw, flesh and skin	1 medium	100	1.4
Raisins, dried, flesh and skin	2 tbs	20	1.4
Figs, green, raw, approximately 9/lb	1	50	1.3
Nectarines, raw, flesh and skin, no stones, medium	1	50	1.2
Fruit salad, canned	½ C	100	1.1
Melon, cantaloupe, raw, flesh only (5 in diameter)	¼ melon	100	1.0
Peaches, canned, fruit halves and 2 tbs syrup	2 medium	100	1.7
Melon, honeydew, raw, flesh only (5 in diameter)	¼ melon	100	0.9
Olives in brine, without stones	3 medium	20	0.9
Pineapple, canned, large fruit slice and syrup	1	100	0.9
Pineapple, fresh, flesh only, no skin or core	½ C, diced	67	0.8
Avocado	⅛	31	0.6
Grapefruit, fresh, flesh only, no skin or seeds	½	100	0
Mandarin oranges, canned, with syrup		100	0.3
Grapes, black, raw, no skin or pits	12 grapes	50	0.2
Grapefruit juice, canned	½ C	120	0
Lemon juice	1 tbs	15	0
Orange juice, strained juice from fresh oranges	½ C	120	0

Continued.

TABLE 11-2

Fiber content of common foods—cont'd

Food	Common measure	Weight (g)	Fiber (g)
Cereal/crackers/flour			
Bran wheat	¼ C	20	8.8
All-Bran	⅓ C	19	5.1
Crisp bread or rye crackers	4	25	2.9
Shredded Wheat biscuits	1	22	2.7
Bread, whole wheat	1 slice	28	2.4
Soy flour, low-fat	2½ tbs	20	2.4
Puffed wheat	1 C	15	2.3
Barley, boiled	½ C	100	2.2
Cornflakes	¾ C	19	2.1
Grapenuts	¼ C	28	2.0
Flour, whole meal	2½ tbs	20	1.5
Graham crackers	2 squares	14	1.4
Sugar Puffs	¾ C	22	1.3
Porridge	½ C	120	1.0
Rice Krispies	¾ C	21	0.9
Special K	1 C	16	0.9
Bread, white	1 slice	28	0.8
Matzo (6 × 6 in)	1 piece	20	0.8
Rice, boiled	½ C	102	0.8
Flour, household	2½ tbs	20	0.7
Cakes			
Fruitcake	1 slice (3 × 3 × ½ in)	40	1.4
Cake, iced	1 slice	50	1.2
Gingerbread	1 piece (2 × 2 × 2 in)	57	0.7
Sponge cake	1 piece (⅒ cake)	50	0.5
Other desserts			
Fruit pie (9-in diameter with double crust, e.g., apple, plum, rhubarb)	¼	160	3.5
Custard, egg, baked from mix	½ C	150	0
Nuts			
Almonds	10	25	3.6
Coconut, dried	2 tbs	15	3.5
Brazil	6-8	28	2.5
Peanut butter, smooth	2 tbs	32	2.4
Chestnuts, small	5	25	1.7
Peanuts	10	9	0.8
Walnuts	3	12	0.6
Hazelnuts	6	8	0.5
Miscellaneous			
Marzipan almond paste	—	100	6.4
Jam, fruit with edible seed (blackberry, black currant, gooseberry, raspberry)	1 tbs	20	0.2
Jam, stone fruit (apricot, plum)	1 tbs	20	0.2
Marmalade	1 tbs	20	0.1
French dressing	—	100	0
Mayonnaise	1 tbs	14	0
Sugar, white	—	100	0

Bran Protocol*

Begin with a clean bowel and proceed gradually:
Add 1 tablespoon† of bran daily for 2 days. If tolerated well but no stool results, then increase to 1 tablespoon two times a day.
If the client still has no results, continue giving 1 tablespoon two times a day for 3 days before advancing to 1 tablespoon three times a day.
When results are obtained, maintain that level of bran.
Give 4 ounces of prune juice at bedtime for defecation to occur after breakfast.
Give 4 ounces of prune juice in the morning for defecation to occur after dinner.

*Incorporation of bran may be considered by an institution as the responsibility of either the dietary or the pharmacy department. In either case a physician's order is usually necessary.
†1 tablespoon = 4 g of dietary fiber. Fiber should never be taken dry but may be added to a variety of foods, such as hot or cold cereal, soup, pureed foods, gravy, and sauces. Fiber can also be used in baking and cooking.

ing agent. An isotin derivative of phenolphthalein is the active cathartic agent in prune juice.[1]

Adequate fluids are essential to avoid and manage constipation. It is often necessary for the nurse to be creative in assisting the client to meet the necessary fluid intake. The nurse also must be fully aware of all aspects of the client's rehabilitation plan, including bladder rehabilitation and therapy schedules, so as not to jeopardize but rather to enhance and facilitate the comprehensive plan for rehabilitation.

Exercise

Diet alone is not sufficient to alleviate constipation. Physical activity is essential and can be easily accomplished in a rehabilitation setting by incorporating therapy sessions as a means of accomplishing needed exercise. The nurse needs to realize that movement or physical activity can greatly assist in defecation and that if the bowel program includes a morning bowel movement after breakfast, the client needs to have sufficient time to attend to the bowel schedule before going to therapy. Episodes of fecal incontinence can be embarrassing and discouraging to an individual trying to cope with a new disability, new body image, and life-style change; therefore accidents should be avoided. The activity of ambulating short distances may be sufficient to stimulate defecation.

Timing

The timing of the bowel program should be considered when establishing the therapy schedule. Ignoring the urge to defecate is a major cause of constipation, and the individual should not be given the impression that defecating is less important than any other part of the rehabilitation plan.

Laxatives

Laxatives are beneficial in the treatment of *acute* constipation but are not recommended for chronic problems. Cathartics cause a rapid evacuation of the colon, whereas laxatives are less pronounced in their action, although the exact mechanism of action is unknown.[14] According to the *American Hospital Formulary Service Drug Information*,[14] laxatives are divided into six categories, including bulk-forming, hyperosmotic, lubricant, saline, and stimulant laxatives, and stool softeners (Table 11-3). The types, action, cautions, and interactions of these categories of laxatives are discussed briefly. For more detailed information, the reader should refer to a pharmacology text.

Bulk-forming laxatives include cellulose derivatives, karaya, malt soup extract, psyllium, and dietary bran. These laxatives are natural and semisynthetic polysaccharides and cellulose derivatives that are nondigestable and nonabsorbable. They stimulate intestinal motor activity and absorb water, helping to lubricate and ease the passage of stool. When treating hypotonic constipation with bulk-forming laxatives, a mass of soft feces may form in the sigmoid colon and can be avoided by adding a stimulant laxative. This type of laxative binds orally with digitalis, nitrofurantoin, salicylates, and oral anticoagulants in the GI tract.

Hyperosmotics include glycerin and sorbitol and are administered rectally. These cause a local irritation and may produce rectal discomfort or burning.

Mineral oil acts as a lubricant and emulsifier, augmenting fecal bulk and softening stool. Mineral oil may impair absorption of fat-soluble vitamins and should not be used with stool softeners. Stool softeners are surface-active wetting agents that enhance the systemic absorption of the oil. Mineral oil should not be given to persons with an impaired gag reflex or elderly persons, since it can be aspirated easily and lead to lipid pneumonia.

Saline laxatives are those which contain magnesium cations or phosphate anions. Lactulose is included because its action is similar to saline laxatives. The salts in these laxatives are absorbed in the intestine, which produces a laxation be-

TABLE 11-3
Laxatives

Category examples*	Actions/uses	Nursing considerations
Bulk forming *Powders* Unprocessed bran Fiberall (sugar free) Metamucil Hydrocil Instant Modane Bulk	Stimulate intestinal motility and bulks stool by absorbing water; usually begin to act in 12-24 hr but delay of 3 days is not unusual	Dose should be taken with at least 8 oz of fluid; interfere with absorption of digitalis, nitrofurantoin, salicylates, anticoagulants; always mix powders as directed by manufacturer; unprocessed bran can be mixed with food
Granules Periden Plain Serutan		
Miscellaneous Naturacil (soft chewable pieces) Fiber Med Crackers		
Hyperosmotic *Rectal* Glycerin (solution or suppository)	Cause local rectal irritation	May produce rectal discomfort, irritation, burning
Oral or rectal Sorbitol (solution or powder)		
Lubricant *Oral* Mineral oil	Lubricant and emulsifier; augments fecal bulk and softens stool; acts in 6- to 8 hr after oral or rectal administration	Plain mineral oil should be given on empty stomach at bedtime to avoid reflux aspiration; emulsions may be given at mealtimes; helpful in clients who should avoid straining; seepage from rectum may occur with either oral or rectal route; should not be given to elderly clients or those with impaired gag reflex, since aspiration can occur with subsequent lipid pneumonia; do not give with stool softeners
Emulsion Agoral Plain (sugar free) Zymenol (sugar free) Kondremul Plain (sugar free) Petrogalar Plain (sugar free)		
Rectal Fleet Mineral Oil Enema Saf-Tip Oil Retention Enema		

Data from Carnevali DL and Patrick MP, editors: Nursing management for the elderly, Philadelphia, 1979, JB Lippincott Co., Iseminger M and Hardy P: Geriatr Nurs 3:402, 1982; Nivatvongs S and Hooks VH: Postgrad Med 74:313, 1983; Nursing 85 drug handbook, Springhouse, Pa, 1985, Springhouse Corp.
*This is not an all-inclusive list but rather highlights the most commonly used laxatives. Additionally, combination laxatives were not addressed to avoid a cumbersome and confusing table. Please refer to a pharmacology text for such agents.

cause of the osmotic attraction for water. The water increases the bulk, softens the stool, and increases peristalsis. These laxatives can cause electrolyte imbalance, especially hypermagnesemia.

Stimulant laxatives are indicated to treat acute constipation and include anthraquinone, diphenylmethane derivatives, castor oil, and dehydrocholic acid. These laxatives cause local irritation of mucosa or selective action on nerve plexi, which causes increased motility. Abdominal dis-

TABLE 11-3
Laxatives—cont'd

Category/examples	Actions/uses	Nursing considerations
Saline *Oral* Phillips Milk of Magnesia Haley's M-O Fleet Phospho-Soda (sodium biphosphate, sodium phosphate, potassium phosphate) Evac-Q Mag Lactulose *Rectal* Evac-Q-Sert Fleet Enema Phosphate Enema	Salts contained in these agents have osmotic attraction for water; absorbed water produces laxation; should be used infrequently and in single doses; oral doses produce watery stool in 3-6 hr or less, whereas rectal enemas cause evacuation in 2-5 min	For short-term therapy, should not be used for more than 1 wk, magnesium retention possible in client with poor renal function, which can cause CNS depression; dehydration possible with hypertonic solutions of sodium
Stimulants *Oral* Prune juice Cascara sagrada Nature's Remedy Modane Liquid Dorbane Senokot (granules or tablets) Castor oil Bisco-Lax Dulcolax Feen-A-Mint Ex-Lax Evac-U-Lax *Rectal* Senokot Bisco-Lax Dulcolax	Causes local irritation of mucosa or selective action on nerve plexi, which causes increased motility, oral bisacodyl agents act in 6-8 hr and within 15-60 min when given rectally; cascara sagrada and senna agents act in 6-24 hr	For short-term therapy, should not be used for more than 1 wk; stimulant laxatives are ones most often abused and are habit forming
Stool softeners *Oral* Surfax Colace Doxinate Bu-Lax Laxinate Modane Soft	Act as detergents and allow water to enter feces; only soften stool and have no effect on peristaltic movements; usually given in combination with stimulant laxative; usually begin to act in 1-3 days	Should not be given with mineral oil agents; should be given to prevent constipation and not to resolve existing constipation

comfort, nausea, mild cramps, and fluid and electrolyte imbalance are associated with stimulants. Stimulants are habit forming, and long-term use may result in laxative dependence and loss of normal bowel function.

Calcium, potassium, and sodium salts of docusate are types of stool softeners. These laxatives act as detergents, tend to lower surface tension, and allow water to penetrate feces. No serious side effects are associated with stool softeners, but as stated previously, these should not be used in conjunction with mineral oil.

The Client with Diarrhea

When a client experiences diarrhea, an investigation for impaction should first be conducted. If the bowel is impacted, then the basic components of bowel management and the nursing interventions explained for the client with constipation should be instituted. If diarrhea is treated without assessing for impaction, then a more complex problem could arise, namely, bowel obstruction.

Diarrhea is managed most easily by treating or eliminating the cause. If it is the result of disease, then the pathological condition should be managed. As stated previously, if antibiotics are the cause, then other antibiotics should be tried. Yogurt can be beneficial in managing the diarrhea. Foods also may cause diarrhea, and the offending foods should be discovered and eliminated. In the process of juggling the diet, nutritional adequacy should be monitored.

Electrolyte imbalance is a potentially serious problem when diarrhea occurs. The client should drink 2 to 3 quarts of fluid a day and also supplement for fluid lost. Excessive use or an excessive dosage of laxatives can result in diarrhea. In addition, diarrhea can occur in the initial phase of dietary supplementation with bran. The following medications may cause diarrhea as a side effect:

1. Broad-spectrum antibiotics
2. Ferrous sulfate
3. Magnesium-containing antacids (Gelusil, Maalox, Mylanta, Riopan)
4. Guanethidine sulfate (Ismelin)

If the client experiences incontinence as a result of diarrhea, the nurse should offer assurance and emotional support. The client can become anxious, frustrated, and embarrassed by uncontrollable diarrhea, and the nurse can help the client deal with the situation effectively and positively. Additionally, the nurse can assist the individual in avoiding future episodes, thereby alleviating or decreasing anxiety.

The Client with Incontinence

Management of bowel incontinence in a rehabilitation setting is an independent nursing function. The physician, however, orders the medication and establishes protocols, whereas the nurse makes the necessary adjustments within the protocols according to the client's circumstances. The nurse must continually evaluate the client's status and alter the bowel program when necessary. Any changes in a bowel program should not be made before at least a 1-week trial. Daily changes in a bowel control program could result in modifying a program blindly without learning the response to the previous bowel program.

Accurate documentation of the results of any bowel program is absolutely vital. Unfortunately, management of bowel control for many clients is approached on a trial-and-error basis. The effectiveness of the program can be evaluated only if accurate records are kept (Figure 11-5).

Uninhibited neurogenic bowel

In general, the following measures should be taken in establishing a bowel program for a client with an uninhibited neurogenic bowel:

1. Follow a consistent schedule. Assist to toilet 30 minutes after meals to take advantage of gastrocolic reflex.
2. Provide a nutritious diet with adequate fiber.
3. Give fluids adequate to stimulate reflex activity and to promote soft stool.
4. Begin program with an enema to ensure that the rectum is not filled with stool
5. Obtain a physician's order for stool softeners in the early stages of program. Colace, Surfac, and Doxidan are examples of often used emollient fecal softeners. When the client's condition improves so that the diet, fluid intake, and physical activity are well tolerated, these medications may be unnecessary.
6. Give a daily glycerin suppository to initiate the defecation reflex. Glycerin is generally strong enough to be effective in the unin-

		WEEK 1				WEEK 2				WEEK 3				WEEK 4		
	DATE	11-7	7-3	3-11	DATE	11-7	7-3	3-11	DATE	11-7	7-3	3-11	DATE	11-7	7-3	3-11
SUN BM																
MED																
SUPP																
DIET																
MON BM																
MED																
SUPP																
DIET																
TUES BM																
MED																
SUPP																
DIET																
WED BM																
MED																
SUPP																
DIET																
THURS BM																
MED																
SUPP																
DIET																
FRI BM																
MED																
SUPP																
DIET																
SAT BM																
MED																
SUPP																
DIET																

BM

Lg = Large
M = Medium
Sm = Small
L = Loose
W = Watery
S = Soft
H = Hard
0 = No BM
I = Incontinent

MEDICATION

S = Stimulant
BF = Bulk forming
SS = Stool softener
O = Osmotic
E = Enema

SUPPOSITORY

G = Glycerine
V = Vacuetts
B = Bisacodye

DIET

P = Prune juice
UB = Unprocessed
     bran
HF = High fiber
     meals

Figure 11-5
Record of bowel movements.

hibited bowel. If glycerin is not successful on the first day, allow the client to rest and insert another suppository the next day. If glycerin is successful, continue with the program. If there has been no bowel movement after 2 days with glycerin, obtain an order for a Dulcolax suppository and continue the program. If the program is unsuccessful, give an enema and begin the program over again with Dulcolax suppositories. Digital stimulation is *not* recommended for clients with uninhibited bowel function because many clients have intact sensation, making stimulation painful.

Accurate documentation is necessary to determine progress and to make appropriate changes in the bowel program. Depending on the client's condition, it may take a week or longer to establish a satisfactory pattern. Staff should be alert to verbal and nonverbal efforts by the client to communicate the need to eliminate. In the absence of functional speech, such behavior as restlessness or picking at the anal area may indicate awareness of rectal sensation. Praising the client for communicating the need to defecate helps the client to recognize success. The frequency of toileting may be decreased when the need to eliminate can be reliably communicated.

Frequency of suppository administration can be decreased as the client demonstrates an awareness of the need to eliminate and has consistent bowel movements. By complying with the basic components of all bowel programs, continence and control can be achieved without the need for medication in most cases.

Reflex neurogenic bowel

During the acute stage of spinal cord injury, spinal shock is responsible for tonic paralysis of the GI tract and flaccid tone of the anal sphincter. Small, properly administered enemas are given to stimulate the bowel until spinal shock subsides.

In general, the following measures should be taken to establish a bowel program for a client with a reflex neurogenic bowel:

1. Once bowel sounds are present, physical activity increases, and oral food, including high fiber, is tolerated, administer a Dulcolax suppository daily to trigger reflex elimination. Administration time should be consistent with the establishment of preonset habits and anticipated future life-style.

2. Once a reliable bowel pattern is observed, suppository administration may be decreased to every other day or every third day as long as the stool consistency remains soft. Be alert for signs of fecal impaction that may develop with infrequent elimination.
3. Progress from Dulcolax to a glycerin suppository and finally to digital stimulation alone to stimulate a reflex bowel movement after the program has been effective for 3 weeks. The program may or may not be successful during the client's stay in the rehabilitation setting. Hopefully, digital stimulation may be the only stimulus necessary to produce reflex stimulation. Digital stimulation also may be used as an adjunct to the suppository program when the suppository has not produced results within 15 to 20 minutes.
4. Stool softeners and bulk agents may be necessary to assist elimination when abdominal muscles are weak or paralyzed. Obtain an order for these medications and administer according to the client's needs.

Documentation of progress remains important to detect reliable patterns of elimination and to initiate appropriate changes.

For individuals with spinal cord lesions above the T6 vertebral level (above the splanchnic outflow), autonomic dysreflexia is a potential problem. *Autonomic dysreflexia* (hyperreflexia) is an abnormal hyperactive reflex activity as a result of an interrupted spinal cord and is set off most often by stimuli arising from a distended bladder, but rectal distention, stimulation, and passage of feces also may precipitate this sympathetic response. This syndrome constitutes a medical emergency that can result in death if not treated promptly (Chapter 10). Nupercainal ointment applied to the rectum 10 minutes before suppository insertion or digital stimulation is helpful in preventing symptoms in susceptible individuals.

Autonomous neurogenic bowel

Management of autonomous neurogenic bowel is extremely difficult. Enemas may be used until spinal shock subsides, but continued use is not recommended because of the potential for mechanical injury to the colon. Manual removal of stool may occasionally be necessary for an impaction, but routine continuous use of this procedure further decreases tone of an already incompetent anal sphincter. Since the S2-4 reflex arc is absent, rectal suppositories are theoretically ineffective. However, clinical experience has demonstrated that suppository use does result in control.

In general, the following measures should be taken in establishing a bowel program for the client with an autonomous neurogenic bowel:

1. Develop a stool consistency that is firm yet not hard by providing dietary fiber and using bulk-forming agents such as Metamucil and Dialose Plus.
2. Administer a suppository daily based on preonset habits and anticipated future lifestyle. Dulcolax and Vacuett suppositories are often used to effectively stimulate defecation (Table 11-1). Once a reliable pattern is established, the frequency of suppository administration may be decreased to every other day or perhaps every third day.
3. Teach the client to perform the Valsalva maneuver (see discussion on defecation) to augment effectiveness of the bowel program.

Because of the lack of sphincter tone, some individuals may experience prolonged oozing of stool following suppository administration. This residual action may be counteracted by inserting a small amount of Nupercainal or Dibucaine ointment into the rectum. Clients with autonomous bowel function are fearful of embarrassing incontinence. Consequently, they strive for a hard stool consistency, which often develops into constipation and fecal impaction. The rehabilitation nurse must help the client understand that a hard stool risks impaction and atony of the colon.

The most sensible way to prevent incontinence is through use of suppositories to evacuate the distal section of the colon. Table 11-4 provides a summary overview of the types of neurogenic bowel dysfunction discussed above. A successful bowel routine for the client with incontinence resulting from any type of neurologic bowel dysfunction requires effort and consistency for both the client and the nurse. Table 11-5 summarizes the problems encountered in planning a successful bowel program with the incontinent client. Again, documentation is extremely important.

Client and Family Education

The details of client education should parallel the individualized bowel program. Education should begin early during hospitalization to give the client sufficient time and opportunity to discover and clarify problems or concerns. The nurse should teach the client about diet, fluid intake, exercise, and timing, as well as stress the importance of adhering to the established program. The client who experiences problems with the program or a change in stool consistency or regularity should be urged to contact the nurse or physician before attempting to alter the program. The client might find it easier to purchase over-the-counter laxatives. To avoid this practice, the nurse should communicate that assistance is readily available after the individual returns home. Consistency is an important factor in success. Any variance from the established program could have untoward effects.

During the educational experience, the client should be given reassurance and emotional support as well as information. As the person's self-confidence is enhanced and the life situation improves, symptoms of constipation may become less evident or less troublesome. The client may feel overwhelmed at discharge with all the information presented and anxious at the thought of leaving the security of the rehabilitation setting. It is helpful to give the client an outline or fact sheet that details the instructions and can be used as a reference at home (Figure 11-6). It is often necessary for the family to be involved, since some clients require assistance with the bowel program at home.

Discharge Planning and Follow-up

Referrals are essential for any client with a disability and should not be overlooked when developing a lifetime bowel program. Consider the gentleman with a stroke who returns home to face problems with incontinence and constipation. Functionally he may have been successfully rehabilitated and have little difficulty coping with residual deficits. However, he may have become dependent on adaptive equipment routinely available on the nursing unit to achieve bowel control and regularity. Armrests on the toilet provide the extra position leverage for security and comfort when evacuating the bowel in the hospital setting. Other members of the team have determined that it will not be necessary to provide armrests on the toilet for safe transfer but rather a grab bar on the wall. The rehabilitation nurse,

TABLE 11-4 _____

Neurogenic bowel dysfunction

Dysfunction	Level of lesion	Possible etiology	Pattern of incontinence	Bowel program
Uninhibited	Brain	Cerebrovascular accident; multiple sclerosis; tumor	Frequent or infrequent; urgency	Consistent habit and time; physical exercise; high fluid intake; high-fiber foods; prune juice; stool softener, suppository as needed
Reflex	Spinal cord above T12 to L1 vertebral level	Trauma; tumor; vascular disease; syringomyelia; multiple sclerosis; pernicious anemia	Infrequent; sudden; unexpected	Consistent habit and time, physical exercise, high fluid intake, high-fiber foods, suppository program, digital stimulation, stool softener as needed
Autonomous	Spinal cord at or below T12 to L1 vertebral level	Trauma, tumor, spina bifida, intervertebral disk	Frequent; may be continuous or induced by exercise or stress	Consistent habit and time, physical exercise continuous, high fluid intake, high-fiber foods, prune juice, suppository program, Valsalva maneuver

From Staas WE and DeNault PM: Am Fam Phys 7:96, Jan 1973.

BOWEL ELIMINATION

Client's name: _____

1. Maintain the diet recommended. Allow for sufficient time for each meal.
2. Schedule a regular time to go to the bathroom.
3. The urge to defecate is a natural process. DO NOT IGNORE IT.
4. Allow sufficient time for defecation.
5. Notify _____ of any change in bowel habits or if there is any change in color, consistency, or regularity of stool.
6. Drink _____ glasses of fluids each day.
7. Do not strain or use excessive effort to defecate.
8. Exercise on a regular basis as recommended.

SPECIAL INSTRUCTIONS: (Include here any schedule of supplemental bran, prune juice, use of suppositories or medication.)

Figure 11-6
Bowel program.

TABLE 11-5

Incontinence: problems associated with bowel programs

Problem	Nursing management
Constipation	Increase fluids; review diet, increase intake of soft, high-fiber foods as needed; give prune juice; use stool softeners or bulking agents that may be of additional benefit
Diarrhea	Rule out impaction; try to eliminate causes; if antibiotic, add yogurt; if secondary to certain food, eliminate irritant
Suppository does not work within expected time of 15-30 min	Make sure suppository is at room temperature; make sure it is in contact with wall of rectum; remove stool if necessary; perform digital stimulation
Abdomen distended	Rule out impaction
Patient complains of "bloated" feeling	Review diet; remove gas-forming foods; introduce fiber gradually
Poor results during scheduled bowel routine	Ensure consistency of program (time, day, method); expect change with alteration in lifestyle, diet, etc.; allow time for routine to become reestablished
Continued results from suppository throughout day	Review diet; increase bulk formers. Consult with physician about adding senna to assist stool into lower part of bowel for complete emptying; if problem continues, Dibucaine ointment inserted in lower section of rectum after completion of bowel routine will counteract continued action of suppository
Autonomic dysreflexia	Initial actions are to lower blood pressure immediately; place person in upright position; monitor blood pressure every 3-5 min; notify physician; after symptoms subside, insert Nupercainal ointment into rectum 10 min before doing manual evacuation to minimize further stimulation

From Staas WE and LaMantia JG. In Ruskin AP, editor: Current therapy in physiatry, Philadelphia, 1984, WB Saunders Co.

when teaching the client, discovers the need for armrests as part of the bowel program. Since it is the nurse who is intimately involved with the client on a daily basis, the client often feels most comfortable in divulging personal "rituals." In this particular case, the installation of armrests on the toilet at home is an important part of the discharge plan.

The rehabilitation nurse plays a major role in coordinating the discharge plan and community referrals. Each client's needs are different and require different community services, but there are basic considerations when any client with impaired bowel elimination is discharged. The nurse should give attention to the following items:

1. Cost and availability of supplies needed at home
2. Location of supplier and availability and cost of delivery service
3. Availability of support groups
4. Location of the bathroom in the home
5. Family or agency assistance needed at home to carry out the bowel program

REHABILITATION TEAM INTERVENTIONS

Although the nurse is the primary team member involved in planning and implementing a successful bowel program with the client and family, other members of the interdisciplinary team offer important input for the successful management of impaired bowel elimination. The physician, nutritionist, occupational therapist, and physical therapist collaborate with the nurse to plan interventions based on individual needs.

The physician prescribes treatments and medications. The nutritionist assists the rehabilitation team in meeting the nutritional needs of the client. The occupational therapist designs adaptive devices to help the individual in managing the bowel program. Also, the occupational therapist and sometimes other team members perform a home assessment to determine if any bathroom modifications or adaptive equipment are needed to carry out the bowel program at home. The physical therapist assists the client in developing an appropriate exercise program.

OUTCOME CRITERIA

The following outcome criteria are related to bowel management:

1. In the maintenance and restoration of bowel function and control:
   a. Bowel regularity and continence are maintained.
   b. Bowel regularity and continence are restored.
   c. The client and family (as needed) assume responsibility for the bowel program.
2. In the area of safety, the client and family incorporate safe techniques in the bowel program.
3. In the area of education:
   a. The client and family understand the rationale for the bowel program.
   b. The client and family understand causes and prevention of alterations in bowel elimination.
   c. The client and family demonstrate techniques of bowel management.
4. In the area of discharge planning and follow-up:
   a. The client and family use community resources appropriately.
   b. The client and family request assistance if problems in bowel management occur.

SUMMARY

The rehabilitation nurse is the member of the team who is in constant contact with the client. The nurse has the opportunity to assess continually all segments of the comprehensive rehabilitation plan in dynamic interaction. When assisting the client to maintain or restore bowel function, the bowel program cannot be isolated or unrelated to the entire rehabilitation plan. Bowel habits are highly personal and if not managed effectively can have untoward effects on the client's ability to cope with a disability and give full effort to the rehabilitation program.

TEST QUESTIONS

Circle the correct response.

1. Which one of the following statements is *true* regarding normal bowel function?
   a. The sigmoid, rectal, and anal regions of the large intestine are supplied with sympathetic fibers that function to inhibit the defecation reflexes.
   b. Stimulation of sympathetic nerve fibers originating in T8 to L2 cord segments results in increased activity of the GI tract.
   c. The myenteric plexus nerve supply controls secretion and sensory functioning of the GI tract.
   d. The two primary functions of the colon are to absorb water and electrolytes and to store fecal material until it can be expelled.
2. The process of defecation takes place when:
   a. Reflex relaxation of the rectum and contraction of the internal and external anal sphincters occur.
   b. Both autonomic and somatic systems are involved.
   c. Sensory nerve fibers in the sigmoid colon are stimulated by the presence of fecal material.
   d. The S2-4 reflex mechanism initiates peristaltic waves via parasympathetic nerve fibers.
3. Of the following statements, all are true regarding impaired bowel elimination *except:*
   a. In hypotonic constipation, there is an increase in activity of the segmental contractions but not of the propulsion type.
   b. The greatest hazard of diarrhea is the loss of water and electrolytes needed for normal cell function.
   c. A common cause of diarrhea and flatulence may be an insufficiency of the enzyme lactose, which digests milk sugar.
   d. Immobility seems to be a crucial factor that predisposes the older client to constipation.
4. In *uninhibited neurogenic bowel:*
   a. There is damage to the lower motor neurons at or below the T12 to L1 spinal level.
   b. Involuntary bowel elimination occurs when the sacral reflex is activated.
   c. There is increased cerebral awareness of the need to defecate.
   d. Bowel sensation is absent, and the bulbocavernosus reflex is decreased.
5. In *autonomous (flaccid) neurogenic bowel:*
   a. Sensation is increased, and the bulbocavernosus reflex is present.

b. Activity of the spinal reflex arc is intact.
c. The lesion directly involves the S2-4 spinal segments.
d. There is reflex emptying of the bowel.

6. A *reflex neurogenic bowel:*
   a. Occurs with spinal cord lesions below the T12 to L1 level
   b. Is characterized by an increased bowel and saddle sensation
   c. Is classified as an upper motor neuron lesion
   d. Results in voluntary control of defecation

7. In performing an initial, comprehensive nursing assessment for the client with impaired bowel elimination:
   a. Realistic goals are set jointly by the client and nurse.
   b. Discharge goals are not planned until the client is past the spinal shock stage.
   c. The age of the client will determine the bowel program to be implemented.
   d. The client's suggestions and preferences are not incorporated into the care plan at this time.

8. In setting goals that foster maximum bowel independence, the nurse emphasizes:
   a. Having a bowel movement daily without the need for stool softeners
   b. Eliminating or minimizing accidents as a result of incontinence
   c. Achieving control on a daily basis with the aid of laxatives or enemas
   d. Minimizing complications of diarrhea, constipation, and impaction with daily use of suppositories

9. A factor that is common to all bowel programs is to:
   a. Establish a "clean" bowel with the use of soapsuds enemas.
   b. Introduce fiber rapidly into the diet to provide for bulking action.
   c. Provide bedpans for clients with spinal lesions to assure a sitting position for elimination.
   d. Schedule elimination to accommodate the client's preonset routine.

10. A rehabilitation nursing intervention to assist the client in maintaining bowel elimination might be to:
    a. Encourage physical activities to increase muscle tone and return of bowel function.
    b. Administer laxatives and enemas routinely to prevent constipation.
    c. Keep suppositories refrigerated before insertion to prevent melting.
    d. Administer bran concurrently with salicylates to promote absorption from the colon.

11. In establishing a bowel program for a client with an *uninhibited neurogenic bowel*, the rehabilitation nurse:
    a. Changes the program if not successful after a 3-day trial period
    b. Gives a daily glycerin suppository to initiate the defecation reflex
    c. Performs digital stimulation to initiate the defecation reflex
    d. Restricts fluid intake to prevent diarrhea and incontinence

12. In caring for a client with a spinal cord lesion above the T6 vertebral level, the nurse is aware that autonomic dysreflexia:
    a. Is an abnormal hypoactive reflex activity resulting from an interrupted spinal cord
    b. May be set off by stimuli arising from a distended bladder or rectum
    c. Constitutes a medical emergency that can result in permanent paralysis if not treated promptly
    d. Is preventable by having the client perform the Valsalva maneuver to augment bowel elimination

13. Which one of the following statements is *true* of an *autonomous neurogenic bowel* as opposed to a *reflex neurogenic bladder?*
    a. Daily continual enema use is recommended to prevent fecal impactions.
    b. Management of this type of bowel dysfunction is extremely easy.
    c. The S2-4 reflex arc is absent, with resultant lack of sphincter tone.
    d. Digital stimulation may be the only stimulus necessary to produce the defecation reflex.

14. Which statement is *true* regarding the primary role of a rehabilitation team member?
    a. The nurse is responsible for determining and prescribing the client's treatments and medications.
    b. The physician is the team member responsible for planning and implementing a successful bowel program for the client.

c. The occupational therapist assists the client in developing an appropriate exercise program.

d. The nurse plays a major role coordinating the client's discharge planning and community referrals.

Answers: 1. d, 2. b, 3. a, 4. b, 5. c, 6. c, 7. a, 8. b, 9. d, 10. a, 11. b, 12. b, 13. c, 14. d.

LEARNING ACTIVITIES

1. List three factors that contribute to the development of constipation.
2. List two factors that may cause diarrhea.
3. List seven factors that the rehabilitation nurse assesses before developing a bowel program.
4. List the basic components of management for alterations in bowel elimination.
5. Describe the three types of neurogenic bowel commonly seen in rehabilitation settings.
6. Discuss nursing interventions that should be considered when assisting a client experiencing constipation.

REFERENCES

1. Brandt LJ: Gastrointestinal disorders of the elderly, New York, 1984, Raven Press.
2. Cann PA and others: What is the benefit of coarse wheat bran in patients with irritable bowel syndrome? Gut 25:168, Feb 1984.
3. Carnevali DL and Patrick MP, editors: Nursing management for the elderly, Philadelphia, 1979, JB Lippincott Co.
4. Connell AMC and others: Variations of bowel habit in two population samples, Br Med J 2:1095, 1965.
5. Davenport HW: Physiology of the digestive tract: an introductory text, ed 4, Chicago, 1977, Year Book Medical Publishers, Inc.
6. Devroede G: Dietary fiber, bowel habits, and colonic function, Am J Clin Nutr 3:S157, Oct 1978.
7. Goldberg SM and others: Essentials of anorectal surgery, Philadelphia, 1980, JB Lippincott Co.
8. Gordon M: Nursing diagnosis: process and application, ed 2, New York, 1987, McGraw-Hill Book Co.
9. Graham DY and others: The effect of bran on bowel function in constipation, Am J Gastroenterol 77:599, 1982.
10. Hanlon D and others: Management of constipation in the elderly patient. Unpublished clinical evaluation, Buffalo, NY, 1982, The Buffalo General Hospital.
11. Hull C and others: Alleviation of constipation in the elderly by dietary fiber supplementation, J Am Geriatr Soc 28:410, 1980.
12. Iseminger M and Hardy P: Bran works! Geriatr Nurs 3:402, 1982.
13. Jones VA and others: Food intolerance: a major factor in the pathogenesis of irritable bowel syndrome, Lancet 2:1115, 1982.
14. McEvoy GK and other editors: American hospital formulary service drug information, Bethesda, Md, 1984, American Society of Hospital Pharmacology.
15. Nivatvongs S and Hooks VH: Chronic constipation: important aspects of workup and management, Postgrad Med 74:313, 1983.
16. Nursing 85 drug handbook, Springhouse, Pa 1985, Springhouse Corp.
17. Physician's desk reference, Oradell, NJ, 1987 Medical Economics Co.
18. Staas WE and LaMantia JG: Bowel function and control. In Ruskin AP, editor: Current therapy in physiatry, Philadelphia, 1984, WB Saunders Co.
19. Wrick KL and others: The influence of dietary fiber source on human intestinal transit and stool output, J Nutrition 113:1464, 1983.
20. Zimring JG: High-fiber diet versus laxatives in geriatric patients, NY State J Med 78:2223, 1978.

ADDITIONAL READINGS

Anderson BJ: Tube feeding: is diarrhea inevitable? Am J Nurs 86:704, 1986.
Brocklehurst JC: Disorders of the lower bowel in old age, Geriatrics 35:47, May 1980.
Cannon B: Bowel function. In Martin N, Holt N, and Hicks D, editors: Comprehensive rehabilitation nursing, New York, 1981, McGraw-Hill Book Co.
Conrad KA and Bressler R, editors: Drug therapy for the elderly, St Louis, 1982, The CV Mosby Co.
Cornell SA and others: Comparison of three bowel management programs, Nurs Res 22:321, 1973.
Guyton AC: Basic human physiology, ed 3, Philadelphia, 1981, WB Saunders Co.
Luckmann J and Sorenson KC: Medical surgical nursing: a psychophysiologic approach, ed 3, Philadelphia, 1987, WB Saunders Co.
Martin N, Holt N, and Hicks D: Comprehensive rehabilitation nursing, New York, 1981, McGraw-Hill Book Co.
Mendeloff AI and others: Modified fiber diets. In Walser M and others, editors: Nutritional management: the Johns Hopkins Handbook, Philadelphia, 1984, WB Saunders Co.
O'Brien MT and Pallett PJ: Total care of the stroke patient, Boston, 1978, Little, Brown & Co.
Wolf S: Functional G.I. problems: insights into the psychosocial components at work, Consultant 23:129, Aug 1983.

CHAPTER 12

Sleep and Rest

Sandra Chenelly

OBJECTIVES

After completing Chapter 12, the reader will be able to:

1. Describe the role of sleep and rest in physical and mental restoration.

2. Discuss the events in each of the five stages of sleep.

3. Explain the changes in sleep patterns in the elderly.

4. List factors that can cause sleep interruptions for the rehabilitation client.

5. Conduct a nursing assessment pertinent to the client's sleep/rest pattern that includes a sleep history, description of the client's sleeping and waking behaviors, and assessment of the environment in which sleep occurs.

6. Formulate a nursing diagnosis for a client experiencing difficulties in sleeping.

7. Develop goals with the client experiencing difficulties in sleeping.

8. Describe nursing interventions for sleep pattern disturbances related to illness or disability, for providing an environment conducive to sleep and rest, and for clients taking prescribed sleep medications.

9. Teach a client and family techniques for promoting adequate sleep and rest.

10. Identify ways rehabilitation team members and community resources may assist the client in the management of sleep pattern disturbances.

11. List outcome criteria for the client with a sleep pattern disturbance.

> . . . sleep, oh gentle sleep
> Nature's soft nurse! how have I
> Frightened thee,
> That thou no more wilt weigh my
> eyelids down
> And steep my senses in forgetfulness?
> —William Shakespeare, *King Henry IV*

FUNCTIONS OF SLEEP

In these lines written centuries ago, Shakespeare aptly described an essential function of sleep and linked the promotion of sleep with the activities of the nurse. Sleep has been described as a state of rest for the body and mind in which consciousness, voluntary activities, and certain body functions are completely or partially suspended.[32] Although the scientific catalogue of sleep's beneficial effects has only recently begun, it is increasingly evident that sleep of sufficient quality and quantity is important in maintaining physical and emotional well-being.

Sleep is a normal, patterned physiological phenomenon involving an altered state of awareness characterized by profound relaxation and reduced levels of overtly manifested physical and cognitive activity.[33,39] Although the functions of sleep and the amount of sleep needed for optimum function are as yet unclear, it is recognized as a basic physiological need.[5] Experimental evidence indicates that body growth and cellular renewal are faster during sleep than during the waking state. Growth hormone is released in larger amounts during sleep. This substance enhances amino acid incorporation into protein molecules and promotes both ribonucleic acid synthesis and red blood cell production.[37] Sleep may serve to remove unnecessary data accumulated and stored during wakefulness from the nervous system. It also may facilitate categorization and integration of new data in the brain's organizational system. Senses "steeped in forgetfulness" are allowed to escape from the continual bombardment of stimuli experienced during the day. It is believed that this respite may foster better problem solving and decision making.[22]

Sleep, like many other body functions, appears to be cyclical. Both sleep and waking are active processes dependent upon interaction of antagonistic brainstem areas. The maintenance of wakefulness is generally attributed to the action of the reticular activating system located in the upper brainstem region and to the secretion of adrenaline. Sleep production is often attributed to the secretion of serotonin by nuclei of the raphe sleep system in the pons and medial forebrain regions.[7,18,34] Sleep and wakefulness also are influenced by impulses received from the higher centers, peripheral receptors, and limbic system.

The benefits of maintaining regular sleep and rest patterns have been documented by several studies. Belloc and Breslow[1], in a famous study, investigated seven life-style variables and found that obtaining 7 to 8 hours of sleep each night was correlated positively with longevity and favorable health status. Subjects in their study who slept 9 or more hours or 6 or fewer were less healthy and had an increased mortality.

Sleep Stages

Normal sleep can be divided into two main phases: rapid eyeball movement (REM) and non-REM (NREM). NREM sleep consists of four stages. In stage 1, the transitional stage from wakefulness to sleep, the person becomes progressively more relaxed and inattentive to outside stimuli. After a few seconds, the person enters stage 2. This is a deeper level of sleep, but one from which the individual may still be easily aroused. Stages 3 and 4 represent the deepest levels of sleep. Arousal becomes more difficult; movements are few; and pulse rate, respiration, and blood pressure levels drop. Stage 4 sleep is associated with physical repair and restoration. Persons who have experienced significant physical stress, such as heavy exercise, pain with muscular contraction, or surgery, probably have a greater need for stage 4 sleep.[22]

The interval between the onset of stage 1 sleep and the completion of stage 4 sleep is roughly 90 minutes for the young adult. At the end of this period, the sleeper gradually drifts back up through the stages to stage 1 and then enters REM sleep.

REM sleep constitutes 20% to 25% of sleep time and is divided into tonic and phasic stages. Rapid eye movements occur during the phasic stage. REM sleep is characterized by voluntary muscular relaxation so profound it resembles paralysis.[43] Tendon reflexes are suppressed; heart and respiratory rates are erratic; airway resistance and gastric secretion rise; and penile erections occur.[22,43] REM sleep also has been associated with adrenal hormone release.[12]

Although the muscular state suggests profound relaxation, in REM sleep there is considerable autonomic and mental activity. This is the stage in which most dreaming occurs.[6] Dreaming is believed to be necessary for learning, memory, and psychological adaptation to stress. Just as stage 4 sleep physically restores the body, REM sleep provides mental renewal.

Individuals experiencing psychological stress or adaptation to new situations may require more REM sleep.[22] Unfortunately, many preparations used to enhance sleep onset, such as alcohol and most hypnotics and sedatives, suppress REM sleep. After a period of REM deprivation, a phenomenon called *REM rebound* occurs. The body attempts to make up for lost REM sleep by increasing the amount of time spent in this stage. However, for certain individuals, extended periods of REM sleep may hold risks. Seizures are much more likely to occur during REM sleep than at any other stage. Sleep apnea and hypoxemia are more evident during REM sleep, especially in elderly persons or those with chronic obstructive pulmonary disorders.[29] Individuals with angina or cardiac rhythm disturbances may be at increased risk during REM sleep. As far back as the late 1800s, two studies reported that the most common time of death was between 4 and 7 AM, a period coinciding with the greatest amount of REM sleep for most people.[37]

A number of studies have helped determine the functions of sleep by exploring what happens to human function when persons are deprived of sleep. Although total sleep deprivation rarely occurs, reduction in total sleep time by interruption or fragmentation of sleep is common. Hartmann[19] summarizes the data on sleep deprivation by stating that "most researchers report that sleep-deprived subjects become increasingly angry, irritable, unfocused, and antisocial." Most of the physiological changes occurring as a result of sleep deprivation indicate impairment of the central nervous system.[41] Brewer[4] identifies these symptoms as nystagmus; ptosis; hand tremors and clumsiness of the fine movements of the fingers; slowed response times; brief losses of equilibrium; decreases in word memory; decreases in reasoning, judgment, and association; decreases in auditory and visual vigilance; decrements in hypoxic and hypercapnic ventilatory responses; cardiac arrhythmias; and loss of strength of neck flexion.

When persons are deprived of sleep, the amount of recovery sleep needed seems to be inconsistently associated with the amount of sleep lost. Highly individualized sleep pattern changes occur following prolonged wakefulness, including changes in total sleep time, sleep latency, arousal thresholds, and wakefulness during recovery sleep.[38]

Sleep Pattern Changes with Aging

Aging causes significant changes in the character of sleep. Total sleep time changes from about 16 hours per day at birth to 6 to 7 hours per day in those over 50 years old.[15] The amount of time awake while attempting to reach the sleeping state (sleep latency) increases nine times from young adulthood to age 60, reaching 20 minutes or longer at the latter age.[22,39] Stage 4 sleep at 50 years of age is only half that experienced by young adults, although the amount of REM sleep appears to remain constant throughout adult life. The elderly have almost no stage 4 sleep. These changes result in a number of sleep-related complaints from older individuals, including spending more time in bed, taking longer to fall asleep, experiencing daytime drowsiness, and needing longer to adjust to changes in their usual sleep-wake schedule.[25] The ill, elderly individual also may be disturbed by pain, the frequent need to void, and shortness of breath. Older persons may awaken earlier in the morning than young adults.[22] Contrary to popular opinion, older persons have sleep requirements similar to younger people. However, since their sleep patterns tend to be more fragmented, they may obtain more sleep through daytime napping and may require a longer period in bed to obtain sleep amounts equivalent to those of young adults. There is some evidence that the "old old" (75 years and above) may require more total sleep time.[21]

FACTORS ALTERING SLEEP AND REST PATTERNS

Sleep can be altered by a number of circumstances. Among these are environmental and psychological factors, illness and disability, and specific sleep disorders.

Environmental and Psychological Factors

Individuals undergoing an illness or stressful life experience, such as hospitalization or extended institutional care, are exposed to many threats to normal sleep. Most of us have difficulty sleeping in a strange environment, and illness exacerbates such difficulty. Most persons facing loss of functional ability because of these circumstances feel anxiety, a state that further impairs their capacity for obtaining adequate sleep and rest. The unfamiliar sights, sounds, and smells of an institution frequently intrude on the sleep of many rehabilitation clients. Most people have developed lifelong rituals for sleep behavior that are not readily available to them in the foreign atmosphere of the health care facility.

Studies in hospitals have focused primarily on the effects of sleep deprivation in intensive care units. Findings suggest that factors which interfere with sleep are pain, interruptions for assessment procedures such as vital signs, interruptions for medications and treatments, general discomfort (for example, an uncomfortable position in bed, bright lighting during the night, an uncomfortable room temperature, noise made by nurses), daytime sleeping or boredom, confused or noisy roommates, hyperthermia, and anxiety or depression.[11,17,24,42] Most of these factors could affect a person with a disability whether residing in a hospital, long-term care facility, or home.

Clapin-French[8] studied the sleep/wakefulness patterns of 102 elderly persons residing in long-term care facilities. She found that nocturnal awakenings associated with elimination showed a marked increase following admission, that the proximity of other people increases in significance as a cause of nocturnal awakenings, and that traffic noises are a less significant cause of awakening after admission. Of these residents, 71% were receiving some type of sleep medication. Although nursing sleep histories had been taken for a little over half of these persons, minimum information was recorded. Only 65 records had some mention of sleep, usually entered under the heading "rest and sleep patterns," on the nursing care plans, and 37 records had no mention regarding sleep. The author concluded that individuals in these facilities may be receiving sleep medication inappropriately without investigation into factors promoting their insomnia.[8] Given the multitude of factors operating to prevent normal

sleep in the person separated from home it is remarkable that the client in a hospital or long-term care facility obtains adequate sleep to meet physiological and psychological requirements.

Illness and Disability Factors

Several illnesses are associated with sleep impairment. Approximately two thirds of individuals over 65 years of age have one or more chronic illnesses.[9] The discomfort and stiffness of arthritis may disrupt sleep. Polyuria and nocturia caused by diabetes mellitus also may be troublesome. Since gastric secretion increases during REM sleep, ulcer pain may occur. Anginal pain often follows a similar pattern. Dyspnea caused by conditions such as chronic obstructive pulmonary disease and congestive heart failure with pulmonary edema may be exacerbated by the supine position assumed for sleep. Those with Parkinson's syndrome may have episodes of greater rigidity during nocturnal awakenings, and the amount of REM sleep also may be diminished. Muscle spasticity accompanying multiple sclerosis or a cerebrovascular accident may disrupt sleep. Depression is often manifested by difficulty falling asleep and early morning awakenings.[31] Benign prostatic hypertrophy, prostatic disease, and urethritis (especially in older women) can lead to frequent awakenings during the night to void.[25] All of these conditions deprive the rehabilitation client of the sleep critical to supply physical and mental energy needs.

Psychological factors contributing to sleep pattern disturbances include losses of job, physical capabilities, material belongings, and loved ones. These losses lead to depression and anxiety, which in turn may cause a delay in falling asleep the earlier appearance of REM sleep, frequent awakenings, feelings of sleeping poorly, and early morning awakenings.[9] As individuals age they develop less tolerance for stress and take longer to return to baseline functioning, causing alterations in sleep patterns.[2] A decrease in sleep time, less REM sleep, and more frequent awakening have been associated with organic brain changes such as those found in Alzheimer's disease.[36]

Specific Sleep Disorders

Although anyone may experience a sleep pattern disturbance as a result of environmental or illness factors, some persons also may suffer from specific sleep disorders. Nearly 15% of persons living in industrialized nations suffer from these serious sleep disorders.[43]

Insomnias

The *insomnias* are probably the most common sleep disorders. Insomnia may be defined as difficulty falling asleep, multiple awakenings during the night, or awakening early in the morning and being unable to return to sleep. Insomnia can be situation related or persistent. Persistent insomnias can be caused by a wide range of abnormalities, including physical or mental pathological conditions, stress, and personality changes. Insomnia also is common during alcohol or drug withdrawal and with indiscriminate use of hypnotic medications.[43]

Situational insomnias are associated with a significant life change and exist for 3 weeks or less. These situations can be pleasant, such as a marriage, or grim, such as the death of a loved one. When insomnia lasts longer than 3 weeks, it is said to be persistent. Some specific causes of persistent insomnia are biological rhythm disturbances, drug dependency, psychophysiological abnormalities, psychiatric disturbances, sleep apnea syndrome, miscellaneous "normal" conditions, such as snoring, and nocturnal myoclonus.[30] Nocturnal myoclonus has no known cause. It is characterized by periodic leg movements during sleep at precise intervals of 20 to 40 seconds.[20]

Nightmares

Nightmares affect about 10% of the population. These occur during REM sleep, usually later in the night when REM sleep periods increase in frequency and duration.[27] Approximately half of the adults with this problem relate the onset as occurring before age 10 years.[3] Common themes of nightmares are falling, being attacked, and dying. Persons who experience nightmares often talk and walk in their sleep, wet the bed, and have night terrors. Nightmares also are associated with delirium in adults, particularly in those who are elderly or chronically ill.[28] Withdrawal of treatment with certain barbiturates may cause nightmares.

Sleep apnea syndrome

Sleep apnea syndrome has received much attention in recent years. In this condition, there is an interruption of the normal inspiration/expiration cycle. Normally individuals experience fewer than six periods of apnea each night. Those persons with prolonged and recurrent apnea are said to experience sleep apnea syndrome. This syndrome can be central or obstructive. Persons with central apnea exhibit an absence of any expiratory effort and immobility of the diaphragm. In obstructive apnea, airflow is impeded by varying degrees of oropharyngeal airway collapse. The incidence of sleep apnea appears to rise with age.[29]

NURSING ASSESSMENT

Because of the multiplicity of physical problems and psychological adjustments facing the rehabilitation client, it may be difficult for the client or nurse to attribute impairments in function to the effects of sleep pattern disturbance. The client may complain of feeling tired or depressed, without identifying disruption of normal sleep patterns. The nurse may note changes in energy level or irritability, without linking these changes to impaired sleep patterns. It is best to assume that every client attempting to cope with physical disability or a new environmental situation is at high risk for sleep pattern disturbance. An organized assessment of sleep patterns should become part of every rehabilitation nurse's comprehensive client assessment. The assessment should include a sleep history, observation of sleeping and waking behaviors, and an environmental assessment.

The Sleep History

The first step in the assessment of a sleep pattern disturbance is to obtain a comprehensive sleep history. The following guidelines are helpful in eliciting detailed information regarding former sleep habits and current problems with achieving or maintaining sleep[39]:

1. Ask the client to describe his or her sleep patterns (for example, usual bedtime, naps, use of medications for sleep) in as much detail as possible. Find out what previous sleep habits have been and when the current problem was first noticed.
2. Explore any current life change or crises the client is undergoing, and attempt to determine the degree of anxiety this change may be causing. Find out if the client has

reacted to previous life changes with an altered sleep pattern.

3. Ask about the client's primary problem with sleep. Is it one of prolonged latency, frequent awakenings, or earlier-than-usual arousal? Is the client confusing normal age changes in sleep style with a true sleep pattern disturbance?
4. Try to determine whether the sleep pattern disturbance affects other aspects of functioning. For example, does it affect interpersonal relationships or result in an inability to think clearly?
5. Be sure to ask about any concurrent illnesses. Consider whether any of these illnesses normally result in altered sleep patterns, whether there is a problem of self-medicating with excessive alcohol, or if any prescribed medications are known to affect sleep patterns. Some medications may contribute to nightmares. Administration or withdrawal of certain drugs may cause marked changes in the frequency and intensity of dreams.[26]
6. List those activities the client generally finds most relaxing and use them in the future as potential interventions for the sleep problem.
7. Find out what the client does at home to facilitate sleep.
8. Request that the client keep a sleep log, with a daily record of:
   a. Daytime physical activities
   b. Daytime mental activities
   c. Mealtimes and intake (for example, food, beverages, caffeine, alcohol)
   d. Recurring worries
   e. Presleep ritual
   f. Presleep state of mind
   g. Time of retiring
   h. Estimated length of sleep latency period
   i. Quality of sleep
   j. Nature of dreams or nightmares
   k. Number of times awakening
   l. Time of awakening

Observation of Sleeping and Waking Behaviors

Observe the client (or have a family member do so) during sleep. The following behaviors may indicate that physical discomforts are causing a sleep pattern disturbance:

1. *Impaired respiration.* Watch for use of accessory muscles of breathing, frequent coughing, increased respiratory rate, cyanosis, and use of two or more pillows for comfortable sleep.
2. *Impaired elimination.* Watch for frequent trips to the bathroom or repeated use of the commode, urinal, or bedpan.
3. *Pain.* Watch for frequent requests for pain medication at night. Also, observe for restlessness, facial grimacing, or moans that may indicate inadequately managed pain.
4. *Restlessness.* Many people, especially elderly persons with peripheral neuropathy caused by diabetes or chronic alcohol abuse, experience the sensation of "restless legs" at night. Nocturnal leg cramps also may be troublesome. In addition, spastic movements may be observed when the client is at rest.

The rehabilitation nurse should observe the client during the day, or ask a family member to observe the client's waking activities. Does the client appear somnolent or inattentive or doze off easily while sitting quietly? Does the client exhibit slowed movements or increased clumsiness? Is there evidence of irritability, tearfulness, or withdrawal? The presence of these behaviors may provide subtle clues to the existence of a sleep pattern disturbance.

Environmental Assessment

If the client is currently residing in an institution, the environment should be evaluated by the nurse for factors contributing to sleep impairment. A similar assessment of the client's home environment can be performed by a family member. Some considerations include the following:

1. Is the client situated in a noisy, high-traffic area, such as near the television, bathroom, elevator, or nursing station?
2. What is the level of light in the room?
3. Is the room excessively warm or cold?
4. Are there disturbing smells in the room?
5. Do roommates create unusual noises, sights, illumination, or odors?
6. Does the client have adequate and comfortable sleepwear, bedding, mattress, and pillows?

NURSING DIAGNOSIS

The complete elaboration of a client's sleep problem includes the nursing diagnosis, the etiological factors, and the manifestation of the problem. Data collected from the previously described nursing assessment can be used to determine whether the client's problem is manifested by difficulty in attaining the sleeping state, achieving optimum quality of sleep, or obtaining an adequate amount of sleep. The nursing assessment also may yield clues regarding the cause of the disturbance. An example of a nursing diagnosis for a client experiencing frequent awakenings is *sleep pattern disturbance*.[16] The complete nursing diagnostic statement would include the etiological factors and the manifestation of the problem. The complete statement is useful in determining appropriate and measurable goals and provides direction for planning nursing interventions.

GOALS

Once the complete nursing diagnosis of the client's sleep problem is made, client goals can be projected. These projected outcomes are related to the third part of the nursing diagnosis, the *manifestations* of the problem. The goals or projected outcomes are mutually determined by nurse and client and are stated in observable or measurable terms. Each goal also should include an estimate of the time frame for achieving the desired outcome. For example, a projected client outcome for a client with a sleep pattern disturbance related to diabetic nocturia might be stated as follows: "Client will awaken no more than once per night for toileting." Generally, goals for clients with a sleep pattern disturbance might be as follows:

1. To obtain enough sleep to supply physical and mental energy to engage in normal activities of daily living
2. To obtain enough sleep to engage in those physical and intellectual pursuits necessary for well-being
3. To sleep at least 7 hours per night
4. To return to sleep rapidly following awakenings to fulfill physiological needs for mobility, elimination, and respiration
5. To feel refreshed and rested on awakening

REHABILITATION NURSING INTERVENTIONS

A number of nursing interventions can be implemented for the client with a sleep disturbance. Included are interventions related to the illness or disability, providing an environment conducive to rest and sleep, and administering medications to promote sleep.

Sleep Pattern Disturbances Related to Illness or Disability

The statement in the complete nursing diagnosis that identifies the cause of the client's sleep pattern disturbance serves as a guide for nursing interventions. If the nurse's assessment indicates that the illness or disability is the cause of the client's sleep pattern disturbance, efforts are directed toward relieving the specific physical discomfort that prevents the client from obtaining sleep of adequate quality and quantity.

Some people experience arthritic pain at night because analgesic medications taken before retiring may wear off during sleep. Pain may be managed by administering time-released forms of aspirin or by applying heat or cold to the joints immediately before bedtime. Careful attention to positioning and room temperature also may be helpful. Similar approaches may decrease sleep interruptions caused by spasticity. Clients with muscle spasticity may obtain more restful sleep if appropriately prescribed resting splints are applied at bedtime. Clients who suffer from nocturnal angina may benefit from long-acting forms of nitroglycerin (Nitrodur Paste, Transderm Nitro) or from the knowledge that a bottle of nitroglycerin is available for use at the bedside should chest pain occur during sleep.[31]

Clients with chronic obstructive pulmonary disease frequently develop important individual adaptations for achieving and maintaining sleep. Sensitive nursing assessment should elicit information regarding the successful practical techniques developed by the client in response to illness. Insofar as possible, the nurse should use these approaches in planning care. Similar techniques may be appropriate for clients with congestive heart failure complicated by pulmonary congestion.

Clients with pulmonary dysfunction may be unable to sleep in a prone position because it inhibits chest wall expansion and proper inspiratory effort. They may sleep best with the head of the bed elevated or even sitting in a comfortable easy chair or recliner. Often they will need several pillows to elevate the head and chest. Teaching the client to perform pulmonary toilet before retiring and administering bronchodilators before bedtime may help. Many clients with pulmonary dysfunction do not use oxygen during the day. They may sleep better if low-flow oxygen is administered continuously during the night, since lying in bed promotes pooling of secretions in the lungs and consequent decreases in pulmonary ventilation and perfusion. Reduction of anxiety also is critical for promoting sleep in the pulmonary client, because anxiety leads to increased oxygen requirements and respiratory effort. Nursing interventions to decrease anxiety may include relaxation training, timely administration of anxiolytic medication, and provision of opportunities to discuss concerns and fears. Clients with respiratory impairment also may need to alter sleep habits, for example, by obtaining sleep during planned daytime naps and having shorter nighttime sleep periods.

Clients awakened by the need for frequent voiding, such as those with diabetes mellitus or renal disorders, may benefit from restriction of fluids after the evening meal. If polyuria is related to diuretic medication, scheduling diuretic administration during the early part of the day may reduce nighttime elimination. Beverages such as coffee, cola, tea, or hot chocolate have a natural diuretic effect and also act as central nervous system stimulants. These drinks should be avoided by any client suffering from sleep pattern disturbance.

The provision of comfort measures to clients before retiring has long been a standard part of nursing practice. The soothing tactile sensations of a partial bed bath or a tub bath may relax the client and therefore enhance sleep. A skillful back rub may ease muscular tension. Positioning may help induce sleep. Even the traditional glass of warm milk has gained some scientific credibility as a soporific. Research indicates that the neurotransmitter serotonin may induce and maintain sleep. Milk contains the amino acid L-tryptophan, a biological precursor of serotonin.

Recently nurses have added relaxation training to their repertoire of skills used to promote sleep and rest. Jacobson was the first to outline a technique aimed at teaching clients skills to attain total muscular relaxation. He also postulated that muscle tension is a result of anxiety or pain and that the resultant muscle tension can exacerbate discomfort.[13] Since the discovery of the association between discomfort and muscle tension in the 1930s, numerous relaxation techniques have been proposed by practitioners in psychology, psychiatry, and nursing. These include slow deep breathing and rhythmic contracting and relaxing of muscles.

The most commonly used relaxation technique involves tensing and relaxing specific muscle groups. The client is instructed to successively tense each group, focusing on the sensation of tension, and then to consciously relax the muscles, contrasting the feelings of relaxation and tension. Eventually the client becomes aware of how tension feels and what to do to eliminate that tension.[14]

Providing an Environment Conducive to Rest and Sleep

Nursing interventions designed to provide a relaxing sleep environment are indicated whether the client's sleep pattern disturbance is caused by physical or situational factors. The rehabilitation nurse's challenge is to determine what the client's previous sleep routine has been and then to duplicate this routine as much as possible, given physical and environmental constraints.

Over the years most people acquire characteristic, idiosyncratic ways of preparing for sleep. Data obtained from the sleep history should give a picture of what has worked for the client in the past. For the client to attain and maintain sleep, it may be necessary for the nurse to use certain objects or rituals that serve as "triggers" for normal sleep behavior.[40] A typical presleep and sleep ritual might be as follows:

10:00-11:00 PM	Read newspaper
11:00-11:30 PM	Watch late news on television
11:30-11:40 PM	Wash face, brush teeth, void
11:40 PM	Go to bed; use two feather pillows, a lightweight cotton blanket and a night-light
3:45 AM	Arise to void and then return to sleep

In the preceding example, each step in the ritual serves as a trigger for the next step, and collectively these steps act as signals that it is time for the body and mind to succumb to sleep. If a client with a normal sleep ritual such as this was experiencing a sleep pattern disturbance, knowledge of the sleep ritual could be used to plan nursing interventions. Pillows and a cotton blanket could be brought from home and a night-light provided. The nurse also could schedule the client's care so that the period of time from 10:00 to 11:40 PM could be reserved for the client to perform the usual presleep activities of reading and watching television. At the usual time of arising to void, the nurse could be available if necessary to assist with ambulation to the toilet or commode. Normal sleep patterns would be promoted through use of the client's own tried and true sleep habits.

The institutional environment is not usually supportive of sound and restorative sleep. One study of hospitalized individuals found that the chief deterrents to sleep, in order of importance, were noise and activity, pain and physical discomforts caused by the condition, nursing procedures, lighting, and hypothermia.[11] A study involving sleep patterns of elderly hospitalized subjects found that these individuals consistently awakened earlier in the hospital than they did at home.[35]

The environmental stimuli of a health care facility generally are under some degree of nursing control. Nurses can plan procedures to ensure long periods of uninterrupted sleep. Lighting and noise levels can often be manipulated, and hospital routines such as delivery of breakfast trays and visits from laboratory personnel can be adjusted to fit the client's usual sleep habits. Compatibility of sleep habits can be used in making roommate assignments. Room selection can be planned so that the client with a sleep pattern disturbance is placed in an area with lower noise, activity, and light levels.

Medications to Promote Sleep

Although prescribed and administered frequently, sleep medications present problems in terms of both safety and efficacy. An understanding of the physiological effects of commonly used sleeping medications enables the nurse to use these drugs intelligently in the management of a sleep pattern disturbance.

Many hypnotics, sedatives, and antidepressants suppress or alter REM sleep. The alcoholic nightcap, in amounts as small as 1 ounce, may shorten sleep latency but ultimately yield deleterious effects by reducing REM sleep. These drugs may lead to daytime grogginess or confusion and predispose the client to the hazards of immobility by decreasing body movements during sleep. Misuse or abuse of hypnotics and sedatives can lead to habituation, dependency, falls, and incontinence.[13] Most hypnotic medications lose their effectiveness after continual use for 14 days or longer.[10]

Despite these drawbacks, judicious use of hypnotic and sedative medications can be part of a comprehensive nursing plan for the rehabilitation client with a sleep pattern disturbance. Chloral hydrate (500 mg), flurazepam (30 mg), chlordiazepoxide (50 mg), and diazepam (10 mg) have all been shown to have no REM-suppressant effects.[23] These medications may be indicated for the client who is restless, wandering, or confused or for the client troubled by early morning awakenings associated with depression. Depressed clients also may exhibit improved sleep patterns when treated with appropriate doses of antidepressant medications.

No sleep pattern disturbance should ever be managed with medications alone. There is always a place for well-designed nursing interventions in the management of this problem, and sleep-inducing drugs should serve as an adjunct to these interventions.

Client and Family Education

A comprehensive nursing care plan for the rehabilitation client with a sleep pattern disturbance includes education of the client and family regarding normal sleep, deviations from normal, and techniques for promoting adequate sleep and rest. The following guidelines may be used in teaching sleep management to clients and families:

1. Every individual has different sleep needs and habits. Most adults require an average of 7 hours of sleep per day, but it is not unusual for people to function well with as little as 5 hours or as much as 12 hours of sleep. Previous sleep needs are the best guide to the client's current needs. Keep in mind that illness or stress may increase an individual's need for sleep.

2. As much as possible, former presleep habits and routines should be used to reestablish normal sleep patterns. These in-

clude consideration of clothing, bedding, mattress, lighting, noise level, and room temperature.

3. Much restful sleep can be obtained in daytime naps. If one has difficulty sleeping 7 hours at night, regular naps can be scheduled as a part of the daily routine. Morning naps tend to provide more physical restoration; afternoon or evening naps tend to enhance mental restoration.[22]

4. Caffeine should not be ingested after the evening meal because it tends to stimulate the nervous system and prevent the onset of sleep.

5. Alcohol should not be ingested before bedtime because it also tends to stimulate the nervous system after initially depressing it.

6. For minor aches and discomforts, a small amount of aspirin or acetaminophen taken ½ hour before bedtime may help to promote sleep. For more serious pain, pain medication should be taken so that its maximum effect will occur during the attempt to fall asleep.

7. Dreams are a normal and necessary part of sleep. Unusually vivid dreams or extended periods of dreaming may indicate a person's need to obtain more of the kind of sleep necessary for mental restoration. One is likely to have more dreams when facing a new situation or when called upon to make an important decision. Unless vivid dreams begin to cause frequent awakenings, they are probably harmless and will abate by themselves within a short period of time.

8. Over-the-counter drugs for sleep can be dangerous and should be avoided. They can cause confusion, change in heart rate, and vision problems. One should always check with the primary care provider before using these medications.[31]

9. Consider the safety of the sleeping environment. A night-light may be useful for those with diminished vision. A clear, uncluttered path from the bed to the bathroom should be available. If the bathroom is located far from the bedroom, a urinal or commode should be kept near the bed to avoid full arousal and overstimulation that may occur while walking to the toilet.[31]

10. Regular times for retiring and arising should be established. This schedule should be maintained as closely as possible, even on weekends. A set bedtime will help establish a regular rhythm of sleep and wake time and promote sound sleep habits.

11. If the client has difficulty falling asleep or awakens during the night and is unable to return to sleep, lying in bed tossing and turning is not recommended because it encourages a "conditioned" insomnia.[2] Instead the client should get up and engage in some quiet, restful activity such as watching television or reading. Returning to bed and relaxing as completely as possible may help prevent associating bed with the discomfort of being unable to sleep.

12. Daytime exercise can improve muscular relaxation and joint mobility, making it easier to get a good night's sleep. However, heavy exercise in the evening hours before bedtime should be avoided.

Referral

Depending on the cause of the client's sleep pattern disturbance, it may be desirable to use an interdisciplinary approach to diagnosis and intervention within the institution and within the community. Generally sleep pattern disturbance caused by environmental factors may be handled exclusively through nursing interventions aimed at manipulating the sleep setting so that it is conducive to rest and relaxation.

Referral within the institution

Other team members may provide input to the management of sleep pattern disturbance.

Physician. The physician's skills in illness diagnosis are needed to rule out physical problems contributing to sleep pattern disturbance. A thorough diagnostic workup to determine the existence of respiratory and renal disorders, congestive heart failure, angina, arthritis, multiple sclerosis, and sleep apnea may be essential in detecting the underlying physical cause of insomnia or frequent awakenings. When indicated, the physician may prescribe an appropriate hypnotic or sedative medication to be used as one component of the treatment of the client's sleep pattern disturbance.

Psychologist. Referral to a psychologist may be useful in determining whether depression, anxiety, or emotional disturbances are contributing to deviations from a normal sleep pattern. In addition, the psychologist may teach the client self-help skills for relaxation using specific behavioral and relaxation training. These skills may include the use of biofeedback techniques.

Physical therapist. If pain from arthritis or spasticity is implicated as a cause of sleep pattern disturbance, the physical therapist may be instrumental in managing the client's pain using appropriate exercise programs, heat and cold therapy, or transcutaneous electrical nerve stimulators.

Chaplain. If the client's sleep pattern disturbance involves emotional or psychological discomfort because of a difficult life situation, pastoral counseling may be indicated.

Social worker. Many clients must cope with severe social, familial, and financial changes. These problems are a common source of anxiety and can be a significant etiological factor in sleep pattern disturbance. The social worker can help the client deal with these very real threats to the social world, thus making it possible for the client to achieve the relaxation necessary for reestablishing a normal sleep pattern.

Referral within the community

In recent years there has been an explosion of knowledge regarding normal and abnormal sleep states. Several university medical centers have established sleep disorder clinics for the study and treatment of serious sleep pattern disturbances. The client whose sleep pattern disturbance fails to respond to the interventions of the rehabilitation team is a prospective candidate for referral to one of these sleep disorder clinics.

Sleep disorder clinics employ in-depth history taking and psychological testing in the diagnosis of sleep pattern disturbance. The clinic usually has facilities for sleep observation and recording of physiological indices of sleep function, including brain-wave monitoring (electroencephalography), recordings of eye movements (electrooculography), respiratory movements and airflow monitoring, electrocardiography, leg movement monitoring, penile tumescence, and oxygen saturation level.[43]

The following national organizations also may provide useful information or referral for nurses or clients dealing with sleep pattern disturbance[43]:

1. Project Sleep: National Program on Insomnia and Sleep Disorders, U.S. Department of Health and Human Services, Washington, DC
2. Association of Sleep Disorders Centers Department of Psychiatry, T-10, HSC State University of New York Stony Brook, NY

Other resources that may be recommended to the client with a sleep pattern disturbance include the following books, cassettes, and equipment:

1. *Easing into Sleep: Putting the Day to Rest*. A cassette available to help anyone fall asleep. Produced by Dr. Emmett E. Miller, the cassette features ways to relax the body and the mind on side 1, and side 2 is to be used on nights when sleep is difficult. This tape is available from the Source, PO Box W. Stanford, CA 94305. The telephone number is 1-415-328-7171.
2. *Marsona 1200 Sound Conditioner*. High-technology sound producer-generator that reproduces tranquil sounds of nature (surf, rainfall, waterfall) to induce a state of calm. This resource has been used in many hospitals and is available for $130 from Sharper Image, 406 Jackson St, San Francisco, CA 94111. The telephone number is 1-800-344-4444.
3. *Wal-Pil-O Neck Pillow*. A clinically tested cervical support pillow to help individuals with a variety of conditions sleep better. It provides the proper support to reduce pain and allows those using it to wake in a more refreshed and relaxed state. It is available from Roloke Co., 9400 Brighton Way, Beverly Hills, CA 90210.
4. *Space Music*. A catalog of relaxing music available from Narada Distributing, 1804 E. North Ave, Milwaukee, WI 53202. The telephone number is 1-800-8-Narada.
5. Good information on sleep can be found in the following publications:
   a. Goldberg P and Kaufman D: Natural sleep: how to get your share, New York, 1980, Bantam Books, Inc.
   b. Hales D: The complete book of sleep: how your nights affect your days, Reading, Mass, 1981, Addison-Wesley Publishing Co, Inc.

c. Maxman JS: A good night's sleep: a step-by-step program for overcoming insomnia and other sleep problems, New York, 1981, WW Norton & Co, Inc.

d. Drugs and insomnia: the use of medications to promote sleep, NIH Consensus Conference Statement, JAMA 251:2410, 1984. A clinical review of literature pertaining to appropriate use of sedative-hypnotics in the management of insomnia. This article provides advice on when sleep-promoting medication may be considered, what medications to use, what pharmacological factors should be considered in selecting such medication, and what treatment strategies should be employed.

OUTCOME CRITERIA

Successful interventions for a sleep pattern disturbance should result in a reduction of those specific behaviors described in the third part of the nursing diagnostic statement as *manifestations* of the client's sleep pattern disturbance. In general terms, the following broad outcome criteria indicate resolution of the client's sleep problem:

1. The client has adequate energy to perform normal activities of daily living.
2. The client has energy to engage in those physical and intellectual pursuits necessary for well-being.
3. The client sleeps at least 7 hours per night. The client may obtain additional sleep in daytime naps if needed.
4. The client is able to return to sleep rapidly following a minimum number of awakenings required to fulfill physiological needs for mobility, elimination, and respiration.
5. The client reports feeling refreshed and rested on waking.

SUMMARY

Sleep of sufficient quality and quantity is a basic human need that is often threatened by physical and psychological discomfort experienced by the rehabilitation client. The nurse has a central role in the management of sleep pattern disturbances.

Management begins with a thorough nursing assessment of the sleep pattern disturbance. The disturbance is usually one of difficulty in attaining and maintaining the sleeping state. The causes may be related to illness or disability factors; the environment; or a variety of other situational, social, or psychological imbalances. Nursing interventions are focused on helping the client identify and reestablish methods formerly successful for achieving adequate sleep. Special attention is directed toward controlling the environmental elements implicated in the sleep pattern disturbance.

A coordinated team approach may be most beneficial in resolving a sleep pattern disturbance of complex and multifaceted etiology. The client with a specific sleep disorder may require referral to a specialized sleep disorder clinic.

TEST QUESTIONS

1. All of the following statements about the role and function of sleep are true *except:*
   a. Sleep is a basic physiological need.
   b. Sleep is a state of rest for body and mind.
   c. The sleep/wake pattern is cyclical.
   d. All persons need at least 7 hours of sleep for optimum function.
2. Individuals who have experienced psychological stress or adaptation to a new situation require more of what type of sleep?
   a. Stage 1 sleep
   b. Stage 4 sleep
   c. REM sleep
   d. Daytime naps
3. Physical repair and restoration are associated with _____ sleep.
   a. Stage 1
   b. Stage 2
   c. Stage 3
   d. Stage 4
4. Which of the following statements about the sleep of older people is true?
   a. Older people require more sleep than younger people.
   b. Older people require less sleep than younger people.
   c. Older people generally have a decrease in the sleep latency period.
   d. Older people obtain approximately the same amount of REM sleep obtained by younger people.
5. Factors that cause sleep interruption for clients with a disability include:

a. Depression
b. Pain
c. Spasticity
d. All of the above

6. The most common sleep disorder is:
   a. Insomnia
   b. Nightmares
   c. Enuresis
   d. Sleep apnea

7. When assessing the client with sleep pattern disturbance, the nurse explores the client's:
   a. Previous sleep habits
   b. Current life changes
   c. Prescribed and over-the-counter medications
   d. All of the above

8. The use of two or more pillows for sleep may indicate:
   a. Pain
   b. Impaired respiration
   c. Impaired elimination
   d. Restlessness

9. Nursing interventions to decrease anxiety may include:
   a. Relaxation training
   b. Administration of anxiolytic medications
   c. Provision of opportunities for the client to discuss worries and fears
   d. All of the above

10. Clients who are awakened by the need for frequent voiding would benefit from all of the following nursing interventions *except:*
    a. Restriction of fluids after the evening meal
    b. Avoidance of coffee, cola, tea, and hot chocolate
    c. Administration of prescribed diuretic medications before the evening meal
    d. All of the above

11. The nurse is responsible for controlling:
    a. The client's ingestion of alcohol
    b. Environmental stimuli
    c. The client's and family's sleep and rest pattern
    d. Physical and psychological stress caused by a disability

12. All of the following statements are true *except:*
    a. Sleep medications should be administered to anyone who has difficulty falling asleep.
    b. Hypnotics, sedatives, and antidepressants alter or suppress REM sleep.

c. Hypnotics, sedatives, and antidepressants decrease body movements during sleep.
d. Alcohol reduces REM sleep.

13. The client and family should understand all of the following *except:*
    a. Over-the-counter drugs for sleep can be dangerous and should be avoided.
    b. The sleeping environment should be safe.
    c. Dreams are abnormal.
    d. Presleep habits and routines should be used to help reestablish normal sleep patterns.

Answers: 1. d, 2. c, 3. d, 4. d, 5. d, 6. a, 7. d, 8. b, 9. d, 10. c, 11. b, 12. a, 13. c.

LEARNING ACTIVITIES

1. Using yourself as a subject, systematically tense and relax your major muscle groups. What are the sensations you experience as you go through the exercise?
2. Make a list of your personal presleep rituals. Ask family members or friends to describe their personal rituals. What are the similarities and differences?
3. Listen to three different relaxation tapes on three consecutive nights before bedtime. On the basis of your review of these tapes, decide which one you would recommend for a client experiencing sleep pattern disturbance. Explain why you chose the particular tape.

REFERENCES

1. Belloc NB and Breslow L: Relationship of physical health status and health practices, Prev Med 3:405, 1972.
2. Birren JE and Sloane RB, editors: Handbook of mental health and aging, Englewood Cliffs, NJ, 1980, Prentice-Hall, Inc.
3. Bixler EO and others: Prevalence of sleep disorders in the Los Angeles population, Am J Psychiatry 136:1257, 1979.
4. Brewer MC: To sleep or not to sleep: the consequences of sleep deprivation, Crit Care Nurse 5:35, Nov/Dec 1985.
5. Carter D: In need of a good night's sleep, Nurs Times 8(46):24, 1985.
6. Cherniak NS: Breathing disorders during sleep, Hosp Pract 21(2):81, 1986.
7. Chuman MA: The neurological basis of sleep, Heart Lung 12:177, 1983.
8. Clapin-French E: Sleep patterns of aged persons in long-term care facilities, J Adv Nurs 11(1):57, 1986.

9. Colling J: Sleep disturbances in aging: a theoretic and empiric analysis, Adv Nurs Sci 6(1):36, 1983.

10. Davignon D and Bruno P: Insomnia: causes and treatment, particularly in the elderly, J Gerontol Nurs 8:333, 1982.

11. Dlin B and others: The problems of sleep and rest in the intensive care unit, Psychosomatics 12:155, May-June 1971.

12. Fensebner B: Sleep deprivation in patients, AORN J 37:35, 1983.

13. Flaherty GG and Fitzpatrick JJ: Relaxation technique to increase comfort level of postoperative patients, Nurs Res 27:352, 1978.

14. Fletcher DJ: Coping with insomnia: helping patients manage sleeplessness without drugs, Postgrad Med 79:265, 1986.

15. Goldman R and Rockstein M, editors: The physiology and pathology of human aging, New York, 1975, Academic Press, Inc.

16. Gordon M: Nursing diagnosis: process and application, ed 2, New York, 1987, McGraw-Hill, Inc.

17. Grant D and Klell C: For goodness sake—let your patients sleep, Nurs '74 4:54, 1974.

18. Guyton AC: Textbook of medical physiology, ed 6, Philadelphia, 1981, WB Saunders Co.

19. Hartmann E: The functions of sleep, Chicago, 1974, University of Chicago Press.

20. Hauri PJ: Current concepts: the sleep disorders, Kalamazoo, Mich, 1982, Upjohn.

21. Hayter J: Sleep behaviors of older persons, Nurs Res 32:242, July-Aug 1983.

22. Hayter J: The rhythm of sleep, Am J Nurs 80:457, 1980.

23. Hemenway J: Sleep and the cardiac patient, Heart Lung 9:453, 1980.

24. Hilton B: Quantity and quality of patients' sleep and sleep-disturbing factors in a respiratory intensive care unit, J Adv Nurs 1:453, 1976.

25. Hoch C and Reynolds C: Sleep disturbances and what to do about them, Geriatr Nurs 7(1):24, 1986.

26. Kales A, Constantin R, and Kales J: Sleep disorders: insomnia, sleepwalking, night terrors, nightmares, and enuresis, Ann Intern Med 106:582, 1987.

27. Kales A and others: Nightmares: clinical characteristics and personality patterns, Am J Psychiatry 137:1197, 1980.

28. Karacan I and others: The effect of fever on sleep and dream patterns, Psychosomatics 9:331, 1968.

29. Krieger J and others: Breathing during sleep in normal young and elderly subjects: hypopneas, apneas, and correlated factors, Sleep 6:660, 1983.

30. Lareau SC and Bonnet MH: Sleep disorders: insomnias, Nurs Pract 10:13, Aug 1986.

31. Lerner R: Sleep loss in the aged: implications for nursing practice, J Gerontol Nurs 8:323, 1982.

32. McCullough K, editor: Dorland's pocket medical dictionary, ed 23, Philadelphia, 1982, WB Saunders Co.

33. Morrison AR: A window on the sleeping brain, Sci Am 248:94, April 1983.

34. Nicholson AN and Marks J: Insomnia: a guide for medical practitioners, Boston, 1983, MTP Press.

35. Pacini C and Fitzpatrick J: Sleep patterns of hospitalized and nonhospitalized aged individuals, J Gerontol Nurs 8:327, 1982.

36. Reynolds CF and others: Sleeping pills for the elderly: are they ever justified? J Clin Psychiatry 46:9, Feb 1985.

37. Roberts SL: Behavioral concepts and the critically ill patient, Englewood Cliffs, NJ, 1976, Prentice-Hall, Inc.

38. Rosa RR, Bonnet MH, and Warm JS: Recovery of performance during sleep following sleep deprivation, Psychophysiology 20:152, 1983.

39. Schirmer MS: When sleep won't come, J Gerontol Nurs 9:16, Jan 1983.

40. Senn B and Steiner J: Don't tread on me: ethological perspectives on institutionalization, Int J Aging Hum Dev 9(2):177, 1978-1979.

41. Vein AM and others: Physiological and psychological consequences of single sleep deprivation, Hum Physiol 8:392, 1982.

42. Walker B: The postsurgery heart patient: amount of uninterrupted time for sleep and rest during the first, second, and third postoperative days in a teaching hospital, Nurs Res 21:164, 1972.

43. Walsleben J: Sleep disorders, Am J Nurs 82:936, 1982.

ADDITIONAL READINGS

Allen RM: Tranquilizers and sedative/hypnotics: appropriate use in the elderly, Geriatrics 41:75, May 1986.

Bliwise DL and others: Risk factors for sleep disordered breathing in heterogeneous geriatric populations, J Am Geriatr Soc 35(2):132, 1987.

Cummiskey J and others: The effects of flurazepam on sleep studies in patients with chronic obstructive pulmonary disease, Chest 84:143, Aug 1983.

Feinberg I and Floyd C: Systematic trends across the night in human sleep cycles, Psychophysiology 16:283, 1979.

Goodemote EJ: Sleep deprivation in the hospitalized patient, Orthop Nurs 4:33, Nov/Dec 1985.

Kavey NB and Anderson D: Why every patient needs a good night's sleep, RN 49:16, Dec 1986.

McNeil BJ, Padrick KP, and Wellman J: I didn't sleep a wink, Am J Nurs 86:26, 1986.

Orr W: Physiological sleep patterns and cardiac arrhythmias, Am Heart J 97:128, Jan 1979.

Pappenheimer J: Nature's soft nurse: a sleep-promoting factor isolated from brain, Johns Hopkins Med J 145:49, Aug 1979.

Maintaining Skin Integrity

Sharon S. Dittmar
Theresa P. Dulski

OBJECTIVES

After completing Chapter 13, the reader will be able to:

1. Explain the anatomy and physiology of the skin.
2. Describe impairments in skin function.
3. Assess a client's skin condition and ability to care for the skin.
4. Formulate nursing diagnoses associated with maintaining and restoring skin integrity.
5. Develop goals with the client and family to foster maximum independence in skin care activities.
6. Determine nursing interventions to assist the client in maintaining and restoring skin integrity.
7. Identify the interventions of other rehabilitation team members in assisting the client to maintain and restore skin integrity.
8. List the outcome criteria used to evaluate the effectiveness of planned intervention for maintaining and restoring skin integrity.

Maintaining skin integrity is a major consideration in rehabilitation. Skin acts as a biological barrier between a person and the environment and also as a psychosocial mediator between a person and society. Failure to maintain skin integrity extends the length of stay in a rehabilitation facility and interferes with an individual's ability to perform self-care tasks and resume social roles. In some instances, loss of skin integrity can be life-threatening. Therefore, helping the client maintain and restore skin integrity is a major responsibility of the rehabilitation team. The rehabilitation nurse is the team member primarily responsible for assessing skin and teaching the client and family techniques and interventions to assure maintenance of skin integrity.

Anatomy and Physiology

The skin is composed of two main layers: the epidermis and the dermis, or corium (Figure 13-1). Underneath these layers is a third layer of subcutaneous fatty tissue.

Epidermis. The epidermis consists of stratified squamous epithelial tissue. Blood vessels do not reach into this outer layer of the skin. Melanin,

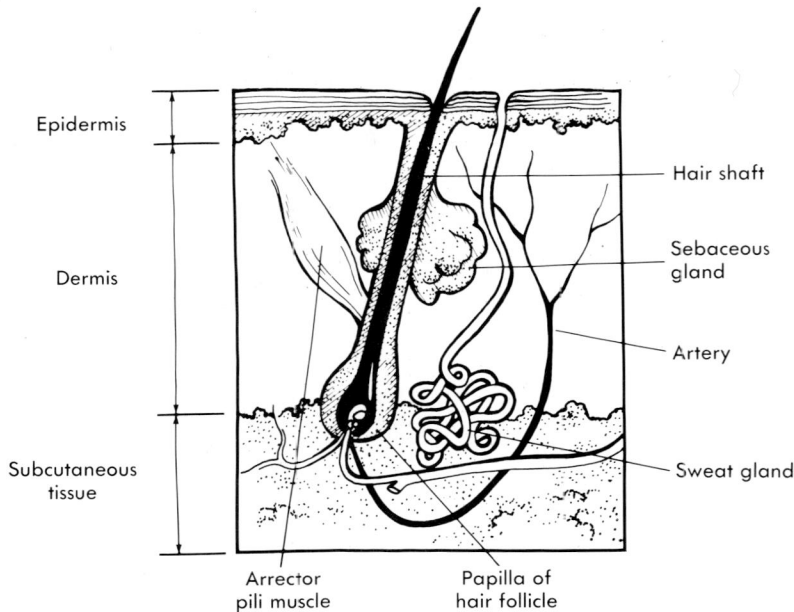

Figure 13-1
Cross section of skin and hair follicle.

which gives skin its pigment, is deposited in the epidermis. Exposure to the sun stimulates the melanocytes (special cells) to produce melanin. Certain races have more active melanocytes; therefore some individuals have darker pigmentation of the skin.

Dermis. The dermis, the inner, thicker layer of the skin, consists of fibrous connective tissue that supports the epidermis.[4] It is tough, elastic, and flexible. The dermis is well supplied with nerves, blood vessels, sweat glands, sebaceous glands, and hair follicles. Millions of nerve endings keep the body informed of changes in pain, temperature, touch, and pressure sensations. Blood vessels found in this layer give the skin a pink tint. Sweat glands are located on all body skin surfaces except the lips and parts of the genitalia. When the sympathetic nervous system is stimulated sweat is discharged from these glands, resulting in lowered body temperature caused by evaporation. Sebaceous glands secrete *sebum*, an oily substance that lubricates the skin and inhibits the growth of bacteria. When an individual shivers, muscles that attach to the hair follicles contract, giving the skin a goose flesh appearance.[16]

Subcutaneous fatty tissue. Adipose or subcuta-

neous fatty tissue acts as a body insulator and as a cushion between skin and bony prominences.

Major functions of the skin are[17]:

1. *Regulation of body temperature*. Evaporation of moisture on the skin through the sweat glands lowers body temperature. Constriction and dilation of blood vessels in the skin regulate body temperature according to environmental temperature.

2. *Protection of underlying tissue from injury*. Varied thicknesses of the skin protect underlying tissue and organs from injury.

3. *Biological barrier protection*. The skin prevents passage of harmful microorganisms and chemicals into the body. Sebum protects the hair follicle from infection and lubricates the skin. Oiliness and low permeability of the skin act as protection against harmful elements.

4. *Protection provided by nerve receptors*. Survival and everyday safety depend upon transmission and interpretation of pain, temperature, touch, and pressure sensations received through these nerve receptors. Responses to these sensations protect the body from impending injury.

5. *Vitamin D production.* Vitamin D is produced when the skin is exposed to ultraviolet light. This vitamin is necessary for metabolism of calcium and phosphorus used in building strong bones and teeth.

6. *Excretion.* Salt and water losses through the skin are factors in maintaining fluid and electrolyte balance in the body.

7. *Expression.* Since the skin contributes to appearance and nonverbal communication, it serves as a means of conveying feelings and projecting body image. Therefore, disfigurement of the skin affects an individual's feelings about self.

Normally differences exist between light- and dark-skinned people. Since the sun's rays do not easily penetrate darker skin, the aging effects of the sun are reduced. Thus black persons retain a youthful appearance longer than lighter skinned individuals.[31]

Some normal impairments in function also occur as the individual ages. Exposure to sunlight contributes to dryness, wrinkling, and loss of elasticity and durability. Progressive vascular changes alter the response of the integument to physical trauma, cold, and infection. Pigmentary changes are common, especially on exposed areas of the body. There are also diminished sensations and interpretations of pain, temperature, touch, and pressure. The skin tends to thin and gradually lose the layer of subcutaneous fat. Production of sweat and sebum also tends to decrease. All of these changes make the skin more susceptible to trauma.[14]

Impaired Function

The degree to which the skin protects the underlying structures depends on the general health of the cells. A number of skin lesions may interfere with the ability of the skin to perform its functions. Poorly nourished skin is dry, cracks easily, and is prone to wounds and infection. Sensory receptors, when subject to prolonged stimulus such as pressure, adapt and can no longer perceive the sensation.[16] If subcutaneous tissue over bony prominences is lost, skin may break down when pressure is exerted on these areas.

Skin Lesions

A number of primary and secondary lesions can be observed by the rehabilitation nurse. Primary lesions are the signs of basic cutaneous responses to pathophysiological responses or stressors. These lesions include the following[17]:

macule A flat, circular discoloration of the skin less than 1 cm in diameter and not raised above the skin.

nodule A raised, solid lesion palpated deeper in the skin than a papule. When larger than 1 cm it is called a *tumor*.

papule A raised, solid lesion up to 1 cm in size. A similar lesion over 1 cm is called a *plaque*.

vesicle A fluid-filled, superficially elevated lesion of the skin or mucous membrane less than 1 cm in size. If it is larger than 1 cm it is called a *bulla*.

wheal An irregularly shaped, elevated area on the skin caused by edema.

Secondary lesions develop from the primary lesions and are called[17]:

crust Dry exudate over lesions.

erosion A moist, depressed area extending the full thickness of epidermis and resulting from a ruptured bulla or vesicle.

fissure A deep lesion split through the epidermis and dermis.

hyperkeratosis Thickening of the keratin layer of the epidermis.

plaque Result of a papule developing into a flat-topped layer.

scale Flaky, dry cells seen on the skin surface.

scar Nonelastic tissue resulting from damage to the dermis.

ulcer An irregularly shaped excavation resulting from necrotic tissue. An ulcer can completely destroy the dermis. All ulcers have scar tissue when healed.

Since black skin has greater pigmentation, pathological signs may differ from those seen in lighter skin. Skin lesions observed in black persons include the following[31]:

dermatosis populosa nigra Characterized by brown to black lesions over the body. These lesions may vary from a few to hundreds. In some instances, these lesions create cosmetic problems and may have to be removed.

hyperpigmentation Increased pigmentation occurring after inflammation of the skin or mucous membrane. An increase in production of epidermal melanin causes the pigment to enter the dermis.

keloid A hard plaque that forms scar tissue. It may be caused by excessive amounts of collagen formed by connective tissue healing.

vitiligo Hypopigmentation. Loss of pigmentation leaves areas of the skin white and very noticeable. The cause is unknown but may result from trauma.

The following skin lesions are commonly seen in aging individuals[6]:

acrochordons Flesh-colored, pedunculated or stalklike lesions that occur around the neck, eyelids, and axillary areas. These small skin lesions consist of collagen with small amounts of subcutaneous tissue.

actinic keratosis Calluslike growths common in persons with fair skin. Calluses are localized areas of hyperkeratosis. These lesions appear in areas most exposed to the sun, such as bald scalp, ears, cheeks, lips, nose, hands, and arms. The lesions are red, yellow, or flesh-colored papules or plaques that feel gritty and are sometimes surrounded by an erythematous ring. These lesions are considered premalignant and should be removed.

corns Hard masses of keratin. Corns can result from pressure and shearing forces, often resulting from irritation of shoes.

leukoplakia Thick, white leathery or fissured lesions found on mucous linings of the mouth, tongue, lip, or palate. These lesions are often associated with irritation from smoking, poor mouth care, ill-fitting dentures, or excessive alcohol ingestion. Leukoplakias are often accompanied by *perlèche*, candidiasis characterized by deep fissures at the corners of the mouth. Perlèche also can be caused by drooling in persons with Parkinson's disease or who have had a stroke.

rhinophyma An irregular, lobulated, bulbous thickening of the distal part of the nose. The enlarged and purplish red nose is called *cobblestone nose* and is a result of vasodilation, increased sebaceous gland production, increased connective tissue, and chronic inflammation.

senile angiomas Pinpoint, bright red papules that are usually scattered over the trunk or extremities. These are sometimes removed for cosmetic reasons.

senile lentigo Pigmentation change that occurs as melanocytes increase at the junction of the dermis and epidermis. These spots are pale to dark brown, flat macules that appear mainly on the dorsum of the hands and on the face.

These age spots seem to increase with sun exposure.

senile purpura An extravasation of blood into skin or mucous membranes. These lesions may be caused by capillary fragility from low vitamin C or such diseases as thrombocytopenia. Vessel walls may rupture in the elderly with minimum trauma.

stasis dermatitis, ulcers Lesions caused by circulatory impairment in persons with chronic heart failure and peripheral venous insufficiency.

xanthelasma A tumorlike, fatty deposit on the eyelid. This lesion is often related to abnormal lipid metabolism, which may occur with diabetes and high lipid levels. Although benign, individuals may have them surgically removed to improve appearance.

Some of these skin lesions may be a result of ingesting multiple prescribed drugs. Use of multiple drugs makes differential diagnosis of skin lesions difficult.

Wounds and Wound Healing

Open or closed wounds of the skin may be caused by blows, cuts, prolonged pressure, and burns from heat, chemicals, or radiation. Invasion of bacteria can lead to infection of these wounds. Stasis dermatitis and ulceration of the lower limbs are often seen as a result of stagnation of blood caused by arteriosclerosis or poor peripheral circulation. In aging persons the skin becomes fragile, particularly on the dorsal surfaces of the hands and arms, and is subject to easy bruising and tearing.

Wound healing can be classified as primary, secondary, and tertiary. Wound healing occurs by primary intention when the wound edges are closely approximated, by secondary intention when the wound is left open, and by tertiary healing when there is delayed primary closure. In all three types there are three phases of healing: (1) the inflammatory phase, (2) the proliferative phase, and (3) the differentiation phase. These phases overlap, but each phase does occur in sequence.

Inflammatory phase

Skin healing begins with inflammation and is characterized by local increase in heat, redness, and edema. Initially, damage to the microcirculation at the area of injury results in vasoconstriction lasting from 5 to 10 minutes. Local clotting occurs with resultant hypoxia and tissue acidosis. It is believed that these occurrences stimulate the inflammatory process. White blood cells engage in phagocytosis or engulfment of bacteria and foreign substances. These cells dispose of microorganisms and foreign material and help prepare the tissue for healing.[29] The exudate formed from the increased vascularity and foreign material can be serous (clear, sterile fluid as seen in a blister), sanguineous (hemorrhagic), or pustulent (puslike) if the wound is infected. The collection of exudate causes swelling and pain, leading to possible loss of function.

New epithelial cells form granulation tissue covering the surface of the wound. Wounds that result only in skin loss begin epithelialization within 12 hours after injury. Wounds that are sutured have a watertight seal within 24 hours. Deeper wounds require collagen formation and granulation before epithelialization. Epithelial cells grow rapidly in healthy tissue but have delayed growth in chronic wounds such as pressure ulcers. Biopsy specimens taken from pressure ulcer tissue demonstrate less than 70% growth rate by the fourteenth day. Optimum epithelial migration occurs in a moist, protected wound that is free of necrotic tissue.[24]

Proliferative phase

This phase begins about 48 hours after the wound occurs. During this phase, the activity of fibroblast cells is stimulated by macrophages and platelets. Fibroblasts, in the presence of vitamin C, begin to synthesize collagen on the fifth or sixth day after injury. Collagen synthesis occurs rapidly for 2 or 3 weeks. Collagen acts as the support matrix for the new tissue.

A vascular bed to nourish the new tissue is necessary for wounds such as pressure ulcers that heal by secondary intention. Macrophages activate the production of capillary beds from existing blood vessels, which grow and combine with other capillary beds to form capillary vessels called *granulation tissue*. This tissue is vivid red and forms a capillary bed over which epithelial cells must grow. When proliferation is complete, this vascular bed recedes.

Contraction occurs when a large wound with tissue loss is reduced in area by the inward migration of normal tissue. It begins on about the fifth day after injury, and along with granulation and epithelialization may produce wound closure.[29]

Differentiation phase

Differentiation begins about 21 days after the wounding. During this phase there is a decrease in fibroblasts, and the collagen deposition continues in a more refined pattern.[29] Beneath the surface, fibroplastic cells begin to form scar tissue. This new fibrous tissue is soluble, very fragile, and prone to breakdown. During the last stage of healing, the scar matures, becomes thicker, and shrinks.[15] Scars remain dark scarlet red for approximately 4 months, but then gradually fade and become silvery-white.

Influencing factors

Many factors influence healing, including age, nutrition, circulation, endocrine function, the presence of foreign bodies, infection, steroid therapy, fluid collection in dead space, radiation, wound separation, and concomitant medical diagnoses such as diabetes mellitus.[29] Tissue repair takes longer in the elderly because of impaired circulation. Each year as persons age, approximately 1% of body collagen is lost; therefore as we age we become more susceptible to skin damage.

A diet high in protein and vitamin C is essential for normal growth and healing. The depletion of vitamin C contributes to capillary fragility and susceptibility to trauma. Anemia decreases the blood's oxygen-carrying capacity. Persons who smoke further decrease oxygen available to wounds because carbon monoxide from cigarette smoke has greater affinity for the hemoglobin molecule than for oxygen.[13] Obese individuals have a poor oxygen supply to wounds and are prone to wound dehiscence because adipose tissue has poor blood supply.[29] Turgor of the skin is maintained and infection prevented by adequate hydration. Arteriosclerosis interferes with blood flow to the skin, causing metabolic disturbances that affect the healing process.

Pressure Sores

Pressures sores, also referred to as ischemic ulcers, decubiti, and bedsores, are localized areas of cellular necrosis, or death. The term decubitus is derived from the Latin verb "decub," which means lying down. Pressure sore is the most accurate term because it more closely conveys the underlying problem.[10] According to Seiler and Stahelin,[27] tissue necrosis that leads to ulcer formation can occur with small amounts and durations of pressure, such as the "repeated pressure-induced reddened sacral skin area in an immobile patient or inadequate massage treatment."

In addition to the physical and psychosocial impact of these complications, the economic impact of prolonged hospitalization is a grim reality. It is estimated that 5% to 10% of hospitalized patients develop pressure ulcers. The cost expended for pressure ulcers ranges from $3.5 to $7 billion annually, and the nursing time required for these persons doubles.[18,28,30] Prevention is easier than cure; therefore preventive measures are a major focus for the nurse working in rehabilitation settings.

Risk factors

Persons at risk for developing pressure ulcers include those individuals who:
1. Are thin or obese
2. Have limited mobility and sensation
3. Have lowered body resistance from poor nutrition, metabolic disturbance, or systemic infection
4. Have interrupted skin integrity because of skin lesions
5. Have psychosocial problems that prevent them from using preventive practices or seeking treatment for early skin lesions
6. Take medications that place them at risk for pressure sore formation, for example, anticoagulants may result in skin hemorrhages; sedative and pain medications reduce mobility[8]
7. Have diminished mental status
8. Are advanced in age; when accompanied by a decrease in elasticity, rate of cell replacement, and healing rate, as well as an increased risk of tissue trauma because of impaired peripheral sensation[11]

Contributing factors

Factors contributing to pressure sore formation include the following:
1. *Shearing force*. Compression placed on sacral tissue when the head of the bed is el-

evated more than 30 degrees. In this situation the body tends to slide to the foot of the bed.
2. *Moisture*. From perspiration, incontinence, or body discharge.
3. *Friction*. Sheet burns caused by pulling instead of lifting the individual across the sheet.
4. *Poor nutrition and hydration*. Poorly nourished cells lack protein for new cell growth. Loss of subcutaneous tissue decreases the padding between the skin and bony prominences, resulting in increased susceptibility to pressure.
5. *Anemia*. Decreased hemoglobin diminishes skin oxygenation and increases the chance of tissue necrosis.
6. *Atrophy*. Disuse of muscles reduces mass. Reduction in muscle mass occurs when an individual experiences long periods of immobility or muscle disease. Muscle atrophy decreases padding over bony prominences and subjects the area to increased pressure.[16]
7. *Loss of sensation*. Decreases the individual's awareness of discomfort from prolonged pressure.
8. *Circulatory dysfunction*. Decreased blood supply diminishes oxygen and nutrients to the skin, predisposing to tissue breakdown.

Sites

Pressure sores usually are formed over bony prominences and develop when these areas are subjected to pressure in excess of capillary pressure for extended periods of time. They are a particular concern for the rehabilitation nurse caring for a client who is immobilized and has loss of sensation.

When lying in a bed or sitting in a chair, an individual's bony prominences exert pressure against the skin, squeezing soft tissue until blood vessels and capillaries collapse. Without adequate blood flow, tissue cells die from lack of oxygen and nutrients. Poorly nourished tissue often does not have sufficient subcutaneous tissue for protection. Although the mean capillary pressure is 25 mm Hg, the pressures exerted on support surfaces can be much greater.[23] Sitting and lying cause more than 32 mm Hg of capillary pressure. Redfern and others[23] studied the pressure exerted by 10 types of support surfaces. They found pressures ranging from 26 mm Hg for the low–air loss bed to greater than 260 mm Hg for a Plaistow operating table. Other pressure readings of interest were 58 mm Hg for a water bed and 122 mm Hg for a ripple mattress. The question of how much pressure leads to pressure sores in an individual is highly complex and subject to nursing judgment.

Normally when individuals experience discomfort from sitting or lying for a prolonged period of time they adjust position. When they are unable to change position, the sensory receptors in the skin, which are subject to the stimulus, adapt, and discomfort is no longer felt. In addition, alteration in sensation affects perception, such as the client who is paraplegic experiences, and pain may not be felt or interpreted in the usual manner.[16]

Bony prominences commonly susceptible to pressure are the ischial tuberosities, sacrum, greater trochanters, heels, and lateral malleoli. Less common sites are knees, heads of the fibula, iliac crests, elbows, spinous processes, occiput, scapulae, and tibial tuberosities (Figure 13-2).[16]

Stages

The four stages of pressure sore formation follow:

Stage I: A bright flush that blanches to the touch and lasts more than 24 hours. The skin and underlying tissues are soft.

Stage II: Persistence of redness and the formation of blisters and fissurelike cracks accompanied by edema and induration. The edges are distinct and the epidermis and dermis are involved.

Stage III: Superficial ulceration involving epidermis, dermis, and subcutaneous tissue. There is frequently exudate. Fascia may be seen at the base of the ulcer.

Stage IV: Penetration of deep fascia and muscle, which may progress to penetration of deeper tissue, including muscle and bone. This situation is extremely toxic and can result in septicemia and death.[26] Periosteitis, osteitis, and osteomyelitis can result from bone destruction.[7]

NURSING ASSESSMENT

The health history obtained before the physical assessment provides insight into past and present skin problems experienced by the client. Information is needed concerning the client's ability to participate in self-care activities to maintain and restore skin integrity.

General history questions related to the skin should include the following:

1. What are your health concerns related to your skin?
2. Are you able to care for your skin?
3. What medications do you currently take?
4. What is your usual daily diet?

Assessment of the client's skin enables the nurse to identify beginning skin problems and evaluate the response to treatment.

Specific questions related to the skin and asked during history taking include:

5. Have you had any past or present skin problems (lesions, dryness, tumors)?
6. Have you noticed changes in skin pigmentation (change in size of moles or dark spots)?
7. Have you noticed excessive dryness, moisture, or odor?
8. Have you noticed changes in the texture of your skin?
9. Do you inspect your skin daily?
10. What do you do to take care of your skin?
11. How often do you bathe?
12. What are your bathing preferences (shower, tub, time of day)?
13. Do you have problems obtaining bath equipment or using your bathing facilities?
14. What bath and skin care products do you use (soap, lotions, creams)?

Questions asked to identify a knowledge deficit concerning safety precautions needed while performing bathing and skin care activities are:

15. Have you had accidents or received injuries while bathing?
16. What safety measures do you take to prevent injuries while bathing?

After obtaining a history, the nurse inspects and palpates the skin. Observations are made of color, pigmentation, wrinkling, hygiene, lesions, masses, and bites. Any lesion noted should be measured, described, and documented in the client's record. The skin is palpated for texture, dryness, elasticity, and turgor.

Pressure points should be checked each time the client is turned or shifts position. Norton, McLaren, and Exton-Smith[20] have devised a valuable method of assessing the client's risk for pres-

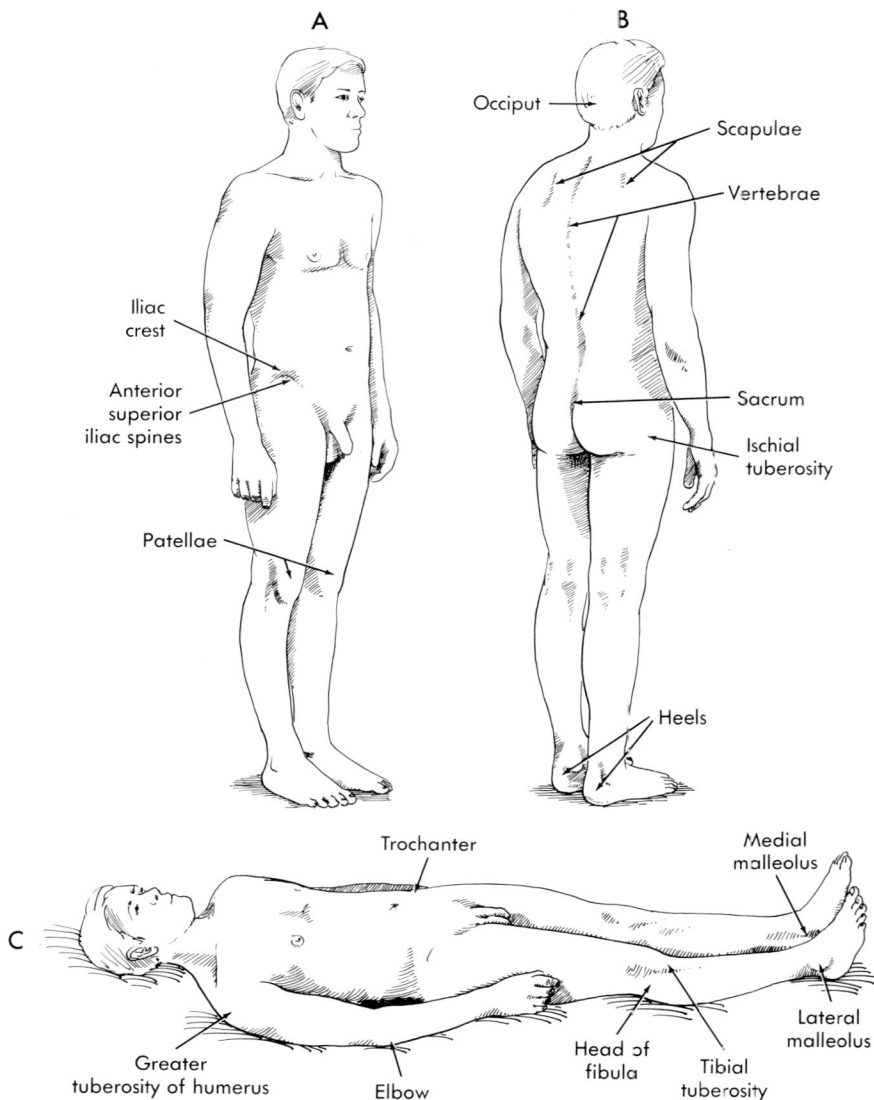

A

B

Occiput

Scapulae

Vertebrae

Iliac crest

Anterior superior iliac spines

Sacrum

Ischial tuberosity

Patellae

Heels

C

Trochanter

Medial malleolus

Greater tuberosity of humerus

Elbow

Head of fibula

Tibial tuberosity

Lateral malleolus

Figure 13-2
A and **B**, Common sites of pressure. **C**, Pressure sites when client is supine.

sure sore formation. This method is now known as the Norton pressure sore risk rating scale. Clients scoring 14 or below are deemed at risk. A score below 12 indicates great risk. The scale assesses physical condition, mental condition, activity, mobility, and incontinence. Gosnell[10] expanded this scale to include nutrition (Table 13-1). She found a downward pattern and a total score probably less than 11 at the time of occurrence of a pressure sore.

Bathing provides an excellent opportunity for inspecting the client's skin, as well as observing the client's mobility, coordination, gross and fine hand movement, and needs associated with skin care activities. Mental and emotional status also are assessed. This assessment enables the nurse to determine the client's ability to perform skin care adequately and safely.

NURSING DIAGNOSES

Data concerning the skin and skin care activities are gathered from the client's health history and physical assessment. Analysis of the data and conclusions about nursing interventions are influenced by current nursing knowledge and past nursing experience. The nursing diagnoses reflect identification of the client's strengths and limitations. Identification of strengths and limitations assists the nurse in determining interventions.

Nursing diagnoses accepted by the North American Nursing Diagnosis Association related to the skin are as follows[9]:

1. *Impaired or potential impaired skin integrity:* Inability of the client to take responsibility for performing activities to prevent skin breakdown or restore skin integrity. Planning is directed toward interventions to encourage maximum client responsibility and performance of activities to maintain or restore skin integrity.
2. *Self-care deficit:* Lack of ability to care for the skin because of impaired motor or cognitive function. The individual may be unable or unwilling to inspect the body for pressure sore areas, wash the body or body parts, obtain a water source, or regulate water temperature and flow. Planning should incorporate strategies to assist the individual in performing these tasks with optimum responsibility and minimum assistance.

Other related nursing diagnoses include[9]:

3. *Activity intolerance:* Inability to carry out activities because of fatigue. Planning should incorporate rest periods as the individual relearns the component steps of these activities.
4. *Knowledge deficit:* Lack of knowledge regarding skin care. The individual may have never known how to care for the skin properly or because of the disease condition, may have perceptual, motor, or sensory impairments that interfere with the ability to perform these functions adequately. Planning should incorporate strategies that will allow a person to perform these activities as independently as possible.
5. *Potential for injury:* Related to sensory or motor deficit or to lack of awareness of skin care practices or environmental hazards. Planning should incorporate use of assistive and adaptive devices and safe practices in the client's and family's performance of bathing and other skin care activities.

GOALS

Goals established with the client include provisions for teaching self-care and involvement of the family when self-care is not possible. Nursing judgment concerning self-care of the skin is based on the client's physiological, psychological, and physical ability.[25] The nursing theory postulated by Orem[21] focuses on self-care as a process whereby individuals contribute to their own health.

Self-care is behavior that evolves from social and cognitive experiences and is learned through interpersonal relationships and culture. Self-care contributes to self-esteem and self-image and is directly affected by self-concept.[21]

Generally goals mutually established with the client and family for maintaining skin integrity could include plans to:

1. Maintain and restore skin integrity.
2. Prevent damage to the skin.
3. Understand the cause and prevention of pressure sores and the rationale for prevention.
4. Inspect the skin and incorporate skin care tasks in daily care with optimum responsibility, safety, and minimum assistance.
5. Identify and correct environmental hazards posing a danger to the skin.
6. Use assistive and adaptive devices in bathing and other skin care activities if appropriate.
7. Use community resources for assistance if needed (for example, skin care equipment, nursing services).

REHABILITATION NURSING INTERVENTIONS

Rehabilitation nursing interventions to maintain and restore skin integrity are designed to provide adequate nutrition, keep the skin clean and dry, eliminate or minimize pressure to bony prominences, and treat interruptions in skin integrity promptly.

TABLE 13-1

Assessing a client's potential for pressure sores

Date of assessment	Mental status	Continence	Mobility	Activity	Nutrition	Total score	Skin appearance	Skin tone	Skin sensation
	1. Unconscious 2. Stuporous 3. Confused 4. Apathetic 5. Alert	1. No control 2. Minimally controlled 3. Usually controlled 4. Fully controlled	1. Immobile 2. Very limited 3. Slightly limited 4. Full	1. Bedfast 2. Chairfast 3. Walks with help 4. Walks independently	1. Poor 2. Fair 3. Good		Dry, oily, wrinkled, scaly, flaccid, etc.)	1. Loose 2. Moderate 3. Hard	1. None 2. Slight 3. Moderate 4. Great

Rater's Guide

Mental status

Response to environment

1. *Unconscious:* Nonresponsive to painful stimuli

2. *Stuporous:* Totally disoriented; no response to name, simple commands, verbal stimuli

3. *Confused:* Partial and intermittent disorientation to time, person, place; purposeless response to stimuli; restless, aggressive, irritable, or anxious

4. *Apathetic:* Lethargic, passive, drowsy, depressed; can obey simple commands; may be disoriented to time

5. *Alert:* Oriented to time, person, place; responds to all stimuli

	1.	2.	3.	4.
Continence Control of urination and defecation	*No control:* Incontinent of urine, feces	*Minimally controlled:* Often incontinent of urine; occasionally incontinent of feces	*Usually controlled:* Incontinent occasionally or has catheter and is occasionally incontinent of feces	*Fully controlled:* Total control of urine, feces
Mobility Amount and control of body movement	*Immobile:* Cannot change position without help; depends on others for movement	*Very limited:* Offers minimum help in changing position; may have contractures, paralyses	*Slightly limited:* Can control and move extremities, but still needs help changing position	*Full:* Can control and move extremities at will; may need device, but can lift, turn, pull, balance, and sit up at
Activity Ability to walk	*Bedfast:* Confined to bed	*Chairfast:* Walks only to chair with help or confined to wheelchair	*Walks with help:* Can walk with help of another or with crutches, braces; may not be able to handle stairs	*Walks independently:* Can rise from bed and walk without help or can walk without help of another using cane or walker
Nutrition Quality of food intake	*Poor:* Rarely eats complete meal; is dehydrated; has minimum fluid intake	*Fair:* Occasionally refuses to eat or leaves large portions of meal; must be encouraged to take fluids	*Good:* Eats some food from each basic food category every day; drinks 6-8 glasses of fluid a day; eats major portions of each meal or receives tube feedings	
Skin appearance Observed skin characteristics	Degree of turgor and tension determined by pinch at high-risk sites for pressure sores	**Skin sensation** Response to tactile stimuli	**Comments:**	

From Gosnell D: An assessment tool to identify pressure sores, Nurs Res 22:55, 1973.

General Considerations

General considerations in assisting the client and family to maintain and restore skin integrity include nutrition, possible drug reactions, relief of pressure, administration of prescribed medications and treatments, and psychosocial reasons for lack of attention to the skin and skin responses.

Nutrition

A number of nutritional factors may increase susceptibility to pressure sores. Obesity creates a risk factor for pressure formation because adipose tissue has poor blood supply. On the other hand, small amounts of adipose tissue tend to cushion the bony prominences from pressure. Some experts believe that obesity after the age of 75 may be helpful in preventing injury from pressure.[19]

Poor nutrition contributes to negative nitrogen balance, thus increasing a client's risk for the development of pressure sores. Hypoproteinemia, low vitamin C levels, and zinc deficiencies seem to contribute to this risk. The client's appetite is often poor because of inactivity, institutional food, and stomach upset as a side effect to medication. The elderly population is at particular risk for poor nutritional practices and consequent skin problems because of lack of money, reduced chewing ability, lack of storage and preparation facilities, and lack of energy to prepare nutritionally adequate food.[19]

Clients at risk for and those who already have pressure sores should receive diets high in protein, moderate in fat, high in vitamin C and zinc supplements, and adequate calories. The nurse collaborates with the nutritionist and consults with the client to determine food preferences and prescribe nutritional meals. It is particularly important that young adults, who often prefer junk food, and the elderly, who have long established eating habits, receive food that is nutritious and appealing. Dietary supplements may be introduced when all efforts to provide nutritional and adequate food intake fail.

Drug reactions

Because of close contact and continual assessment of the client, the nurse is usually the first to observe a skin rash or hear the client complain of an itch. The nurse also is aware of any new drug the client may be taking and therefore is usually the one to initiate an investigation to determine

whether the rash is drug related. Collaboration with the physician in this investigation and regulation of drug therapy usually alleviates this problem.

Relief of pressure

The nurse teaches the importance of maintaining skin integrity. Clients with limited mobility are made aware of the importance of changing position frequently to avoid pressure sores. A client confined to bed should be turned and positioned regularly at least every 2 hours, sometimes more often. The turning schedule should be established after determining the client's skin tolerance for pressure. Shearing force should be avoided by lifting clients in bed rather than dragging them across the bed sheet. Clients should be encouraged to move about in bed and to get out of bed as soon as possible to prevent the hazards associated with immobility. A wheelchair client must relieve pressure over the ischial tuberosities by shifting weight or doing pushups regularly every 10 to 15 minutes.[22] Good alignment should be maintained when the client is in bed or a chair. Pillows between the legs and bony surfaces help minimize pressure. Skin areas prone to pressure sore development should be checked for redness each time the weight is shifted or position changed. Clients should be instructed to inspect susceptible areas daily. A hand mirror may be used to view areas not readily visible (Figure 13-3).

Administration of prescribed medications and treatments

The rehabilitation nurse administers prescribed medications and treatments for skin lesions and teaches the client and family about application, purposes, and side effects of prescribed therapies.

Psychological considerations

Lack of attention to the skin sometimes occurs when a client is denying a disability. Consequently, preventive measures are ignored or given little attention when the person is adjusting to a disability, often resulting in a pressure sore.

The occurrence of a pressure sore or skin lesion can be frightening and demoralizing to a client. It may reinforce feelings of helplessness and loss of control. Often fear and helplessness affect fam-

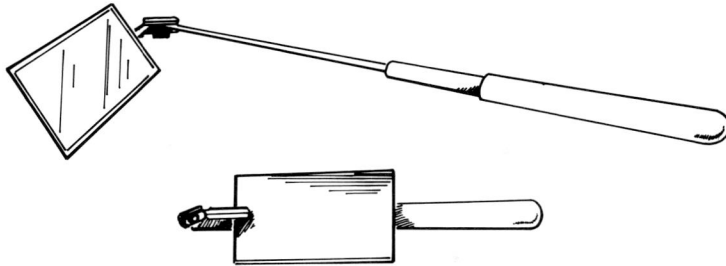

Figure 13-3
Long-handled skin inspection mirror.

ily members and rehabilitation personnel. The idea that skin is decomposing can be repulsive to the affected individual, and the odor associated with infected pressure sores may be repugnant to the client and others.[26] Dressings, salves, cushions, special beds, and equipment create additional inconveniences and expense. The rewards for prevention of a pressure sore may not be apparent to clients who have no sensation, because they do not experience the pain or discomfort associated with the lesion.

Skin Care

The skin should be kept clean and dry. The major purpose of bathing is to rid the skin of dirt, bacteria, and dead epithelial tissue. Washing with soap lowers the surface tension of water on the skin and aids in the emulsification of bacteria-entrapping sebum. Comfort, relaxation, increased circulation from vigorous scrubbing, and exercise of muscles and joints are less obvious benefits of bathing. A warm bath also dilates the superficial arterioles, bringing more blood and nourishment to the skin.

Elderly persons may not require bathing more than once or twice a week. In fact, daily bathing for the elderly may do more harm than good by increasing skin dryness already compromised by a reduction of oil and perspiration. A partial bath, including the face, hands, axillae, and pubic area, may be all that is needed to maintain cleanliness.[14] Lubricants applied to dry areas and special attention to the feet are beneficial. Aging skin is fragile; therefore extra care is needed to protect it from trauma or injury during the bath.

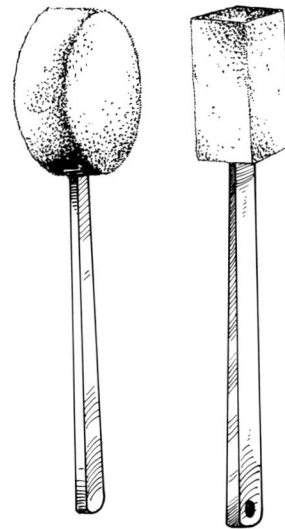

Figure 13-4
Long-handled bath sponge.

Cracking skin from dryness can be avoided by applying water before topical application of an emollient. Many emollients are hydrophilic and can aggravate dry skin. Bath oil is an example of an emollient that should be applied to moistened skin.

The nurse should collaborate with the occupational therapist to devise modified bathing techniques and adaptive and assistive devices that allow the client to be as independent as possible in performing skin care (Figure 13-4). Assistive bathing devices are used according to the individual's need. A client needing total assistance in skin care may require a bath or shower stretcher, whereas a client with some sitting balance may use a shower chair. Clients who have difficulty standing or lowering themselves into a bathtub may need a tub bench or grab bars (Figure 13-5). A shower hose attached to the faucet or permanently installed also assists the client or caregiver (Figure 13-6). The nurse should collaborate with the client, physical therapist, and occupational therapist in modifying tub transfers so the client can be as independent as possible and avoid injury to the skin.

Safety is a major concern in caring for the skin. Care should be taken when clients with diminished sensation are exposed to the sun. Sunscreen and protective clothing should be used. Decreased skin sensation should be considered and care taken to avoid injury to the skin from car mufflers, heaters, appliances, heating pads, heat lamps, and bath water. Hot water should be tested on the inner wrist before the client climbs into the tub or shower. Getting into the tub before filling it and emptying it before getting out will help prevent slipping. Slipping also can be prevented by placement of a nonskid bath mat or strips on the tub or shower surface.

Prevention of pressure is the best approach to the problem of pressure sores. Beds should be wrinkle and crumb free. Skin beneath any cloth-ing or devices creating pressure should receive special attention. Toilets and commodes should be padded for clients at risk for pressure sore development. Skin beneath splints, braces, and casts should be monitored at regular intervals for redness. Clothing and shoes should fit well, not too tight or too loose. Bony prominences should be inspected every time the client changes position. If redness appears, pressure should be alleviated in that area.

Management of Pressure Sores

Nursing intervention begins with identifying the client at risk. Intervention continues with the management of the actual or potential skin problems and includes alleviating pressure; administering prescribed treatments; providing consistent information to the client about causes, prevention, and rationale for skin care; planning for discharge; and referring the client to appropriate agencies for follow-up care. Interventions should be individualized according to client need. No single treatment will be effective for all persons with pressure sores. Nothing can take the place of frequent skin inspection, turning and positioning to allow the blood to perfuse the tissue, and gentle massage, around but not including reddened areas, to stimulate circulation. Nursing in-

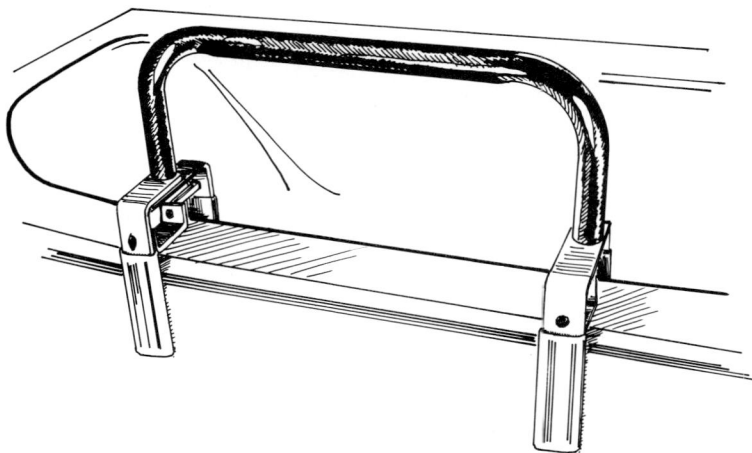

Figure 13-5
Bathtub with grab bars.

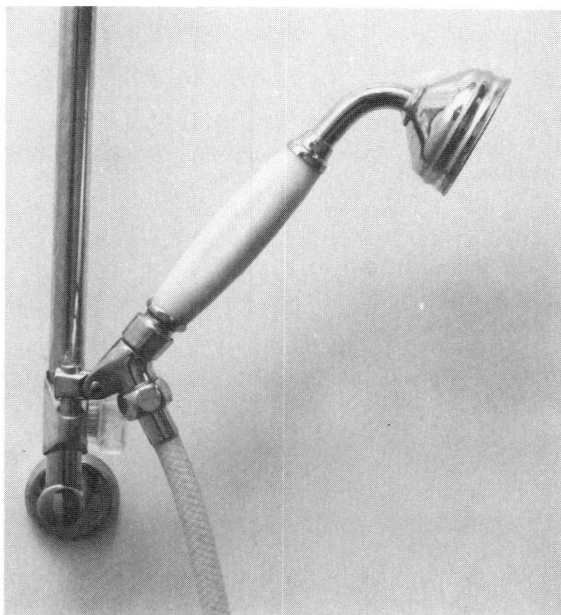

Figure 13-6
Shower hose.

tervention is adjusted as the client's condition changes and as response to treatment is evaluated.

Alleviating pressure

Pressure should be relieved at regular intervals. Position changes are essential because body weight is sufficient to obstruct blood flow wherever the weight is concentrated. Whenever a person is unable to change position or cannot sense the need for turning, constant occlusion of local circulation can cause tissue destruction and a pressure sore.[5] A turning schedule should be established and adhered to when the client is in bed. The client should be taught to shift weight or to push up to relieve weight when in bed or a wheelchair.

A number of devices are available to help relieve pressure. Pads that decrease friction include body pads, heel and elbow pads made of sheepskin, and convoluted pads. Pads must be protected if the client is incontinent. Although these devices decrease friction, they do not relieve pressure. Sheepskin pads have the disadvantage of matting with washing and need to be changed frequently. Heel and elbow pads are sometimes difficult to keep in place. Other pads are not cleaned easily and therefore have to be replaced frequently.

Devices that roll, move, or turn the client include turning frames such as the Stryker Wedge Frame* and Roto Rest.†[12] These beds minimize self-motivated movement. All too frequently nursing staff members rely on special beds to manage pressure sores rather than adhering to a turning and positioning schedule that allows for assessment of the skin at regular intervals.

Devices that equalize pressure and distribute weight include water beds, intermittent water or airflow beds, Clinitron therapy,‡ and mud beds. These devices are expensive and bulky but are regarded highly for pressure sore prevention. Their design permits the largest skin area possible

---

*A turning frame manufactured by Stryker Corporation, Kalamazoo, Mich.
†An oscillating hospital bed manufactured by Kinetic Concepts, Inc., San Antonio, Tex.
‡An air-fluidized support system used in place of a bed, Support Systems International, Charleston, SC.

to be in contact with supporting equipment. The Clinitron bed can be used for incontinent clients or those with heavy wound exudate. However, some clients may complain of "seasickness" in the water bed.

Administering prescribed treatments

Reddened areas (stage 1) are protected by covering them with a transparent film such as Op-Site or a skin barrier such as Duoderm. Adhesive foam is then applied over the dressing to help relieve pressure.[7] Topically prescribed products such as solutions and salves and the application of dressings may be prescribed for the management of stage II to stage IV pressure sores. Surgical and chemical debridement of wounds and Hubbard tub baths also are ordered for management of stage III and stage IV pressure sores. If eschar is not removed, the underlying tissue will continue to break down. Surgical debridement is fast but introduces the risks of sepsis and bleeding. Chemical debridement may take 10 days or longer. When the eschar disappears, the debridement should be stopped so that healthy granulation tissue is not removed.[7]

A number of topical preparations are used. The indications, limitations, and precautions of commonly used topical treatments are described in Table 13-2.[1]

The type and kind of dressings ordered for pressure sores are a medical decision. An open wound, however, should generally be covered since the skin is already broken. Care should be taken to pad and protect the area from further injury and to prevent bacterial invasion. A moisture balance which promotes healing also is created by covering the wound.[26]

Enzymatic ointments are used to remove superficial fibrinous debris. Necrotic tissue in small pressure sores may be removed by the physician at the client's bedside. Larger pressure sores require surgical debridement in the operating room. Cleansing around the sore with a bland antiseptic soap and warm water should be done at least twice daily, and then the area should be rinsed with normal saline. Daily Hubbard tank or whirlpool baths are more effective for larger pressure sores. Systemic antibiotics are ordered for clients who are septic or have cellulitis and are given as an adjunct to surgical treatment.[22] Skin grafting sometimes becomes necessary to assist in the healing process.

Teaching the client and family

The educational program for clients with pressure sores should emphasize the importance of skin care problems; good nutrition; skin care information, including the causes and prevention of pressure sores; safety precautions; preventive techniques; problem-solving techniques and management of any existing pressure sores. Families should be included in the educational program, and stress placed on the need for individual responsibility for skin care.[3] Individualized needs for equipment, medications, pressure relief, and diet should be taught on a one-to-one basis. The importance of psychological problems, such as depression, should be addressed as a contributing factor to pressure sore formation. Depression may interfere with a person's ability to maintain a skin care program. Verbal instruction should be supplemented with printed materials. The client's understanding of material presented and ability to demonstrate techniques of skin care should be documented in the record.

Allen,[2] a nurse specializing in rehabilitation of persons with spinal cord injury, found that treatment of pressure sores often necessitated multiple hospital admissions and surgical procedures. Nursing care had been directed to maximizing medical interventions and did not include an assessment or teaching plan for the paralyzed client. To decrease the number of readmissions, the nursing care plan was revised to incorporate a social and nursing assessment, reeducation of the client about methods of preventive skin care, and discharge planning with community follow-up by appropriate community agencies. This plan emphasized the importance of a comprehensive nursing approach to skin care problems.

Discharge planning and follow-up

A community nurse, along with a physical therapist and occupational therapist, may visit the client's home before discharge to evaluate the availability of indoor plumbing, heating arrangements, and wheelchair accessibility. The client and family are the final decision makers in any adjustments or modifications made in the home. Whenever possible, predischarge conferences should be held with the community agency representatives who supply equipment, medications, or rehabilitation services to the client to facilitate

TABLE 13-2 _____

A comparison of topical preparations for the treatment of pressure ulcers

Preparation	Indications	Limitations	Precautions
Antacids	Superficial wounds	Apply frequently	Not reported
Antibiotics			
Local	Not useful		May destroy normal flora; watch for superinfection
Systemic	Systemic infections only	Sensitivity of infecting agent	
Antiseptics			
Povidone-iodine	Draining infected wounds; clean wounds	Hard necrotic eschar; dress frequently	Watch for allergy to iodine; protect surrounding skin; stop if no results in 7 days
Helafoam	Same as above; severely undermined ulcers	Hard necrotic eschar; dress frequently	Same as above
Dextran beads (Debrisan)	Draining wounds	Dry ulcers or hard necrotic eschar; possible frequent dressings	Discontinue use when drainage ceases if no further healing is evident; can cause bleeding, burning; mix with sterile glycerin on shallow ulcers
Enzymes			
Collagenase (Santyl)	Soft or hard necrotic tissue; crosshatch first with surgical blade	Clean healing tissue; dress daily	Manufacturer recommends discontinuation when necrotic tissue is removed; avoid hexachlorophene, tincture of iodine, merthiolate, nitrofurazone (Furacin), Burow's solution
Fibrinolysin and desoxyribonuclease (Elase)	Soft necrotic tissue on hard necrosis after deep crosshatching	Clean healing tissue; dress three times a day	Discontinue when necrotic area is removed; keep away from skin and granulation tissue
Gelfoam (powder, sponges)	Small to medium size clean wounds; daily to weekly dressing changes	Draining or hard necrotic ulcers; dress every 1-7 days	Debride and clean wound before use; do not cleanse between applications; inspect wound daily; if purulent, debride and start over

From Ahmed MC: Choosing the best method to manage pressure sore, Special Report, Nurses' Drug Alert 4(15), Dec 1980.   *Continued.*

TABLE 13-2

A comparison of topical preparations for the treatment of pressure ulcers—cont'd

Preparation	Indications	Limitations	Precautions
Gold leaf	Clean wounds only; dress two times a day	Draining or hard necrotic ulcers; wound edges undermined; wound ringed by scar tissue	Prevent excessive friction; keep hemoglobin level above 12 g/100 ml
Insulin	Superficial wounds; drainage wounds	Deep or hard necrotic ulcers	Watch for hypoglycemia; apply at mealtimes; no better than usual methods
Op-Site (polythene film)	Superficial ulcers; selected deep, draining, or necrotic ulcers	Skin must be dry; *Pseudomonas aeruginosa* infection; dress every 3-7 days	Remove only nonadherent portion or skin may tear; cut hole in center of Op-Site, clean, and reapply; film may stick to fingers or patient's skin if not applied carefully
Sugar			
Granulated	Clean ulcers	Not reported; dress daily	Therapeutic range unknown
Paste	Clean ulcers	Stasis, radiation, or scleroderma-associated ulcers	Improvement should occur within 14 days
Egg white	None found	Not recommended	Procedure may retard normal healing
Vegetable gums			
Karaya	Clean, draining, superficial, deep ulcers	Hard necrotic eschar; dress daily	Watch for possible skin allergy; do not remove any karaya left on wound after gentle irrigation; reports of use are limited; if seepage or odor develops, remove Stomahesive, clean, and reapply new piece; round off edges so they do not cut into skin
Peristomal covering (Stomahesive)	Clean, draining, superficial, deep, hard necrotic ulcers; may be left in place 5-7 days	None reported	

the transition from the rehabilitation facility to the community. Communication systems should be established between rehabilitation facility nurses and the client and family so that any complications can receive prompt attention. Appointments are made for return visits when appropriate. (See Table 13-3 for nursing interventions according to nursing diagnoses.)

REHABILITATION TEAM INTERVENTIONS

An interdisciplinary approach is vital to the maintenance of skin integrity. Other rehabilitation team members who work closely with the client and family in areas of skin care are the physiatrist and surgeon, occupational therapist, physical therapist, nutritionist, social worker, and biomed-

TABLE 13-3 _____

**Examples of nursing diagnoses and nursing interventions for the client
with actual or potential skin impairment**

Nursing diagnosis	Nursing intervention
Impaired or potential impaired in skin integrity	Eliminate pressure at regular intervals: turning schedule, assist and teach turning techniques (specify)
	Eliminate shearing forces
	Inspect skin several times daily (specify)
	Control incontinence
	Keep sheets dry and wrinkle free
	Provide cleansing bath, lubrication
	Massage areas at risk
	Teach good skin care
	Encourage mobility
	Increase activity
	Maintain and teach good nutrition
	Provide protective devices (pillows, pads, cushions, mattresses)
	Administer topical preparations as ordered
	Educate client and family in preventive measures
Self-care deficit: bathing/ hygiene	Provide adaptive bathing devices, such as bath brush, bath mit, bath bench, shower chair, and grab bars
	Teach safety precautions
	Involve family
	Refer to occupational therapist and other disciplines for assistance
Activity intolerance	Specific activity schedule planned with client, nursing staff, and other team members according to client's abilities (physical, physiological, psychosocial)
Knowledge deficit	Consider client's abilities, values, developmental level, interest, past experience, readiness to learn (planned according to area of deficit)
	Involve family
	Plan time to teach
	Plan method of teaching according to client's learning ability (audiovisual, illustrations, brochures, demonstrations, groups or individual teaching)
	Collaborate with other team members to plan and implement client teaching
Potential for injury	Individual at risk for injury because of perceptual or physiological deficit, lack of awareness of potential hazards
	Provide for bathroom safety (grab bars, bath bench, nonskid floors and bathtub)
	Teach safe bathing procedures: test water, safe transfer techniques
	Collaborate with other team members to plan and implement safe use of assistive and adaptive bathing devices

ical engineer. Interventions are designed to meet the individual needs of the client through a collaborative team effort.

The physician prescribes medication and treatment. Debridement and surgical interventions also are ordered and performed by the physician. The occupational therapist designs adaptive devices and develops techniques of skin care to suit individual needs. The physical therapist helps the client strengthen muscles for weight shifts and pushups, selects alternatives such as a reclining wheelchair to alleviate pressure when weight cannot be shifted, administers whirlpool treatments, assists the client in increasing endurance for performing skin care activities, and recommends adaptive equipment. The nutritionist collaborates with the rehabilitation team, including the client and family, to meet the client's nutritional needs.

The social worker assists the client and family in obtaining financial resources for needed equipment and supplies and lends emotional support. A biomedical engineer may be called upon to design or adapt equipment used for relief of pressure and maintenance of skin integrity.

OUTCOME CRITERIA

Outcome criteria of skin care for the client include the following:

1. Maintenance and restoration of skin integrity:
   a. Skin integrity is maintained.
   b. Skin integrity is restored.
   c. The client and family assume responsibility for the maintenance and restoration of skin integrity.
2. Area of safety:
   a. The client incorporates safe practices while engaging in skin care.
   b. The family incorporates safe practices while assisting the client in skin care.
3. Area of education:
   a. The client and family understand the rationale for skin care.
   b. The client and family understand the causes and prevention of pressure sores.
4. Area of discharge planning and follow-up:
   a. The client and family use community resources appropriately.
   b. The client and family call for assistance if problems occur and return for follow-up visits if scheduled.

SUMMARY

The condition of the skin is an indicator of general health and to a great extent contributes to physical appearance and self-concept. The skin serves to control body temperature, protects the body from injury and infection, assists with metabolism, and acts as a means to convey emotions. Interruptions in skin integrity can seriously affect the total function of an individual and hinder any rehabilitation efforts. Meticulous preventive care on a daily basis and early detection of any skin problems are essential in maintaining and restoring optimum function to the individual with a disability. The rehabilitation nurse plays a major role in the continual assessment of skin condition and in teaching the client and family methods to prevent skin problems. When skin integrity is compromised, a rehabilitation team effort is necessary to restore physical, social, psychological, and vocational gains lost during treatment for skin problems.

TEST QUESTIONS

1. Of the following statements, which one is accurate regarding the anatomy and physiology of the skin?
   a. The dermis is supplied with nerve endings that inform the body of changes in pain, temperature, touch, and pressure sensation.
   b. The epidermis consists of fibrous connective tissue that acts to support the dermis and subcutaneous fatty tissue.
   c. Stimulation of the sympathetic nervous system causes decreased sweat secretion with a resultant elevation in body temperature.
   d. The subcutaneous fatty layer consists of stratified squamous epithelium tissue deposited with melanin responsible for skin pigmentation.
2. A major function of the skin is to:
   a. Produce vitamin A necessary for calcium and phosphorus metabolism.
   b. Regulate body temperature by preventing moisture evaporation on the skin.
   c. Constrict and dilate blood vessels to protect underlying tissue from injury.
   d. Contribute to appearance and feelings about self.
3. The inflammatory phase of wound healing is characterized by local:
   a. Increase in heat, redness, and edema
   b. Damage to the macrocirculation followed by vasodilation lasting 1 to 2 hours
   c. Bleeding with resultant hypoxia and tissue necrosis
   d. Formation of new fibroblast tissue from epithelial cells
4. In comparing the proliferative and differentiation phases of wound healing, the nurse is aware the differentiation phase is characterized by:
   a. Synthesis of collagen in the presence of vitamin A
   b. Production of capillary beds from existing blood vessels

c. Formation of new fibrous tissue that is prone to breakdown

d. An increase in fibroblast production and loss of collagen

5. In assessing a client's skin, the nurse performs all of the following activities *except* to:

a. Use the Norton pressure sore risk rating scale to identify those at risk.

b. Check pressure points weekly for signs of pressure sore formation.

c. Observe mobility, coordination, gross and fine finger movement.

d. Palpate for texture, dryness, elasticity, and turgor.

6. A nursing goal mutually established with the client and family for maintaining skin integrity is to:

a. Discourage use of assistive and adaptive devices during bathing.

b. Incorporate daily skin care tasks with maximum nursing assistance.

c. Understand the causation and prevention of pressure sores.

d. Encourage dependence on the family for self-care activities.

7. A rehabilitation nursing intervention in maintaining and restoring skin integrity is to:

a. Encourage clients to eat a diet low in protein, vitamin C, and calories.

b. Turn and position immobile clients every 4 hours.

c. Encourage wheelchair clients to shift weight or perform pushups every 2 hours.

d. Determine if the client's itching or skin rash is drug related.

8. In providing skin care for clients, the rehabilitation nurse is aware that:

a. Elderly clients require daily bathing to cleanse the body of oil and perspiration.

b. Cracking from dry skin can be avoided by applying water before applying a topical emollient.

c. Clothing and shoes should fit tightly to prevent slipping and pressure sore formation.

d. Clients needing total assistance in skin care may require a shower chair or tub bench.

9. Nursing management of pressure sores includes:

a. Establishing a turning schedule when the client is confined to bed.

b. Implementing a standardized treatment plan for all clients.

c. Massaging and applying heat to the client's reddened areas.

d. Substituting devices for a client's positioning and turning schedule.

10. In administration of prescribed treatments in the management of pressure sores, the nurse knows to:

a. Leave an open wound uncovered to promote drying and healing.

b. Apply enzymatic ointments to remove necrotic tissue from small areas.

c. Cover an open wound to provide a moisture balance and promote healing.

d. Treat stage II pressure sores with Hubbard tub baths.

11. Which statement is *true* in describing the role of a rehabilitation team member in maintaining the client's skin integrity?

a. The nurse performs debridement and whirlpool interventions.

b. The physical therapist prescribes medicine and treatments.

c. The occupational therapist assists the client in obtaining financial resources.

d. The biomedical engineer designs pressure relief equipment.

12. An outcome criterion of skin care for the client would be for the:

a. Nurse to assume full responsibility for maintenance and restoration of skin integrity

b. Client and family to understand rationale for skin care

c. Client to be self-sufficient and not need follow-up visits to the rehabilitation center

d. Client to be independent and not require use of community resources

Answers: 1. a, 2. d, 3. a, 4. c, 5. b, 6. c, 7. d, 8. b, 9. a, 10. c, 11. d, 12. b.

LEARNING ACTIVITIES

1. Identify skin impairments.
2. List the general nursing interventions for prevention of pressure sores.
3. Describe the stages of pressure sore formation.
4. Discuss nursing interventions that should be considered when assisting the elderly client with skin care.
5. **Case study:** Bob is a 19-year-old with C7 quad-

riplegia who has just been admitted to a rehabilitation facility from an acute care hospital. Bob's appetite is poor. Up to this time, he has been completely dependent in skin care. His goals are to return to his parent's home and resume his college education.

  a. Identify nursing interventions to assist him in achieving a higher level of independence in skin care activities.
  b. Identify ways in which other rehabilitation team members can assist him in achieving his goals.

REFERENCES

 1. Ahmed MC: Choosing the best method to manage pressure ulcers, special report, Nurses' Drug Alert 4(15), Dec 1980.
 2. Allen MS: Nursing care of the spinal cord patient with recurrent pressure sores, Rehabil Nurs 9:34, Jan/Feb 1984.
 3. Andberg MM, Rudolph A, and Anderson TP: Improving skin care through patient and family training, Top Clin Nurs 5:45, July 1983.
 4. Anthony CP and Thibodeau GA: Textbook of anatomy and physiology, ed 10, St Louis, 1983, The CV Mosby Co.
 5. Baron MC: The skin and wound healing, Top Clin Nurs 5:11, July 1983.
 6. Berliner H: Aging skin. II, Am J Nurs 86:1259, 1986.
 7. Cassell BL: Treating pressure sores stage by stage, RN 49:36, Jan 1986.
 8. Feustel D: Pressure sore prevention, aye, there's the rub, Nurs '83 12:78, April 1983.
 9. Gordon M: Nursing diagnosis: process and application, ed 2, New York, 1987, McGraw-Hill Book Co.
10. Gosnell D: An assessment tool to identify pressure sores, Nurs Res 22:55, Jan/Feb 1973.
11. Gosnell DJ: Assessment and evaluation of pressure sores, Nurs Clin North Am 22:399, 1987.
12. Hargast T: Understanding pressure sores, Rehabil Nurs 6:23, May/June 1981.
13. Hotter AN: Physiologic aspects and clinical implications of wound healing, Heart Lung 11:522, 1982.
14. Hudson M: Safeguard your elderly patients' health through accurate physical assessment, Nurs '83 13:58, Nov 1983.
15. Lindberg J, Hunter M, and Kruszewski A: Introduction to person centered nursing, Philadelphia, 1983, JB Lippincott Co.
16. Long BC and Woods NF: Essentials of medical-surgical nursing: a nursing process approach, St Louis, 1985, The CV Mosby Co.
17. Luckmann K and Sorensen K: Medical surgical nursing—a psychophysiological approach, Philadelphia, 1980, WB Saunders Co.
18. Maklebust JA and others: Pressure relief characteristics of various support surfaces used in prevention and treatment of pressure ulcers, J Enterostomal Ther 13:85, May/June 1986.
19. Natow AB: Nutrition in prevention and treatment of decubitus ulcers, Top Clin Nurs 5:39, July 1983.
20. Norton D, McLaren R, and Exton-Smith AN: An investigation of geriatric nursing problems in hospital, Edinburgh, 1962, Churchill Livingstone, Inc
21. Orem DE: Nursing concepts of practice, New York, 1971, McGraw-Hill Book Co.
22. Reddy MP: Decubitus ulcers: principals of prevention and management, Geriatrics 38:55, July 1983.
23. Redfern SJ and others: Local pressure with ten types of patient support systems, Lancet 2:277, 1973.
24. Robson M: Infection in the surgical patient: an imbalance in the normal equilibrium, Clin Plast Surg 6:493, 1979.
25. Rogers S: The spirit of independence: the evaluation of a philosophy, Am J Occup Ther 36:709, 1982.
26. Rowell G and Steffl B: Pressure ulcers: prevention and treatment. In Steffl B, editor: Handbook of gerontological nursing, New York, 1984, Van Nostrand Reinhold Co.
27. Seiler WO and Stahelin HB: Recent findings on decubitus ulcer pathology: implications for care, Geriatrics 41:47, Jan 1986.
28. Shanon ML: Pressure sores. In Norris C, editor: Concept clarification in nursing, Rockville Md, 1982, Aspen Systems Corp.
29. Sieggreen MY: Healing of physical wounds, Nurs Clin North Am 22:439, 1987.
30. Staas WE Jr and Lamantia JG: Decubitus ulcers and rehabilitation medicine, Int J Dermatol 21:437, 1982.
31. Stykes J: Black skin problems, Am J Nurs 79:1092, 1979.

ADDITIONAL READINGS

Barnes SH: Patient/family education for the patient with a pressure necrosis, Nurs Clin North Am 22:463, 1987.
Bergstrom N, Demuth PJ, and Braden BJ: A clinical trial of the Braden Scale for predicting pressure sore risk, Nurs Clin North Am 22:417, 1987.
Black JM and Black SB: Surgical management of pressure ulcers, Nurs Clin North Am 22:429, 1987.
Bobel LM: Nutritional implications in the patient with pressure sores, Nurs Clin North Am 22:379, 1987.
Bristow JV, Goldfarb EH, and Green M: Clinitron therapy: Is it effective? Geriatr Nurs 8:120, May/June 1987.
Chagares R and Jackson BS: Sitting easy: how six pressure-relieving devices stack up, Am J Nurs 87:191, 1987.
Cooper DM: Pressure ulcers: unpublished research 1976-1986, Nurs Clin North Am 22:475, 1987.
Dimant J and Tanael L: Decubitus ulcers: when to suspect osteomyelitis, Geriatrics 42:74, June 1987.

Fowler EM: Equipment and products used in management and treatment of pressure ulcers, Nurs Clin North Am 22:449, 1987.

Jones PL and Millman A: A three-part system to combat pressure sores, Geriatr Nurs 7:78, March/April 1986.

Knust S and Quarn J: Integration of self-care theory with rehabilitation nursing, Rehabil Nurs 8:26, July/Aug 1983.

Nelson A: Correlation of patient motivation and staff motivation, Rehabil Nurs 8:24, May/June 1983.

Ross MC: Healing under pressure, Am J Nurs 86:1118, 1986.

Sebern MD: Pressure ulcer management in home health care: efficacy and cost-effectiveness of moisture vapor permeable dressing, Arch Phys Med Rehabil 67:726, 1986.

Sebern MD: Home-team strategies for treating pressure sores, Nurs '87 17:50, April 1987.

Shannon M: Five famous fallacies about pressure sores, Nurs '84 14:10, Oct 1984.

Stoneberg C, Pitcock N, and Myton C: Pressure sores in the homebound: one solution, Am J Nurs 86:426, 1986.

Stotts NA: Age-specific characteristics of patients who develop pressure ulcers in the tertiary-care setting, Nurs Clin North Am 22:391, 1987.

Wade NP, Lemerman RD, and Mastrioanni EJ: Rehabilitative care and education—practical guidelines for preparing patients to function at home, Rehabil Nurs 8:32, Sept/Oct 1983.

PART III

Promotion of Client Function in Activities of Daily Living Necessary for Participation in Life

Personal Hygiene and Grooming

Theresa P. Dulski

OBJECTIVES

After completing Chapter 14, the reader will be able to:

1. Describe personal hygiene and grooming activities one normally performs for oneself.

2. Identify problems that can affect a person's ability to perform personal hygiene and grooming activities.

3. Recognize the importance of performing personal hygiene and grooming activities in promoting positive body image and self-esteem.

4. Describe conditions that alter the client's ability to perform personal hygiene and grooming activities.

5. Assess the client's ability to perform personal hygiene and grooming activities.

6. Formulate nursing diagnoses associated with impaired ability to perform personal hygiene and grooming activities.

7. Develop goals with the client and family to foster maximum independence and safety while engaging in personal hygiene and grooming activities.

8. Determine nursing interventions to assist the client in achieving maximum independence and safety in performing personal hygiene and grooming activities.

9. Identify the interventions of other rehabilitation team members in assisting the client to achieve maximum independence and safety when performing personal hygiene and grooming activities.

10. List outcome criteria used to evaluate the effectiveness of planned intervention for personal hygiene and grooming activities.

Orem defines self-care as "the practice of activities that individuals initiate and perform on their own behalf in maintaining life, health, and well-being."[15] She identifies the five methods that nurses use to assist clients as doing for, guiding and directing, providing physical and psychological support, providing a developmental environment, and teaching. Furthermore, she divides nursing interventions into three nursing systems: wholly compensatory, partly compensatory, and supportive-educative. The rehabilitation nurse most commonly uses the latter two systems to assist clients to become more independent in self-care.

Self-care activities necessary for participation in everyday life include personal hygiene and grooming. Hygiene has been defined in Webster's New World Dictionary as sanitary practices and cleanliness. Grooming is defined as making neat and tidy. Personal hygiene activities considered in this chapter include bathing, washing hair, caring for the mouth, brushing teeth, cleaning fingernails, and managing menstrual flow for women. Grooming activities discussed include combing hair, shaving, applying deodorant, applying makeup, and dressing.

Performing self-care activities is a very personal matter. The rituals, habits, timing, and methods of carrying out these activities are learned at a young age, usually from immediate family members. Physical conditions in the home such as the availability of toilets, plumbing, water, and the number of family members using facilities all influence the ways in which these activities are approached.

The rehabilitation nurse's role in assisting the disabled client is to encourage self-care and human dignity by capitalizing on the client's abilities to become as independent as possible in self-care activities. Collaboration with the occupational and physical therapist in teaching the client techniques to modify self-care practices, as well as the use of assistive and adapted devices when there is a need is common in rehabilitation nursing practice.[8]

Rehabilitation goals are directed toward helping the client achieve and maintain maximum independence and safe performance of self-care activities. Achievement of some independence in the performance of these skills is one measure of successful rehabilitation.

STRUCTURE AND FUNCTION OF THE HAIR, MOUTH AND TEETH, AND NAILS

Cleaning and grooming hair, brushing and caring for the mouth and teeth, and cleaning and grooming nails contribute to feelings of health and well-being. Even when someone has been sick in bed for a period of time, the person frequently feels better if the hair is washed and the mouth cleaned. Often one of the first requests by a person who has been acutely ill is to have the hair washed. A clean mouth helps one to feel fresh and vibrant. Clean, well-groomed nails enhance the overall feeling of well-being.

Hair

Hair consists of threads of hard keratin that project through the epidermis from epithelial bulbs located in the dermis. Two types of hair appear on the body: (1) vellus, which is pigmented and covers large areas, and (2) terminal hair, which is longer, coarser, and pigmented. The entire body, except the palms of the hands, soles of the feet, and parts of the genitalia, is covered with hair.

Hair grows at varying rates and sheds at varying times. Normally 20 to 100 strands are lost each day. The shaft of the hair can be seen above the dermis. Beneath the dermis, the root is encased in a tube called a hair follicle. Muscles in the dermis attach to the hair follicles. When the body temperature is lowered, these muscles contract to conserve body heat, resulting in a "goose flesh" appearance of the skin.[16]

Characteristics of a black person's hair differ from those of a white person's hair. Although the hair of blacks looks coarse, it is actually quite fragile and requires special care. Because the shaft is flat, the hair twists on itself to form whorls or loops. The relatively dull sheen may be caused by a larger concentration of microscopic air bubbles that diffuse and reflect the light in such a way as to give a matte appearance.[18] *Alopecia* (loss of scalp hair) is often caused by pulling hair back tightly in elaborate styles for long periods of time. Frequent styling in corn rows, pick combing, or hot combs may damage the hair.[18]

Hair changes commonly occur with aging. Generally changes in melanin production cause hair to thin and to turn gray. The male hormone testosterone controls hair distribution in both sexes, and this hormone decreases with age, resulting in diminished pubic and axillary hair.[1] By age 50, the number of hair follicles decreases by one third and continues to decrease. Loss of scalp hair is common in men, whereas hair in other areas of the body increases. Estrogen controls the male hormones in younger years. As estrogen decreases with aging, women often experience increased hair growth around the chin and upper lip.[1] Men often experience increased hair growth on the ears and in the nostrils.[6]

Hair growth patterns and distribution reflect the general health of an individual. Abnormal hair loss, excessive hair growth, or changes in hair texture may be caused by hormonal imbalance, general ill health, infection, chronic liver disease, or drugs.

Lice or nit infestation usually indicates poor hygiene. Nits, the eggs of lice, are usually embedded in hair strands behind the ears. These are observed as small glistening grayish specks along the hair shaft near the scalp.

The Mouth and Teeth

The mucous membrane of the mouth is a continuation of the skin in the body orifices. Mucous membranes secrete mucus, salt, and enzymes to protect the mouth from harmful organisms. Additionally, these membranes absorb nutrients into the body and provide support for the teeth.[16] Each tooth is composed of a crown, a root, and a pulp cavity. The crown, the exposed part of the tooth, is covered with hard enamel. The internal part of the crown, located below the enamel, is dentin. The root of the tooth is embedded in the jaw and covered with bony tissue called cementum. The pulp cavity, located in the center, contains blood vessels and nerves (Figure 14-1). Teeth are needed to masticate food in preparation for digestion in the stomach and intestines. Since the mouth reflects the condition of the body, it requires proper care, nutrition, and frequent inspection.[14]

Two major consequences of poor oral hygiene are dental caries and periodontal disease. *Dental plaque,* a thick puttylike material composed of salivary deposits, food particles, and bacteria, forms around the neck of the tooth. If dental plaque is not regularly removed, bacteria react with sucrose in the plaque to form an acid that attacks the surface enamel of the tooth, causing *dental caries,* or decay. When dental decay

reaches nerves in the pulp of the tooth, pain results. Untreated caries may become infected and cause abscess formation. Irritating effects of plaque on soft tissue may cause inflammation of the gums, or gingivitis, which in turn can destroy soft tissue and supporting bone. The result is loosening and subsequent loss of the teeth.[19]

The oral mucosa of elderly patients is thin and less resistant to disease. Because the elderly often experience tooth loss from neglect or disease, some form of denture may be needed. Dentures are supported by the bones of the jaw, or alveoli dentales. These bones are absorbed slowly throughout life, often causing difficulty with the fit of dentures and consequent problems with speech and mastication. Absence of teeth and loose-fitting dentures contribute to poor nutrition. Chronic illness, lowered resistance, and the use of drugs may make dental treatment for the elderly a hazardous procedure.

Nails

Nails consist of hard flattened keratin cells that help to protect the fingers from injury. Under normal conditions the nail plate grows continuously throughout life at a rate of about 1 ml per week. If the matrix is injured, the nail may grow in a split or distorted manner. When the matrix is destroyed, the nail is permanently lost and replaced by stratum corneum of the epidermis.[16]

Some common problems affecting the nails are paronychia, ingrown toenails, and onychauxis. *Paronychia,* or inflammation of the tissue around the nail, is often the result of an infected "hangnail." Ingrown toenails may result from a familial trait, improper cutting, or wearing tight, ill-fitting shoes. *Onychauxis,* or hypertrophy or thickening of the nails, is associated with aging, nutritional disturbances, repeated trauma, or degenerative diseases. With degenerative disease, the nail plate may become thickened and discolored and is difficult to trim.[10]

Appearance of the nails may change with age and ill health. As aging occurs, nails have a tendency to become thick and brittle and therefore more difficult to manicure. Brittleness, roughness, or a change in shape may be indicative of metabolic disease, nutritional imbalance, or digestive disturbance. *Beau's lines* (temporary

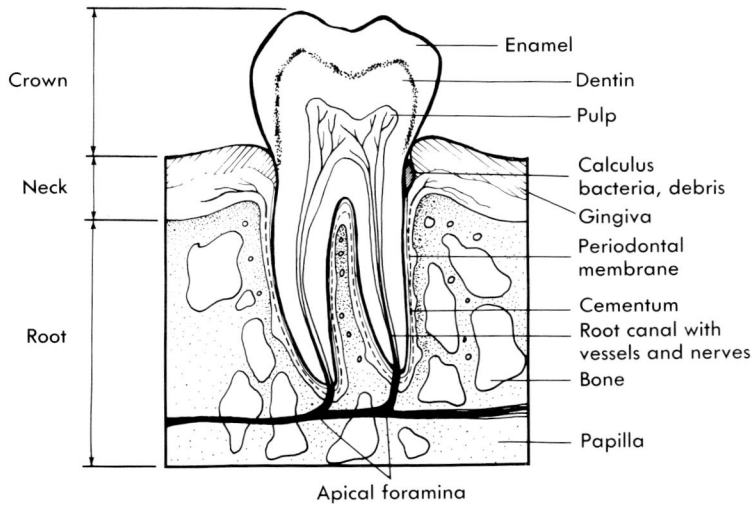

Figure 14-1
Cross section of normal tooth.

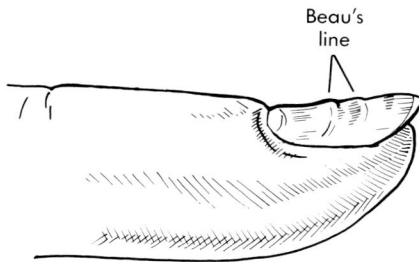

Figure 14-2
Beau's lines.

transverse grooves in the nails) are a clue to an internal disorder (Figure 14-2).

IMPORTANCE OF PERSONAL HYGIENE AND GROOMING

It has long been acknowledged that personal hygiene and grooming, including attractive, clean, well-fitting, appropriate and fashionable clothing contribute to a person's feeling of well-being and positive body image. Conversely, poor hygiene and grooming and ill-fitting, unattractive clothing can contribute to low morale and poor body image. Thus an individual may choose to wear a certain hairstyle or article of clothing to project a desired body image.[12] For example, long hair and hats are often used to project body image and sometimes to divert attention away from disabilities. Appropriate dress for climate and social situation projects body image through nonverbal communication. Choice of hairstyle, makeup, and apparel and adornment is highly personal and is a rich source of information about an individual. An individual who does not maintain an appropriate appearance is often ill, indifferent, or has low self-esteem.

During the rehabilitation process, personal clothing rather than hospital clothing should be worn. Wearing personal clothing and makeup, as well as practicing good hygiene and grooming contribute to a sense of well-being and an optimistic outlook for discharge and return home.

CONDITIONS ALTERING ABILITY TO PERFORM PERSONAL HYGIENE AND GROOMING ACTIVITIES

Alterations in the client's ability to perform self-care in personal hygiene and grooming activities are related to a variety of conditions: (1) paralysis or paresis of a hand, (2) decreased sensation of a hand or arm, (3) incoordination of upper extremities, (4) perceptual deficits such as body image disturbances, spatial disorientation, and apraxias,

(5) hemianopsia, (6) limited range of motion, (7) poor or weak hand grasp, (8) amputation(s) of an upper extremity, and (9) limited endurance. In some instances, a single disease process may hamper ability whereas in other instances, multiple processes contribute to the client's limited self-care ability.

Functional limitations also may be associated with impairment in ability to reason, solve problems, or communicate. Alteration in any area of sensory function may restrict ability to see, hear, and touch and may render the client vulnerable to accidents and injuries.

Poor balance may mean that personal hygiene and grooming activities have to be performed in a lying or sitting position to prevent injury from falls. Clients with reduced stamina caused by impaired respiratory or circulatory function may experience fatigue while performing these activities and may require complete or partial assistance to limit their frustration and conserve energy for other activities.

Clients with limited range of motion and strength may have restricted movement of the head with limited ability to look up, down, or from side to side. Limited range of motion can alter ability to raise or bend the arms and legs. Alteration in coordination may restrict the client's ability to direct movement of the extremities. Limited fine hand movements may restrict use of self-care appliances and manipulation of dressing closures.

Optokinetic nystagmus, an ocular movement reflex, can also affect ability to perform personal hygiene and grooming activities. Dudgeon, DeLisa, and Miller,[3] using upper extremity dressing independence as an indicator of functional skill level, found that persons with defective optokinetic nystagmus who have had right hemisphere brain damage with a stroke were "significantly less independent at admission and at discharge when compared to subjects with intact optokinetic nystagmus . . . those with defective optokinetic nystagmus had a 40% greater inpatient length of stay and were more likely to be discharged to a nursing home or need care by a significant other after rehabilitation."[3]

NURSING ASSESSMENT

The client's presenting appearance gives the nurse information about ability to perform self-care in hygiene and grooming activities. The health history obtained before the physical and functional assessment provides information about current health practices and past and present health problems, as well as elicits the client's estimate of ability in performing these activities.

Subjective Assessment

During the history, information is obtained about the client's hair, nails, mouth and teeth, as well as the client's ability to perform care for these areas of the body. In addition, information about menstrual management is obtained from women of childbearing age. General survey questions that elicit this information are shown in the following lists:

Personal hygiene and grooming

1. Do you have any health concerns related to your hair, nails, teeth, mouth, or menstrual management (if applicable)?
2. Are you able to care for your hair, nails, teeth, mouth, and menstrual management (if applicable)?
3. When was your last dental examination?
4. How often do you shave? What type of appliance do you use? Do you require assistance in shaving or trimming your beard and mustache (if applicable)? Do you require assistance in shaving your legs or under your armpits (if applicable)?
5. Do you use deodorant? Do you have difficulty putting it on?
6. Do you wear makeup? Do you require assistance in applying makeup?

Hair

7. Have you noticed any unusual hair loss or growth?
8. Do you use a hair remover?
9. Do you have any scalp itch or infestation?
10. Have you noticed any change in the texture of your hair?
11. What hair care products do you use (shampoo, dyes, permanents, conditioners)?

12. What are your hair care practices (frequency of shampoo, haircuts)?

Mouth and teeth

13. Do you have any gum soreness, lesions, or bleeding gums?
14. Have you noticed any mouth odor?
15. What are your oral hygiene habits (frequency of cleaning, use of mouthwash, frequency of dental visits)?
16. Do you have any difficulty getting to the dentist?
17. Do you have difficulty chewing?
18. Do you wear dentures? If yes, do you have any difficulty (irritation, clicking, difficulty talking) or with caring for your dentures?

Nails

19. Have you noticed any change in your nails (appearance or texture)?
20. How do you take care of your nails?
21. Do you have any difficulty cutting your nails?

Menstrual management (if applicable)

22. What position do you use to insert tampons or place pads?
23. Do you use any adaptations to your underwear?
24. Do you use any additional equipment such as a mirror to insert tampons or place pads?
25. Do you have any difficulty inserting tampons or placing pads?

Dressing

26. Do you have any difficulty dressing?
27. Do you require any assistance dressing (help of another person, assistive devices)?
28. What type of clothing do you prefer?
29. Do you have any difficulty obtaining or caring for your clothing?
30. Do you have any concerns about your clothes or about dressing?

Safety

31. Have you had any accidents or received any injuries while performing personal hygiene and grooming activities?
32. What safety measures do you take while performing these activities?

Objective Assessment

After obtaining a history, the nurse physically examines the client, and observes the following:

Hair. Cleanliness, odor, texture, color, distribution, and infestations are noted. The scalp is observed for dryness and lesions.

Nails. The nurse observes for cleanliness, color, and texture. Observations are made to determine whether the nails are smooth, brittle, dry, or flexible. The contour is inspected for Beau's lines and clubbing.

Mouth. Observations are made of odor, color, and moisture of lips. The mouth is inspected for *xerostomia*, or dry mouth, and *leukoplakia*, white spots or patches in the mouth. The client is asked to stick out the tongue, and it is observed for edema, coating, inflammation, lesions, tumors, hemorrhagic gingivitis, or purulent drainage.

Teeth. The teeth are inspected for cleanliness, plaque, occlusion, missing teeth, dental caries, restorations, sharp edges, chips, cracks, or looseness. The color may indicate poor personal hygiene practices and health risk habits such as heavy cigarette smoking and frequent consumption of coffee. Dentures and prostheses should be inspected for condition, fit, sharp edges, loose parts, and chips.

Dress. The nurse observes for apparel fit. Loose clothing may indicate weight loss whereas tight clothing may indicate weight gain. The cleanliness, condition, and appropriateness of clothes in terms of climate, as well as the client's age and life-style, finances, and culture are noted.

Movement. The nurse observes for unusual movement such as spasticity and tremors, and tests range of joint motion, strength, and dexterity.

Sensation. The nurse tests for sensation. Lack of sensation can be a barrier to the performance of self-care activities and can present a safety hazard when performing self-care activities.

The nurse assesses the client for self-care ability by observing the client perform personal hygiene and grooming activities and noting mobility, coordination, range of motion, strength, stamina, and gross and fine motor movements. By giving instructions and asking direct questions, the nurse assesses the client's ability to communicate, comprehend, and solve problems. Depending upon interviewer skill, insight may be gained into some of the more personal aspects of the person's self-care activities such as menstrual management. Attention is given to the client's ability to see, hear, discriminate textures, handle objects, and follow simple directions. These observations help the nurse determine the client's ability to perform personal hygiene and grooming activities adequately and safely.

NURSING DIAGNOSES

The nursing diagnoses reflect the identification of the client's strengths and limitations. Data concerning personal hygiene and grooming activities are gathered from the client's history and physical assessment. Analyses of the data and choices of nursing interventions are influenced by accepted nursing knowledge and past nursing experience. Accepted nursing diagnoses from the North American Nursing Diagnosis Association related to personal hygiene and grooming activities include the following[4]:

1. *Bathing/hygiene and dressing/grooming self-care deficits.* The client's inability to perform personal hygiene and grooming activities and the reason for this limitation, whether caused by impaired motor, sensory, or cognitive function or a combination is stated. Is the client unable or unwilling to perform these activities of daily living? Can the client manipulate devices needed to perform hygiene activities (such as a toothbrush, comb, hairbrush, razor). Is the client able to manipulate needed materials (such as toothpaste dispenser, deodorant, makeup, shampoo, tampon, pad)? Is the client able to don, fasten, wash, obtain, and replace articles of clothing? Planning should include strategies to enable the individual to perform these tasks with optimum responsibility and minimum assistance.

Other nursing diagnoses related to the above include:

2. *Activity intolerance caused by fatigue.* Affected individuals may not initially be able to participate in or complete personal hygiene and grooming activities. Planning should include rest periods as the individual relearns the component steps of these activities.

3. *Knowledge deficit.* Affected individuals may lack understanding of good personal hygiene and

grooming, or because of their condition may have perceptual, sensory, or motor impairments interfering with their ability to perform these tasks adequately. Planning should include strategies to help increase knowledge of good personal care and allow persons to develop skill in performing these activities as independently and safely as possible.

4. *Potential for injury.* This diagnosis may be due to perceptual, sensory, or motor deficits; lack of awareness of safe self-care practices; or lack of attention to environmental hazards. Planning should incorporate use of assistive and adapted devices when needed and information about safety.

GOALS

Realistic goals that are mutually determined with the client and family should be established. Success of the client's rehabilitation is influenced by support received from the family; therefore family members should be included in the rehabilitation plan at the beginning of the rehabilitation process. Support and instructions from rehabilitation team members will help the family assist the client in achieving maximum independence throughout life.[7]

Goals for self-care activities in personal hygiene and grooming are based on the nursing diagnoses and define clearly what the client, family, and nurse hope to accomplish. Goals should be prioritized so that the client is able to accomplish one goal and go on to the next. The reward of success in achieving one goal helps motivate the client to continue and attempt the next goal. [7] The client's readiness and ability to strive for another goal is assessed by the nurse and other rehabilitation team members, who use information about and observation of the client's physical, psychosocial, and functional skills.

The following are broad goals for achieving maximum independence in personal hygiene and grooming activities:

1. To perform personal hygiene and grooming activities at the highest level of function possible
2. To understand when and how to use assistive and adapted devices
3. To plan for rest periods before fatigue occurs
4. To understand the role of personal hygiene

and grooming in promoting good health and maintaining and restoring positive self-esteem and body image
5. To practice personal hygiene and grooming activities safely within one's own environment

REHABILITATION NURSING INTERVENTIONS

After the initial client assessment, the nurse is able to develop an individualized plan with the client's strengths and limitations in mind. Interventions are chosen that promote maximum health, independence, and safety and are based on nursing knowledge of biophysical and behavioral sciences, as well as nursing research and past experience.

Therapeutic intervention related to self-care in personal hygiene and grooming may involve teaching the client and family the problem-solving process, supplementing self-care abilities by providing assistive or adapted devices when necessary, and educating the client and family regarding safe and effective performance of self-care skills. According to Mossman,[13] the following principles of teaching should be employed when teaching any activity of daily living:

1. Know the procedure thoroughly before starting to teach the client.
2. Know the client's abilities and limitations and do not expect achievement beyond ability. Expect to provide extended supervision, since the client may forget part of the procedure from one day to the next.
3. Provide encouragement, but do not pressure the client to perform. When difficulty is experienced, provide help to try another activity that can be performed, then return to the first procedure later.
4. Use assistive or adapted devices if the client does not have the use of muscles needed to perform the task. Provide proper equipment for the activity, and allow sufficient time and space so the client does not feel rushed or restricted.
5. Be flexible. Adapt procedures with the help and suggestions of the client and family. If one method does not work, try another.
6. Ensure that everyone who works with the client is aware of what is being taught. Each person involved in teaching should teach the same way, follow the same steps, and use the same terms.
7. Give instructions as simply as possible, using short sentences and repeating them often. If the client has difficulty understanding a sentence it should be reworded. Gestures should be used to clarify directions, especially with clients who have language problems.
8. Repeat the procedure each time the client would normally perform the activity.

Clients should be reminded of safety precautions with each activity they are learning. Frequent repetition of instructions, demonstration of the activity by the nurse or therapist, practice with each step of the activity, and evaluation of performance assists in learning. Limiting distractions in the environment makes it easier for the client to concentrate on the instructions and to practice the component steps of the activity.

Personal Hygiene

As part of good personal hygiene, frequent handwashing should be encouraged, especially before meals and after toilet. Soap and products that interfere with the natural pH of the skin should be avoided. Hand lotion applied after washing prevents chafing and irritation, helping to maintain skin integrity. Individual towels, washcloths, and personal articles should be used, and this practice emphasized as part of good hygiene.[10] Further discussion of bathing and skin care is found in Chapter 13.

Hair

Combing and brushing the hair daily is necessary to prevent tangling and matting. Weekly shampoos are usually adequate to maintain hair cleanliness, but individuals who have a tendency to have oily hair may wish to shampoo more frequently. If the client is unable to sit at a sink or shampoo in a shower, a shower tray or a clean bedpan can be used to catch the water while the person is lying on a stretcher or positioned in bed (Figure 14-3).[21]

Hair infested with lice or nits may be treated with gamma benzene hexachloride (Kwell) shampoo or other medication specific for this problem.

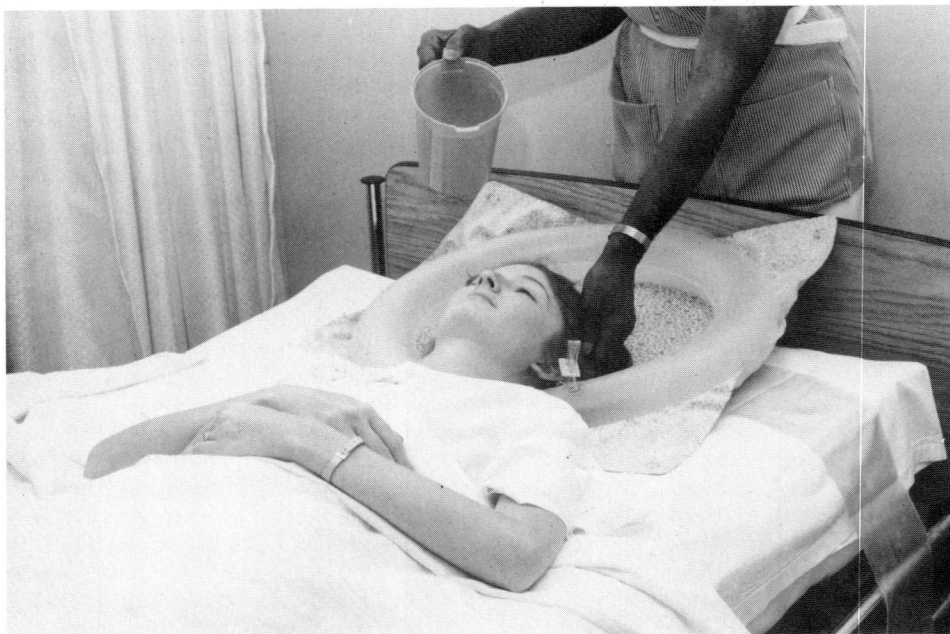

Figure 14-3
Shampoo tray being used to wash client's hair.

A fine-toothed comb may be used to remove remaining nits. Regular shampoos can be used within 24 hours after treatment.[10] To prevent spread of lice or nits, all personal hair care items as well as towels, washcloths, and linens should be washed and used solely for the individual affected.

Mouth and teeth

Good oral hygiene is essential for physical and mental well-being. It includes daily brushing and flossing to prevent plaque formation and help prevent tooth decay. A soft toothbrush with end-rounded bristles should be used to prevent trauma to the gums. Brushing removes food particles and plaque and also stimulates the gum circulation, helping to maintain firmness. Proper brushing and flossing are demonstrated in Figure 14-4.

When a client has limited or absent function in one hand, a toothpaste cap can be removed by grasping the tube close to the top and using the thumb and index finger of the unaffected hand to turn the cap. If the client has minimal grasp, the tube can be stabilized between the knees before removal of the cap.

If a client is unable to perform mouth care, the nurse or family member may give assistance by standing behind the chair when the client is seated. The person is instructed to tilt the head backward or look at the ceiling, while the helper then supports the head in the desired position and performs mouth care activities.

If the client wears dentures, these should be cleaned with a soft brush and dentrifice after eating. When the dentures are taken out, the mouth should be rinsed to remove food particles. Dentures are usually removed at night to allow the oral tissue a chance to recover from any irritation.[20] The mucous membrane should be checked every 6 months and dentures examined for proper fit. Dentures may have to be replaced every 5 to 8 years.

Good oral hygiene should be practiced and taught as part of the rehabilitation process. When toothaches, dental caries, or other mouth problems are present, the client should be referred to

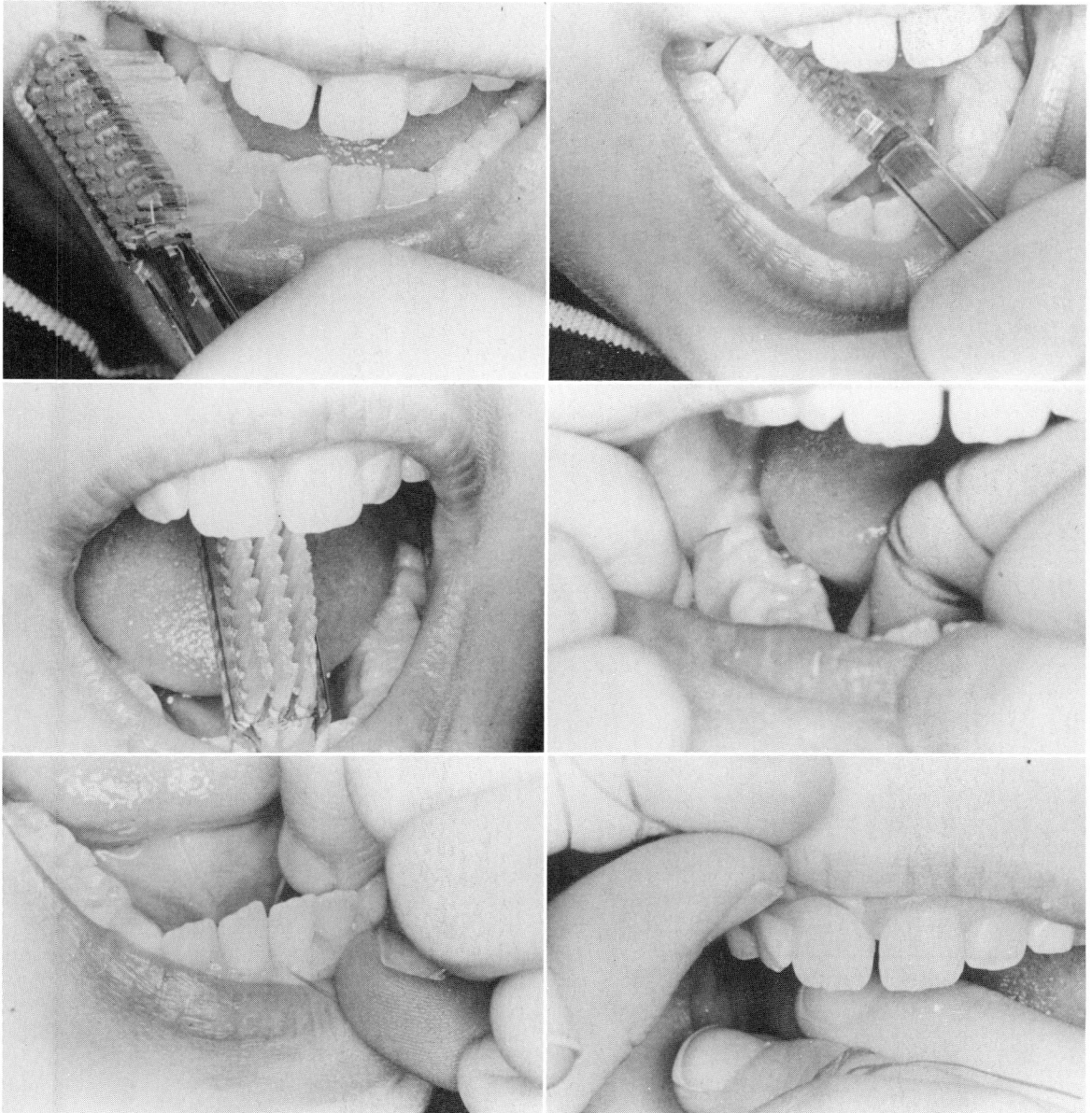

Figure 14-4
Proper toothbrushing and flossing. *(Courtesy American Dental Association, Chicago, Ill.)*

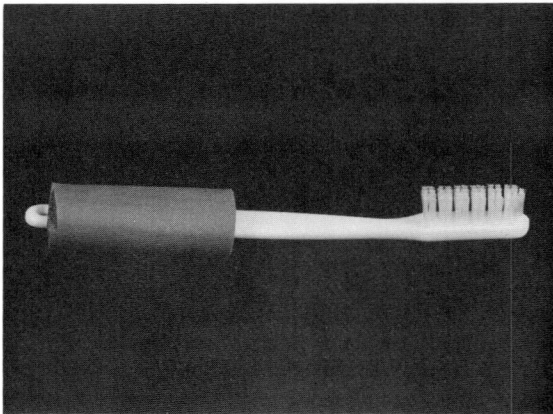

Figure 14-5
Toothbrush with adapted handle.

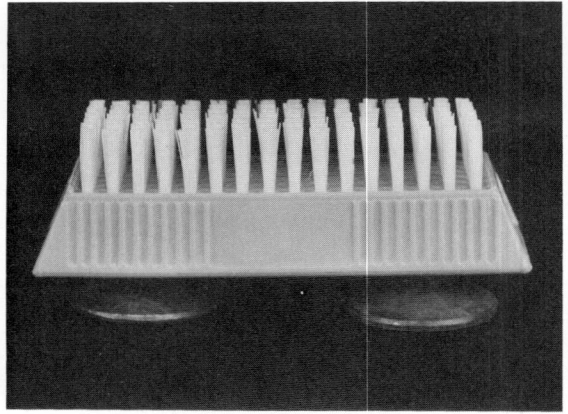

Figure 14-6
Nailbrush stabilized with suction cups.

a dentist. The client should be advised to schedule regular dental examinations. If there is any alteration in the client's ability to perform oral hygiene, the nurse collaborates with a dentist, dental hygienist, and occupational therapist to devise modified procedures or adapted devices, such as a built-up handle on a toothbrush to aid the client in self-care activities (Figure 14-5).

Nails

Nursing interventions for nail care involve observing for predisposing factors that cause alteration in the nails, assisting the client with care, directing self-care, and teaching the client about care of the nails. Special precautions should be taken when cutting the nails. Fingernails should be trimmed in a curved fashion, and rough edges of the nails filed. Toenails should be soaked before trimming and then cut straight across.

When cleaning the nails, an orange stick can be used to gently remove dirt, thus preventing injury to the underlying skin. Particularly dirty nails should be soaked, and a nailbrush used to scrub the dirt from underneath. A nailbrush stabilized with suction cups can be used to clean the nails on one hand when an affected hand cannot be used to hold the brush (Figure 14-6). Only mild soap should be used for scrubbing, because harsh soap may dry the nails and cause them to be brittle. An adapted file can be made from a file board stabilized with suction cups.

Hands that have limited range of motion and

are fixed in a closed, or grasp, position should be carefully opened, washed, and dried to prevent accumulation of dirt and dry skin. Skin between the toes should be dried gently. If these areas remain moist maceration of the skin can occur.[5] Tissue surrounding the nails, and the nails themselves, may need regular lubrication to prevent dryness and cracking. Frequent inspection of the nails is required to identify beginning infections or ingrown toenails and is particularly important when the client has loss of sensation in the extremities.

Clients who have poor eyesight need special assistance with nail care. Adapted clippers can be used successfully when only gross hand motion is present. Persons who have difficulty handling the trimming instrument need assistance. Clients with limited range of motion may have difficulty reaching the toes and may need specific adapted devices or total assistance. Those clients who have thickened nails that are difficult to trim should be referred to a podiatrist.

Menstrual management

One of the most difficult self-care tasks for women with lack of sensation, spasticity, loss of strength and dexterity, or loss of movement is menstrual management. To accomplish the insertion of a tampon or the placement of a pad, the woman must pull her pants down or skirt up, her underwear down, position herself, remove and dispose of the soiled pad or tampon, wipe and wash the perineal area, unwrap a new pad or tampon, place the pad or insert the tampon, get up from the toilet, and pull up underwear and pants or pull skirt down.[2]

Several recommendations can be made to assist the disabled woman in managing menstrual flow. These include adaptations to position, underwear, tampon or pad, and the use of mirrors or knee spreaders. Duckworth[2] recommends the following adaptations of position. For the woman using a wheelchair who can slide her pants down and who has good hand dexterity, sitting right on the front edge of the seat may enable her to manage tampons, but it may be difficult to get pads far enough back. The woman who cannot lean over may need a raised toilet seat with a front opening in order to place the tampon or pad. She also may require a mirror if she lacks sensation or a knee spreader if she cannot abduct her legs. Inserting the tampon will probably increase her spasticity. If balance is poor, she may need to lean sideways and hold onto a bar or wheelchair side. Both positions allow tampon insertion but require transfers from wheelchair to toilet. Pulling pants down and up remains a problem. Some women find it easier to transfer to a bed to change pads or tampons.

Those who have problems with coordination, such as women with cerebral palsy, may have to kneel to stabilize themselves. This position can be quite distasteful if used in public facilities that are littered or unclean, or embarrassing if there are wide gaps underneath the cubicles. Women with spasticity or loss of balance may be able to stand to manage pads or tampons if a grab bar is present.[2]

Underwear may be adapted by replacing the crotch with a crotch flap that has velcro fastening and loops, placing an unsewn flap from the back of the crotch or the back waistband to the front waistband, or sewing loops to the side of underwear to assist the woman with lack of hand dexterity to pull underwear up and down. Persons who lack dexterity will probably have to use pads. Pads with stick-on backs are easier for both disabled and able-bodied women to use because belts are hard to fasten.[2]

Grooming

A number of recommendations can be made to assist the disabled client to gain more independence in grooming hair, shaving, applying deodorant, applying makeup, and dressing.

Grooming hair

Shorter hairstyles can be cared for more easily by both men and women. Using a mirror provides feedback to the client about appearance of the hair when styling. Clients with perceptual problems may need reminders to touch ignored parts of the head and to comb, brush, and style neglected areas. Hair care appliances such as a blow dryer or electric comb can be used by clients with function in one upper extremity. Many women may prefer to have their hair professionally cared for and styled.

Blacks lubricate, stretch, and straighten their hair. Using a wide-toothed comb and combing the hair when wet will help avoid tangling during these procedures. Careful brushing is needed to avoid breaking the hair. Styling also can be accomplished with rolling or braiding.[21] When alopecia is observed as a result of severe hairstyles, the nurse may suggest other ways of fashioning the hair. A variety of adapted devices can be used for combing and brushing the hair (Figure 14-7).

Shaving

Shaving the face is an important aspect of cleanliness and grooming for men. In most instances a daily shave is required, but the frequency also depends on the rate of hair growth and personal habit. Electric razors should be used if the client has restricted movement or loss of sensation on one side. Safety blade razors may be used with supervision or when there is no great danger of nicks or cuts occurring. These razors should not be used when the client is taking anticoagulants. If a beard or mustache is grown, daily washing and frequent trimming are needed to keep facial hair clean and neat. Growing a beard or mustache contributes to body image and may convey a more masculine appearance. Depilatory creams and lotions may be used by men and women to remove excessive hair. Care should be taken to avoid skin irritation with these products. Electrolysis may be used as a permanent method of hair removal. For women who shaved the legs and axillary hair before their disability, continuing these activities during rehabilitation will help foster a more positive body image.

Applying deodorant

Deodorant, either spray or roll on, can be applied with an unaffected hand. When the client is in

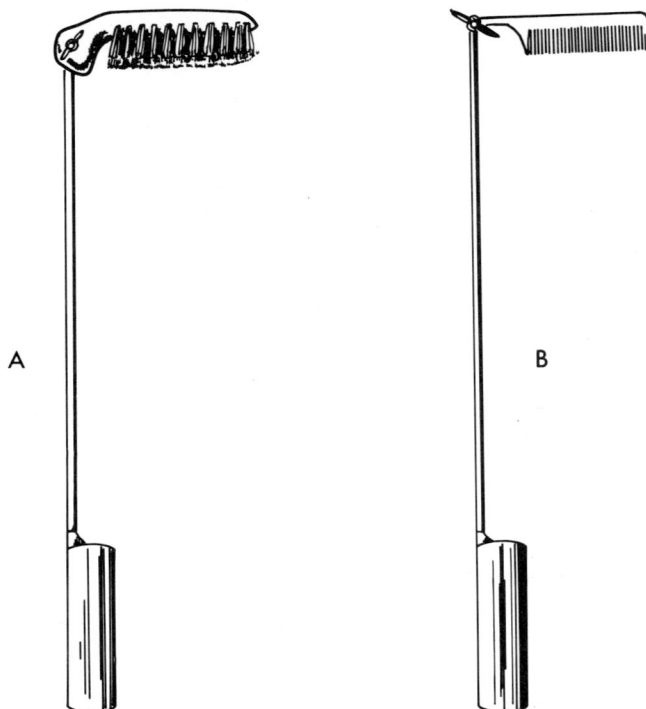

Figure 14-7
Adapted hairbrush (**A**) and comb (**B**).

the supine position and one extremity is flaccid or spastic, the unaffected extremity should be used to raise the affected extremity above the head before deodorant is applied. Alternatively, when the client is in the sitting position, the affected arm should be moved forward on a table surface to facilitate application.

Applying makeup

Application of makeup also is an important consideration in grooming and contributes to body image and feelings of well-being. A light application of makeup enhances appearance and protects the skin. Women who regularly wear makeup should be encouraged to continue to do so during the rehabilitation process. Makeup jars can be opened with one hand if the bottom of the container is stabilized with suction cups. Tubes can be opened by grasping them close to the top with an unaffected hand and using the thumb and index finger to loosen the cap. Motor, sensory, or perceptual deficits influence the success of per-

forming this task. Makeup incorrectly applied can be grotesque. Correctly applied, it enhances the client's appearance. Nurses and therapists should give support and honest feedback until this skill is perfected.

Dressing

Nurses should be aware of the significance of personal clothing and teach and assist the client to put on regular clothes during the rehabilitation process. To assist the client in achieving optimum function in dressing, assessment must be made of the client's range of motion, coordination, finger dexterity, sitting balance, strength, and stamina.[9] Restricted range of motion limits the client's independence in dressing unless modified techniques and assistive or adapted devices are designed for the individual.

Clothing that is attractive, comfortable, and easy to manage contributes to positive body image and promotes feelings of independence. Fabrics should be durable and easy to care for with such additions as gussets, pleats, reinforcements, fastenings, and openings that assure comfort and ease of dressing. Slacks, shorts, or other pants-type clothing should be worn for comfort and freedom during physical therapy sessions. The nurse also can advise the client to obtain loose-fitting, stretch fashions; full shirts to fit over the hips; trousers or slacks with a front zipper and elastic waistbands; and bras with front closures and elastic straps. Reasonably priced garments designed especially for individuals with physical limitations are now available from several distributors. (See Appendix D for listing of distributors.)

Clothing worn by the client before the disability can be altered. Alterations in clothing should be made so openings and fastenings are within easy reach and simple to manipulate. Velcro, larger hooks, large buttons, large snaps, and zippers with large pull loops or extension pulls can be used to adapt clothing to the individual's ability and thereby allow maximum independence in dressing. A Velcro closure is shown in Figure 14-8.

Clients who must spend time in spica casts should buy or make extra large shirts that go on

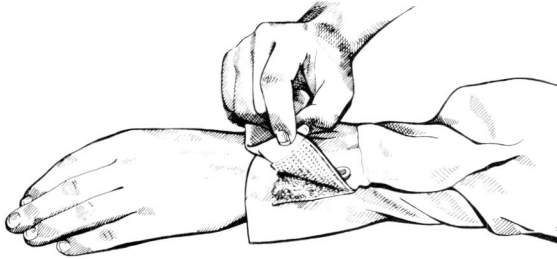

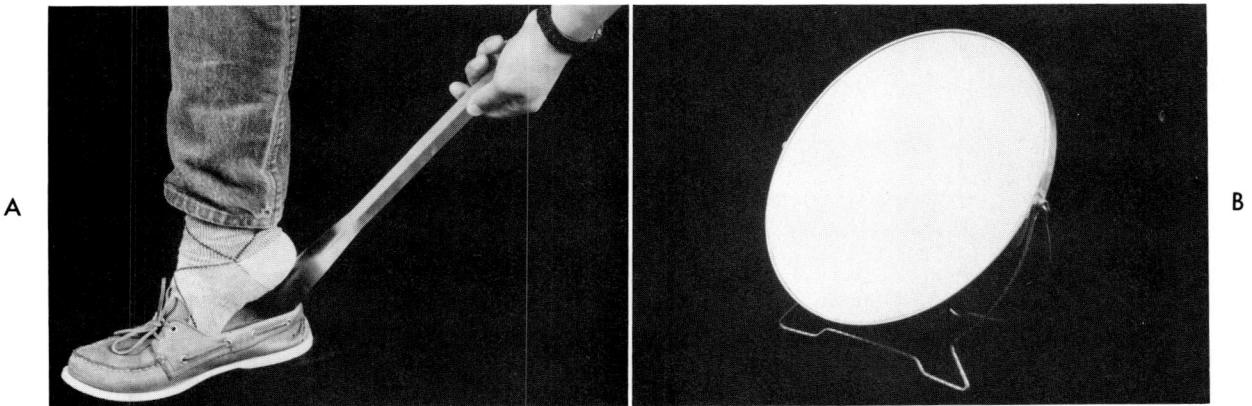

Figure 14-8
Velcro shirtsleeve to facilitate closure.

A

B

C

Figure 14-9
Assistive/adapted dressing devices. **A,** Long-handled shoehorn. **B,** Stand-up mirror. **C,** Zipper pull.

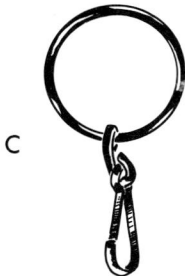

with ease, skirts or pants that have wide tops (hip size plus 10 or 12 inches) and a drawstring or elastic waist. Antiembolic stockings can be worn on the unaffected leg, and a boot for the other foot.[11]

Assistive devices such as long-handled shoehorns, stand-up mirrors, and zipper pulls are some of the items used to aid the client in obtaining maximum independence in dressing activities (Figure 14-9). The nurse and occupational therapist should collaborate in developing modified dressing techniques for the client according to individual needs. Figure 14-10 demonstrates a modified dressing technique for a person with left hemiplegia who is dressing while sitting in a chair. The affected extremity should be inserted into clothing first. Modified dressing techniques also may include dressing while in bed, or using a wall or door jam for support when balance or stamina are altered. When average dressing time exceeds 30 to 40 minutes and the procedure is consistently frustrating for the client, assistance should be given by the nurse, therapist, or family member.

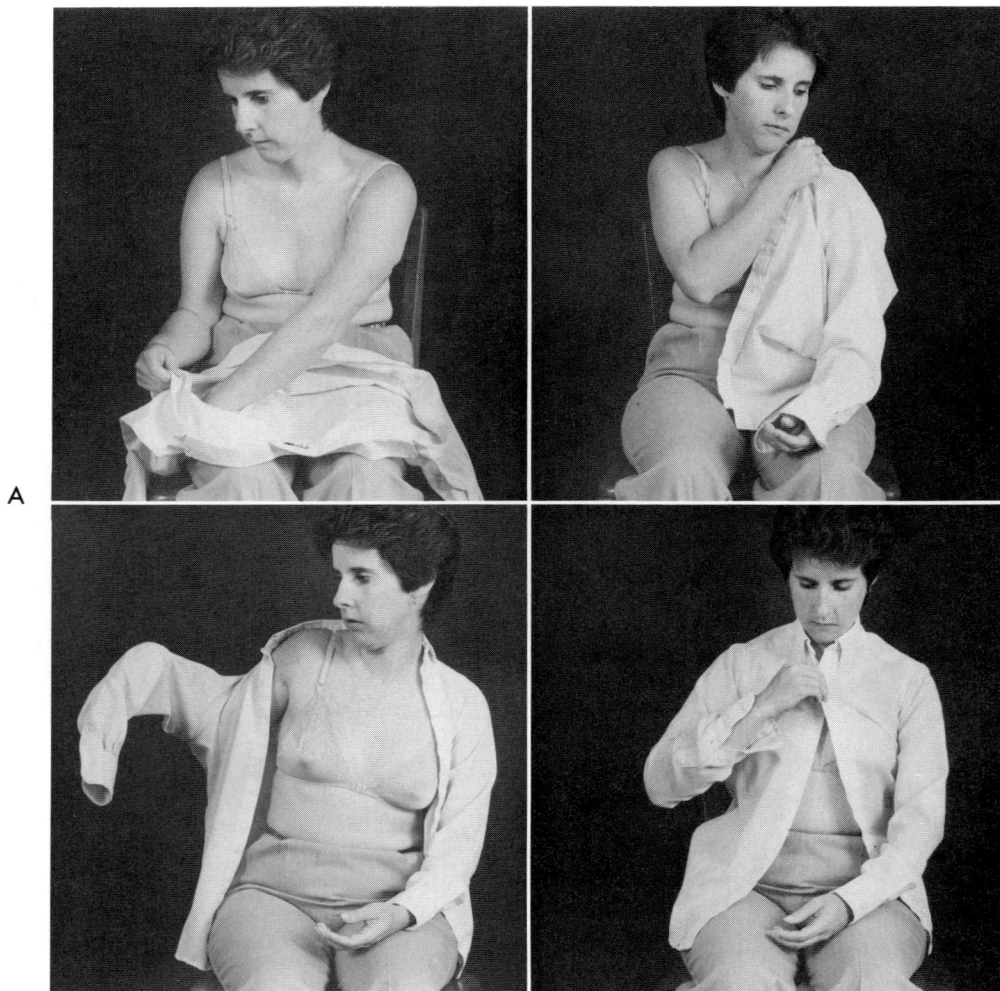

Figure 14-10
A, Putting on shirt when left arm is paralyzed.

Both hypothermia and hyperthermia are a concern when the client has altered sensation. The nurse should advise the client and family of the dangers of hypothermia and instruct them in appropriate dress for inclement weather. Sweaters and warm footwear should be worn inside. The client also should be advised to take fewer baths to avoid lowering body temperature as a result of evaporation. When outside, the client should be instructed to layer clothing and wear a hat and gloves. Exertion in cold weather should be avoided. If money is a problem in maintaining adequate home heating, the client should be advised to contact government agencies for assistance with payment of heating bills.

To avoid hyperthermia the client should be instructed to wear cool, lightweight clothing in the summer, avoid going outside on extremely hot days, wear a hat for head protection, and take plenty of liquids to avoid dehydration. Hyperthermia or increased body temperature is just as damaging to the client as hypothermia because it leads to dehydration. Clients with sensory deficits and their families may not be aware of the physical

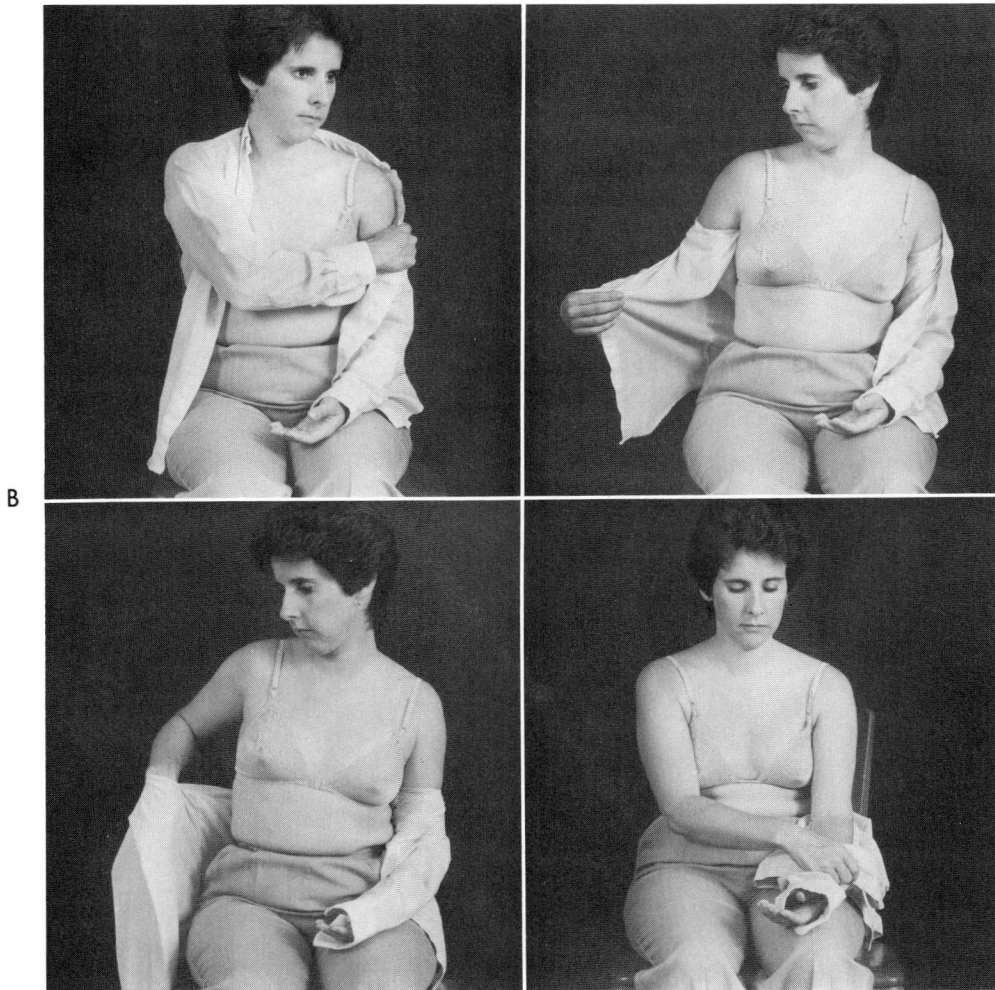

Figure 14-10, cont'd
B, Taking off shirt when left arm is paralyzed.

TABLE 14-1 _____

Examples of nursing diagnoses and nursing interventions for the client with deficits in personal hygiene and grooming activities

Nursing diagnosis	Nursing intervention
Self-care deficit	
Bathing/hygiene	Collaborate with occupational therapist and other disciplines to accomplish goals
Hair grooming	Teach use of adapted devices: long-handled comb, brush
	Teach use of external modifiers: handles, universal strap
	Teach use of assistive devices: around the neck mirror, shampoo tray, shower hose
	Teach use of appliances: hair blower, electric comb, electric razor, battery razor, razor with universal strap
Mouth	Lubricate mouth, use mouthwash
	Teach proper brushing and flossing
	Refer to physician and dentist when lesions found
Teeth	Teach dental hygiene and use of adapted devices: one-handed dental floss holder, handles on toothbrush, modified electric toothbrush, water-Pik, toothpaste squeeze key, toothpaste pump dispenser
	Collaborate with occupational therapist and other disciplines to accomplish goals
	Refer to dentist
Menstrual management	Teach different positions to facilitate insertion of tampon or placement of pad
	Teach ways to adapt underwear
	Teach use of assistive or adapted devices
Dressing/grooming	
Nails	Teach use of adapted devices: external modifiers, handles on clippers
	Refer to podiatrist when necessary
Shaving	Teach to organize equipment in safe area
	Teach use of assistive and adapted equipment when needed
Application of deodorant	Teach different positions to use for ease of application
Application of makeup	Teach one-handed techniques for opening containers, tubes
	Teach use of neck mirrors, stand-up mirrors
	Give appropriate feedback
Knowledge deficit	
Personal hygiene	Plan varies according to area of deficit
	Consider client's abilities, values, developmental level, interest, past experience, readiness to learn
	Involve family
	Plan time to teach
	Use appropriate methods to teach according to client's preference and learning ability
	Collaborate with other team members to plan and implement client and family education
Grooming	Teach use of specially designed equipment, clothing
	Teach use of clothing closure devices: snaps, zippers, Velcro, hooks
	Teach use of assistive devices: spray shoe polish dispenser, electric shoe polisher, buttons, elastic, shoehorn, reacher
	Teach modified dressing techniques
	Refer to occupational therapy
	Collaborate with occupational therapist and other disciplines to accomplish goals
Activity intolerance	Plan specific activity schedule with client, nursing staff, and other team members according to client's physical, physiological, psychosocial abilities
Potential for injury	Teach about safety hazards as result of perceptual or physical deficits
	Involve family as necessary in use of safety measures for personal hygiene, dressing activities
	Collaborate with other team members to plan, teach, and implement safe use of assistive and adapted devices and special techniques

problems caused by extremes in environmental temperature. The client and family members should be alerted to factors that may influence the client's perception of the environment, taught to monitor body temperature, and helped to plan appropriate interventions with regard to dress when alteration in body temperature is an actual or potential problem.

Safety

Safety deserves particular attention during personal hygiene and grooming procedures. An opening under the bathroom sink allows the client to sit while grooming and provides access to the sink from a wheelchair. Exposed hot water pipes under the sink should be insulated or covered to prevent burns. Enough countertop space should be available to accommodate personal care items. Use of electrical appliances such as a razor or hair blower should be avoided over the sink, since resting or dropping these items into a wet sink may cause a shock. To prevent injury, electrical outlets located near the mirror should be positioned away from the sink.

Examples of nursing diagnoses and interventions for deficits in personal hygiene and grooming activities are shown in Table 14-1.

REHABILITATION TEAM INTERVENTIONS

The nurse collaborates with other rehabilitation team members to plan, implement, and evaluate interventions and accomplish goals mutually established with the client and family in relation to personal hygiene and grooming. Other team members who work closely with the client and family in these areas of function are the physiatrist, dentist, occupational therapist, physical therapist, social worker, and prosthetist or orthotist.

Physiatrists diagnose the client's condition and prescribe treatment. They must have knowledge of the biophysical, physiological, and psychological responses to various treatments used by physical and occupational therapists. Prescriptions should be individualized and specific for each client, contain enough detail to inform the therapist about the goal to be accomplished, and include instructions for treatment to be continued by the client upon discharge.

A dentist, when visited regularly by clients and used as a regular source of referral by rehabilitation team members, can help the client prevent oral problems by providing instruction in oral hygiene and treating any problems at an early stage. Problems occurring in the mouth as a result of some medications and problems accompanying the normal aging process can be treated before complications occur.

The occupational therapist carries out training in many of the activities of daily living, designing special assistive and adapted devices to assist the client in these activities. The prescription received from the physiatrist may specify personal self-care areas needing particular attention.

A physical therapist supervises a program of therapeutic exercise. Before carrying out a prescription for therapeutic exercise, the therapist will perform a complete evaluation of the client's function, including a manual muscle test, evaluation of range of motion, assessment of bones and joints, and evaluation of coordination. Depending on the client's diagnosis, physician's prescription, and results of the evaluation, the therapist establishes a program to improve strength, balance, range of motion, coordination, and stamina.

Social workers assist the client in exploring sources for financial aid for equipment and supplies, home modifications, and heating. They also help resolve problems that may interfere with the client's and family's function in activities of daily living.

The prosthetist fits clients who have upper extremity amputations with artificial limbs when loss of limb interferes with independence and threatens body image. Upper extremity prostheses can now be operated with batteries connected to electric motors, allowing these limbs to be functional in performing activities of daily living. A team consisting of the client, prosthetist, physiatrist, rehabilitation nurse, physical therapist, occupational therapist, orthotist, and vocational counselor can best determine the prosthesis suitable for the client's needs. The orthotist designs braces according to individual client needs. Braces are used to apply force to an extremity and assist, resist, align, or stimulate function of the extremity.

The rehabilitation plan for achieving maximum functional independence in personal hygiene and grooming requires assessment and evaluation by all team members, who meet together regularly and reevaluate the plan with the client and family to determine progress in meeting the established goals.

OUTCOME CRITERIA

Outcome criteria for the client diagnosed with functional deficits in personal hygiene and grooming activities include the following:

1. The client and family will perform the client's personal hygiene and grooming activities at an optimum level of function.
2. The client and family know when and how to use assistive and adapted devices when these are prescribed.
3. The client and family will anticipate fatigue and plan rest periods before fatigue occurs.
4. The client will possess positive self-esteem and body image.
5. The client and family will perform personal hygiene and grooming activities safely within their own environment.

SUMMARY

The rehabilitation nurse is in a unique position to assist the client in achieving an optimum level of independence in personal hygiene and grooming activities. Through nursing assessment of the client's ability to perform these activities, the nursing diagnoses are formulated and interventions planned and implemented. The nurse collaborates with other rehabilitation team members to assist the client and family in use of assistive and adapted devices and specialized techniques that allow the client to function safely at an optimum level in these activities. When the client can be independent in performing some or all of these activities, body image and self-esteem are enhanced.

TEST QUESTIONS

1. Identifying the client's personal hygiene and grooming habits is an important part of the nursing assessment because:

   a. This helps the nurse identify areas of health teaching that are needed.
   b. This helps the nurse accomplish nursing interventions as quickly as possible.
   c. The client needs to change personal care habits after experiencing a disability.
   d. The family needs to give the client personal care.
2. It is important that rehabilitation goals for personal hygiene and grooming are directed toward assisting the client to be as independent as possible because:
   a. This makes the job easier for the family.
   b. The client can do it better.
   c. It takes less time if the client does it.
   d. It increases the client's self-esteem
3. Appropriate clothing is an important consideration for the client because of all of the following *except:*
   a. Clients with a sensory deficit may not be able to distinguish extremes in environmental temperature.
   b. Clothes project body image.
   c. Clothes affect the client's feeling of well-being.
   d. Disabled clients shouldn't draw attention to themselves by wearing inappropriate clothing.
4. Clients who are unable to be independent in personal hygiene and grooming activities because of reduced stamina should:
   a. Forget about hygiene; rest is more important.
   b. Have the family do all of the personal care.
   c. Plan care so as to conserve energy.
   d. Ignore the fatigue; hygiene and grooming are more important.
5. When the client has difficulty putting on trousers because of poor balance, an appropriate intervention might be to:
   a. Instruct a family member to help.
   b. Instruct the client to put trousers on while lying in bed.
   c. Instruct the client to put on trousers while sitting on a straight chair.
   d. Instruct the client to wear pajama bottoms because these are easier to put on

Answers: 1. a, 2. d, 3. d, 4. c, 5. b.

LEARNING ACTIVITIES

1. Discuss alterations that can affect ability to perform personal hygiene and grooming activities.
2. Describe assistive and adapted devices and special techniques that allow the client maximum function in personal hygiene and grooming.
3. Describe safety precautions that should be considered when the client is performing personal hygiene and grooming activities.
4. **Case study:** Louise is a 46-year-old housewife who has rheumatoid arthritis. She was admitted to a rehabilitation facility. Her goals are to return home and be as independent as possible in personal hygiene and grooming.
   a. Identify nursing interventions to assist her in achieving a higher level of independence in caring for hair, nails, and teeth as well as in getting dressed.
   b. Identify ways in which other rehabilitation team members can assist her in achieving her goals.
5. **Case study:** Mr. D. is 84 years old and suffered a cerebral thrombosis 3 weeks ago. He has a right-sided paresis but no speech impairment. He wants to resume self-care. His wife has arthritis and is unable to assist with his care. He wants to return home to his ground floor apartment where he lives with his wife.
   a. Describe the nursing interventions you would plan and implement to assist Mr. D. in achieving his goals safely.
   b. Describe the continued services that he may need after discharge.

REFERENCES

1. Berliner H: Aging skin, Am J Nurs 86:1138, 1986.
2. Duckworth B: Overview of menstrual management for disabled women, Can J Occup Ther 53:25, Feb 1986.
3. Dudgeon BJ, Delisa JA, and Miller RM: Optokinetic nystagmus and upper extremity dressing independence after stroke, Arch Phys Med Rehabil 66:164, March 1985.
4. Gordon M: Nursing diagnosis: process and application, ed 2, New York, 1987, McGraw-Hill Book Co.
5. Graham S and Morley M: What foot care really means, Am J Nurs 84:7, July 1984.
6. Hudson M: Safeguard your elderly patients' health through accurate physical assessment, Nurs '83 13:58, Nov 1983.
7. Jacus CM: Working with families in a rehabilitation setting, Rehabil Nurs 6:10, May/June 1981.
8. Joseph L: Self-care in the nursing process, Nurs Clin North Am 15:131, March 1980.
9. Lowman E and Klinger J: Aids to independent living, New York, 1969, McGraw-Hill Book Co.
10. Luckmann J and Sorensen K: Medical-surgical nursing—a psychophysiological approach, ed 2, Philadelphia, 1980, WB Saunders Co.
11. Mather MLS: The secret to life in a spica, Am J Nurs 87:57, Jan 1987.
12. McChoskey D: How to make the most of the body image theory in nursing practice, Nurs '76 6:58, May 1976.
13. Mossman P: A problem-oriented approach to stroke rehabilitation, Springfield, Ill, 1976, Charles C Thomas, Publisher.
14. Normal V and Snyder M: Assessment of self-care readiness, Rehabil Nurs 7:17, May/June 1982.
15. Orem D: Nursing: concepts of practice, New York, 1980, McGraw-Hill Book Co.
16. Phipps WJ, Long BC, and Woods NF: Medical-surgical nursing: concepts and clinical practice, St Louis, ed 3, 1986, The CV Mosby Co.
17. Rogers S: The spirit of independence: the evaluation of a philosophy, Am J Occup Ther 36:709, 1982.
18. Sims N: All about health and beauty for the black woman, New York, 1976, Doubleday & Co, Inc.
19. Urbanska D: Care of the mouth and teeth, Nurs Mirror 144:13, May 1977.
20. Urbanska D: Care of the mouth and teeth—the elderly, Nurs Mirror 145:27, July 1977.
21. Wells R and Trostle K: Creative hairwashing techniques for immobilized patients, Nurs '84 14:84, 1984.

ADDITIONAL READINGS

Bedlack J and Bamford P: Nursing assessment—a multidisciplinary approach, Monterey, Calif, 1984, Wadsworth Publishing Co.
Cassamassimo P: Tooth brushing and flossing: a manual of home dental care for persons who are handicapped, Chicago, 1977, The National Easter Seal Society.
Greenwood A: Dental care for the elderly poses special problems, Geriatrics 31:103, May 1976.
Hinks M: Clothing and the long-term patient, Nurs Mirror 144:39, March 1977.
Knust S and Quarn J: Integration of self-care theory with rehabilitation nursing, Rehabil Nurs 8:26, July/Aug 1983.

Lipsky J: Saving the elderly from the chilling cold, Nurs '84 14:2, 1984.

Lord JP and others: Functional ability and equipment use among patients with neuromuscular disease, Arch Phys Med Rehabil 68:348, 1987.

Nelson A: Correlation of patient motivation and staff motivation, Rehabil Nurs 8:24, May/June 1983.

Parsons LC, Peard AL, and Page MC: The effects of hygiene interventions on the cerebrovascular status of se-vere closed head injured persons, Res Nurs Health 8:173, 1985.

Wade NP, Lemerman RD, and Mastrioanni EJ: Rehabilitative care and education—practical guidelines for preparing patients to function at home, Rehabil Nurs 8:32, Sept/Oct 1983.

Wingerson E: The value of occupational therapy in rehabilitation, Geriatrics 31:99, 1976.

CHAPTER 15

Communication: Speech and Language

Martha F. Markarian

OBJECTIVES

After completing Chapter 15, the reader will be able to:

1. Explain the physiological processes by which speech and language production occur.

2. Discuss the levels of language production.

3. Discuss cerebral dominance and identify the major anatomical areas involved in speech and language production.

4. Identify and discuss the common causes of aphasia and dysarthria.

5. Compare and contrast the speech and communication problems resulting from aphasia and dysarthria.

6. Discuss the components and purpose of a nursing assessment of speech and language capabilities.

7. Identify considerations used when planning for the assessment of speech and language capabilities.

8. Identify areas of function to be considered when preparing for the gathering of assessment data.

9. Formulate nursing diagnoses and develop goals related to speech and language difficulties.

10. Discuss the various facilitation techniques that rehabilitation team members can use to promote speech and language production.

11. Determine alternate forms of communication that clients experiencing speech and language problems might find helpful.

12. Give examples of the special safety problems that can occur when speech and language are not effective.

13. Discuss socialization needs related to speech and language problems.

14. Discuss the purposes, importance, and content of client and family education relative to speech and language problems.

15. Discuss follow-up and maintenance activities frequently required by persons experiencing speech and language difficulties.

16. Explain the contributions of selected rehabilitation team members.

17. List outcome criteria for the client with speech and language problems.

The ability to communicate is so basic to human nature that a reduction or elimination of language skills strains nearly every aspect of an individual's ability to function in everyday life. Social, psychological, and physiological needs cannot be fully expressed. Other persons may not understand the affected individual's communication efforts. In addition, understanding the communication of others may be impaired. Life becomes chaotic.

Speech is the process through which language is communicated via sound. It involves distinct neuromuscular activities necessary for articulation and phonation. Expression of cognitive functions also can take place through writing and gesturing. Normally these activities occur in a coordinated manner.

Language involves the cognitive processes related to the perception of sensory stimuli and the integration of these stimuli with prior experiences. Cognitive functions essential to language are the manipulation and formulation of thoughts, including mathematical calculations, listening, and reading. Language and speech provide humans with well-ordered, rule-bound systems of communication through which thoughts can be exchanged.

Injuries to the brain's speech centers result in varying degrees of loss of the ability to understand and integrate messages received and to formulate and use expressive language. Types of reception and expression affected in varying degrees and combinations are speaking, writing, calculating, gesturing, listening, and reading. Language problems resulting from damage to speech centers are commonly referred to as *aphasias* and are further classified according to the speech areas affected. Disease processes that affect the function of upper and lower motor neurons involved in conveying action potentials to muscles that produce and control sound production are referred to as *dysarthrias*. Dysarthrias are further classified according to the type of motor function deficit experienced.

In most instances, the nurse works closely with the speech/language pathologist when developing a plan of care for the client with speech problems. Speech/language pathologists practice in medical centers, rehabilitation centers, small community hospitals, clinics, and home health care agencies. There are, however, times when the nurse may have to develop and revise the care plan without the benefit of the speech/language

pathologist's input. Two examples are the nurse working in rural areas and the nurse working with the client whom the physician or speech/language pathologist has decided will not benefit from therapy sessions.

Regardless of where the rehabilitation nurse practices, nursing intervention for the person with aphasia must be based on knowledge of the disease process, treatment modalities, and rehabilitation principles. In this chapter, rehabilitation nursing for the client with aphasia and dysarthria is addressed.

FUNCTIONS OF SPEECH AND LANGUAGE

Effective language involves many processes: development of thoughts to be spoken; selection, formulation, and ordering of words; application of rules of grammar; initiation of muscle movements; control of respiratory activity to produce the required sounds; and verbalization. Finally, while speaking, individuals listen to their verbalizations, evaluate them, and correct them when necessary. Optimum use of speech and language requires an intact cerebral cortex, subcortical regions, brainstem, and association fiber tracts that permit communication between sensory and sensorimotor areas of the brain.

The highly ordered and rule-bound system of symbols needed for effective communication requires four major elements: (1) ordering of sounds used to form words, for example, "wa-gon" versus "gon-wa"; (2) application of correct meanings to words (semantics); (3) use of rules to order statements (syntax); and (4) appropriate application of plurality and tense.

The level of effective language production is determined by the degree of complexity with which the brain can function. The three basic levels of language production are[19]:

1. *Automatic speech:* A basic level that consists of habitual responses such as prayers, social responses, curses, and songs
2. *Imitation:* A higher level of language that requires a person to hear what is said, process the message, produce the appropriate response, and evaluate the content of the transmission
3. *Symbolic speech:* The highest level of speech, which is produced without the benefit of a model: an expression of one's own choice; involves the use of words with the

correct meaning, application of rules for ordering sounds and words, and use of appropriate tense and plurality

Broca and Wernicke (late 1800s) and Penfield and Roberts (1959) were noted for their early research on brain function.[10] Their studies revealed a great deal of information about the roles of various areas of the brain in producing speech and language. Traditionally, autopsies have been used to compare areas of brain damage to symptoms experienced by patients and thereby localize speech centers. Currently, computed tomography (CT) and positron emission tomography (PET) scanners are employed to determine abnormalities and correlate symptoms to specific areas of injury within the brain.[5] These diagnostic studies continue to provide data helpful in advancing our knowledge of brain function. Planning of care specific to the particular cerebral trauma also has been facilitated.

Knowledge of anatomy and physiology relative to speech and language enhances the nurse's understanding of the complex cerebral activities that take place to allow individuals to communicate with each other.

Cerebral Dominance

The cerebral hemisphere containing the speech centers is referred to as the *dominant hemisphere*. In approximately 95% of the population, the speech centers are located in the left hemisphere. In the remaining 5%, the right hemisphere is dominant. A correlation has been identified between handedness and cerebral dominance, with more left-handed individuals having right-sided dominance. Not all left-handed individuals, however, have right hemisphere dominance. Similarly, not all right-handed individuals have left hemisphere dominance.

Speech Centers and Their Functions

The frontal lobe contains neuronal tissue responsible for the elaboration of thought, initiation of automatic gestures and facial expressions, and the production of automatic and willed speech. *Broca's area*, located in the premotor area of the left frontal area, is responsible for programming neuronal activation of muscle movements required for the volitional production of speech. Current research suggests that the region surrounding

Broca's area, sometimes described as "big Broca's area," is responsible for the syntactical component of language expression.[6] The area directly above Broca's area has been associated with actions related to written language (Figure 15-1).[6]

The parietal, occipital, and temporal lobes serve as receivers and basic interpreters of somatic, visual, and auditory stimuli, respectively. Each lobe has an interpretive area that feeds into a "general interpretive area" located in the posterior superior portion of the temporal lobe and the anterior portion of the angular gyrus. *Wernicke's area* is that portion of the interpretive area located in the temporal lobe. This entire area of the dominant hemisphere is responsible for the analysis of impulses received from all sensory input and the processing of these impulses into coherent, complex thoughts[8] (Figure 15-1).

The temporal lobe contains several areas involved in speech. Wernicke's area, located in the posterior superior temporal gyrus, in addition to being responsible for auditory comprehension of language, formulates the basic structure of utterances, which are then transmitted to Broca's area for programming into spoken words. Semantic comprehension and syntactical comprehension are believed to take place in the adjacent superior and middle temporal gyri. The *auditory association areas* located in the temporal lobe and the *supramarginal gyrus* are credited with the processing of sentences for semantics and comprehension. The *angular gyrus*, located in the general interpretive area of the temporal lobe, is especially important in the interpretation of visual information[8] (Figure 15-2).

Transmission of messages from Wernicke's area to Broca's area is necessary for programming neurons to initiate speech. The *arcuate fasciculus* (subcortical bands of association fibers) has been credited with the transmission of this information. Recent studies suggest that this activity may instead take place in the left temporoparietal region above and below the posterior sylvian fissure, the primary auditory cortex, Wernicke's area, and sometimes the insula and its subcortical white matter.[6]

The right hemisphere has a role in language activity as it relates to spatial elements and comprehension. In addition, adults who have experienced hemidecortication with damage to the left hemisphere may be able to sing and participate in automatic speech without meaning. They are

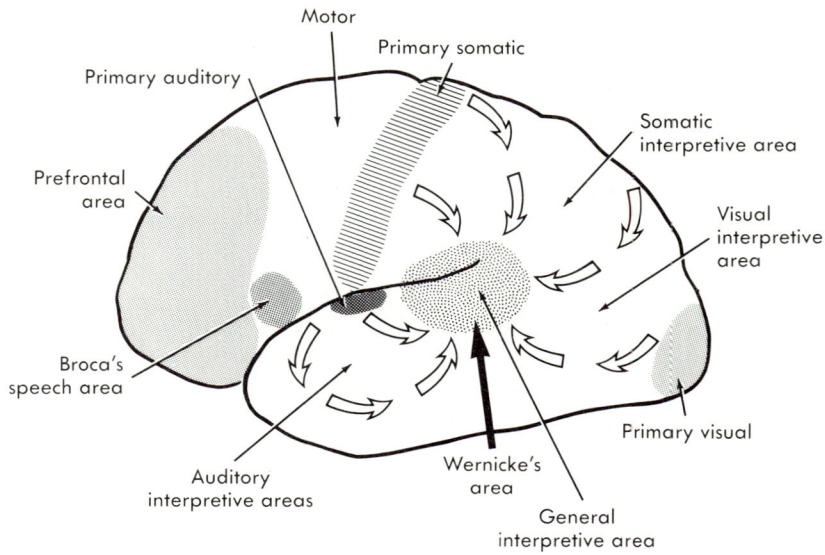

Figure 15-1
General interpretive area. *(Modified from Guyton AC: Human physiology and the mechanisms of disease, Philadelphia, 1982, WB Saunders Co.)*

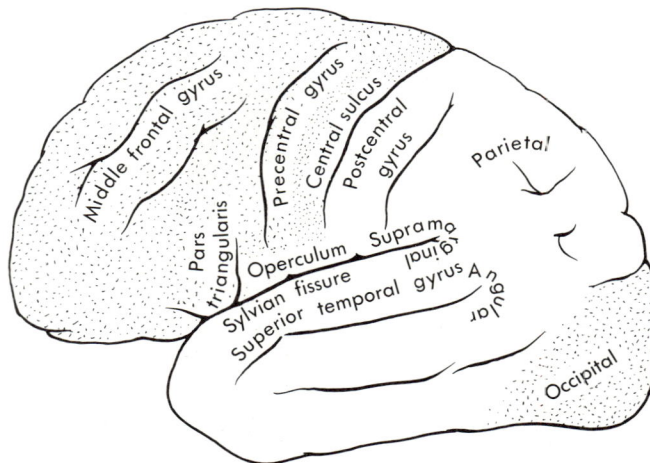

Figure 15-2
Lateral view of cerebral cortex showing areas of brain involved in speech and language function. *(From Davis GA: A survey of adult aphasia, Englewood Cliffs, NJ, 1983, Prentice-Hall, Inc.)*

severely limited, however, in the use of symbolic speech.

Subcortical Structures

The thalamus has many connections within the sensory and motor cortex. Its role in language production is at this point unclear, but it is believed to influence attention and vigilance for speech processes and short-term memory.[6]

The limbic system is believed to play a major role in the emotional component of communication by initiating and influencing internal sensations, drives, motivation, emotions, and communication behaviors.[6] Awareness of this influence helps us appreciate the emotional component of verbal and nonverbal communication and the interpretation of messages.

Damage to pyramidal or extrapyramidal tracts traveling through the brainstem can result in limitations in ability to gesture and assume various postures.

Cranial nerves

Cranial nerves, located in the brainstem, are involved with the transmission of the motor impulses for speech. Cranial nerve VII, the facial nerve, innervates muscles of the eyelids, cheeks, and lips. Cranial nerve IX, the glossopharyngeal nerve, supplies motor fibers in the pharynx. Cranial nerve X, the vagus nerve, innervates muscles of the soft palate, pharynx, and larynx. Cranial nerve XII, the hypoglossal nerve, innervates muscles controlling movement of the tongue. Damage to cranial nerves from trauma, disease, or loss of blood supply can result in difficulties in articulation, production of vocal sounds, and swallowing.[17]

Circulation

Alterations in or loss of particular speech capabilities can often be related to pathological conditions affecting the circulation to speech centers. These centers require a continuous supply of oxygen and nutrients carried to the brain via the internal carotid and vertebral arteries.

The anterior cerebral, middle cerebral, and posterior cerebral arteries branch off the carotid artery and serve as conduction arteries. Penetrating arteries are derived from branches of these arteries. The anterior division of the middle ce-

rebral artery supplies the frontal lobe and the Rolandic cortex, including Broca's area. The posterior division of the middle cerebral artery branches to supply the lateral surface of the parietal, occipital, and temporal lobes, including the angular and supramarginal gyri, Wernicke's area, and the primary auditory cortex.[20]

The vertebral arteries enter the skull at the foramen magnum. The pons receives its nourishment from branches of the basilar artery, which is formed when the vertebral arteries join. The basilar artery bifurcates at the midbrain to form the superior cerebellar and the posterior cerebral arteries. The posterior cerebral arteries pass around the midbrain, supplying it and the medial surfaces and undersurfaces of the temporal lobe and the medial occipital lobe (the visual cortex).[20]

IMPAIRED FUNCTION

More than 1 million persons in the United States suffer from some form of speech problem related to disease processes. Cerebrovascular accidents affecting the dominant cerebral hemisphere are a major cause of impaired function in the production of speech and language. Other causes include trauma, tumor, infection, carbon monoxide poisoning, and multiple sclerosis. The interruption of the anatomical integrity of speech centers in the brain and subcortical structures can produce a variety of permutations in speech and language. Pathological changes resulting from physiological insults such as circulatory infarction, hemorrhage, or gunshot wound result in destruction of neuronal tissue and the formation of edema in adjacent tissues. Severe edema can result in death of involved neurons. Lesser amounts may, however, only temporarily impair neuronal function. Therefore one can expect the degree of disability to decrease as the edema clears.

Aphasias

There are a number of aphasias. Aphasias resulting from damage to Broca's area, the general interpretive areas, Wernicke's area, and any combination of areas concerned with speech and language are discussed below.

Impaired function: Broca's area

Impaired function resulting from damage in Broca's area is referred to as *Broca's aphasia*, or *non-*

fluent aphasia. Injury to Broca's area can result in apraxia manifested by the inability to voluntarily move the muscles of the mouth, throat, and tongue in patterns needed to produce speech. The affected individual may, however, be able to use these muscles for other purposes such as eating.

Problems resulting from damage to Broca's area are deficits in oral expression, especially in spontaneous conversation, and in tasks of naming and repetition. Utterances are produced in a monotone, the rate is slow, and the phrases are short (telegraphic speech). Words may be composed of inappropriate sounds and have inappropriate meanings. Errors in speech are highly inconsistent.

Written expression reflects oral expression. If the injury is confined to Broca's area, no auditory or reading comprehension deficits should be present. People with Broca's aphasia often experience paresis of the right arm, since the damage producing the aphasia may extend into the adjacent major motor area responsible for upper extremity movement on the opposite side of the body.

Impaired function: general interpretive area

Damage within the general interpretive area reduces the brain's ability to analyze various sensory impulses. These impulses may be perceived but not understood. In the adult loss of function in this area leads to inadequate mental function.[8]

Damage to the angular gyrus, located in the general interpretive area of the temporal lobe, results in inability to understand the meaning of words, because the stream of visual information passing from the visual cortex to the general interpretive area is blocked. Clients will be aware of this problem and express concern.

Impaired function: Wernicke's area

Injury to Wernicke's area and the supramarginal gyrus results in deficits in auditory comprehension. If the injury is severe, the affected individual may hear but be unable to interpret correctly. In addition, efforts to express oneself are incorrect. Utterances are effortless, fluent, and of normal rhythm, intonation, rate, and phrase length but do not resemble meaningful language. Because of an alteration in perception of visual sensations, reading comprehension and writing are impaired. Deficits in language resulting from damage in this area are referred to as *Wernicke's aphasia*, or *fluent aphasia*.

Other impairments in function

Interruption of the transmission of messages from Wernicke's area to Broca's area results in effortless, articulated sound substitutions. Errors occur in spontaneous conversations and in tasks of naming and repetition. The client is aware of the problem.

Damage to Broca's area and to the temporal lobe results in both speech production and auditory comprehension problems. The degree of awareness and impaired function depends upon the size of the area involved. Damage to speech centers rarely affects only one area of speech and language function. Usually there is damage to several areas of the brain. Extensive anterior and posterior lesions produce syndromes known as *global aphasia*. With these syndromes, the client experiences little or no auditory comprehension. Utterances are meaningless. Some meaningful words may be used inappropriately. *Perseveration*, the continuous use of a word with or without varying types of stimulation, may occur.[6] Additionally, emotional interjections such as "ah" and "oh" may occur.

Dysarthrias

Neuromuscular diseases such as low brainstem stroke, poliomyelitis, myasthenia gravis, amyotrophic lateral sclerosis, Parkinson's disease, multiple sclerosis, Friedreich's ataxia, head injury, and cerebellar dysfunction can result in dysarthria. An understanding of the pathological basis and treatment of dysarthria allows the establishment of a supportive environment for optimal responses to therapies planned by the speech/language pathologist.

Dysarthria is a speech articulation problem resulting from trauma and various types of neuromuscular diseases that impair neuromuscular control of the muscles of the face, oral cavity, and larynx. Difficulty may be experienced in manipulating the tongue, lips, soft palate, jaw, and vocal cords. This muscle impairment can cause speech to be slurred, labored, sluggish, weak, and hypernasal. Problems with chewing, swallowing, and drooling may occur[22] (Chapter 9).

Comprehension of language is not affected.

The speech dysfunction is a result of faulty motor output of speech. Muscles of respiration, phonation, resonance, *parsody* (rhythm, stress, and intonation),[21] and articulation are affected.[16]

Evaluation of dysarthria includes assessment of the muscles of speech for atrophy, fasciculations, tremors, and other involuntary movements. Voluntary and reflex muscle activities are tested, as well as chewing and swallowing. Muscle movements are evaluated for strength, rate, range, accuracy, and tone. This is done by observing the client close the lips, elevate the tip of the tongue, and rapidly repeat movements while speaking syllables. Muscle tone can be evaluated by checking the resistance to movement. Increased or decreased muscle tone can influence the ability to speak. Accurate assessment of the loudness, nasality, stress, imprecise consonants, and voice quality can be accomplished through the recording of speech.[2]

Types of dysarthria

The type or types of dysarthria experienced depend upon the area of neurological impairment. Types of dysarthria are[9]:

1. *Flaccid:* A result of damage to lower motor neurons. The extent of dysarthria depends upon the amount of cranial nerve involvement. It can be seen in clients with pseudobulbar palsy, cranial nerve palsy, and myasthenia gravis.
2. *Spastic:* A result of an upper motor neuron disorder. Hypertonicity and breakdown of movements are manifestations of this type. Examples of causes are strokes, multiple sclerosis, and brain trauma. With unilateral involvement, dysarthria should not be permanent.
3. *Mixed:* A result of bulbar and pseudobulbar influence. This type can be seen in clients with amyotrophic lateral sclerosis[16] and multiple sclerosis in which multiple and diffuse lesions occur.
4. *Ataxic:* A result of damage to the cerebellum. Causes include multiple sclerosis, trauma, and strokes.
5. *Hypokinetic:* A result of certain disorders in the extrapyramidal system. An example of such a disorder is Parkinson's disease.
6. *Hyperkinetic:* A result of certain disorders in the extrapyramidal system. It can be

manifested as a slow or quick hyperkinetic movement or involve both types.[2] Dystonia and chorea are two types of movement disorders in which it can be manifested.

Treatment of dysarthria

Treatment depends upon the degree of involvement and the client's potential for recovery. Early development of effective communication techniques to compensate for the deficit is desired to help reduce the level of anxiety. The focus of treatment is to maximize effectiveness of speech through exercise, prosthetic devices, or alternate forms of communication.

When the potential for speech improvement is present, treatment is concentrated on muscle strengthening and exercises to develop control of sounds. Next, the training focuses on moving from one sound to another with the goal of sound production that can be distinguished by a listener. When this is accomplished, production of phrases is attempted. Here the emphasis is on sounds and phrases appropriate to daily activities and needs.[2]

Beukelman and Yorkston[2] recommend using an alphabet board and asking the client to point to the first letter of each word as attempts at speech are made. This provides the listener with more information about the word and helps the client communicate before effective speech is possible.

Further treatment focuses on maximizing the intelligibility of speech through specific skill training and prosthetics. This includes controlling speaking rates, emphasizing consonant sounds when appropriate, controlling the number of words in a breath, and stressing important words. Appropriate stress, loudness, and pitch can also be taught.[2]

A prosthetic device is sometimes used to reduce abnormal speech characteristics. It improves the quality of speech by elevating the soft palate, thereby reducing hypernasality and nasal emissions.[2]

Other aids for facilitating speech are breathing exercises, binders, posture supports, stress reduction techniques, and biofeedback devices. Breathing exercises can help with speaking and breath control. Abdominal binders or binders designed to meet a client's unique needs and the support of posture with pillows can help breathing and breath control.[16] Muscle relaxation techniques and stress reduction techniques also may be helpful.[17] A biofeedback device known as a *VISIPITCH* has been manufactured to improve voice production. Its visual display provides the client and the speech/language pathologist with objective information about speech performance.[16]

A number of alternate methods are used to provide or improve communication. These methods vary from sophisticated electronic equipment to simple finger tapping or eye blinking. Morse code, typewriters, magic slates, the Amerind Communication System, and communication boards also are used. Communication systems available for clients are the Zygo Model 100 Scanner, Prentke-Romich Express I, and the Canon Communicator. Most of these devices can formulate and store messages, which are retrieved by the client through light touch. Messages are displayed on some form of screen or monitor.[2] A manually operated electronic device providing an artificial voice is now available and is valued for its wider latitude in communication and its provision for speaking to someone who is not looking directly at the client.[11]

Appropriateness of alternate forms of communication depends upon cost and the ability of the client to manipulate the equipment. The client's level of function is an important consideration, since the disease process or trauma that caused the dysarthria frequently affects motor or mental function or both. Furthermore, success in using the alternate forms of communication requires patience and practice. As technology improves, nurses will have to become more familiar with devices used to help clients communicate.

NURSING ASSESSMENT

A nursing assessment specific for speech and language skills is important because of the frequent interactions with the client and family and the focus of nursing interventions on daily activities to promote health and optimum function. Each client's communication deficits and skills vary greatly because of the differences in extent and location of the damage and the time interval since the initial damage.

Multiple and obvious deficits in communication are often easily identified, but sometimes deficits are subtle and dangerous for the client. Consider, for example, the hazards when the client cannot understand the directions on a prescription bottle and is not able to communicate this lack of understanding. Other examples where a lack of comprehension may be dangerous include the driver who does not understand the word "Stop" on a street sign or the client or visitor who does not understand the signs "No Smoking, Oxygen in Use" or "Emergency Exit." Misunderstood verbal instructions can present hazards too, such as with the following statements: "Put the nitroglycerin tablet under your tongue," or "Do not get this lotion in your eyes," or "Be careful, the floor is slippery."

Preparation

Preparation for the nursing assessment requires consideration of the client's behaviors, fatigue tolerance, and psychological state.

The client's behaviors

The commonly used statement "I don't know where you are coming from" can serve as an excellent guide in preparing for the nursing assessment. The complexity of speech and language production and the functions of the various speech centers may seem to be enough to worry about when performing the assessment. If the client's response to this problem is not considered, however, there will be no true "nursing."

Initial interactions during the admission or while giving care can provide basic information regarding the client's communication status. The nurse should determine what behaviors to look for during the formal assessment and what techniques to use to elicit information about the client's communication function. The techniques used should allow optimum responses, establish rapport, and limit frustration. Trauma to various sensory areas predisposes the client to altered visual, auditory, and tactile sensations. A quiet and uncluttered room helps to control distractions resulting from these altered sensations. Privacy also facilitates responses. Drawing the curtain in a semiprivate room is not sufficient because the client can be overheard, and the presence of others in the room can easily divert the client's attention. Whenever possible, assessment should not be done in the client's room because it can connote sickness and dependence, thereby influencing responses.

Brain damage also can result in physical limitations and mental impairment. Fear and physical discomfort are common. These factors must be recognized and taken into consideration in order to obtain reliable measures of the client's abilities and disabilities.

Fatigue tolerance

Fatigue has a negative influence on communication. The stressors that accompany illness, a decrease in communication skills, and hospital routines all increase fatigue.[24] The time of day also is significant in determining fatigue tolerance, since individuals vary in when their daily energy levels peak and wane. Additionally, health problems, such as cardiac and respiratory diseases, decrease energy levels. Often the assessment must be carried out in small units of time because of fatigue, frustration, or pain.

Psychological state

Knowledge of an individual's psychological makeup facilitates planning for effective nurse-client interactions during the assessment.[15] The rehabilitation nurse should ascertain the client's previous ways of coping with frustrations, reactions to the current illness, and reactions to others on the rehabilitation team. Negative feelings should be suspected if the client retreats or acts embarrassed about speech and language problems. Attentiveness and initiation of interactions may indicate a positive attitude.

Ongoing assessment, carried out while interacting with the client, is valued for its informality. At these times, activities may reduce apprehension, thereby allowing abilities, progress, or previously undiscovered disabilities to surface. Because of their continuous, intimate contacts with clients, nurses frequently discover new ways to successfully communicate with individuals experiencing aphasia. Sharing these techniques with fellow nurses and other members of the rehabilitation team increases opportunities for the client to interact and improve communication skills.

When ready to begin the assessment, the nurse should take time to explain its purpose, acknowledge the client's difficulty in communicating, and describe what will be done and why. Interactions and questions should be invited while keeping in mind that responses may be those of automatic speech or imitation, with little or no comprehension on the part of the client.

Assessment Areas

A comprehensive nursing assessment concerning speech and language function must include an investigation of the health history, evaluations conducted by other rehabilitation team members, developmental level of the client, previous intellectual and communication abilities, and present function in communication. The assessment should identify areas of strength that would help the client cope with the many problems that result from impaired speech and language function.

Health history

A health history is necessary to gain an understanding of the circumstances surrounding the onset of aphasia and the existence of any other health problems that might influence the client's needs and functional progress. The family frequently must be consulted regarding previous or coexisting health problems because of the client's limitations in communication.

Evaluations by other rehabilitation team members

The nurse's initial assessment often may precede evaluations by other team members, and thus the information obtained should be shared formally by means of the client record and team meetings and informally in daily focused interactions. Data collected by other team members are considered when planning nursing interventions. The physician can provide information about the findings of the physical and neurological examination, CT scan when performed, additional diagnostic tests and laboratory findings, reasons for medical prescriptions, and prognosis for recovery of function. Consultation with the physician and review of the medical records can furnish in-depth information on chronic disease processes, such as atherosclerosis, coronary disease, anemia, or diabetes mellitus, that will influence the plans for nursing intervention.

The speech/language pathologist can provide information on the type of speech problem and techniques most effective in improving or encouraging verbalizations and maximizing the potential for recovery. The client's auditory comprehension, speaking capabilities, and language strengths and weaknesses are evaluated to allow development of a treatment plan and to provide information to rehabilitation team members on how to best communicate with the client. The speech/language pathologist may decide to discontinue therapy if the client fails to respond.[1] If, however, the nurse notices changes that may indicate that speech therapy would again be appropriate, the speech/language pathologist should be contacted for further evaluation and possible continuation of therapy. (see discussion on "Rehabilitation Team Interventions.")

Developmental stage

Age and stage of life can affect the aphasic client's response to therapy. Physical stamina and expectations for life may be greater in the younger individual.[9,18] Anticipation of recovery, a disease-free body, and energy needed to participate in therapies can promote functional progress. Conversely, the elderly individual frequently may experience additional health problems. Aphasia and the condition that produced it may be viewed as "a further step toward death" and result in a loss of motivation. Limited stamina, a decrease in rate of mental processing, and sensory impairments associated with aging also can hinder one's ability to respond to therapy.[18] An understanding of the client's developmental stage and aspirations must be considered as the nursing interventions are planned.

Social developmental factors also can serve as positive or negative reinforcers in response to therapy. Personal goals, occupation, hobbies, career goals, financial status, and family role and responsibilities should be assessed as intervention is planned.

Previous intellectual and communication abilities

Background information on previous communication abilities may help to identify communication problems unrelated to the present aphasia but that may affect responses to therapy. Previous speech problems or abilities such as stuttering, difficulty with articulation, command of other languages, primary language, and handedness should be ascertained. The use of foreign-sounding words may be related to fluency in another language but should not be assumed to be correct because aphasia can affect all language capabilities. Also, some jargon can resemble foreign languages. If paresis of an extremity is present because of damage to motor neurons adjacent to a speech center, knowledge of handedness is helpful in determining the potential for communicating through writing.

An understanding of previous intellectual abilities allows planning of therapies appropriate to the client's background. For example, a client who has had advanced university education may have a very different program designed for treatment of the aphasia than a client who has never learned to read and write.

Current functional communication status

Certain principles are important in assessing the current communication status. Performance of communication tests should not be too difficult or too simple for the particular client. Some performance tests at first seem too simple but may be necessary for gathering baseline data about the client's communication abilities. The reason for the test should be explained to the client at the outset.

Often the nurse asks the client to name specific items. Initially, presenting multiple items should be avoided. The client may only be able to identify two or three items. It is important to observe for guessing, because with two items and a little luck, the client may guess correctly.

To test the ability to carry out self-care activities safely, the nurse should ask the client to demonstrate what needs to be done in response to verbal and written instructions. Nonverbal cues should be avoided. The nurse should monitor his or her actions for these nonverbal cues because many gestures become habit. An example of such a cue would be to gesture with your hand when asking a client to roll over.

Motor and auditory speech abilities can be tested by asking the individual to repeat simple sounds such as "ti, ti" or "bo, bo." If these attempts are successful, more complex phrases can be used.

Motor speech and comprehension can be tested by using objects familiar to the client. Examples of objects that can be employed are articles used for activities of daily living, such as eating utensils and money. The nurse should be sure the articles selected are appropriate for the client's level of function.

The client's ability to identify objects can involve various techniques, including identifying the objects in writing, naming objects the nurse points to, asking the client to point to objects the nurse names, or instructing the client to read a card with the name of the object on it. These techniques test the ability to hear, write, verbalize, identify with sight, gesture, and read. The specific techniques selected should be appropriate to the client's abilities in order to limit frustration and encourage successes. These techniques can be used to test many of the areas in which functional communication skills are used. (See box at right.) The assessment form shown can be used as a guide when considering what functions to assess to determine the client's abilities and limitations in communication. Since each client's capabilities and limitations vary, the areas assessed differ with each client.

Photographs of the family, workplace, home, and familiar objects also can be used as props to stimulate language production and determine the client's language and speech capabilities. Pictures of happy, sad, and angry faces may help the client acknowledge the presence of these emotions. Magazines and books are excellent resources for pictures that can be used in assessment of speech and language. When making cue cards for the client, the nurse should print in large, bold letters or design large pictures with only one word or picture to a card. Laminating the cards with clear plastic available at stationery stores prolongs their usefulness.

The nurse should document the results of the assessment in the client's record, including the specific responses, time, and date. Serial assessments should be performed to evaluate progress or lack of progress over time.

NURSING DIAGNOSES

A number of nursing diagnoses may be formulated for the person with impairments in speech and language function. The primary diagnosis is *impaired verbal communication*.[7] This nursing diagnosis affects every aspect of daily living. The nurse must be acutely aware of its pervasiveness and attuned to its presence during all components of nursing care. The cause of the deficit, the severity, and the potential for recovery also must be considered.

With brain damage resulting in communication deficits, assessment also may reveal deficits in mental processes. It is important to keep in mind, however, that the loss of speech does not indicate that mental function has been affected. Should

---

Nursing Assessment of Functional Communication Skills

Basic needs
1. Bathing, toileting, oral care, denture care, and use of objects needed to carry out these activities
2. Eating: where, when, food preferences, special preparations of food, dietary restrictions or supplements, selection of food from the menu
3. Elimination: when, where, assistive devices or objects needed
4. Sleeping: where, when, number of pillows needed, blankets, need for side rails

Safety and awareness
1. Identification of self, current location, home address, telephone number
2. Ability to tell time
3. Ability to read with comprehension, for example, newspaper, magazines, safety signs
4. Ability to handle money, write checks
5. Recognition of physical and mental limitations
6. Understanding of reason for hospitalization, treatment plan, medications

Psychosocial concerns
1. Expression of fear, anger, sadness, and happiness
2. Identification of factors related to stress

Family
1. Identification of relatives and friends, for example, wife, mother, son, daughter, neighbor, roommate
2. Ability to communicate with significant others

Occupation
1. Identification of type of work, workplace, work schedule

Religious needs
1. Religious orientation
2. Religious habits

---

mental function be affected, an appropriate nursing diagnosis is *altered thought process*.[7]

Changes in mental function may be subtle or obvious. The nurse should determine whether the individual can function in a safe manner independently. Often the client's awareness of the deficit causes great concern and discouragement. The nurse also must keep in mind that the family finds altered thought processes difficult because of the changes in the relationship with their loved one and the added responsibility that accompanies these changes.

Many of the problems related to speech and language deficits predispose the client to injury. It may be simply because the client cannot make needs known, or it may be more complex in that the client is not in tune with the environment and its hazards. An appropriate nursing diagnosis is *potential for injury*.[7] Determination of the potential for injury and the creation of a safe environment are needed to help the client compensate for the deficits and still function at an optimum level of independence.

Damage to the central nervous system resulting in loss of or decreased ability to perceive visual, auditory, or tactile sensations greatly hampers an individual's ability to relate effectively with others or with the environment. Central nervous system damage occurs frequently and often results in varying degrees of limitation. An appropriate nursing diagnosis would be *sensory/ perceptual alterations in visual, auditory, or tactile areas*.[7] With these alterations, the client's world becomes confusing and disordered.

Limitations in the most basic independent actions, namely, self-care, can cause severe depression and greatly discourage attempts to overcome the disability. A suitable nursing diagnosis would be *self-care deficit related to impaired communication*.[7] Often clients' self-care needs can be anticipated by the nurse. The development of ways to communicate about needs and the encouragement of participation in self-care activities provide hope and increase rehabilitation efforts.

Frequently the pathological changes that produced the communication problems are accompanied by other physical and mental impairments. These deficits can further compromise the individual's functional ability and interest in participating in activities of daily living.

The causes of anxiety in the person experiencing communication problems are endless. The nursing diagnosis can be simply stated as *anxiety*.[7] Anxiety also can occur in family members and can have a significant influence upon the client. These anxieties can stem from the pathological process that produced the deficit, a concern over the health care being received, and realized or anticipated changes in life-style or societal role. Care should be focused upon anticipated or present anxiety. It also is important to seek out ways to reduce its level and limit causes of anxiety and stress when possible.

Interruption of the "normal" family interactions and roles, stemming from the communication deficits, depends upon the position in the family that the client assumes, such as child, brother, sister, parent, or grandparent. The nursing diagnosis appropriate for this problem is *altered family processes*.[7]

Family roles, although somewhat prescribed by society, are clarified by the particular family unit. No matter what the role or family expectations, one can expect considerable upheaval within the family unit. Family support for the client depends upon the family's ability to support and cope with the crisis.

Human existence requires interactions with others. Individuals vary in the amount of socialization desired, but for most, the ability to communicate is needed to maintain a homeostatic state. Speech and language deficits affect all types of communication and can affect the desire to be with other people. When clients purposefully avoid other people and human interaction, the appropriate nursing diagnosis is *social isolation*.[7] The intimate communications between loved ones and friends may be decreased or lost. Attempted communications with others unaware of the problem may be awkward and embarrassing. A strain is placed upon all interactions.

GOALS

Identification of goals appropriate for the various speech and language problems helps to determine where and how care should be focused for each client. Careful analysis of the client's entire situation will be required to ensure identification of appropriate goals. Speech and language deficits are particularly challenging because of the uniqueness of each client's deficit, the cause or causes, other health problems, the potential for recovery, and the psychosocial factors influencing the client's response to the deficits and therapies.

Many clients improve their communication capabilities over time, so no matter what the level of health care, nursing actions often help the client to gain a higher level of function. Goals established with the client and family may include the following:

1. To assist the client in achieving optimum speech and language function
2. To establish a functional means of communication
3. To limit anxiety and frustration
4. To preserve the client's self-esteem
5. To establish an environment conducive to communication
6. To prevent injury
7. To promote social interaction
8. To assist the client in returning to social roles
9. To provide communication opportunities
10. To educate the client and family regarding the speech and language problem
11. To assist the client and family in establishing effective support systems

REHABILITATION NURSING INTERVENTIONS

Rehabilitation nursing interventions for aphasia and dysarthria depend upon each client's unique needs. These needs vary with level of health care required, the degree of functional recovery, and the pattern of damage in the speech centers. The interventions described in this section can be used as appropriate and adapted as necessary.

Nursing interventions should be designed to provide the client with a mentally and physically supportive climate and include the facilitation of speech and alternate forms of communication. Speech and interpretation of sensory input can be severely limited in some individuals, but this does not mean that all abilities to communicate and understand are completely lost. The methods available for determining the level of understanding when aphasia is present are still limited.[9] The nurse must assume that conversations with or in the presence of the client are understood. Misunderstandings can occur easily because of the alterations in interpretation of sensory input. It is important to monitor for and clarify any misunderstandings. It also is important to keep in mind that the client's ability to understand often improves, sometimes unexpectedly.

Psychological Considerations

Physical impairments and a decrease in the ability to effectively express oneself and understand the communications of others lead to dependence on others. Most individuals take pride in their social roles both at work and at home. Alterations accompanying aphasia and dysarthrias, as well as coexisting physical and mental inpairments, can cause severe depression and lack of motivation for participation in rehabilitation therapies.

Health care workers and family members who assist the client can easily and unknowingly assume a parental role. This role can increase feelings of hopelessness and loss of control. Thus the client's effort to improve language abilities may diminish.

To counteract feelings of dependence, the nurse should determine ways to involve the client in decision making regarding care. The client also should be consistently involved in the decisions about the rehabilitation process. Client involvement should be complimented, but not excessively. All rehabilitation team members who interact with the client should monitor their actions for postures, behaviors, tones of voice, or facial expressions suggesting frustration, annoyance, or impatience that can make the client feel incompetent and discouraged.

Anxiety can motivate or dampen efforts and responses to therapies. A mild to moderate degree of stress can often help the individual focus on therapies, whereas a high level of anxiety can hamper responses. High levels of anxiety can result from worries about the illness, communication, or family responsibilities. Some individuals may have a history of difficulty in dealing with anxiety-producing situations.[26] Recognition of anxiety-producing stressors and attempts to alleviate them are an important part of nursing interventions.

Clients can be depressed because functional improvement is often slow and rarely complete.[13] With extensive paralysis or loss of control over body functions, recovery of speech may be slower, since the client must focus energies on many areas during the rehabilitation process. Progress experienced may wax and wane, thereby creating uncertainty that improvements are truly taking place. When occasional difficulties with communication are experienced, it may be helpful to remind the client that you are aware that the client's verbal expressions do not clearly express thoughts and to offer reassurance that everyone has times when thoughts are not expressed clearly. The client should be encouraged to look to tomorrow. Anticipation of depression and appreciation of its causes help in planning ways to provide a supportive environment for the client and family.

Discouragement arising from slow functional return also can be experienced by rehabilitation team members. Regularly scheduled staff and family-staff support meetings should include time for verbalization of frustrations and problem solving for ways to reduce tensions and to deal with staff and family reactions to the slow or limited progress.

Therapeutic Environment

Both in the institution and at home, clients experiencing aphasia and dysarthria can greatly benefit from an environment that reduces stress and supports communication attempts. All clients with speech and language problems benefit from an environment structured to consider their individual needs.

In the institution, when a room must be shared, the individual with nonfluent or Broca's aphasia and dysarthria benefits most from having a roommate who can understand that verbal communication skills are impaired. The environment most supportive for the individual with fluent aphasia is one that does not cause excessive auditory or visual stimulation. A roommate should not be troubled by spontaneous, inappropriate, and frequent verbalizations.

Decor and supportive equipment also should be considered. Generally, the client's living area should be neat with minimum clutter from plants, cards, stuffed animals, and pictures. Supportive equipment such as wheelchairs, walkers, oxygen, and infusion pumps should be placed in the least distracting areas. Stable positioning of furniture and belongings helps to reduce the physical and mental stressors caused by change, thus allowing more energy for and attention to communication attempts. The nurse's awareness of these client needs helps provide a sense of control over the environment.

Many times aphasia and dysarthria physically and mentally isolate an individual. If this isolation is ignored, confusion and dementia may result. Radios and televisions are frequently used to provide stimulation. In a long-term care facility, another common therapy is to move the individual to the activities room with other residents. These efforts may not help the isolation and can upset the client if the environment produces confusion and frustration. Most individuals, regardless of their physical and mental state, do not like continuous noise or constant interaction with others. Excessive stimulation can cause agitation, fatigue, and decreased ability to effectively use remaining or restored communication skills.

When an individual cannot express reactions to the environment, the nurse should look for behaviors suggestive of the feeling state. Such behaviors may be unique to the affected individual and require attention to posture, gestures, facial expression, and behaviors.

Facilitation Techniques for Clients with Aphasia

Embarrassment about the inability to communicate in a meaningful way can discourage the client from interacting with others and participating in treatment. The nurse, other rehabilitation team members, and family can help reduce embarrassment by demonstrating acceptance and interest. The nurse plays a key role in instructing other staff members and family about ways in which to interact with the client.

Trauma is rarely isolated to one speech area. Degrees and areas of impairment vary with each client. Some of the facilitation techniques presented in Table 15-1 may be helpful in developing and expanding communication skills. Often experimentation with various techniques is necessary to determine what works best for a particular client. The nurse should record which techniques have been tried and the results. Methods used at one time may not be effective but may be appropriate at a later time.

General considerations

Clients with aphasia need time to process incoming statements. If the nurse has trouble eliciting a response from the client, the nurse's own communications should be monitored. Perhaps more time should be allowed for the client to formulate and verbalize the response. Sometimes the client has "lost" the meaning of some words. If this is suspected, key words should be changed to other words with the same meanings. Changing statements frequently should be avoided, however. Repetition of the same statement several times can help the client mentally process it.

TABLE 15-1

Facilitation techniques for clients with aphasia*

Method	Action	Purpose	Example
Self-talk	Speaking about activity as you perform it	Facilitates association of activity with specific words	"I'm combing your hair"
Par-allel talk	Describing aloud activity client is carrying out with you	Promotes association of activity with spoken words	"We are looking at the book"
Expan-sion	Adding substance to statement	Makes verbalizations more complex	Add to statement "Drink of water"; "You want a drink of water"
Cueing	Pronouncing initial syllable of word; showing printed version of word; presenting sentence completion task to fill in missing word (see also techniques for treating apraxia)	Helps client verbalize word not possible to verbalize on own	"We turn on the faucet to get . . ." (water)

*With all facilitation techniques the emphasis should be on speech production. Correcting errors in speech produced should be avoided.

Clients with Broca's (nonfluent) aphasia

Nursing interventions for Broca's (nonfluent) aphasia focus on improving speech through repeated practice of verbalizations. Consultation with a speech/language pathologist provides the best guidance for specific therapies to promote verbalization.

With impaired motor function, all attempts to verbalize should be facilitated. The nurse's acknowledgment of the desire to verbalize and the great effort required for such efforts lets the client know that the nurse is aware of the problems.

Efforts to speak can be facilitated through interactions with the client and the use of the facilitation techniques described in Table 15-1. Automatic speech or imitation can be encouraged by asking the client to say prayers or engaging in social conversations such as "Hello," "How are you," and "I'm fine." Cursing may present a problem for those who must listen but is valuable as a verbal exercise. Singing, which involves right cerebral hemisphere function, also allows verbal expression using the motor components of speech. Furthermore, it is a positive psychological experience for the client and the nurse. Interventions designed to initiate speech should take place while care is given, when activities are performed, and during special times

specifically scheduled for the practice of speech.

Techniques for the treatment of apraxia focus on the practice of sound patterns and speech. The practice sessions should be highly structured and controlled. Cueing and melodic intonation therapy are techniques that speech/language pathologists have found useful. Cueing involves the production of words after having heard and seen the phrase produced.[9] With melodic intonation the therapy progresses from singing in unison to the repetition of phrases with more normal intonation and then sentence production in response to questions.[14] Rosenbeck[21] points out that melodic intonation does not involve true singing and that popular lyrics and melodies should not be used.

Some caution is needed if Wernicke's aphasia accompanies Broca's aphasia because multiple stimuli can cause confusion and frustration. The nurse should provide both quiet times to prevent fatigue and opportunities for spontaneous verbalizations.

Clients with Wernicke's (fluent) aphasia

Individuals with damage to the speech centers responsible for the perception and formulation of language (interpretive area and Wernicke's area) have difficulty interpreting auditory, somatic, and visual input. Consequently, interpretation of their own speech, the speech of others, written messages, and visual and somatic input may be inappropriate or impossible. Usually some input is perceived correctly. Faulty interpretation of stimuli can lead to confusion and frustration. If the motor component of speech is intact but Wernicke's area is damaged, speech may be fluent but inappropriate.

Communication techniques for persons with damage in Wernicke's area and the interpretive areas require that sensory stimuli be controlled to prevent confusion. Control of the environment is especially important.

Sometimes, because of altered sensory perception, written communication, pictures, or gestures can be used to communicate more effectively than verbal instructions. Combining verbal instruction with pantomime has been found to be helpful for many.[3] For some clients, these props can be used to supplement verbal input. The nurse should keep in mind the hazards of sensory overload.

All communications should be clear and brief. Adjectives, adverbs, prepositions should be limited or avoided. The degree of simplicity depends upon the severity of the aphasia and the nurse's ability to effectively communicate. The nurse should look and listen for clues indicating understanding of communications and appropriateness of the client's responses. Appropriate responses should be reinforced.

Alternate forms of communication

Gestures can often clearly express needs and emotions. Cards depicting words or pictures also can be used to declare needs. Communication boards containing a variety of objects and action words can be used for expanding expression. With these boards, the individual points to the appropriate picture or word to communicate. Sometimes spelling boards can be used in the same way. A notebook filled with pictures of objects, persons performing particular actions, and pictures of faces expressing varying moods may be useful to some clients who can thumb through the book to the appropriate page.[4,15]

Some individuals with Broca's aphasia can successfully communicate in writing. The level of writing skill depends upon intact visual and motor centers needed to perform this activity. When an individual is unable to write, use of a typewriter will probably not be useful either.[4]

Clients with Dysarthria

Nurses need to work closely with the speech/language pathologist to understand the specific treatments prescribed and the methods for employing the treatments during nurse-client interactions. Knowledge about the use of prosthetic devices and alternate forms of communication used by the client should be sought.

Some common strategies the nurse uses when interacting with clients experiencing dysarthria include the following:

1. Providing physical and emotional support
2. Attending very carefully to communications
3. Assuming some responsibility for misunderstanding communications[17]
4. Requesting that statements be repeated or rephrased if not understood[17]
5. Encouraging the use of shorter phrases, single words, or slower verbalizations if the client is distressed or fatigued or if verbalizations are misunderstood[9]
6. Reacting with physical actions or verbalizations to convey your understanding of the verbalizations[17]
7. Encouraging the use of gestures and other forms of communication when the client's verbalizations are misunderstood

Safety Considerations

Impaired verbal communication can seriously compromise a person's safety. Careful assessment of each client for any special precautions needed to ensure safety must be done continually.

Damage to the general interpretive area may prevent a person from understanding how to use the call light in the hospital or the telephone at home. This impairment could be constant or occur only at times of stress. Imagine the problems that could occur if a fire broke out in the hospital room or in a bedroom when the person is at home alone. Although recognizing the danger, the person might be unable to call for help.

Difficulty in understanding sensory input can also present hazards if the individual cannot understand verbal instructions or read with comprehension. If the use of side rails or oxygen therapy is not understood, inappropriate behaviors such as climbing over the bed's side rail and falling or lighting a cigarette when oxygen is in use may occur. The potential for injury is endless, and problems must be anticipated to ensure safety.

Two examples illustrate the hazards that clients with aphasia experience.

Case study 1

Mr. Jones, a 65-year-old man with a history of a myocardial infarction, suffered from Broca's aphasia as a result of a stroke. The stroke occurred 6 weeks ago. While ambulating in the hospital corridor, he experienced a severe episode of left-sided chest pain that radiated down his left arm. He became weak, fell to the floor, and remained there rubbing his arm. Initially the staff thought he had injured his arm in the fall. No one could tell why he looked so apprehensive and pale. After taking his vital signs, a nurse found he was hypotensive and was experiencing a severe cardiac dysrhythmia. Fortunately, because the vital signs were taken, early treatment for the cardiac condition was initiated.

Case study 2

Mrs. Brown experienced Broca's aphasia as a result of an automobile accident. She continually rubbed her right eye but never complained (she could not). She was frequently restless and often appeared uncomfortable, but no one could determine the cause. Sometimes when the eye became red, a wrist restraint was applied to stop the irritation of the eye with her hand. The eye became severely inflamed so an ophthalmologist was consulted. Examination revealed that a piece of glass had become embedded in the eye at the time of the accident. Unfortunately, the prolonged irritation left Mrs. Brown's cornea scarred.

Promotion of Social Interactions

As the client regains strength from the trauma that produced speech and language impairment, social interactions should be encouraged. Initially interactions should involve rehabilitation team members with whom the client regularly interacts, family, and close friends. Interactions involving one or two people are usually best because this makes it easier for the client to focus. Visitors or other clients should be instructed regarding appropriate communication techniques. The nurse should monitor visits to ensure that the encounters are pleasant and not too long.

When a client returns home, resumption of a "normal" social life is often difficult. The stress that comes with a limited return of communication skills can reduce the amount of energy available. Frustration and embarrassment about poor communication skills can result in loss of any interest in socializing.

Old friends often feel uncomfortable in initiating interactions because the interests once shared can no longer be pursued. Friends also may be frustrated by their inability to communicate effectively or to help the impaired person. They may be frightened by the changes seen in their friend's health.[4] The nurse and family can teach the client's friends ways to communicate. Friends, like family, need to be encouraged to visit and receive recognition for the support offered. They too need a chance to verbalize their fears and frustrations.

The American Heart Association has facilitated the development of many self-help Stroke Clubs in this country. These organizations fulfill social, supportive, and educational needs. The Stroke Clubs are helpful not only to the client but also to the spouse who is frequently isolated with the affected mate. Today many families live in towns hundreds or thousands of miles from other relatives. Support systems are few, and new friends not always available in times of crisis. The Stroke Club can serve as a source of new friends who understand, share good ideas regarding mutual problems, and seek new friendships themselves. If there is not a Stroke Club in your area to which you can refer clients, the American Heart Association can help you start one.[4]

Client and Family Education

Both the client and family must understand the cause of the speech and language problem and the purpose of treatments, as well as have a realistic view of the potential for recovery. The nurse is well qualified to teach the client and family about the causes of aphasia and the purposes of therapy.

The primary physician, physiatrist, or speech/language pathologist should be responsible for presenting information concerning the prognosis. The nurse must have full knowledge of what the client and family have been told so that support, reinforcement, and teaching plans about aphasia can be knowledgeably implemented.

Realistic hope for the client and family should be supported. This hope can come from the awareness that aphasia is a recognized condition for which therapies have been developed to improve speech. The client must be informed that full recovery is rare. Failure to give this information may lead to loss of trust.[4]

Education should include the promotion of optimum mental and physical well-being. The client should be instructed about ways in which health can be maintained or improved and chronic illness managed and controlled.

The family should be taught the importance of creating an environment that is physically and emotionally supportive. Facilitation techniques found to promote more effective communication should be taught to all persons who interact with the client. The client's need for and readiness for social interaction must be identified and ways to meet this need planned.

Two references especially useful in assisting family members to cope with the problems of aphasia are the booklet entitled "Aphasia and the Family," available upon request for a small fee from the American Heart Association and the article "An Open Letter to the Family of an Adult Patient with Aphasia," published in *Rehabilitation Literature*, vol. 23, May 1962. This literature can serve as handy reference material to give the family and help the nurse in providing support and reassurance.

Referrals

The nurse assumes a key role in the referral of clients to various health disciplines within the institutional and community settings. Close and often long-term interactions with the client provide the opportunity for assessing obvious and subtle behaviors indicating that problems exist. Most referrals made within institutions require a physician's order. To facilitate communication of findings, the nurse should carefully note and record information needed by the attending physician or physiatrist.

Individuals with aphasia often have other major and minor health problems. The physician should be informed of changes in health status. Problems can range from decompensating congestive heart failure to incontinence or skin rashes. Every effort must be made to promote comfort and optimum function so that the client can focus on improving communication ability.

Referral of clients to other health disciplines should include information regarding communication techniques used with the client. Levels of understanding about aphasia vary among health care providers and health disciplines, so the nurse should determine what information is needed for each referral and plan to confer with the health care provider to determine progress of the client in therapy and to gain information about techniques that worked. Clients with aphasia are most often referred to other physicians, speech/language pathologists, physical therapists, occupational therapists, nutritionists, social workers, clergy, and audiologists. The contribution of each of these disciplines to functional communication is discussed in the section on rehabilitation team interventions.

All of the disciplines suggested as possible referrals for the client in the institution can offer services appropriate to those living in the community. Clients also may be discharged to communities or facilities where rehabilitation or supportive care is provided. In preparation for discharge, the nurse must communicate all information to ensure optimum function of the client and continuity of care by those care providers who continue to assist with rehabilitation efforts in the community.

Clients discharged home often benefit from community health nurse visits. These nurses must receive a referral from a physician, but hospital nurses, insurance nurses, and outpatient nurses frequently identify the need and make arrangements for referral. Visiting nurses' associations and other community health agencies often employ speech/language pathologists, physical and occupational therapists, social workers, nutritionists, and homemaker–home health aides who visit clients in the home for continuation of rehabilitation therapies. These services allow discharge sooner, thereby promoting a feeling of well-being when the client returns home. Early discharge also helps to limit medical expenses for clients and insurance companies.

If clients need to visit a physician or therapist on an outpatient basis, wheelchair vans are available when transportation is a problem. Currently expenses for traveling to and from a physician's office are tax deductible.

Follow-Up and Maintenance

Two major areas to be considered in the planning of follow-up care and maintenance of the person experiencing aphasia are the continued focus on improvement of speech and language skills and the promotion of general health and well-being.

Speech therapy is often continued after discharge from the hospital or rehabilitation center. Speech/language pathologists working in clinics and private practice can continue therapy when needed. Often the cost of continued therapy can be prohibitive. Some speech/language pathologists design programs that the family can use with the client. With this arrangement, return visits are scheduled at regular intervals to allow for evaluation of the client's progress and refinement of the therapy program.[4]

To ensure optimum recovery, most clients also need regular appointments with the physician who treated them for the trauma that resulted in aphasia. In addition, if chronic health problems are present, they should be monitored in order to maintain an optimum level of function. Attention can then be focused on continuing the improvement of speech and resuming social roles.

REHABILITATION TEAM INTERVENTIONS

In addition to the nurse, members of the rehabilitation team who most frequently work with the aphasic client are the speech/language pathologist, physical therapist, occupational therapist, audiologist, dentist, social worker, psychologist, nutritionist, and clergy member.

All members of the rehabilitation team should be knowledgeable about speech and language processes and facilitation techniques used to promote effective communication in clients experiencing aphasia and dysarthrias. Team members making diagnoses and implementing specific treatments should also be aware of the client's underlying disease or diseases, physical and mental impairments, and speech and language deficits, as well as the client's responses to these problems. In light of the client's limitations in communication, team members must be especially sensitive to the need for communication about pertinent problems such as heart disease, diabetes, and psychiatric illness, and functional limitations such as decreased vision or stamina. In making referrals or managing team functions, the nurse is often the one who must ensure transmission of this pertinent information.

As a team works together to resolve client problems, significant changes in the client's condition or responses to therapies, changes in health status, and significant psychological issues must be shared so that individual discipline and team plans can be revised to ensure therapeutic interventions. Contributions of team members are discussed below.

The physiatrist manages the care of clients experiencing functional limitations. The physiatrist's training and philosophy promote comprehensive evaluation and the planning of treatments designed to promote optimum function. Pathophysiological processes that result in speech and language disabilities usually also cause multiple, chronic health problems. Obviously, the client facing a number of health problems can greatly benefit from the physiatrist's comprehensive approach. Clients with limited communication abilities are especially in need of the physiatrist's awareness of needs, ability to evaluate responses to therapies, and skills in coordinating medical care.[23]

A physician's order is usually required for speech therapy. Some physicians do not think that speech therapy is necessary immediately after the onset of aphasia and therefore are reluctant to write the prescription. Many speech/language pathologists believe that apraxic speech should be treated immediately, while therapy for aphasia is best begun 1 month after onset. Supportive therapy during that 1-month period is considered valuable because it helps to reduce anxiety.[4] Research findings support the value of initial and ongoing therapy.[25] The speech/language pathologist evaluates the client's ability to understand verbal and written communications, to gesture, to speak spontaneously and upon instruction, and to evaluate his or her own communications. Findings from this evaluation, along with the findings of the physician's physical examination and results of diagnostic tests, are used to determine the type of speech and language problem and to implement appropriate treatment.[12] The American Speech and Hearing Association can provide information on the location of speech/language pathologists. Other agencies that may provide assistance with speech and language impairments are the American Heart Association, the Easter Seal Foundation, and the United Way.[12]

Physical and occupational therapists offer therapies for clients experiencing aphasia along with physical limitations. These therapists plan therapies taking into consideration the client's limitations in understanding directions and expressing needs during treatments. Sensory and motor activities used in conjunction with facilitation techniques can promote the production and use of language and speech. Skills relearned and strength regained in the therapy sessions can provide individuals with the hope and motivation needed to continue working on speech and language impairments, which are often slower to improve.

Optimum hearing is essential for effective communication. Hearing loss in an otherwise healthy person can severely alter one's life-style. Hearing loss in the person experiencing aphasia can discourage efforts to communicate or lead to greater confusion. Trauma resulting in aphasia does not cause loss of hearing, but loss is more common in elderly persons. This group also experiences strokes resulting in aphasia more often than a younger age group. Assessment of hearing should be performed early and the client referred to an audiologist for further assessment, selection of a hearing aid if deemed necessary, and training in use of the aid. Information from the family may be necessary to determine premorbid hearing ability. The nurse may very often be the person to discover this problem.

Social workers often assist the client or family with financial concerns related to hospital costs, dependent family members, and postdischarge needs. Many are trained in counseling and may be helpful in assisting the client and family to cope with changes and losses. When social work counseling is unavailable or the problem is complex, psychologists may be contacted to assist persons coping with disability.

Dental consultations may be needed if dentures do not fit properly or the teeth are in poor repair. Articulation can be difficult with loose dentures or may cause the client embarrassment and thus result in hesitation to attempt speech. Decayed or loose teeth can cause the client pain or discomfort. The client may be unable to inform others of the problem. Observation of chewing ability and assessment of the oral cavity often help to identify problems. Halitosis resulting from caries or poor oral hygiene may be offensive and discourage others from interacting with the client. Referral should be made promptly.

Difficulty in chewing and swallowing is common in clients experiencing brain damage. In addition, depression related to the aphasia or other health problems may cause a loss of appetite. Proper nourishment is essential for healing, mental health, and physical stamina. The nurse should seek consultation with a nutritionist about special meals and supplements. Physicians must order changes in diet related to calories or those specifically related to health problems such as diabetes. General nutritional counseling by the nurse can be provided independently.

Many clients greatly benefit from visits with members of the clergy who can assist them in meeting spiritual and emotional needs. The nurse's understanding of the client's religious practices helps in determining if a clergy member should be actively involved as part of the rehabilitation team. The client and family should be consulted regarding their wishes for visits from a clergy member.

OUTCOME CRITERIA

Outcome criteria for the individual experiencing speech and language problems depend upon the client's unique deficits and resulting problems. The following criteria can be adapted for an individual's specific functional deficits in communication:

1. The client participates in all activities planned to improve communication as demonstrated by:
   a. Participation in speech therapy sessions and periodic evaluations
   b. Interaction and communication with health team members, family, and friends
   c. Explanation, demonstration, or recognition of speech therapy methods and communication techniques designed to improve speech and language
   d. Explanation and use of alternate forms of communication
2. The client safely functions at the optimum level of independence as demonstrated by:
   a. Safe levels of independent function
   b. Searching for and accepting assistance of others as needed
3. The client is free of uncontrolled stress and frustration as demonstrated by:
   a. Participation in speech therapies
   b. Effective expression of anxieties and frustrations via verbalizations or gestures
   c. Communication of needs to others

4. The client demonstrates an attitude of self-worth as evidenced by:
   a. Spontaneous communication to others
   b. An awareness and interest in the environment and others
   c. An expression of interest in appearance
5. The family can provide effective support for the client as demonstrated by the ability to:
   a. Explain the cause of the communication deficits
   b. Explain the expected prognosis for recovery of speech and language skills
   c. Provide realistic and honest support for the client
   d. Explain facilitation techniques, methods for optimum communication, and the purpose and value of alternative methods of communication
   e. Explain the importance of promoting optimum independence
   f. Identify safety needs of the client
   g. Identify methods for promoting optimum health status
   h. Identify the importance of psychological support for the client and themselves
6. The client enjoys social interactions as demonstrated by:
   a. Identification of opportunities
   b. Participation in chosen activities

SUMMARY

The onset of speech and language problems usually results in long-term and often incomplete resolution of communication deficits. Nurses, present in many settings where individuals with communication problems seek assistance, are well suited to facilitate and carry out activities needed to promote optimum recovery of speech and language skills. The nurse's close and cooperative efforts with the speech/language pathologist, physicians, and other rehabilitation disciplines ensure a comprehensive approach to rehabilitation.

TEST QUESTIONS

1. Speech and language production can be affected by injury to which of the following areas?
   a. Left hemisphere of right-handed individuals
   b. Right hemisphere of right-handed individuals

   c. Autonomic nervous system
   d. All of the above
2. Impairment or loss of the ability to use language results from injury to which of the following areas?
   a. Broca's area
   b. Wernicke's area
   c. Right hemisphere
   d. Brainstem
3. Clients may understand the speech of others, but not be able to speak effectively, with injury to which of the following areas?
   a. Broca's area
   b. Brainstem
   c. Cerebellum
   d. All of the above
4. When performing the actual client assessment, it is important to:
   a. Gather all the data as quickly as possible.
   b. Avoid causing excessive fatigue or frustration.
   c. Have a family member present to answer questions to which the client is unable to respond.
   d. Carry out the assessment in the client's hospital room or bedroom.
5. Ongoing nursing assessments of the client experiencing speech and language deficits are appropriate because:
   a. These provide many and varied opportunities to observe the person's ability to understand the environment.
   b. These provide many opportunities to observe changes in the person's ability to communicate.
   c. The nurse's findings are significant to other members of the rehabilitation team.
   d. All of the above.
6. A major goal for the nursing care of the client experiencing speech and language problems is:
   a. The establishment of a functional method of communication
   b. The limitation of social interactions to reduce the risk of frustration
   c. Focusing the client's efforts on learning to use forms of communication not requiring verbalization
   d. Teaching the family the importance of reducing client frustration by communicating for the client

7. When assessing language capabilities of a person who has experienced injury to the speech centers, it is important to realize that:
   a. Deficits will be obvious.
   b. Deficits may be isolated and difficult to identify.
   c. Motor speech limitations will not occur with language formulation deficits.
   d. Language formulation deficits will not occur with motor deficits.

8. An alternate form of communication often useful for the client experiencing Broca's aphasia is:
   a. Writing
   b. Typing
   c. Gesturing
   d. Drawing

9. The environment most helpful for the client experiencing aphasia is:
   a. Uncluttered
   b. Filled with visual stimuli
   c. Filled with auditory stimuli
   d. Frequently rearranged to encourage adjustments to change

10. Communication with the individual experiencing aphasia can often be improved by:
    a. Speaking loudly
    b. Quickly repeating verbalizations
    c. Changing the statement's form if it is not immediately understood
    d. Controlling factors that produce fatigue

11. While encouraging speech in a client experiencing dysarthria, the nurse should:
    a. Discourage attempts to rephrase or repeat mistaken verbalizations.
    b. Encourage the client to speak more quickly.
    c. Assume some responsibility for not understanding communications.
    d. Discourage the use of gestures or writing as compensatory ways to communicate.

12. To ensure that all members of the rehabilitation team can communicate with the client experiencing aphasia, the nurse should:
    a. Direct professionals to seek needed information from current literature.
    b. Provide information on communication techniques that have been successful with the client.
    c. Serve as spokesperson for the client while therapies are provided.
    d. Ask the family to serve as spokesperson for the client while therapies are provided.

Answers: 1. a, 2. b, 3. d, 4. b, 5. d, 6. a, 7. b, 8. c, 9. a, 10. d, 11. c, 12. b.

LEARNING ACTIVITIES

1. The following activities are designed to increase your awareness of the mental processes involved in speech and language.
   a. Monitor your own behaviors related to speech and language.
   b. Identify elements in your environment that stimulate speech and language.
   c. Observe your own communications for "slips" of the tongue (when you do not say what you intended to say). How did you know you made the slip? How did you respond?
   d. Identify times when slips are more likely to occur (for example, when a person is fatigued, anxious, hurried, or in a noisy environment).

2. The following instructions are planned to help you become more attuned to nonverbal communications. This awareness may help you understand the client's nonverbal communications. It may also help you to use nonverbal communication with clients who have trouble understanding verbal messages. Gestures also may be encouraged or taught to clients who have problems with the verbalization of language
   a. Monitor yourself and others for behaviors such as postures, gestures, and facial expressions that influence messages conveyed verbally. Further appreciation for the influence of nonverbal communications can be gained by observing their use in advertisements, on billboards, in magazines, and on television.
   b. Consider the problems that can occur if gestures and facial expressions are missing, as might occur in individuals with facial paralysis, hemiplegia, or Parkinson's disease. What are some of these problems? Awareness of these restraints upon speech and language will help you to be less biased in your responses to the communication attempts made by clients experiencing these limitations.

3. The following exercise is planned to help you begin to understand some of the frustrations experienced by individuals who have speech and language problems: Increase your awareness of the frustrations experienced when the ability to verbalize is lost by not using verbal communication during a 2-hour period. This exercise should take place when you are with others. Note

how you compensate for the lack of ability to verbalize. Did you resort to writing messages to convey your thoughts? Was writing effective? What would you do if you could not write? How did you want others to help you with communication needs?

4. To gain comfort with your new understanding of communication problems, identify the types of clients in your practice and study that are likely to experience communication limitations. In your clinical practice, evaluate the communication of clients with communication deficits and the effectiveness of communications initiated by health team members.

REFERENCES

1. Basso A and others: Influence of rehabilitation on language skills in aphasic patients, Arch Neurol 36:190, April 1979.
2. Beukelman D and Yorkston K: Speech and language disorders. In Kottke F, Stillwell GK, and Lehmann JF, editors: Krusen's handbook of physical medicine and rehabilitation, ed 3, Philadelphia, 1982, WB Saunders Co.
3. Beukelman D and others: Effectiveness of three instruction modalities, Arch Phys Med Rehabil 61:248, June 1980.
4. Broida H: Coping with stroke: communication breakdown of brain injured adults, San Diego, Calif, 1979, College Hill Press.
5. Corria J and others: PET measurement of cerebral blood flow and metabolism in stroke patients, Appl Radiol 12(6):147, 1983.
6. Davis G: A survey of adult aphasia, Englewood Cliffs, NJ, 1983, Prentice-Hall, Inc.
7. Gordon M: Nursing diagnosis: process and application, ed 2, New York, 1987, McGraw-Hill Book Co.
8. Guyton A: Human physiology and mechanisms of disease, ed 3, Philadelphia, 1982, WB Saunders Co.
9. Halper A and Glistra S: Speech and language disorders of neurological origin in adults. In Martin N, Holt N, and Hicks D, editors: Comprehensive rehabilitation nursing, New York, 1981, McGraw-Hill Book Co.
10. Harden W and Merson R: The higher-order dysfunctions: apraxia, agnosia, and aphasia. In Eliasson S and others, editors: Neurological pathophysiology, ed 2, New York, 1978, Oxford University Press.
11. Held J: Rehabilitation of head injury patients. In Ruskin A, editor: Current therapy in physiatry: physical medicine and rehabilitation, Philadelphia, 1984, WB Saunders Co.
12. Howland A: Treatment of aphasia following stroke, Stroke 10(4):475, 1979.
13. Joelson K: Speech and language problems associated with cerebrovascular accidents. In Ruskin A, editor: Current therapy in physiatry: physical medicine and rehabilitation, Philadelphia, 1984, WB Saunders Co.
14. LaPointe L: Aphasia therapy: some principles and strategies for treatment. In Johns D, editor: Clinical management of neurologic communicative disorders, ed 2, Boston, 1985, Little, Brown & Co.
15. Louis M and Povse S: Aphasia and endurance: considerations in assessment and care of the stroke patient, Nurs Clin North Am 15(2):265, 1980.
16. Manly C: The role of the speech-language pathologist in the care of patients with respiratory insufficiency. In Ruskin A, editor: Current therapy in physiatry: physical medicine and rehabilitation, Philadelphia, 1984, WB Saunders Co.
17. Menikheim M and Leon M: Impairments in verbal communication. In Snyder M, editor: A guide to neurological and neurosurgical nursing, New York, 1983, John Wiley & Sons, Inc.
18. Palmer E: Language dysfunction in cerebrovascular disease, Primary Care 6(4):827, 1979.
19. Piotrowski M: Aphasia: providing better nursing care, Nurs Clin North Am 13:543, 1978.
20. Raichle M and others: Disorders in cerebral circulation. In Eliasson S and others, editors: Neurological pathophysiology, ed 2, New York, 1978, Oxford University Press.
21. Rosenbek J: Treating apraxia of speech. In Johns D, editor: Clinical management of neurologic communicative disorders, ed 2, Boston, 1985, Little, Brown & Co.
22. Rosenbek J and LaPointe L: The dysarthrias: description, diagnosis and treatment. In Johns D, editor: Clinical management of neurologic communicative disorders, ed 2, Boston, 1985, Little, Brown & Co.
23. Ruskin A: The physiatrist, physician to the disabled. In Ruskin A, editor: Current therapy in physiatry: physical medicine and rehabilitation, Philadelphia, 1984, WB Saunders Co.
24. Tompkins C and others: Aphasic patients in a rehabilitation program: scheduling speech and language services, Arch Phys Med Rehabil 61:252, June 1980.
25. Wertz R and others: Veterans Administration Cooperative Study on aphasia: a comparison of individual and group treatment, J Speech Hearing Res 24:580, 1981.
26. Wilson H and Kneisl C: Psychiatric nursing, ed 3, Menlo Park, Calif, 1983, Addison-Wesley Publishing Co, Inc.

ADDITIONAL READINGS

Beukelman DR and others: Expressive communication disorders in persons with multiple sclerosis: a survey, Arch Phys Med Rehabil 66:675, 1985.

Blanco KM: The aphasic patient, J Neurosurg Nurs 14:34, Feb 1982.

Boss BJ: Dysphasia, dyspraxia and dysarthria: distinguishing features. I, J Neurosurg Nurs 16:151, June 1984.

Boss BJ: Dysphasia, dyspraxia and dysarthria: distinguishing features. II, J Neurosurg Nurs 16:211, Aug 1984.

Bryere SM and others: Electronic communications in rehabilitation: the future is now, J Rehabil 48:49, Oct/Dec 1982.

Bush PG and Drummond SS: Comprehension and production of idioms in dysphasia, Arch Phys Med Rehabil 66:697, 1985.

Cardinale SP: Lend 'n ear: a therapeutic tool for speech rehabilitation . . . volunteers listen and repeat what patients say and answer questions, Rehabil Nurs 7:25, Nov/Dec 1982.

Chalmers C: Talking to stroke patients, Nurs Times 81:41, Aug 7-13, 1985.

Cole J: A word in your ear, Nurs Times 82:53, Sept 10, 1986.

Fried-Oken M: Voice recognition device as a computer interface for motor and speech impaired people, Arch Phys Med Rehabil 66:678, 1985.

Kumin L and Rysticken N: Aids to bridge the communication barrier . . . people who lose the ability to speak, Geriatr Nurse 6:348, 1985.

Miller M and others: Stop, look and listen . . . stroke patients, Nurs Mirror 158:40, Jan 18, 1984

Ozuna J: Alterations in mentation: nursing assessment and intervention, J Neurosurg Nurs 17:66, Feb 1985.

Pimental PA: Alterations in communication: biopsychosocial aspects of aphasia, dysarthria, and right hemisphere syndromes in the stroke patient, Nurs C in North Am 21:321, 1986.

Reedy DF: The client with aphasia: the nurse's assessment of language abilities, Top Clin Nurs 8:67, April 1986.

CHAPTER 16

Communication: Sensation and Perception

Susan M. Evans

OBJECTIVES

After completing Chapter 16, the reader will be able to:

1. Recognize barriers to communication.

2. Distinguish between internal and external stimuli that influence communication behavior.

3. Understand the role of sensation and perception in the communication process.

4. Identify impairments in sensation and perception.

5. Conduct a nursing assessment specific to sensation and perception.

6. Formulate nursing diagnoses associated with impaired sensation and perception.

7. Develop realistic and attainable goals with the client who has impaired sensation and perception.

8. Determine nursing interventions appropriate for the client with impaired sensation and perception.

9. Identify rehabilitation team interventions appropriate for the client with impaired sensation and perception.

10. List outcome criteria on which to base evaluation of interventions for the client with impaired sensation and perception.

"Poor communication" has been the target of blame in most instances of relationship breakdowns. Marital problems, labor disputes, or generation gaps are some of the reasons people fail to communicate effectively. Nurses, however, rarely consider communication to be the factor responsible for inadequate or ineffective nursing care. Clients are sometimes labeled as noncompliant, poorly motivated, or deviant, and a true understanding of the problem is not discovered.

COMMUNICATION

Communication, a dynamic intrapersonal and interpersonal process, takes place within, between, and among individuals and their environments.

All communication occurs within a context. Intrapersonal communication depends upon receptors within the body and an intact nervous system. Visceroreceptors within body organs receive and transmit hunger, nausea, and pain sensations to the brain for interpretation. Proprioceptors within muscles, tendons, joints, and the inner ear receive and transmit position, vibration, deep pressure, and pain sensations.[6]

Interpersonal communication relies upon exteroceptors to enhance and ensure information exchange between and among individuals. Exteroceptors are located in the skin and mucosa and are responsible for touch, pressure, temperature and pain sensations.[6] Special receptors in the eyes, ears, nose, mouth, and tongue enable individuals to see, hear, smell, and taste. These sensations, referred to as visual, auditory, olfactory, and gustatory sensations, are carried to the brain where they are interpreted according to each individual's perception. Perceptions are based upon accuracy of reception and past knowledge and experience. The individual's perceptions are reflected in verbal and nonverbal communication behaviors that are indicative of response to internal and external environments.

Many senses contribute to effective communication between individuals. The message sender relies upon vision, hearing, smell, taste, and touch to transmit information and emotional states. The message receiver also must rely on the senses to provide appropriate feedback to the message sender. The state of the internal and external environments of both the sender and receiver can negatively or positively affect message transmittal and the success of the communication effort.

Communication Barriers

A number of barriers interfere with communication transactions. Problems in the internal environment, such as impaired sensation and perception, can hamper reception and expression of messages. Distractions within the external environment, such as poor temperature regulation, inadequate lighting, extraneous noise, and foul odors, can affect communication between individuals.

Distractions in the external environment are recognized through the senses. For example, when a nurse responds to a young man's question about future sexual function after a spinal cord injury, noise from other clients and the nurse's nonverbal communication behaviors affect the reception and perception of the message. The smell of an infected pressure ulcer affects communication between the client and others.

Perceptual differences are obstacles in relating messages. Each person possesses a distinct mental filter, so it is quite common for different people to interpret a single message in totally different ways. When this happens, miscommunication frequently results.[5] For example, when an elderly man fell as he was being transferred back to bed from a wheelchair, the nurse and the aide helping him had different accounts of the accident. Different knowledge bases and experiences influenced their perceptions. Both viewpoints need to be acknowledged and respected.

Emotions and personalities also affect the ways people communicate. A person who is emotionally upset may be uncooperative, belligerent, withdrawn, or noncompliant. Someone who is not respected or liked may have difficulty in transmitting messages that are accepted. An awareness of the selectivity, biases, tendencies, and difficulties encountered in perception may help to increase the understanding level during the communication process.

Communication as a Response to Sensory and Perceptual Stimuli

Communication behavior, like other behavior, is an observable reaction to stimuli. A stimulus is anything that acts to elicit a response. It may be internal and consistent with need states of the body or external and influenced by the environment.

People are constantly bombarded by all sorts of internal and external stimuli in their daily lives. These stimuli are received by at least one of the sensory or afferent nerve pathways and then converted from physical energy to neural energy by receptors such as the eyes, ears, nose, skin, and mouth and tongue. These senses are the initial point for attributing meaning to stimuli. Without continuous exposure to internal and external stimuli, growth, development, and survival would be inhibited.

Internal stimuli arise from within the body and include visceral sensations such as hunger, pain, temperature, and peristaltic movement. Other examples of internal stimuli are the sensations of position and balance that are responsible for sitting and walking skills. External stimuli are found outside the body and can be seen, heard, smelled, tasted, and touched. If one considers all of the changing stimuli with which persons are constantly in contact, it becomes apparent that it is impossible to respond to all of them at any one time. In responding to multiple stimuli, a human's basic needs of food, oxygen, and rest are given highest priority. Through automatic nervous system activity, specialized receptors monitor inner body functions and react accordingly. Basic spinal reflexes also elicit responses over which persons have little control. Subliminal stimuli can elicit responses even without conscious awareness.

Neural tissue receptors detect stimuli that are sensitive to sights, sounds, tastes, smells, and touch. Impulses received by the skin, subcutaneous and deep tissues, and viscera are transmitted over afferent pathways to the spinal cord. From there, the impulses synapse in reflex action or are transmitted to the brain. Impulses received by the eyes, ears, taste buds, and nose are transmitted over afferent pathways to the brainstem. As impulses from these general and special senses pass through the brainstem on the way to the cortex, they come into contact with the reticular activating system.

The reticular activating system, a diffuse collection of interlacing fibers and nuclei forming the central core of the brainstem, is important in the integration of sensory data. Ascending paths from the brainstem travel to the thalamus and from there to all parts of the cerebral cortex where interpretation and arousal take place.[6] The interpretation of sensory input in the brain is accomplished by a complex process not yet understood completely. The firing of neurons within the cortex itself also could activate the reticular system and influence or alter the perception of external stimuli. It is hypothesized that the reticular activating system regulates input and output levels of sensory stimuli. When the reticular activating system is stimulated, a state of arousal results; when stimulation is lacking, drowsiness and sleep occur.

Before a response actually takes place, a person reacts to the stimulus. Through cortical interpretation, stimuli are transferred into thoughts. Whether or not a stimulus is acknowledged depends upon a number of factors, including intensity or power, size, changes, repetition, and relevance.[33] Intensity refers to the degree the stimulus is made known. For example, a loud fire alarm bell is effective in notifying everyone that a fire is present. Size of a stimulus helps determine choices. If a person was very hungry and received two offers, one for a banana split and the other for a carrot, there would be no question as to the choice that would be made. A change in stimulus would bring about a change in response. If a client suddenly developed a change in respiratory pattern, the nurse would be stimulated to act. Repetition of a stimulus makes one experienced, proficient, and comfortable in interpretation. The last factor, relevance, relates to the fact that a stimulus is more easily perceived if it has relevance for a specific person. For example, a nursing student would find it easier to retain knowledge of a specific disease entity if a close friend or relative had that same diagnosis.

ROLE OF SENSATION AND PERCEPTION

Under normal circumstances, body sensations connect a person with self and with the environment. These sensations are interpreted and perceived through neural mechanisms. The functions of sensation and perception are discussed below.

Sensation

Humans are able to identify with and understand themselves, other individuals, and the environment through their sensory systems. They are able to receive each stimulus through the senses and afferent pathways of the nervous system. As sensations are interpreted and perceived in the cortex, meanings are attached to objects and persons in the environment, and reactions occur according to the meanings assigned. The senses also give cues to learned behavior. For example, when we hear the telephone ring, we pick up the receiver to take the call. Individuals also have the ability to block out selected stimuli. For example, we may be able to carry on a personal conversation with another despite a noisy room.

Smell

Compared to other animals, a human's sense of smell is rather limited and is not relied on as much as other senses. Most people, however, are able to recognize, detect, and decipher a wide variety of odors.

The olfactory receptors are located in the upper part of the nasal cavity. This surface consists of many free nerve endings embedded in supporting structures and covered by a watery fluid. The presence of olfactory hairs increases the effectiveness of the olfactory epithelium.[11] Efferent axons of the peripheral olfactory sensory cells are unmyelinated and terminate in the olfactory bulb, which is a direct extension of the central nervous system. The olfactory cortex is located in a small region of the anterior portion of the temporal lobe.[10]

Smells enter the nasal passage in the form of a gas and dissolve in the secretions, forming a chemical solution. This solution stimulates the sensitive peripheral receptors to transmit impulses via the olfactory nerve. These impulses are then transmitted to the cerebrum where interpretation takes place.[3]

Certain substances can be smelled very easily and, within Western society, have been connected with specific places and activities. A print shop, florist, brewery, bakery, lumberyard, stockyard, farm, and a number of other places can be distinguished by their smells. An opened can of coffee, a cedar closet, freshly cut grass, and flowers have smells with pleasant associations. Poor personal hygiene, infection, and stale whiskey have smells with unpleasant associations. Unlike taste, however, there is as yet no agreement as to the basic qualities of smell.

Taste

Taste and smell are closely interrelated. Taste is also influenced by pain and tactile receptors of the mouth and temperature of ingested substances. Therefore, the sense of taste depends upon the sensory receptors for taste, smell, pain, texture, and temperature. Upon closer examination, some tastes are found to be odors. For example, vanilla cannot be tasted in the mouth until it can be smelled.

The taste receptors are located in the taste buds. These are small cellular areas found in the mucous membrane of papillae located in the edges and the upper rear surface of the tongue. Although the number varies greatly in different papillae, it is believed that there are 4,000 to 10,000 taste buds. Other sensitive areas in the mouth that contain taste buds include the pharynx and soft palate.[14]

When food dissolves in the saliva, taste bud cells are stimulated and form a chemical substance. Stimulated by this action, afferent nerve fibers then transmit impulses through the facial and glossopharyngeal nerves to the medulla oblongata, where they synapse with ascending tracts. The impulses are then transmitted from the medulla oblongata to the thalamus and cerebrum, where they are interpreted. Cranial nerve VII (facial) innervates the anterior two thirds of the tongue; cranial nerve IX (glossopharyngeal) innervates the posterior third of the tongue and part of the pharynx; and cranial nerve X (vagus) innervates the pharynx and larynx.[11]

Taste buds are sensitive to sweet, sour, salty, and bitter substances. The anterior portion of the tongue is sensitive to sweet and salty, the lateral portion to sour, and the posterior portion to bitter stimulation. Substances with these tastes include sucrose (sweet), sodium chloride (salt), tartaric acid (sour), and quinine sulfate (bitter). Characteristics of taste that greatly influence how these substances are perceived include color, appearance, temperature, texture, flavor, and quality.

Touch

Touching involves skin contact and is a form of nonverbal communication that conveys a message and stimulates a central nervous system response. Culturally determined universal responses to touch include a handshake, a pat on the back, an arm around a shoulder, a kiss on the lips, and a slap on the bottom.

The sense of touch is made possible by countless nerve receptors in the skin, the largest organ of the body. The body is divided into specific areas called dermatomes. Each dermatome is supplied by a nerve root. When external stimulation is applied, a receptor neuron in that dermatome carries sensory impulses to the posterior horn of the spinal cord to synapse with a secondary neuron. The fibers from this neuron then cross to the contralateral side of the spinal cord and continue upward along the ventral spinothalamic tract. Upon reaching the thalamus, the nerve fibers synapse with a third sensory neuron and finally terminate in the sensory cortex.[32]

Touching is a valuable, effective, and intimate

sense. By touching something a person can identify its texture, size, density, consistency, shape, hardness, sharpness (or dullness), and temperature. Although the eyes may give false impressions, touch is not so easily fooled. Touching is powerful. When an individual touches another, attention is gained. A touch in the form of a punch elicits even more attention. Touch also expresses feelings. It communicates affection, pain, acknowledgment, support, and condolence.

Nursing care requires a great deal of touching. A nurse's touch during conversation or performance of nursing tasks portrays feelings. A soft, gentle touch may indicate care and acceptance; a rough, quick touch may indicate lack of concern or preoccupation. A person can often communicate true feelings more effectively by using touch alone or as a complement to verbal messages. Treatment modalities that make use of touch include massage, rolfing (a method of working with the body to achieve a realignment of body structure), and acupressure.

Pain

Pain is a concept that is difficult to describe qualitatively. More difficult, however, is its quantification. A true definition of pain can only be made by the person suffering from it. McCaffery, a nurse who has devoted much time to the study of pain, states that "pain is whatever the person experiencing it says it is and that the pain exists whenever that individual says it does."[24] The difficulty in clearly defining pain lies in the fact that pain is a highly complex phenomenon having two nearly inseparable components: sensation and reaction. Pain arises when tissue integrity is threatened or actually damaged. A noxious stimulus leads to two responses: (1) physical perception of the damage and (2) affective response to the threat of damage.[4] The dual response mechanism involved in the experience of pain includes sensory dimensions, such as time, space, and intensity, as well as emotional, cognitive, and motivational aspects. Receptors in the skin most closely associated with pain are called nociceptors. Pain messages travel from the spinal cord to the brainstem via the spinothalamic tract and then move on to the thalamus in the brainstem. When the pain messages leave the brainstem, they enter the cerebral cortex.[9] The cerebral cortex and brainstem send descending fibers to the spinal cord that

influence incoming pain impulses. A number of theories of pain causation have been proposed, two of which are discussed here.

Gate control theory. In 1965 Melzack and Wall[27] proposed the gate control theory of pain causation. This theory attempts to integrate the roles of physical sensation, motivation, and psychological factors in the experience of pain. Basically, the gate control theory suggests that the intensity of painful stimuli is modulated through a gating mechanism at the level of the spinal cord. The gating mechanism is in the substantia gelatinosa, located in the dorsal horn of the spinal cord. Small-diameter, unmyelinated C nerve fibers and large, myelinated A-delta nerve fibers carry pain impulses to the substantia gelatinosa. A-delta fibers may carry the first sharp pain sensation associated with a pinprick, whereas C fibers may carry the later aching or burning pain sensations from the same pinprick. According to Meinhart and McCaffery,[25] the "C-fiber system is excitory and carries the largest percentage of potentially painful impulses. When the gate is open, impulses travel from the periphery through the dorsal column fibers to the cortical level of awareness. Excitation of C fibers inhibits the activity in the substantia gelatinosa. This results in opening the gate even more and thus allowing more nociceptive impulses through."[25] If the large-diameter A-delta fibers originating in the peripheral nervous system are stimulated, there is an activating effect on the substantia gelatinosa and pain impulses would be stopped at the level of the spinal cord, not reaching the brain or level of awareness.

Endogenous pain control theory. More recently, much attention has been focused on a new theory of pain modulation called the endogenous pain control theory. This theory is based on the discovery of certain endogenous compounds, namely, endorphins and enkephalins, peptides with opiate-like qualities that can alter pain perception, mood, respiration, and release of pituitary hormones. Enkephalin is manufactured in the nerve cells and the posterior pituitary. The related neurohormone beta-endorphin is manufactured by the anterior and intermediate lobes of the pituitary and was named endorphin for *endogenous morphine*.[9] Although endogenous opiates have been detected in many areas of the body, these are concentrated in body areas associated with the nerve transmission of noxious stimuli. Receptors for the endorphins and enkephalins are found in heaviest concentrations in the thalamus, the major center for pain perception.

When the endogenous opiate occupies a receptor site, the action of the cell bearing the receptor is depressed. The ultimate effect of this opiate-receptor combination is the reduction of pain perception and an elevation of pain threshold and tolerance.[40] Research into the role of endogenous opiates continues at a rapid pace and is expected to have a major impact on our understanding of pain and its management.

Temperature

Body temperature is the balance between heat generation of the energy-producing cells and heat-loss mechanisms of the body. The temperature-regulating centers in the hypothalamus control reflex responses such as sweating and shivering. Temperature receptors in the skin are responsible for adaptation to environmental temperature conditions. Temperature sensation is transmitted via the lateral spinothalamic tract along with pain sensation.

Environmental conditions of heat or cold above or below the average of 72°F (22°C) cause sensations of discomfort for many individuals. If environmental temperature variation persists long enough, discomfort manifests itself by shivering or perspiration, eventually progressing to the severe physiological reactions accompanying hypothermia and hyperthermia (Chapter 8). Clients particularly at risk for discomfort from environmental temperature variations include the person with a spinal cord injury or the person with a cerebrovascular accident who has impaired autonomic nervous system regulation.

Proprioception

Proprioception concerns position and movement of body parts. Sense organs, called *proprioceptors*, are located in subcutaneous tissues, deep tissue walls, muscles, tendons, and bones. These organs are stimulated by various actions of the body and receive impulses from muscle spindles and Golgi tendon organs. When stimulated, the proprioceptive impulses travel via the dorsal columns of the spinal cord and then to the cerebellum and cortex.

Perception

Communication involves not only the use of the senses, but also the interpretation of these senses in the cortex. When a person has contact with another individual, an impression is formed. This impression involves the selection, organization, and interpretation of various sensory stimuli. A person's appearance, dress, voice, mannerisms, vocabulary, and gestures are all clues to the impression that is made. The responses generated from this interaction are based on perception. These perceptions may not always be correct, because misinterpretation may occur, even under normal circumstances.

Description

Perception is a result of a complex, integrative system that is responsible for deciphering stimuli into recognizable and meaningful information. It is the ability of the mind to interpret internal and external sensations into thought processes. Through perception, everything is assigned meaning; without it one could not appreciate the wonders of the world or understand the environment.

Ability to perceive is the result of combined activity of end organs, peripheral nerve tracts, ganglia, and the sensory cortex. It is the responsibility of the parietal lobe of the brain. Blood supply to the parietal lobe is provided by the middle cerebral, anterior cerebral, and posterior cerebral arteries. Consequently, obstruction of this arterial blood flow caused by an embolism, thrombus, or the pressure of a tumor would result in perceptual difficulties.[30]

Perception is influenced by a number of variables, including age, education, culture, past experiences, beliefs, customs, rituals, attitudes, motivation, psychological state, expectations, and goals. A person's identity is determined by perceptions.

As the body is bombarded with multiple stimuli, an individual tends to be very selective. Those stimuli that have some relevance or are consistent with a person's beliefs are the ones on which attention is focused. For example, the "cocktail party phenomenon" occurs when a man selectively hears and perceives his own name above the general level of conversation. To cite another example, studies of grocery shoppers have demonstrated the influence of basic biological needs for food on perception. Hungry shoppers buy more food than nonhungry shoppers, because they perceive themselves as needing more food.

Another feature of perception involves the placement of knowledge into categories. Through the process of putting things together, a person can more easily make sense out of pieces of information. This not only allows for comfort and organization but also eliminates elements of surprise and chaos. Individuals can deal with something much easier if it is familiar.[7]

Along with individual perceptions come inevitable distortions. Although people rely on their sensory systems to gain information, assumptions made from past experience, present emotions, and knowledge are often filled in. For example, stereotyping is a way of making assumptions and defining characteristics of people with similar traits. In other words, individuals who stereotype fill in what they expect a person of a particular race, belief, or religion to be. Disabled individuals are frequently perceived as helpless by others who have had little experience in interacting with them. This behavior encourages fixed judgments and impressions that are highly resistant to change.

Regulating perceptual input

Feedback regulates communication and enables individuals to clarify information transmitted in messages. It allows the listener to relay perceptions of the message back to the sender.

Feedback may be internal (from within the person) or external (from others) and may produce positive or negative reinforcement. Internal feedback consists of a self-perception of how one measures up to one's own expectations. For instance, a woman may taste a cake that she has just baked and perceive whether or not it is good. External feedback is obtained through responses of others. Through the questions of an audience or administration of a posttest, a speaker can tell the effectiveness of a speech. The woman who baked the cake may receive compliments from persons who eat the cake. A smile or encouraging word also can act as a positive reinforcement. Conversely, a frown or grimace can act as negative feedback. Positive feedback reinforces a successful effort, whereas negative feedback requires a modification or change in course of action.

IMPAIRED SENSATION

Because of the complexity and uniqueness of the sensory system, any deviation from the norm can result in wide-ranging consequences. Congenital conditions, trauma, and local and systemic diseases may be responsible for these deviations. The problem may involve the sense organ itself, the nerve pathway, or part of the brain. The physician is concerned with locating the source of the problem in order to make a diagnosis and prescribe an appropriate medical regimen. The nurse, on the other hand, uses data from the sensory assessment to determine the effects of any problems on the person's performance of activities of daily living. The nurse also considers the effect of the problem in relation to the person's growth and development. Knowing whether the deficit is temporary or permanent will give the nurse guidance in determining actual and potential problems and in helping the client cope for a short time or make permanent adjustments.

Smell

The following terms have been used to describe different impairments of smell[10]:

anosmia The complete loss of the sense of smell, may be unilateral or bilateral.

hyposmia Impairment of smell.

cacosmia or **parosmia** A distorted or perverted sense of smell.

phantosmia Hallucination of smell.

heterosmia Inappropriate inability to distinguish between certain odors.

agnosia Inability to classify or contrast smells, although able to detect odors.

Unilateral anosmia and hyposmia may not be noticed by the person affected. People who have a congested upper respiratory tract may have experienced anosmia and may complain of a taste deficit because of the close relationship between these two senses. Anosmia by itself is usually viewed as an annoyance and not as a major health problem. It becomes a major problem if it interferes with the performance of such occupations as baker, perfume manufacturer, or wine maker.

The single most common cause of olfactory impairment is an upper respiratory tract infection. Some other possible causes of absent or impaired smell include intranasal obstructions such as polyps or neoplasms, injury to the olfactory nerve, intracranial lesions, tumors of the temporal lobe, trauma, infectious meningitis, and abscesses.[41] A decreased sense of smell has been found in persons with viral hepatitis, but this subsided once the illness disappeared.[15] Anosmia also may be congenital or psychogenic in origin. Impairment of the sense of smell may be caused by malfunction of the olfactory receptors (as with the common cold), the olfactory nerve, or the part of the brain concerned with olfaction. Onset of the problem may be acute, as with an inflammatory process or injury, or gradual, as with a slow-growing tumor or poisoning from toxic fumes.[37] The duration of anosmia may be quite short, as seen after some types of head injury, or it may be permanent, after more extensive destruction of nerves with massive injuries.

A frontal lobe contusion may produce anosmia; an occipital blow because of a contrecoup effect when the brain is driven to the opposite side of the skull may also produce this problem. Both of these injuries may cause damage to olfactory filaments because of shearing, contusion, or tearing as the nerves pass through the cribriform plate. Temporary anosmia may be caused by edema or pressure on the olfactory nerve.[37] The loss of the sense of smell is more likely to be found in persons who have experienced amnesia after injury and in those who have had a fracture of the frontal skull base.[38]

Renal disease, diabetes, and cirrhosis have been associated with olfactory disorders. They also have been found in persons with malnutrition, dietary deficiencies, and autoimmune disorders.[10] In addition, a number of different drugs, industrial chemicals and pollutants, and tobacco can produce disorders of smell.

Medical intervention for the client who has anosmia is directed toward alleviating the source of the problem. Measures may be necessary to decrease intracranial pressure or surgically remove an obstruction. If the cause is unknown or cannot be treated, nursing interventions to assist the individual in making adjustments are needed.

Taste

Most taste abnormalities are, in fact, disorders of the sense of smell, such as experienced with the common cold. The loss of taste may be restricted to one portion of the tongue or to areas innervated by one of the cranial nerves. An individual will experience a loss of taste over the anterior two

thirds of the tongue with a diseased facial nerve, such as in mastoid canal lesions.[32] If taste is present in the remainder of the tongue, this disorder may go unnoticed.

Taste sensation also is influenced by hormones, as demonstrated in pregnancy and in menstruation.[39] There are also taste changes in diabetes mellitus believed to be caused by neuropathy.[1] Taste acuity increases in adrenal cortical insufficiency but reverts to normal with steroid therapy.[16] Central nervous system tumors and pontine cerebrovascular accidents can affect the taste centers in the brain and the major relay tracts to the peripheral end organs.[13]

Touch

Alterations in touch are varied and depend upon the pathological process involved and the location and extent of any lesion in the brain, spinal cord, or peripheral nervous system. Terms related to abnormal sensations of touch include:

anesthesia Loss of touch sensation.
paresthesia Abnormal sensation.
hypoesthesia Decreased sensation.
hyperesthesia Increased sensation.
Complete anesthesia below the lesion level results when there is a complete transection of the spinal cord. Peripheral nerve pathways also may be involved.

Symptoms of paresthesia include tingling, crawling, and burning sensations. Frequently, paresthesia accompanies demyelinating diseases such as multiple sclerosis or incomplete peripheral nerve damage such as is seen with tumor or injury.[8] Abnormal sensations also are referred to as *dysesthesias*.

Pain

The sense of pain involves a degree of discomfort caused by a potentially harmful stimulus. Pain serves a protective purpose by warning the individual of a body malfunction. Nerve endings for the sense of pain are found in almost every tissue of the body. These pain receptors may be stimulated by chemical, thermal, electrical, or mechanical agents. The transmission of pain impulses is similar to that of touch, but pain impulses ascend in the lateral, rather than the anterior, spinothalamic tract to the thalamus.

Pain is the primary symptom that prompts one to seek medical attention. It may be acute or chronic, and treatment is determined by specific signs and symptoms. The onset of acute pain is usually immediate, temporary, and characterized by a pattern of reactions consistent with the epinephrine-norepinephrine responses of the sympathetic nervous system. These reactions include an elevation in blood pressure, pulse, and respiratory rate. Increases in peripheral blood flow, muscle tension, palmar sweating, and anxiety also are experienced.[37]

Clients with chronic pain are highly represented among the rehabilitation population; these are the individuals with rheumatoid arthritis or osteoarthritis, trigeminal neuralgia, postherpetic pain, low back pain, unsuccessful laminectomy, muscle tension or migraine headache, poststroke dysesthesias, or persistent phantom limb pain, to mention a few causes. Their pain becomes an illness in itself and requires different intervention measures and communication about pain. Chronic pain responses depend upon autonomic nervous system involvement and include insomnia, headache, anorexia, irritability, apprehension, and verbal complaints.

Temperature

Extreme *hyperthermia* (very high body temperature) is harmful to neurons and may damage the central nervous system. Causes include severe infection and inflammatory processes, hypothalamic disturbances, spinal cord injuries, brain tumors, or brain injuries. Damage to the brain may result in states of confusion, delirium, disorientation, hallucinations, and seizures. A *hypothermic* condition (very low body temperature) results in diminution of the basal metabolic rate and clinical signs of lethargy, decreased sensorium, diminished reflexes, pallor from capillary restriction, and lowered vital signs.

Proprioception

Disorders of the dorsal column produce ataxia or incoordination. Loss of proprioceptive pathways occurs in tabes dorsalis, right parietal lobe lesions, advanced pernicious anemia, and Brown-Séquard syndrome.

IMPAIRED PERCEPTION

Without intact pathways to interpret data, a person cannot make use of the information received by the senses. Sensory stimuli are distorted and cannot be organized into meaningful data. With changes in sensory perception, reality is distorted and errors are made in the meanings assigned to sensory data. This situation leads to unexpected behavior and confusion.[33]

Perceptual disturbances may take many forms, including disorders relating to perception of self, body image, illness, and the environment. Judgment of space, distance, and movement also can be altered.[30] Sensory perceptual alterations are seen frequently in clients with neurological conditions, especially those who have experienced a cerebrovascular accident or head injury.

Disorientation

Disorientation is a decreased awareness of reality. The confusion demonstrated may be temporary when the responsible cause is alcohol or drugs, metabolic malfunction, or anxiety. Reversible neurosurgical trauma such as subdural hematoma or neurological conditions such as central nervous system infections also may produce confusion. Disorientation may be progressive or permanent when it is caused by congenital anomalies, cerebrovascular disease, normal-pressure hydrocephalus, cerebral degenerative disease, and dementia.

Under normal conditions, persons are able to adjust the flow of sensory stimuli. One can seek human contact by going out, using the telephone, or turning on a radio, record player, or television. Increasing physical activity through work, exercise, and play, or withdrawing into a book are ways of manipulating the amount of incoming stimuli. With sufficient and varied input, individuals are able to perceive the environment appropriately and behave accordingly.

Sensory underload

If for some reason there is a deficiency of informational input, a stressful situation exists that results in a disruption of normal function. Some causes of sensory underload or deprivation include inadequate stimulation, sense organ impairment, and damage to the cerebral centers responsible for processing stimuli.

Many laboratory studies have concluded that with limited sensory input, subjects experience some abnormal behavior. In a study conducted by Downs and reported in Collins,[7] young healthy adults placed in social isolation under conditions simulating semiprivate hospital rooms reported symptoms of anxiety, irritability, drowsiness, disorganized thinking, and hallucinations. In less than 3 hours, auditory, visual, olfactory, kinesthetic, and tactile distortions were observed.

The chronicity and rehabilitation of many disabilities necessitate long periods in a health care institution. The use of Stryker frames, traction equipment, body casts, oxygen, or wheelchairs leads to additional sensory restrictions. People most prone to sensory underload include elderly, handicapped, retarded, depressed, psychotic, and invalid persons.

Boredom and loneliness also can lead to sensory distortions. Symptoms of disorientation, confusion, and hallucinations may be the result of sensory deprivation and not impaired mental function. The use of central nervous system depressants such as narcotics and alcohol may diminish sensations and perceptions further.

Sensory overload

Just as a diminished sensory level can cause alterations in normal thought processing, high-intensity stimuli also can disrupt normal cerebral function. Noise pollution, use of machinery, and too many visitors may all cause sensory overload. A person who lives alone or usually has limited human contact would be more susceptible to sensory overload when exposed to noise and many people such as other rehabilitation clients and rehabilitation personnel. This person also would fatigue easily, and fatigue greatly hinders rehabilitation. The client may be unable to retain new information, so teaching efforts would be in vain.

Certain conditions make a normal sensory environment intolerable. People who are extremely anxious or who are afflicted with migraine headaches, meningitis, or encephalitis are agitated easily by normal lights, sounds, and other everyday stimuli. The use of central nervous system stimulants such as amphetamines can alter or distort perceptions and result in sensory overload.[32]

Agnosia

Agnosia refers to the inability to recognize objects using one of the senses, even though the sense is intact. The disorder may be visual, auditory, tactile, or proprioceptive, depending on the affected area of the cerebral cortex. Agnosia may be seen in clients with progressive dementia or cerebrovascular accidents.[36]

Visual agnosia is generally the result of damage to the visual association areas in the parietal and occipital lobes. A person with this problem who is asked to identify an object will usually describe its parts or its properties but will be unable to identify the object completely as a whole.[21]

Auditory agnosia occurs when a person can no longer recognize the sounds that are heard. The individual can still read and understand words but cannot identify the same words when spoken even while possibly being able to recognize the voice as a voice and recognize language without understanding it. Lesions exist in one or both temporal lobes.

Individuals with tactile agnosia cannot recognize objects placed in the hand. Touch is perceived in the thalamus, but recognition and localization of the sensation occur in the parietal cortex. Tactile agnosia results when the cortical area or the connections between the thalamus and the cortex are destroyed.[30]

An individual feels proprioceptive sensation in the joints, joint capsules, and ligaments. This sensation helps determine where the extremities are in space. With some neurological deficits, the person may not be able to place extremities appropriately or identify their location in space.

Apraxia

Apraxia is the inability to perform a learned action voluntarily, even though comprehension and movement are intact. Although unable to perform a task on demand, the client may unconsciously perform the same task at another time.[29] There seems to be an integrative breakdown while cognition and execution of action function normally. Apraxia may occur as a result of a cerebrovascular accident, encephalitis, or other focal lesions of the brain such as a tumor.[35] Lesions affect the left parietal lobe, precentral gyrus, parietooccipital region, and corpus callosum.[28]

Disturbance of Body Image

A person with a disturbed body image has a distorted view of self. The individual may totally ignore one side of the body (unilateral neglect). With a lack of awareness of use of certain body parts, injury, lack of care and attention, or weakness from disuse may occur.[17] A disturbance of body image may occur in persons who have sustained a head injury or who have experienced a cerebrovascular accident.

Disturbances of Space, Distance, and Movement Perception

Disturbances of space, distance, and movement perception are common deficits and involve difficulties recognizing and understanding the position of objects in relation to one another. The client who has these symptoms usually has a lesion in the nondominant hemisphere. The person also may have difficulty distinguishing right from left, up from down, and inside from outside and in identifying a vertical axis.[30] These symptoms may occur in persons who have sustained a head injury or who have experienced a cerebrovascular accident.

NURSING ASSESSMENT

Testing of sensation and perception is done to identify problem areas. The primary method used to assess sensory and perceptual impairment is observation. When the nurse determines that sensory or perceptual impairments are present, nursing diagnoses can be formulated.

Sensation

The senses of smell, taste, and touch are easily overlooked, and their importance is frequently misunderstood. Through a sensory assessment, the nurse can obtain valuable information about the client's needs and limitations. The nursing assessment should include attention to the sensations of smell, taste, touch, pain, temperature, and proprioception.

Smell

The rehabilitation nurse can discover important information about the client's use of the sense of smell. Some odors are readily discernible such as those from smoking, drinking, and eating highly seasoned food. Certain smells indicate a specific dysfunction such as acetone in diabetic acidosis, stale urine in uremic acidosis, and garlic in arsenic poisoning.

The nurse should be concerned with odors characteristic of infections or poor hygiene. Foul body odor or the use of heavy perfumes and deodorants to mask smells should alert the nurse to the need for teaching personal hygiene and self-care. Halitosis, or bad breath, may be the result of poor oral hygiene, which would necessitate dental health teaching and care. Gingival inflammation or stomatitis may be an underlying cause. Upon investigation, odors can be traced to secretions from body orifices and wounds. A nasal malodor may result from pharyngitis or another infection with a postnasal drip. An infected pressure ulcer hidden under old stained dressings will have odors associated with the growth of specific organisms.

The client may not be aware of odors given off by the body. Over a period of time, reaction to odor lessens, making way for new smells. In Western culture, many scents are obscured with the use of deodorants, powders, air fresheners, and perfumes. The sooner abnormal smells are recognized and diagnosed, the sooner appropriate treatment can be instituted.

An evaluation of the client's olfactory status is important, because it may indicate an underlying problem. Unfortunately, quantification of olfactory or gustatory impairments has been limited by the absence of precise types of measurement to diagnose these disorders. In addition, a standard vocabulary to assign meaning to most odors and tastes is lacking.[34] The nurse should note a lack of client response to odor-producing smells such as those of flowers and foods. If anosmia is suspected, the nurse should conduct a neurological assessment, including inspection of the nose. In assessing the client's sense of smell, the subjective report is not adequate. The client may not be aware of absent or impaired smell unless the loss has been sudden or dramatic. To test olfaction, nonirritating substances that have distinctive smells, such as soap, coffee, tobacco, and alcohol, are used. Ammonia or acetic acid odors are not used, because their pungency can stimulate nerve endings in the mucosa and give a false-positive result. The client may think that he or she is smelling the testing agent but he or she is actually tasting dissolving vapors of the substance. The nurse should test each nostril separately and ask the client to identify odors while the eyes are closed.

Nutritional status also must be assessed and monitored. Foods are not tasty if one cannot smell them. Follow-up health care supervision and support should be part of the intervention, especially if the cause of the anosmia is unknown.

Taste

Sweet, salty, sour, and bitter substances are used for testing taste. The client should be able to recognize these substances on the parts of the tongue used for these tastes if function is normal. Taste is usually not a routine part of a physical examination, and unless a client complains of a related disturbance, it is often not tested. Taste will sometimes be tested during tests of the cranial nerves, because it involves the facial, glossopharyngeal, and vagus nerves.

A person's culture determines, to an extent, the development of taste. The use and importance of food provide clues to one's life-style. Habits such as drinking coffee, using tobacco, drinking alcohol, and preparing food give insights into the social conduct and economic status of an individual. The nurse should observe for a decrease in the client's tasting ability, including any lack of response to foods that are known to produce strong tastes.

Touch

A wisp of cotton is used to test touch. Both sides of the body are tested and responses compared. The client must be given clear instructions and be able to understand to cooperate fully during the testing procedure, or results will be altered. The stimulus is applied distally and then proximally to various parts of the body. With eyes closed, the client is asked to acknowledge the presence and location of the stimulus.

Pain

Nursing assessment of pain may be difficult because pain is subjective. The attitudes of the client with pain and the nurse regarding the language of pain and the proper display and causation of pain are likely to be widely divergent, especially if their cultural experiences have been significantly different.

Another problem in pain assessment that poses a particular challenge is the common lack of recognition by client and nurse of the real differences between acute and chronic pain. Most laypersons and health care professionals base their expectations of the pain experience on the model of acute pain that is experienced immediately after an injury or surgery. Acute pain is viewed by both as severe discomfort of relatively short duration (hours, days, or a few weeks), usually attributed to an identifiable cause that can be effectively managed with potent analgesic medications. Chronic pain, on the other hand, is characterized by an ongoing experience of discomfort, quite often of neuromuscular etiology, that fails either to dissipate naturally or respond to common pain interventions.[20] Because of the extended duration of chronic pain, physiological indices found in acute pain are usually absent or blunted. In addition, the client experiencing chronic pain quickly learns that verbal and nonverbal techniques used to communicate acute pain soon become too exhausting or provoke negative responses from others. Thus the client with chronic pain may have affective signs of depression and hopelessness, which may affect every aspect of performing activities of daily living and social roles. The absence of pain cues featured in acute pain makes assessment of chronic pain problematic.

The starting point in any pain assessment is the client's verbal report. Attention to the onset, nature, duration, intensity, site of origin, radiation, relationship to other circumstances of daily living, control, and emotional responses is helpful in determining nursing interventions. There are three broad categories of pain sensations: pricking, burning, and aching. Pricking pain is associated with cuts, needle pricks, or rashes. Burning pain is found in certain neuromuscular disorders or in thermal injuries from sun, fire, chemicals, or hot water. Aching pain usually arises from the viscera or bones and joints.[2] The nurse should check for objective signs such as sweating, tachycardia, muscle tension, restlessness, crying, and clenched hands.

Several tools have been developed to assist the nurse and client in communicating clearly about the nature of the client's pain experience. One of the most commonly used pencil-and-paper tools for pain assessment is the McGill-Melzack Pain Questionnaire. This tool helps the client to describe pain location, sensation, temporal quality, and strength.[25] Self-report devices for describing pain intensity include pain rating scales consisting of a straight line drawn on a piece of paper with one end representing the greatest possible amount of pain and the other end representing the absence of pain. Clients are asked to draw a line intersecting the pain line at the level corresponding with the intensity of their pain.[2] This technique has the advantage of simplicity of administration and the potential for use in repeat measurements over a period of time to determine the efficacy of comfort interventions.

Despite the fact that the client's self-report of pain is the best indicator of pain experience, there are problems with relying solely on client verbalizations as a measure of pain experience. For a multitude of reasons, people may deliberately or unintentionally exaggerate or downgrade the amount of discomfort they are feeling.[17] Persons who derive substantial benefit from "owning" pain may distort the degree of discomfort they report. Persons from cultures that prize stoicism and endurance may be reluctant to openly share the hurt with which they are attempting to cope. Individuals with poorly developed verbal skills may lack the ability to convey accurately their discomfort. For these reasons, it is useful to incorporate observation of nonverbal behaviors and physiological indicators in any nursing assessment of pain. Nonverbal clues include grimacing, restlessness, withdrawal, teeth clenching, muscle tensing, repetitive movements, groans, crying, vomiting, and sleep disturbance. Physiological indicators of pain include increases in blood pressure, heart rate, and respiratory rate, as well as the physical evidence of weight loss and muscular atrophy.

In certain neurological disturbances, a client may experience altered perception of painful stimuli. Using a pin, the client is asked to distinguish the sharp and dull edges. The areas of sensation and diminished or absent sensation are identified with the use of a dermatome chart. The nurse can test an unconscious individual for response to pain by exerting pressure over the nail bed, supraorbital notch, or sternum or by pinching a skin fold above the elbow. The individual may indicate sensation by pushing the stimulus away or by flexing or extending the extremities. No response to pain indicates total lack of pain sensation. These responses give an indication of the extent of brain damage.

Temperature

Nursing assessment begins with subjective client reports and observation of clinical signs, including frequent temperature checks. The same nerve tracts carrying pain sensations also control temperature sensations, so specific temperature tests need not be done. Ability to perceive temperature changes is assessed by asking the client to close the eyes and identify temperature and position of warm and cold tubes of water held against the body.

Proprioception

Upon observation, the individual with impaired proprioception may appear to be intoxicated. Upper and lower extremities and the trunk may be involved. Testing for proprioception involves grasping the sides of the client's finger or toe and moving it up and down. The client is asked to close the eyes and state the direction of movement when this test is performed.

Perception

In assessing perception, observation of the client during activities of daily living gives the most useful information. Factors that influence the assessment include mental status, comprehension, verbal abilities, motor function, sensory function, vision, and attention span.[41] The client's disabilities, the medical diagnosis, experiences with other clients with the same diagnosis, and progression of the problem are other considerations. The response of the client's family will be influenced by cultural attitudes about the specific disability and previous coping styles and abilities. Family members may expect the client to be helpless and therefore may promote dependency.

Disorientation

The nurse should observe for sensory distortions, including confusion, disorientation, drowsiness, and hallucinations. Assessment should include observation for anxiety reactions, restlessness, headaches, insomnia, fatigue, irritability, and anger.

Agnosia

To determine the existence of agnosia, the nurse asks the client to use all the senses and evaluates the appropriateness of the responses in relation to normal. It may be necessary to repeat the requests to elicit certain responses. To assess visual agnosia, the nurse may ask the client to identify certain objects by sight alone. The nurse should test the client's hearing in both ears and if necessary, question the family to determine the client's previous hearing ability. In assessing tactile agnosia, the client is asked to identify objects by feeling them while the eyes are closed.

Apraxia

The nurse may find that the client cannot perform simple tasks when requested or performs them inappropriately. A client with this condition may be seen combing hair with a toothbrush or pouring milk in the ice cream. In addition, the client may be physically capable of performing a self-care activity but incapable of interpreting the movements to be formed to accomplish the activity. The nurse may observe spontaneous appropriate performance of the task at another time. When appropriate as well as inappropriate performance occurs, the task performed is usually a habit.

Disturbance of body image

Disturbed body image commonly takes the form of one-sided neglect in which the client completely ignores the affected side of the body. The nurse may notice the client's affected arm and leg dragging along the body or that only one side of the meal is eaten. The client also may dress and bathe only one side of the body or read only half of the page of a book.

Disturbance of space, distance, and movement

The nurse observes the client's movements and may find that these are clumsy and that the client is prone to injuries. The individual may bump into objects, collide with doorways when propelling a wheelchair, miss a step and fall down the stairs, or spill liquids as the table is missed.

NURSING DIAGNOSES

A number of nursing diagnoses are associated with alterations in communication because of sensory and perceptual problems. The nursing diagnoses appropriate for each diagnosis follow[12]:

1. *Sensory/perceptual alteration because of neurological damage, sensory underload, or sensory overload.* Damage to nerve tracts may lead to sensory perceptual alteration in visual, auditory, kinesthetic, olfactory, taste, tactile, or temperature sensation. Sensory underload can lead

to confusion, disorientation, and hallucinations. Sensory overload can lead to anxiety, restlessness, insomnia, and fatigue.

2. *Body image disturbance because of sensory/perceptual alteration.* One-sided neglect results in the client ignoring one side of the body.

3. *Impaired thought processes because of sensory perceptual alteration, or disorientation.* The client's perceptions may be inappropriate. With apraxia, the client may not remember what to do. The disoriented client may be unaware of surroundings.

4. *Self-care deficit in feeding, bathing/hygiene, toileting, or dressing/grooming because of sensory perceptual alterations or disturbance in body image.* Clients who have apraxia cannot conceptualize what they want to do. With proprioceptive disorders, the client is uncoordinated in performing activities of daily living. When there is a disturbance of body image such as in one-sided neglect, the client does not perform self-care on the affected side.

5. *Pain or abnormality of temperature sensation.* This diagnosis may occur when there is pain from acute or chronic conditions or abnormality of temperature sensation such as is present in hyperthermia, hypothermia, or inability to interpret temperature sensation.

6. *Altered nutrition: less than body requirements, because of anorexia or limited intake.* Anorexia may be a result of altered taste sensation or olfactory sensation. Limited intake may be caused by disorientation in which the client is unaware of nutritional needs or by pain such as is experienced in trigeminal neuralgia. Additionally, limited intake can occur when there is one-sided neglect in which the client is not aware of the food placed on the affected side of the mouth.

7. *Diversional activity deficit because of sensory underload or overload.* There may not be enough or there may be too much stimulation or activity.

8. *Potential for injury because of alteration of temperature, taste, auditory, olfactory, or tactile sensation; disorientation; confusion; disturbances of space, distance, and movement; and ataxia.* When taste is altered, the client may not recognize spoiled food. A consequence of auditory agnosia is that the client does not recognize warning sounds such as a smoke detector, horn, or police siren. When olfactory sensation is altered, the

client may not be warned of harmful smells such as smoke or gas leakage. The client with altered tactile sensation is prone to injury from bumping, burning or pressure. The client who is disoriented may wander into an unsafe environment. The confused client may be unaware of harmful substances, actions, or surroundings. The client with a disturbance of space, distance, and movement relationships is unsure of the relationship of self to the environment, resulting in falls. Alterations in touch and pressure sensation may result in the wearing of ill-fitting clothes or shoes, or the client may roll out of bed. With ataxia, incoordination may lead to falls.

9. *Ineffective individual coping because of sensory underload or sensory overload*. A client experiencing sensory underload can become confused, bored, and unable to deal with the environment. A client with sensory overload is subjected to multiple stimuli and cannot make proper judgments or decisions.

10. *Social isolation because of sensory underload or body image disturbance*. The client may have restricted stimuli and limited contact with others.

GOALS

Goals for the client, family, and nurse are to:
1. Reduce anxiety and promote rest.
2. Improve body image.
3. Maintain and restore orientation.
4. Achieve maximum self-care function.
5. Alleviate the pain.
6. Achieve and maintain good nutrition.
7. Obtain and provide sufficient environmental stimuli.
8. Promote safety in the environment.
9. Help the client and family cope with the disability.
10. Increase social contacts.

REHABILITATION NURSING INTERVENTIONS

The nursing interventions for impaired sensation and perception are many and varied. Often the nurse must experiment to find the intervention most appropriate for a particular client. Nursing interventions for impaired smell, taste, touch, pain, proprioception, and temperature sense are

discussed, as well as for selected alterations in perception such as disorientation; agnosia; apraxia; disturbance of body image; and disturbances in space, distance, and movement.

Sensation

Nursing interventions for the client with impaired sensation are planned when the client has an alteration in smell, taste, touch, pain, temperature, or proprioception.

Impaired smell

Nursing interventions for altered olfactory sensation include provisions for the detection of spoiled and extremely spicy foods. The client should be instructed to visually inspect food for spoilage and to read food labels for the expiration date. Foods should be discarded when the expiration date passes. Spices should be restricted. If possible, an electric stove should be used for cooking, since a gas leak may go unnoticed. The client should be cautioned to remain in the kitchen when food is cooking. Smoke detectors should be hung in the house. Follow-up health care supervision and support should be arranged if there are unresolved problems.

Impaired taste

The client's nutritional status is assessed and monitored. Plans are made to improve nutritional state and prevent nutritional problems. Nursing interventions include (1) teaching the client to use other senses to compensate for the loss of taste by preparing food in an attractive and appealing manner, (2) considering the client's likes, dislikes, customs, and special diet requirements, and (3) providing pleasant, neat surroundings free of disturbing sights and odors. Health teaching should include explanations of the importance of a balanced diet. The client should be encouraged to use spices, such as lemon juice, mint, cinnamon, and basil, to help improve the taste and aroma of food.

Impaired touch

Little can be done in the form of nursing intervention to alleviate abnormal sensations such as tingling, crawling, or burning feelings of the body. A massage with lotion is sometimes soothing and comforting. The client may be more comfortable with clothes and bed linen removed from the affected area. Diversional activities also may help. Nighttime is especially difficult when clients are experiencing abnormal sensations, and the use of analgesics and sedatives may be warranted to provide rest and relief.

A client with an altered sense of touch needs instruction regarding ways in which to substitute other senses to promote safety in activities of daily living. The individual should be taught to depend more on the sense of sight to observe skin integrity, as well as to change position frequently to prevent pressure ulcers and to wear loose clothing and shoes to prevent undue pressure on the body surface.

Pain

Kim[18] has suggested that all pain-relieving nursing interventions fall into one of the following seven categories:

1. The nurse's support and reassurance
2. Discussion with the client about the nature and strength of the discomfort
3. Reduction of client apprehension and family concern
4. Distraction and suggestion
5. Physical relaxation and comfort
6. Reduction of stimulus
7. Following physician's orders for administration of analgesics and placebos

All but the last of these intervention categories belong within the unique province of nursing practice. The nurse must be open to the client's verbal and nonverbal pain communication and accept the client's definition of pain as the one most relevant to treatment. Every nurse should examine personal beliefs about pain and its "appropriate" expression. Knowledge of one's own social and cultural biases in regard to pain may help the nurse to refrain from inadvertently stereotyping the client or applying personal tenets of pain to the client's unique pain experience. Real support and empathy can then be given to the suffering client. The nurse's attitude toward pain-relieving interventions may strongly influence their efficacy. Kim states that "the effectiveness of positive statements about pain relief is dependent in part on the quality of the nurse-patient relations."[18] In view of the impact past experiences with pain have on the client's perception of and reaction to current discomfort, the nurse's support and reassurance also may help significantly in reducing anticipatory fear or anxiety that can exacerbate the client's discomfort.

Nursing research regarding the effect of enhancing the client's cognitive control over pain suggests that distress can be decreased by providing clients with a description of painful sensations they might experience.[19] Such descriptions of potential sensations of discomfort should be routine nursing practice in the preparation of clients for procedures such as wound debridement, therapeutic bathing for burns, colonoscopy, endoscopy, bronchoscopy, suctioning, enemas, cancer chemotherapy, rectal and pelvic examinations, and surgery of most types in which pain is anticipated.

An important way in which the nurse can facilitate pain relief is through the identification and promotion of the client's own previously successful methods of coping with discomfort. Most people consciously or unconsciously use some form of motor behavior or cognitive control to cope with pain. Clearly, nurses working with clients in pain need to focus attention on encouraging the expression and use of clients' tried-and-true pain reduction strategies.

A number of specific nursing techniques are often helpful in providing relief from pain symptoms. A change in position, straightening the linen, fluffing pillows, administering back rubs and massages, giving warm baths, touching, talking, maintaining a quiet, calm environment, and massages are some approaches that can be tried. Clients should be taught to avoid specific aggravating factors. For example, in trigeminal neuralgia, foods of extreme temperatures may precipitate an attack. To avoid this, the client must be taught to check the temperature of food, chew food on the unaffected side of the mouth, and choose semisolid or liquid foods. Efforts to decrease noise and unwelcome intrusions may be beneficial, especially in discomfort related to muscle tension or stress.

The administration of prescribed analgesics may be necessary to alleviate pain. The nurse is often the health care provider who ultimately decides on the quantity and timing of pain medication. Many nurses have an inordinate fear of creating addiction through what they regard as "overadministration" of analgesic drugs to the client in pain. McCaffery[23] reported that in studies of hospitalized clients who received potent narcotic analgesics for 10 days, less than 1% became addicted. Furthermore, taking narcotics for even longer periods (weeks or months) did not appreciably raise the risk of addiction in the sample studied.[23] Such clients may develop drug tolerance (increasingly higher doses needed for pain relief) or physical dependence (appearance of withdrawal symptoms when the drug is stopped). It is important to note, however, that addiction is not synonymous with tolerance or dependence. Addiction results when the client has an "overwhelming involvement with obtaining and using a drug for its psychic effects rather than for its medically approved reasons."[23] Administration of analgesic medication before activities anticipated to cause pain should continue to be standard nursing practice.

Because of the diurnal pattern of pain, all pain relief measures should be more intense at night. In addition, there is less distraction at night to remove thoughts of pain. The nurse should also be aware that hypnotics do not relieve pain and that there is potentiation between hypnotics and analgesics that can lead to accidental overdoses.[9]

The following guidelines may be useful in teaching individuals and their families to successfully cope with pain:

1. Administer pain medication in the early stages of discomfort. Unrelieved discomfort often develops into frank pain because it causes anxiety and muscle tension, which further increase distressing sensations. Many times, smaller amounts of analgesic medication are needed if pain is to be dealt with effectively as it begins.
2. Constipation is an annoying side effect of many pain-relieving medications. Increased intake of fresh fruits and vegetables and other high-fiber foods may help maintain normal bowel habits while the client is taking these drugs.
3. Distraction may be useful in minimizing attention to uncomfortable sensations. Conversation, television, music, reading, prayer, and handcrafts may be helpful. Conversely, discomfort from muscle tension may respond best to a quiet, calm atmosphere.
4. Maintenance of physical activity to the degree allowed by the pain is desirable. Immobility leads to joint stiffness and muscle weakness, which can make disability more pronounced.

Impaired temperature

Nursing interventions are directed toward promoting safety. The client should be taught ways to prevent burns and frostbite. Any extremes in temperature should be avoided. Using a bath thermometer helps the client determine the safe temperature for bathing. Precautions also should be taken when using an iron or heating pad. Pot holders should be used when moving hot foods. In cold weather, the client should wear very warm clothing and should be encouraged to wear a hat, since the head is an area of great heat loss. (See Chapter 8 for further discussion of body temperature regulation.)

Impaired proprioception

The client with alterations in proprioceptive sense may experience difficulties in performing activities of daily living and is prone to falls. The nurse should adapt interventions to meet individual needs and modify the environment as necessary. Plates equipped with a side guard, suction cups, and drinking cups with spouts may alleviate frustration and spillage while eating. The client can be encouraged to use a typewriter to make correspondence more legible. A four-point cane or walker promotes stability when walking. The physical therapist, occupational therapist, and nurse often will work together closely in assessing, planning, implementing, and evaluating interventions with the client.

Perception

Nursing interventions for impaired perception are individualized according to the client's perceptual problems. These problems may include disorientation, agnosia, apraxia, disturbance in body image, and disturbances in space, distance, and movement. Mutual understanding of problems and participation of the family in planning approaches are important in dealing with perceptual problems. Through informal teaching and planned conferences, the family's understanding of these problems expands and better relationships evolve.

Disorientation

The families of clients experiencing disorientation are disturbed and frightened by mental changes and inappropriate, unacceptable behaviors. These clients need support and reinforcement for reality-based behaviors. Reality orientation can be helpful. Calendars and clocks in the room help the client with orientation to date and time. Holidays and dates of special happenings can be highlighted. Pictures of family and friends in the room help provide familiar perceptual supports. By discussing current events, the nurse can promote orientation. If hearing aids or glasses are necessary, these should be placed where they can be reached. The client's environment should be maintained in a consistent and structured fashion.

Nursing interventions for the confused individual are designed to help the client comprehend. The nurse should face the client and speak in slow, short sentences while using gestures. Restricting noise and allowing adequate time for response also are helpful interventions. Repeating and rephrasing words may be necessary.

Providing assistance as necessary with activities of daily living is very important. The confused client may be unable to assume responsibility for self-care and may require help with personal hygiene, eating, and elimination. The mobile client may become lost or wander into a restricted or dangerous area. The nurse should be sure the client is wearing an identification band with home location marked. If the client must remain in bed, restraining jackets may prevent falls but should be used only when necessary and ordered for protection. Movement should be as unrestricted as possible to prevent secondary complications such as pneumonia and pressure sores.

The client who is experiencing sensory underload should be provided with adequate stimuli. Meaningful, frequent visits and conversation introduce added stimuli. Volunteer groups also may provide this kind of service. The client should be encouraged to use a hearing aid or glasses if these are needed. A radio, television, or cassette player offers sensory stimulation. The room should be well illuminated and a night-light turned on when dark.

Clients must receive sufficient sensory input during the rehabilitation process if they are to respond to rehabilitation therapies. Clients and their families should be encouraged to bring in personal belongings, newspapers, and pictures of loved ones. Wearing their own clothing, frequent human contact, and liberal visitation hours all help clients to maintain enough stimulation for optimum perceptual response.

Unless action is taken to resolve a problem of sensory overload, rehabilitation attempts will be futile. Nurses play an important role in reducing sensory overload. The nurse coordinates appointments and therapies to allow for adequate rest periods and to prevent excessive fatigue. Using eye contact while speaking to a client can lessen the impact of overstimulation. In addition, privacy should be provided by keeping the client's door closed and restricting unwanted visitors.

Agnosia

To compensate for agnosia and to aid in identification of environmental stimuli, the client must be taught to use all of the senses. The environment should be simplified to eliminate hazards such as unnecessary furniture and objects. The client with visual agnosia should be encouraged to use touch to identify objects and to rely on voices and familiar mannerisms of staff, family, and friends for identification. Only one food at a time should be given, and the client should be told what is being eaten. The client should be encouraged to touch extremities and attend to the position of the affected limbs. The client with auditory agnosia may be able to respond appropriately to written words or to lip-reading cues. Equipment should be explained and client needs anticipated. The client with tactile agnosia should be approached gently to assess response to touch, temperature of water, or any other stimuli that may inflict pain. When response to pain or temperature is impaired, precautions must be taken to avoid burns, frostbite, bruising, and pressure to insensitive areas.[30]

Apraxia

The most important nursing intervention for the client with apraxia is to recognize that this condition exists and not to confuse it with lack of cooperation, belligerence, paralysis, or aphasia.[31] Nursing interventions for the client with apraxia include measures aimed at minimizing distractions and using very simple, repetitive instructions. An organized, uncluttered environment should be maintained and simple instructions given for performing self-care tasks. Daily routines and instructions from different staff members should be consistent. The client should be reminded to slow down self-care activities when necessary and should be guided through these tasks with slow, clear directions. Touch should be relied upon more than vision when arranging objects.

If a client has a dressing apraxia, it is sometimes helpful to sew colored labels or other kinds of visual clues on the neck or sleeve of a garment.[30] Persons who have difficulty in performing voluntary movements on request may have preservation of axial movements. Although unable to respond to such requests as "Brush your hair" or "Eat your food," the client may be able to respond to "Walk" or "Bend over."[31] Eventually, when and if apraxia improves, assistance should be withdrawn.

Disturbance of body image

Clients who have alterations in body image need encouragement in recognizing and attending to neglected body parts. They should be reminded to touch and look at the body part along with reminders to bathe, shave, put on makeup, or dress this area. The nurse can provide sensory stimulation during activities of daily living such as performance of personal hygiene and grooming. Washcloths, rough pieces of cloth, sheepskin, soap, and metal safety pins can be used. The potential for injury also is a major concern, and clients must be encouraged to remember to protect affected parts. Frequent monitoring for injuries and proper positioning are important nursing interventions.

Disturbances in space, distance, and movement

Nursing interventions are directed toward providing a safe environment for the client. The room should be kept simple, uncluttered, and well lighted. Unnecessary furniture, decorations, or equipment should be removed so that the client can feel walls and doorways. Items used regularly by the client should be visible, since the client may not remember where these are located. To deal with depth perception difficulties, the client should be taught to reach for objects slowly and cautiously and to handle at the base to avoid tipping.[8] Because of difficulties in perception in space, the client should not be sent anywhere alone on a new route. Within the client's own territory, there should be familiar landmarks to help determine direction.[30]

REHABILITATION TEAM INTERVENTIONS

Through the expertise of the members of the rehabilitation team, the client may benefit greatly in the management of sensory and perceptual impairments. The primary goal of the entire rehabilitation team is to help the client achieve an optimum level of function.

The physician is responsible for the overall medical care of the client. By performing a thorough neurological examination, the physician makes the diagnosis and prescribes the therapeutic regimen. The physician monitors the client's progress and determines the prognosis, as well as prescribes appropriate analgesics and muscle relaxants.

The physical therapist is able to evaluate sensory level and proprioception and develops a plan for maintaining and restoring these areas of function. Methods used include heat or traction when appropriate to relieve painful joints or spasticity and instruction and assistance in the performance of therapeutic exercises to improve coordination. Physical therapists have pioneered the use of transcutaneous electrical nerve stimulation (TENS) for the relief of certain kinds of intractable pain. The TENS device consists of electrodes, usually applied over the site of pain sensations, and a power source for transmitting electrical current at adjustable voltage and pulse widths. It is believed that TENS therapy works by stimulating large-diameter afferent nerve fibers that "close the gate" to pain transmission from the smaller A-delta and C fibers. TENS appears to be most efficacious in acute postoperative or posttraumatic pain, phantom limb pain, peripheral neuralgias, and low back pain.[22]

The occupational therapist, skilled in helping the client with activities of daily living, evaluates sensation and perception, teaches safety precautions, makes and applies splints to support the arm and hand in functional positions, and designs and implements therapies to help the client overcome or compensate for sensory and perceptual alterations. The occupational therapist may provide hot or cold pack treatments to decrease pain in affected joints. Paraffin baths are often useful for the client with arthritis. The occupational therapist also may provide the client with self-help devices to make movement easier. These devices include button hooks, reachers, specially adapted eating utensils, and other tools that make possible continued independence in the face of persistent pain.

The psychologist may determine emotional and motivational factors involved in a client's sensory and perceptual impairments. Psychotherapy may be particularly useful in chronic pain where the disabling effects of discomfort cause severe distress to the client and family. The psychologist also may teach the client sophisticated relaxation techniques or use biofeedback to help the client attain control over autonomic responses contributing to discomfort.

The dietitian can be helpful when the client has altered smell or taste by giving nutritional counseling, which may include instruction about specific nutritional requirements, the importance of good nutrition to general well-being, and the purchase and preparation of appropriate foods.

The social worker helps the client cope with social changes and social roles by counseling the family in dealing with the disability, investigating financial resources and opportunities with the client, helping the client and family make plans for long-term care, and exploring other possibilities for residence when home care is not feasible.

The chaplain may assist clients who suffer from chronic, unremitting pain. Many of these clients have had a succession of disappointments in their search for relief using the traditional approaches offered by health care providers. The problem is exacerbated when no clear-cut physical cause for the pain can be found. In this situation, the client's religious convictions may help to attribute a meaning and purpose to pain, as in the Christian view of suffering as a way of testing, strengthening, and purifying the sufferer.[20] The chaplain may help the client to cope successfully with continued pain and to marshal the emotional energy necessary to continue to search for pain relief.

Rehabilitation is a team effort. Team members working together toward common goals can assist the client in reaching maximum potential in coping with sensory and perceptual impairments.

OUTCOME CRITERIA

Outcome criteria for the person with sensory and perceptual impairments include the following:
1. The client and family obtain adequate rest.
2. The client compensates for disturbed body image.
3. The client is oriented to self, time, place, and person.
4. The client and family function at their optimum level.
5. The client and family demonstrate comfort measures and knowledge about pain relief.
6. The client maintains good nutrition.
7. The client and family provide sufficient environmental stimuli and use appropriate diversional activities.
8. The client and family exercise safety precautions and avoid injury.
9. The client and family use effective coping mechanisms to reduce stress.
10. The client and family experience acceptable levels of social interaction.

SUMMARY

An understanding of sensory and perceptual impairments that affect communication and the rehabilitation plan is necessary to deliver knowledgeable rehabilitation nursing intervention. The client, family, nurse and nursing staff members, and other rehabilitation team members work together to promote understanding of the client in personal efforts to deal with these frustrating problems.

TEST QUESTIONS

1. In establishing relationships with clients, the rehabilitation nurse knows:
   a. Hearing and vision are the primary senses used in communication.
   b. Emotions and personalities have little impact on transmission of messages.
   c. Inadequate knowledge is rarely a factor hindering the communication process.
   d. Perceptual differences of an event may result in miscommunication.
2. In distinguishing between internal and external stimuli that influence communication, external stimuli are classified as those that:
   a. Can be seen, heard, smelled, tasted, or touched
   b. Arise from within the body and include visceral sensations
   c. Are concerned with sensation of position and balance
   d. Are consistent with need states of the body
3. All of the following statements regarding the role of sensation in the communication process are true *except:*
   a. Taste buds are sensitive to sweet, sour, salty, and bitter substances.
   b. The sense of smell is the most relied upon of all the senses.

c. A nurse's touch during conversation portrays feelings.

d. Proprioception concerns position and movement of body parts.

4. In communicating with clients, the nurse is aware that perception is:
   a. Unimportant in forming impressions and beliefs
   b. Controlled by the temporal lobe of the brain
   c. Interpretation of senses in the sensory cortex
   d. Unaffected by age, education, culture, or attitudes

5. Of the following statements, which one is *true* regarding an impairment of sensation?
   a. Hyposmia refers to a distorted or perverted sense of smell.
   b. Paresthesia is the loss of touch sensation.
   c. Anosmia refers to the complete loss of taste.
   d. Pain warns the individual of a body malfunction.

6. Which of the following definitions is *true* regarding an impairment of perception?
   a. Apraxia is the inability to recognize objects using one of the senses.
   b. Agnosia is the inability to perform a learned action voluntarily.
   c. Tactile agnosia is the inability to identify objects completely as a whole.
   d. Auditory agnosia is the inability to recognize sounds that are heard.

7. In conducting a nursing assessment specific to sensation, the nurse knows:
   a. Ammonia is used to test olfaction, since its pungency can produce an immediate positive result.
   b. A pinprick is used to test touch on both sides of the body.
   c. No response to pain indicates a total lack of pain sensation.
   d. Temperature is assessed by placing tubes of scalding water or ice water against the body.

8. In assessing the client for perceptual impairments, the nurse is aware the following statement is *true:*
   a. Observation of the client during activities of daily living will give the most useful information.

b. Tactile agnosia is assessed by asking the client to identify certain objects by sight alone.
   c. Fixating on the affected side of the body indicates a disturbance in the client's body image.
   d. Apraxia is assessed by asking the client to perform several complex tasks.

9. Which of the following statements about chronic pain is *true?*
   a. Chronic pain is best managed by use of narcotic and sedative medications.
   b. Chronic pain can always be traced to a definite traumatic etiology.
   c. Physiological indices for acute pain are absent or decreased in chronic pain.
   d. All clients with chronic pain have a preexisting personality problem.

10. A realistic goal for the client with sensory and/or perceptual problems is to:
    a. Reduce social contacts until perception is restored.
    b. Increase the anxiety level to promote decision-making ability.
    c. Promote safety in the environment.
    d. Decrease environmental stimuli to improve body image.

11. A rehabilitation nursing intervention for the client with impaired sensation is to:
    a. Provide nighttime analgesics and sedatives for those experiencing pain.
    b. Teach the client to chew on the affected side in the presence of trigeminal neuralgia.
    c. Suggest use of a gas stove if there is altered olfaction.
    d. Advise use of heating pads to prevent heat loss for those with temperature alteration.

12. In caring for the client with impaired perception, the nurse performs all of the following interventions *except* to:
    a. Teach the client with agnosia to use all of the senses to identify environmental stimuli.
    b. Close the door and restrict unwanted visitors for the client experiencing sensory overload.
    c. Minimize distractions and use simple repetitive instructions for clients with apraxia.
    d. Change the disoriented client's environment frequently to promote orientation and reality.

13. Which of the following statements explains the way in which TENS works to relieve pain?
    a. It promotes progressive relaxation of specific muscle groups.
    b. It stimulates release of neurotransmitters to block pain transmission.
    c. It causes the thalamus to release endogenous opiates.
    d. It "closes the gate" to pain transmission by stimulating large A-delta nerve fibers.
14. Of the following statements, which one is *true* regarding the function of a rehabilitation team member?
    a. The occupational therapist applies heat or traction to the client experiencing pain.
    b. The dietitian counsels the client on the importance of good nutrition for general well-being.
    c. The social worker develops plans for maintaining and restoring sensory and proprioceptive function.
    d. The nurse performs a thorough neurological examination and prescribes a therapy regimen.
15. An outcome criterion for the client with sensory and/or perceptual impairments is to:
    a. Deny an alteration in body image.
    b. Experience low levels of social interaction.
    c. Demonstrate knowledge about pain level.
    d. Reject the need for diversional activities.

Answers: 1. d, 2. a, 3. b, 4. c, 5. d, 6. d, 7. c, 8. a, 9. c, 10. c, 11. a, 12. d, 13. d, 14. b, 15. c.

LEARNING ACTIVITIES

1. During one day, pay particular attention to your own senses of smell, taste, touch, pain, temperature, and proprioception. Record everything you would have missed if these senses could not be experienced.
2. When meeting a new person, notice the sensory stimuli that contribute to your impressions of that person.
3. Look closely at a person you know very well. Distinguish between your impressions and the initial impressions that you believe that person would make to a stranger.
4. Cover one eye with a patch, and using a mirror, comb your hair. What perceptual alterations do you experience?

REFERENCES

1. Abbasi AA: Diabetes: diagnostic and therapeutic significance of taste impairment, Geriatrics 36:73, 1981.
2. Alyn IB: Pain as a result of physical impairment. In Martin N, Holt N, and Hicks D, editors: Comprehensive rehabilitation nursing, New York 1981, McGraw-Hill Book Co.
3. Bickerton J and Small J: Neurology for nurses, Baltimore, 1982, University Park Press.
4. Bishop B: Pain: its physiology and rationale for management. I. Phys Ther 60:13, Jan 1980.
5. Ceccio J and Ceccio C: Effective communication in nursing: theory and practice, New York, 1983, John Wiley & Sons, Inc.
6. Chusid JG: Correlative neuroanatomy and functional neurology, ed 19, Los Altos, Calif, 1985, Lange Medical Publications.
7. Collins M: Communication in health care, ed 2, St Louis, 1983, The CV Mosby Co.
8. DeYoung S: The neurologic patient: a nursing perspective, Englewood Cliffs, NJ, 1983, Prentice-Hall, Inc.
9. Dolphin NW: Neuroanatomy and neurophysiology of pain: nursing implications, Int J Nurs Stud 20(4):255, 1983.
10. Estrem SC and Renner G: Disorders of smell and taste, Otolaryngol Clin North Am 20:133, Feb 1987.
11. Gardner E: Fundamentals of neurology, Philadelphia, 1975, WB Saunders Co.
12. Gordon M: Nursing diagnosis: process and application, New York, 1987, McGraw-Hill Book Co.
13. Goto N and others: Primary pontine hemorrhage and gustatory disturbance: clinicoanatomic study, Stroke 14:507, 1983.
14. Guyton A: Structure and function of the nervous system, Philadelphia, 1972, WB Saunders Co.
15. Henkin RI: Olfaction in human disease. In English GM, editor: Otolaryngology, vol 2, Philadelphia, 1985, JB Lippincott Co.
16. Henkin RI and others: Studies on taste threshold in normal man and patients with adrenal cortical insufficiency, J Clin Invest 42:727, 1963.
17. Jacox AK: Assessing pain, Am J Nurs 79:895, May 1979.
18. Kim S: Pain: theory, research and nursing practice, Adv Nurs Sci 2:43, Jan 1980.
19. Kim S: Preparatory information, anxiety, and pain: a contingency model and nursing implications. Doctoral dissertation, 1978, Boston University.
20. Kotarba JA: Perceptions of death, belief systems and the process of coping with pain, Soc Sci Med 17(10):681, 1983.
21. Lizak MD: Neuropsychological assessment, New York, 1976, Oxford University Press.
22. Lloyd JW: Pain perception and the control of intractable pain, Practitioner 227:413, 1983.

23. McCaffery M: Patients shouldn't have to suffer: how to relieve pain with injectable narcotics, Nurs 80 10:34, Oct 1980.

24. McCaffery M: Nursing management of the patient with pain, ed 2, New York, 1979, JB Lippincott Co.

25. Meinhart NT and McCaffery NT: Pain: a nursing approach to assessment and analysis, Norwalk, Conn, 1983, Appleton-Century-Crofts.

26. Melzack R and Torgerson WS: On the language of pain, Anesthesiology 34:50, Jan 1971.

27. Melzack R and Wall PD: Pain mechanisms: a new theory, Science 150:971, 1965.

28. Nielson JM: Agnosia, apraxia, aphasia, New York, 1965, Hafner Press.

29. Nolte J: The human brain: an introduction to its functional anatomy, St Louis, 1981, The CV Mosby Co.

30. O'Brien M and Pallett P: Total care of the stroke patient, Boston, 1978, Little, Brown & Co.

31. Ozuna J: Alterations in mentation: nursing assessment and intervention, J Neurosurg Nurs 17:66, Feb 1985.

32. Phipps W, Long B, and Woods N, editors: Medical-surgical nursing: concepts and clinical practice, ed 3, St Louis, 1987, The CV Mosby Co.

33. Rambo B: Adaptation nursing, Philadelphia, 1984, WB Saunders Co.

34. Schiffman SS: Diagnosis and treatment of smell and taste disorders (editorial), West J Med 146(4):471, 1987.

35. Sharpless JW: Mossman's a problem-oriented approach to stroke rehabilitation, ed 2, Springfield, Ill, 1982, Charles C Thomas, Publisher.

36. Siev E and Frieshtat B: Perceptual dysfunction in the adult stroke patient, Thorofare, NJ, 1976, Charles B Slack, Inc.

37. Sparks RK: Sensory-perceptual impairments due to anosmia. In Snyder M, editor: A guide to neurological and neurosurgical nursing, New York, 1983, John Wiley & Sons, Inc.

38. Sumner D: Post-traumatic anosmia, Brain 87:107, 1964.

39. Westerman ST and Gilbert LM: Mastication, deglutition and taste. In English GM, editor: Otolaryngology, vol 3, Philadelphia, 1985, Harper & Row, Publishers, Inc.

40. Wilson RW and Elmassian BJ: Endorphins, Am J Nurs 81:722, 1981.

41. Wyness MA: Perceptual dysfunction: nursing assessment and management, J Neurosci Nurs 17:106, April 1985.

ADDITIONAL READINGS

Bradley J and Edinberg M: Communication in the nursing context, Norwalk, Conn, 1982, Appleton-Century-Crofts.

Brown IA: The widespread influence of olfaction, J Neurosci Nurs 17:273, Oct 1985.

Burt M: Perceptual defects in hemiplegia, Am J Nurs 70:1026, 1970.

Cherry C: On human communication, Cambridge, Mass, 1977, The MIT Press.

Edwards B and Brilhart J: Communication in nursing practice, St Louis, 1981, The CV Mosby Co.

Hein E: Communication in nursing practice, Boston, 1980, Little, Brown & Co.

Hirschberg G, Lewis L, and Vaughan P: Rehabilitation, ed 2, New York, 1976, JB Lippincott Co.

Kozier B and Erb G: Fundamentals of nursing: concepts and procedures, Menlo Park, Calif, 1983, Addison-Wesley Publishing Co.

Seiden M: Practical management of chronic neurologic problems, New York, 1981, Appleton-Century-Crofts.

Taylor J and Ballenger S: Neurological dysfunctions and nursing intervention, New York, 1981, McGraw-Hill Book Co.

Wallhagen M: The split brain: implications for care and rehabilitation, Am J Nurs 79:2118, 1979.

CHAPTER 17

Communication: Vision and Hearing

Linda M. Janelli

OBJECTIVES

After completing Chapter 17, the reader will be able to:

1. Identify the three layers of the eye and their primary functions.
2. Distinguish the treatment modalities used in glaucoma, cataracts, diabetic retinopathy, and retinal detachment.
3. Identify ways in which multiple sclerosis and hemianopsias can affect visual function.
4. Assess a client's visual status by obtaining both subjective and objective data.
5. Formulate nursing diagnoses associated with visual impairment.
6. Develop goals with the client and family that foster maximum visual function.
7. Determine rehabilitation nursing interventions that can be used with a client experiencing a visual dysfunction.
8. Describe at least three specific rehabilitation nursing interventions that can enhance the communication and mobility of a newly blind person.
9. Identify rehabilitation team members who assist the client in achieving maximum visual function.
10. List outcome criteria used to evaluate the effectiveness of planned interventions to assist the client in achieving maximum visual function.
11. Identify the component parts of the external, middle, and inner ear and their primary functions.
12. Describe the order of events for the transmission of sound waves.
13. Discuss the etiology of the four major types of hearing loss.
14. Assess a client's hearing status by obtaining both subjective and objective data.
15. Formulate nursing diagnoses associated with hearing impairment.
16. Develop goals with the client and family that foster maximum hearing function
17. Describe rehabilitation nursing interventions that can be used to enhance communication with hearing impaired persons.
18. Identify rehabilitation team members who work with the client with a hearing impairment.
19. List outcome criteria used to evaluate the effectiveness of planned intervention to assist the client in achieving maximum hearing function.

No matter where one is along the life span, communication is essential for social interactions and for developing feelings of competency in dealing with the environment. Communication involves the transmittal of information through writing, reading, listening, and speaking. Communication occurs between individuals, between groups, and through the media via television, radio, books, magazines, and newspapers. Barriers to receiving and sending messages can result when there are alterations in seeing or hearing.

NORMAL VISUAL FUNCTION

Throughout history, the eye has been associated with both evil and good—a human glance was thought to inflict harm as well as to heal. The physician whose treatment caused the loss of a person's eye could expect severe punishment in return, or so it was documented in 2100 BC in the code of Hammurabi.[12]

Through the eyes, one comes to learn about and appreciate the surrounding environment. Aesthetically, our vision allows us to feel pleasure when viewing a symphony of colors, for example, a sunset or the changing colors of the fall leaves. Vision affords us the opportunity to learn about our environment through books, magazines, newspapers, and television. It also serves as a protective mechanism by which we are warned of environmental hazards, whether a flashing red light at a railroad crossing or a bottle labeled "Dangerous if Ingested."

Layers of the Eye

The eyeball is composed of three layers. The protective *outer layer* consists of the *sclera*, or white part of the eye, and the *cornea*, a transparent structure covering the iris and pupil. The *limbus* is the juncture where the sclera and cornea come together. The sclera contains dense bands of parallel, interlacing tissue bundles arranged in a nonuniform pattern. The cornea, often called the window of the eye, allows light to enter the eye in its route to the retina. The cornea's clarity is the result of its relatively dehydrated state and the uniform arrangement of the collagen fibers.[15]

The cornea serves three protective functions: (1) it acts as a physical barrier, (2) it causes tearing and blinking when foreign bodies come into contact with it, and (3) it selectively resists microorganisms and chemicals by virtue of its five different layers. The latter function can affect the penetration and absorption of optical medications.[3]

The *middle layer*, or uvea, is composed of the choroid, ciliary body, and iris. The *choroid* contains a rich supply of blood vessels, thus providing nutrition to the outer half of the retina. Anatomically, the choroid lies between the sclera and retina (Figure 17-1). Pressure from the vitreous body holds the choroid in place. The *ciliary body* is part of a smooth muscle structure called the ciliary muscle and is responsible for altering the shape of the lens when the eyes focus. Contraction of the ciliary muscle causes the *zonule* (tissue strands attached to the lens) to relax. As a result, the lens takes on a more spherical shape and optical power increases. When the ciliary muscle relaxes, the zonule becomes taut and the optical power decreases.

The *iris*, the colored portion of the eye, surrounds the pupil. It adjusts the pupil size so it can accommodate to brightness and darkness. The pupil dilates in the dark and constricts when there is bright light. There are two muscles in the iris that allow it to change the diameter of the pupil: (1) the iris sphincter, which encircles the pupil and creates constriction when it contracts, and (2) the iris dilator, which extends from the pupil to the iris periphery and creates dilation when it contracts.

The *retina, the innermost layer of the eyeball*, resembles a pink net and is barely the thickness of onionskin paper. Nutrients and oxygen are delivered to the retina by the choriocapillaris and the central retinal artery. Interference with this blood supply can lead to damage or death of the retina.

The retina is predominantly a neuronal layer. It contains two types of visual cells, referred to as *rods* and *cones*. Rods and cones are the photoreceptors of the eye and communicate the light stimulation they receive to the optic nerve fibers. The cones are used to recognize colors and are responsible for fine discrimination and daylight vision, while the rods respond to dim light and are responsible for peripheral vision. The number of cones has been estimated to be 7,000,000, with rods numbering 10 to 20 times as many.[1]

The *macula lutea*, located in the center of the

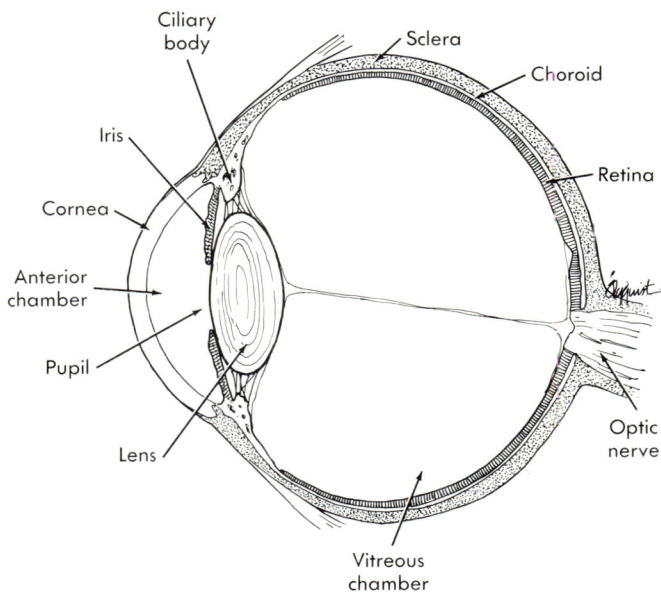

Figure 17-1
Cross section of human eye.

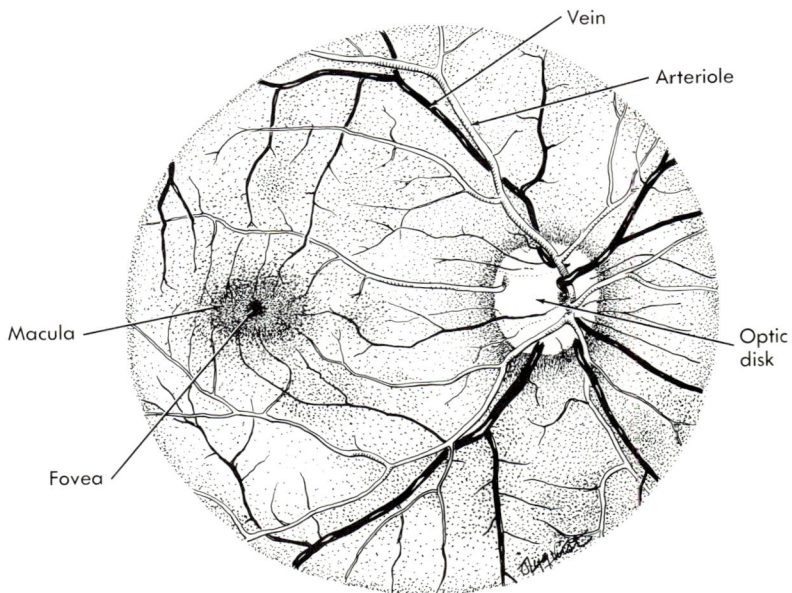

Figure 17-2
Fundus of eye showing optic disk, fovea macula, and blood vessels.

TABLE 17-1

Layers of the eye

Layer	Component parts	Characteristics
Outer layer	Sclera, cornea	Serves protective function; acts as physical barrier; selectively resists microorganisms
Middle layer (uvea)	Choroid, ciliary body, iris	Provides nutrition; contains rich blood supply
Innermost layer	Retina, rods, cones	Contains neuronal tissue; communicates light stimulation to optic nerve

retina, has a yellowish hue when viewed through an ophthalmoscope because fewer blood vessels feed into this area (Figure 17-2). The *fovea centralis* is a small depression in the macula and is the thinnest portion of the retina. Damage to the fovea can result in permanent loss of central vision.[3,17] Table 17-1 summarizes the layers of the eye.

Supporting and Accessory Structures

The supporting and accessory structures of the eye include the eyelids, conjunctiva, lens, anterior and posterior eye cavities, and the lacrimal apparatus. The *eyelids* and *eyelashes* protect the eyeball against intrusion of foreign objects. The skin of the eyelid is the thinnest in the body. The lids are loose and elastic, a quality that allows for some swelling to take place without damage occurring. The upper and lower eyelids join at the *canthus*. The *conjunctiva*, a mucous membrane, lines each lid and also covers the surface of the eyeball. This transparent structure contributes mucus to the tear film.[12]

The *lens*, a semitransparent structure located behind the iris, is primarily composed of water. No pain fibers, nerve endings, or blood vessels are contained in the lens. The focusing process of accommodation is a result of the action of the ciliary muscle and the zonule. The lens brings light rays to a focus on the retina. According to Helmholtz's theory, the ciliary body and choroid are pulled forward toward the lens when the ciliary body contracts. Consequently, the lenses bulge for near vision and remain comparatively flat for far vision.[1,3]

The *anterior cavity*, which is divided into an anterior and a posterior chamber, lies in front of the lens and contains a clear, watery substance called *aqueous humor*. Aqueous humor serves to maintain pressure inside the eye and bathes and nourishes the iris and the posterior aspect of the cornea. It flows through the anterior chamber, is filtered through the *trabeculum*, which acts as a sieve, and then passes into the canal of Schlemm. From there, it passes directly into the bloodstream. *Vitreous humor*, a soft gelatinous material, is contained within the posterior cavity, where it helps to maintain pressure in the eyeball to prevent collapse.[17]

The *lacrimal apparatus* is composed of the lacrimal glands, lacrimal canals, lacrimal sacs, and nasolacrimal ducts. The *lacrimal glands* are responsible for tears of emotion, as well as responding to irritants such as dust and odors. These glands are shaped like almonds and are located in the frontal bone of the upper outer margin of each orbit. The *lacrimal canals* empty into the *lacrimal sacs* located in a groove of the lacrimal bone. Tears then drain into the nasal cavity through the *nasolacrimal ducts*. For this reason, a runny nose can often accompany tearing. With a common cold, the lacrimal sacs can become plugged so that tears, instead of draining into the nose, overflow from the eyes. Tears not only provide nourishment to the cornea but also help to dilute microorganisms. Tears contain immunoglobulins (IgG and IgE), which inhibit microbial growth.[1]

Physiology: Vision

The eye has often been compared to a camera to help illustrate its complex function and structure. The iris acts like a shutter on a camera and controls the amount of light entering the eye through the pupil. The light rays travel to the retina, which responds similarly to film in a camera. Chemical and physical changes take place in the retina and eventually lead to the discharge of electrical impulses. The impulses are conducted along the optic nerve fibers to the occipital lobe of the cortex. The brain interprets what has been seen.

IMPAIRED VISUAL FUNCTION

Many young and older adults have normal visual function. It is usually not until 61 years of age or above that most (over 59%) visual impairments occur. This section briefly presents an overview of the more common eye alterations: injury, glaucoma, cataracts, diabetic retinopathy, and retinal detachment. Visual impairments that occur in multiple sclerosis and hemianopsias also are described.

Injury

Occupational hazards account for a large percentage of eye injuries. A small piece of metal from a piece of equipment can penetrate the eyeball, or a splash of caustic acid can easily damage vision. In both instances, the nurse should be able to perform a quick assessment and take action. Hemorrhage from outside or inside the eyeball indicates that an injury has occurred. Ecchymosis or a black eye from a fist or an object such as a ball may indicate internal damage. Serious injury can be ruled out only by examining the eyes with an ophthalmoscope. Absence of pain does not necessarily mean that damage did not occur. Damage to the surface of the eye is usually painful, whereas damage to the inside of the eye is generally pain free. The individual with altered vision, such as blurring, should be referred to an ophthalmologist for further evaluation.

Chemical burns require prompt treatment to prevent permanent scarring. Regardless of the chemical agent, initial treatment is always the same—prolonged washing of the eyeball for 15 to 20 minutes with plain water. After this immediate response, a physician should be contacted.[23]

Glaucoma

Glaucoma is the third leading cause of blindness and can slowly damage the eye without any awareness by the person. Glaucoma occurs when there is a buildup of intraocular pressure because of blockage of aqueous humor. This condition can

progressively destroy the optic nerve. There are two major forms of glaucoma: open angle and closed angle. In *open-angle* glaucoma, the most common form, the outflow of aqueous humor is reduced. This form of glaucoma is hereditary and is the most difficult to diagnose. Some early signs of open-angle glaucoma are frequent changes of glasses without any improvement in vision, inability of the eyes to adjust to darkened rooms, loss of side vision, and rainbow-colored rings around lights. Eyedrops (miotics) such as pilocarpine and timolol maleate are usually prescribed for open-angle glaucoma. These work by constricting the pupil and the ciliary muscle, helping to relax and open the outflow channels and reducing pressure. Eyedrops do not cure open-angle glaucoma or return previous vision, but if used daily as prescribed they prevent further damage.[5]

Closed-angle glaucoma occurs when the iris is displaced in the periphery of the anterior chamber and blocks the aqueous filtration network. As a result, the intraocular pressure rises quickly, causing severe eye pain and even nausea and vomiting. Physiologically, the cornea becomes edematous, and the pupil dilates. Medical management requires surgery in which part of the iris is removed (iridectomy).[6]

Cataracts

An opacity or clouding of the lens that blocks the passage of light needed for vision is a *cataract*. A cataract forms slowly with age. The exact etiology of cataract formation is still unknown. Cataracts can result from trauma, such as a foreign body that penetrates the lens, or from exposure to certain poisons, such as naphthalene, an ingredient in mothballs. Symptoms develop gradually and may not be noticed. Clients commonly complain of blurred vision, obliteration of parts of images, double images, and distorted images. When vision is decreased to the point that it interferes with a client's occupation or activities of daily living, surgical removal of the lens is indicated.[20]

Intracapsular and extracapsular techniques are the two basic surgical methods used to remove cataracts. The intracapsular approach involves removing the lens intact. The extracapsular method involves removing the lens in pieces with an instrument called a *phacoemulsifier*. This instrument uses ultrasound waves to break up the hard lens and suck it out of the anterior chamber. Following the extraction of the lens, an intraocular lens is implanted or cataract glasses or contact lenses are required to compensate for the loss of focusing power.[24]

Diabetic Retinopathy

Diabetic retinopathy refers to a noninflammatory process in which the eye undergoes vascular changes. Almost all persons with diabetes experience some retinal vascular alterations with increasing longevity. If complications develop, then blindness can result. Persons with uncontrolled diabetes or those who have been dependent on insulin for 20 years or more are at higher risk for developing diabetic retinopathy.

There are two types of diabetic retinopathy: nonproliferative (background) and proliferative. *Nonproliferative retinopathy* is the milder of the two forms and need not be treated except by maintaining good diabetic control. Nonproliferative retinopathy includes microaneurysms, blot hemorrhage, and retinal edema. If macular edema occurs, then fluorescein angiography is used to determine the potential for return of vision. If the macular capillaries are leaking fluid, then laser treatment may be beneficial. If the capillaries are occluded, vision is unlikely to return.

Proliferative retinopathy refers to neovascularization or fibrosis. The cause of these abnormal blood vessels is unknown. One theory postulates that the retina may be trying to compensate for poor blood perfusion. As with nonproliferative retinopathy, laser treatment is used. A laser photocoagulator burns minute openings on the surface of the retina to coagulate new vessels and prevent the formation of other vessels.[24]

Retinal Detachment

The separation of the retina from the choroid is referred to as *retinal detachment*. Atrophy and damage to the rods and cones can occur because the separation prevents nourishment to the outer portion of the retina. There is no pain associated with retinal detachment, but usually the client complains of lack of vision. Individuals who have had cataract surgery, trauma to the eye, or some form of myopia are at risk for detachment of the retina.

There are two classifications of retinal detachment: rhegmatogenous and nonrhegmatogenous. *Rhegmatogenous*, which means ruptured in Greek, occurs when holes form in the retina. *Nonrhegmatogenous* can be caused by the development of fibers within the vitreous. The fibers can adhere to the retina and when they contract, begin to pull the retina away from its normal attachment. Generally in this case, treatment would consist of surgery called a *vitrectomy*.[24]

Chorioretinal bond and scleral buckling are two of the techniques used to seal most holes in the retina. A *chorioretinal bond* brings the choroid and retina together by inducing inflammation. When this inflammation resolves, the structures fuse together. *Scleral buckling* is a silicone sponge or band that indents the retina so that it comes in contact with the choroid.

Multiple Sclerosis

Multiple sclerosis can affect vision. Often persons with this disease describe visual problems as their initial symptoms. These symptoms may include blurred vision, blind spots, and diplopia (double vision) in one or both eyes. Some individuals even have reported losing total sight in one eye for several hours to several days. The basis for these visual disturbances is optic neuritis.[19]

Hemianopsias

Hemianopsia is defective vision or blindness in half of the visual field and usually refers to bilateral defects. It can result from brain damage caused by cerebrovascular disorders, trauma, or tumors.

Hemianopsias are classified as homonymous, bitemporal, and attitudinal. Homonymous hemianopsias are the most common, especially in older persons. *Homonymous hemianopsia* refers to loss of vision in the temporal field of one eye and the nasal field of the other. A client with a right-sided brain lesion would have a left homonymous hemianopsia with loss of vision in the nasal half of the right eye and the temporal half of the left eye. Many times persons with homonymous hemianopsia are unaware of their condition until the deficit is pointed out to them. The individual may psychologically fill in an image while actually seeing only half of it.[10] A more severe visual impairment for reading occurs in a client with a right homonymous hemianopsia, because it is impossible to see the letters or words in advance of the one on which the client is fixating.

Bitemporal hemianopsias are usually produced by tumors whose progression is slow. They are not considered great handicaps if the person's vision is 20/100 or better.

Attitudinal hemianopsia usually affects only one eye and is most often caused by vascular occlusion. It often affects the lower field, making it a more severe disability than bitemporal hemianopsia.[4]

Blindness

At least 498,000 Americans are legally blind. Legal blindness in the United States is defined as vision of 20/200 or less in the better eye with correction, or a visual field limited to 20 degrees or fewer. Currently the most common cause of blindness is macular degeneration. The fastest rising cause of blindness is diabetic retinopathy.[4] However, blindness from industrial accidents remains common, with about 1,000 workers losing the sight of one eye and 100 losing the sight of both eyes annually.[25]

NURSING ASSESSMENT

Information about a client's visual status is obtained by gathering both subjective and objective data. Subjective data are obtained when the health history is taken and are based on what the client can tell the nurse. Responses to the following questions can provide a framework for a more in-depth investigation:

1. Do you wear glasses or contact lenses? If so, how do they help you?
2. Have you noticed any recent change(s) in your ability to see? If so, have these changes affected your activities at home or work?
3. Do you have pain, burning, itching, or blurred or double vision?
4. Have you noticed swelling around your eyes or tearing or spots before your eyes?
5. Have you noticed any difficulty in near or far vision or problems with driving at night? Does glare create problems?
6. Have you been aware of any peripheral vision loss?
7. Have you ever been told that you have cataracts or glaucoma?
8. When was your last eye examination, and by whom was it done?

The next phase of the assessment elicits objective data through inspection and performance of visual acuity measurements. Inspection, like taking a history, can provide further clues to any visual alteration. The first part of the inspection involves inspecting the exterior of the eye (Table 17-2).

The position and color of the eyelids should be observed. Normally the upper eyelid covers part of the iris but not the pupil. If the lid extends over the pupil, this is referred to as *ptosis*. Ectropion and entropion eyelids are two other variations from normal. An *ectropion* eyelid occurs when the eyelid is everted, exposing the mucous membrane lining the eye. The client may experience tearing, with tears running down the cheeks, since they cannot drain into the nose. An *entropion* eyelid occurs when the lower lid is turned in. The lashes can rub against the cornea and lead to a corneal ulcer. Normally, the color of the eyelids matches the skin color. Redness of the margins of the lid could indicate an infection such as a hordeolum.

The color of the conjunctiva, sclera, and iris, as well as the size of the pupils also should be observed when performing the exterior assessment. The color of the conjunctiva can be determined by pulling the lower eyelid down gently with the thumb. The conjunctiva lining the lids should be pink. Paleness could indicate anemia. The conjunctiva covering the anterior surface of the eyeball is usually thin and transparent. Congestion or generalized redness most often indicates an infection such as conjunctivitis.

The sclera is normally white with perhaps some slight yellow coloring because of fat deposits below the sclera. A yellowed or reddened sclera is abnormal. The color of the iris should be noted. In most individuals, the iris is the same color in both eyes. A difference in color is referred to as *heterochromia iridis*, which may or may not be normal. The shape of the iris is round and its appearance is clear.

The size of the pupil varies with the color of the iris and with age. Individuals with brown eyes have smaller pupils than those with blue eyes. Those who are farsighted and older will probably also have smaller pupils. The equality of the pupils can be assessed by determining reaction to both direct and consensual light. Using a pen-

TABLE 17-2

Exterior assessment of the eye

Structure	Normal observations	Variations from normal
Eyelids		
Position	Upper eyelid does not extend	Ptosis: Drooping of eyelid
		Ectropion: Lower lid turned out
		Entropion: Lower lid turned in
Color	Matches skin color	Redness; could indicate infection, for example, hordeolum; inflammation; chalazion
Conjunctiva		
Color	Lining of eyelids pink	Paleness; could indicate anemia
	Anterior surface thin and transparent	Congestion/generalized redness: infection, for example, conjunctivitis
Sclera		
Color	White	Yellowed/reddened
Iris		
Color	Both eyes same	Heterochromia iridis: difference in color
Shape	Round	Irregular, for example, iridectomy
Clarity	Clear	Pus in anterior chamber; could obscure clearness
Pupils		
Size	Varies with color (brown eyes smaller than blue), age (smaller in older adults), and whether nearsighted or farsighted (farsighted smaller)	Unequal in size
Equality	Equal response to light; constriction	Unequal, absent, or sluggish response

light, the nurse can detect the client's reaction to direct light by moving the penlight from the temporal to the nasal side of the eye. The nurse should observe the presence and speed of pupil constriction. Consensual constriction can be tested by shining the penlight into one pupil and observing for constriction of the opposite pupil.[2]

The *Snellen chart* is generally used to measure *visual acuity* for distance (Figure 17-3). Professor Herman Snellen first developed this chart in 1864.[13] The chart is available in numbers or in letter Es, which can be used with non-English-speaking persons. The Snellen chart is usually hung on a wall at eye level 20 feet from the person tested. Visual acuity should be tested with the client's glasses or contact lenses in place. Each eye is tested separately, first the right and then the left. The client is asked to read the smallest line that can be seen on the chart. Normal vision is 20/20. The numerator is always 20 to indicate the distance away from the chart, and the denom-

inator is the distance at which a person with normal vision can read the line. Vision of 20/200 means the client sees at 20 feet what a person with normal vision can see at 200 feet. If the client cannot read all the letters on a line, this should be recorded. For instance, if three letters on the fifth line are missed, it should be documented as 20/40 −3.

Anyone with a visual acuity of less than 20/30 in either eye should be referred to an ophthalmologist. In some cases, the client may not be able to see the largest letter on the chart (usually the 20/200 letter). If this happens, the nurse should hold up two or three fingers and slowly move toward the person until the number of fingers held up can be identified. This is done to determine what can and cannot be seen and should be recorded as C/F (counting fingers) at the distance when perception occurred.[2,18]

Many persons suffer from low vision because of an underlying pathological condition. *Low vi-*

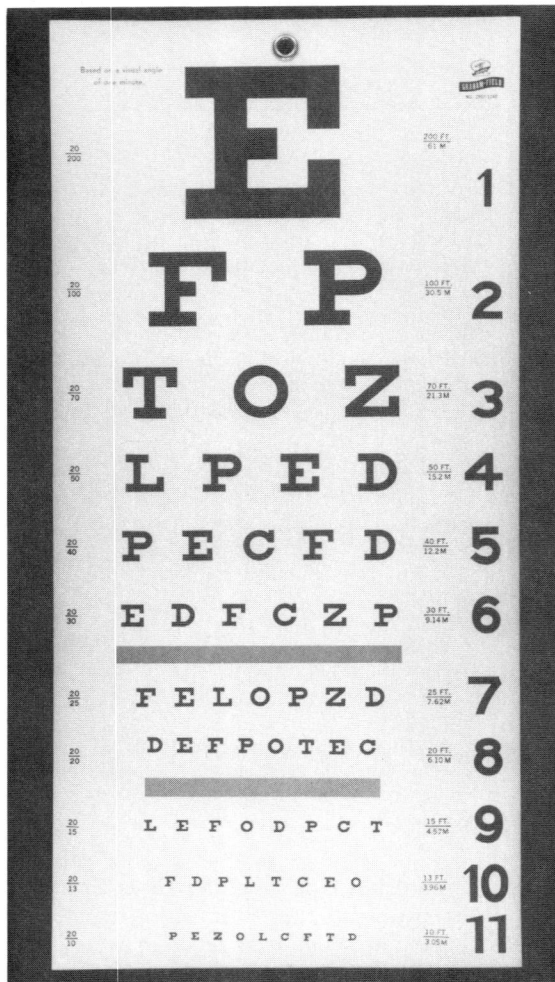

Figure 17-3
Snellen chart.

sion cannot be corrected with conventional eyeglasses or contact lenses. Affected individuals may complain of distorted or blurred images, inability to see objects at certain angles, or inability to recognize objects at certain distances. Low vision aids such as magnifying lenses, telescopic lenses, and closed-circuit television monitors developed especially for reading can help these persons.[24] One does not have to be legally blind to receive low vision care. Legal blindness has been defined as corrected vision of 20/200 or worse in the bet-

ter eye. The ophthalmologist should make the diagnosis of legal blindness when indicated, not only so the client receives the proper follow-up, but also to ensure that the client can receive a tax deduction.

Many of the Snellen charts have two color bars, one red and the other green, to help in assessing individuals with color deficits. Color blindness occurs more frequently among males, since it is a recessive trait carried on the X chromosome. The most common form of color blindness involves the red-green hues.[17]

A *pinhole test* also can be done if one notices diminished visual acuity. The client should be instructed to hold up a piece of cardboard with a pinhole in the center and read the chart. If vision improves significantly, the acuity problem is most likely caused by refraction.[17]

The Snellen chart measures only central vision. An assessment of peripheral vision is necessary because deficits in this area could indicate glaucoma or a partially detached retina. The *confrontation test* can be performed by the nurse to provide a rough measurement of peripheral vision. During this test, the client is seated 3 feet from the nurse, asked to close one eye as the nurse closes the same eye, and instructed to focus on the nurse's uncovered eye. The nurse then moves a small object such as a pencil inside and outside the client's visual field until this object is seen. With normal peripheral vision, the nurse and client should be able to see the pencil at the same time. As previously indicated, this test is not very precise, but in many instances, the client's blind spot can be detected.[2]

Examination of the ocular fundus, or back portion of the eye's interior, is generally performed by the ophthalmologist. Often the pupils are dilated with mydriatic drops. The ophthalmologist may use the following equipment: (1) ophthalmoscope for magnification, (2) slit lamp to evaluate cataracts and corneal disease, (3) ophthalmometer to measure the curvature of the cornea, (4) fluorescent staining to detect abrasions, and (5) tonometer to measure intraocular pressure for the presence of glaucoma.[17]

In some cases, the nurse may assist the ophthalmologist in performing Schiøtz' tonometry. The cornea is prepared by instilling an anesthetic; then the tonometer is placed over the eye. The tonometer measures the indentation or

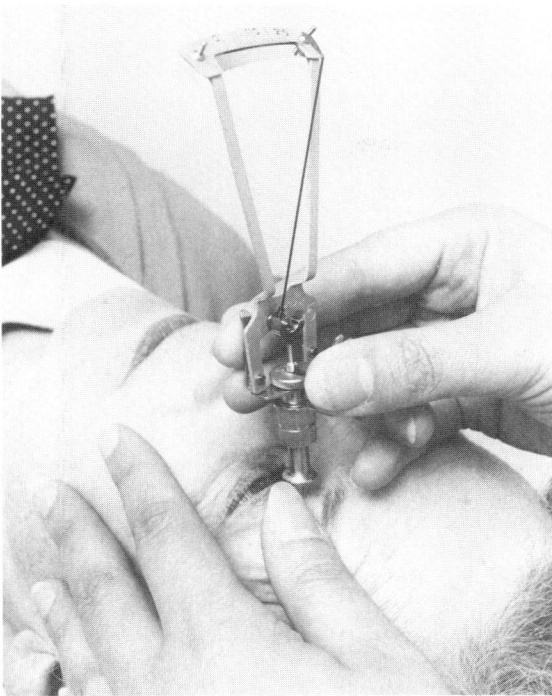

Figure 17-4
Schiøtz tonometer being placed over client's pupil to measure intraocular pressure.

pressure (Figure 17-4). Normal intraocular pressure ranges from 12 to 22 mm Hg.[2]

NURSING DIAGNOSES

Once the nurse has acquired all the information pertinent to the client's visual status, the nursing diagnoses are identified.[24] Although the client may have optimum visual function, the potential for *visual sensory/perceptual alterations* exists.[7] Inadequate eye care, carelessness, or ignorance can lead to a visual alteration. The following three cases illustrate potential situations for eye damage. A college freshman who wears contact lenses is so busy studying for final examinations that he does not properly clean his lenses. Might he be a good candidate for developing an eye infection? What about the industrial worker who forgets to put on protective goggles when pipetting acids? And last, what about the person who wakes up one morning unable to see from the right eye and attributes this to reading too much? The potential for temporary or permanent visual alteration is present in each of these cases.

Visual sensory/perceptual alterations can occur in conjunction with primary disease processes such as multiple sclerosis and cerebrovascular accident. In both of these instances, the nurse needs to be aware that assessment is necessary during both the acute and rehabilitation stages. The individual experiencing a cerebrovascular accident, for example, may be apprehensive and confused as a result of diminished peripheral vision or difficulty interpreting images. How much total visual field loss is experienced? What potential is there for teaching about this loss? These questions will only be asked when visual perceptual alterations are suspected in clients who have other disease processes occurring.

Two secondary functional problems might develop from the initial nursing diagnosis. Certainly once a person is diagnosed with a particular disease entity such as a detached retina, *anxiety* is likely. Not knowing what to expect from treatment, worry over finances, and interruptions in work routine can all lead to anxiety. *Potential for injury* is also present as a result of a visual alteration. The progressive development of low vision may make a person more vulnerable to environmental hazards. Injury could result from inability to see a raised pavement or a car zooming around a corner.

GOALS

Goals are based on the nursing diagnoses and are formulated in collaboration with clients. Nursing diagnoses and goals also provide direction for nursing interventions. Generally the goals are as follows:

1. To improve knowledge regarding normal eye function
2. To encourage precautions to protect vision from hazards present in the home and workplace
3. To give instructions regarding the appropriate methods of caring for eyeglasses and contact lenses
4. To establish compensating mechanisms appropriate to the individual client with low vision

5. To educate the client and family regarding eye care in relation to intraocular implants and prostheses
6. To obtain maximum client and family participation in and responsibility for care of the eyes

REHABILITATION NURSING INTERVENTIONS

The nurse may become involved with a person with visual sensory/perceptual alteration at different levels of prevention. Health screening, direct care, health education, and referral to other service agencies are within the nurse's responsibilities. Psychological support by the nurse is important in dealing with a client with a visual alteration. The client may be anxious and frightened over temporary or permanent loss of vision. The client who requires bilateral eye patches may experience sensory disorientation. The client as well as the family may experience feelings of guilt over carelessness in protecting the eyes.

Direct Care

The nurse's role in gathering data for health screening and emergency care interventions has been previously discussed. Nurses should be aware of the proper method of instilling eyedrops or applying eye ointments, since they may often be in a position of actually carrying out these procedures or assisting the client and family in doing so.

When administering eye medications, the nurse should be sure that the correct medication is placed in the prescribed eye. The client should be asked to tilt the head back and look upward. The nurse should gently pull downward on the lower lid with a cotton ball or gauze square, thus exposing the conjunctiva and forming a small pocket. The drop should be placed on the surface of the conjunctiva. The tip of the dropper should not touch the eye or the bottle cap, since the medication is considered sterile. Natural blinking of the eye will spread the medication so that it can be absorbed.

The same principles apply to the instillation of eye ointments. Only a thin line of ointment is required. It should be placed along the conjunctival surface of the retracted lower lid. When the client closes the eye and rotates the eyeball from side to side, the ointment will be dispersed over its entire anterior surface.[6] All eye procedures should be carried out gently. Hands should be washed before and after performing each procedure.

Client and Family Education

Client and family education is a crucial component of the nurse's role. The public often has misconceptions about visual alterations. Through misunderstanding, a person may associate glaucoma with hypertension, since both conditions are characterized by increasing pressure. Another common misconception is that eyesight can be saved in the person experiencing progressive visual deterioration if the person does not engage in reading or sewing. Avoidance of visual pleasures will not postpone eye damage.

Education directed toward prevention of eye damage is the most beneficial. Clients need to know what eye symptoms should be reported to their ophthalmologist. They should be instructed to have their eyes checked immediately if they experience pain, discomfort, chronic headaches, discharge from the eye, or poor vision. Clients and families may require guidelines in proper eye care. Some of these guidelines are:
1. Avoid glare, and make certain that there is adequate light when engaging in close work such as reading.
2. Wear prescribed glasses, and keep them clean and accessible.
3. Clean contact lenses with special solutions, since the mucus on them may harden and interfere with vision.
4. Use sunglasses in bright or very windy environments. Adaptation to the dark may be affected by prolonged exposure to bright light.
5. Use caution when working with household cleaners such as ammonia, which can cause damage if splashed into the eyes.
6. Make use of large print books and magazines, for example, *Reader's Digest*, or talking books, available upon request from any library.
7. Designate light switches with fluorescent tape.
8. Use special dials that enlarge numbers and glow in the dark for telephones.
9. Avoid the use of white against white to

distinguish objects. Make good use of red and orange colors, since these can be seen more vividly. Yellow increases depth perception so that printed material on a yellow background can be more easily seen.

10. Place soft night-lights in the bathroom and kitchen to help with navigation and prevent falls.

11. Caution family members against moving furniture or objects without telling you.

Additional sensory aids

There are both travel and reading aids that can assist a client to better adapt to the social and physical environment.[15] A *path sounder*, a boxlike device used to aid travel, can be placed over the client's chest. The path sounder produces a low-pitched buzz if an approaching object is between 3 and 6 feet away. Another mobility aid that is widely used is the laser cane. The cane sends out three different beams, providing the traveler with information that an ordinary cane cannot. One beam warns the traveler of drop-offs such as a curb; the second beam indicates obstacles that are straight ahead; and the third beam indicates objects that are head high in the person's path.

The two major devices that can help the visually impaired client with reading are the *Optacon* and the *Kurzweil Reading Machine*. The Optacon converts printed characters into sounds or vibrations. It has a tactile display that allows the individual to feel the shape of the letters. The Kurzweil Reading Machine is even more sophisticated in that it uses a computer-controlled camera that can scan a printed page and transcribe it into synthetic speech. The Kurzweil Reading Machine is available in many public and university libraries.

Hemianopsias: special considerations

Once a client has been diagnosed with a hemianopsia, the nurse needs to be aware of the extent of the client's visual field loss. The nurse in the acute or rehabilitation setting can be instrumental in assessing the client's ability to compensate for this loss. The client's behavior may provide the nurse with important clues. The person who is not compensating adequately may be observed walking into other people or walls, only eating food on one side of the tray, demonstrating inability to participate in self-care, and ignoring environmental stimuli and activities occurring on

the affected side.[10] Persons who have brain lesions of the right hemisphere may experience additional problems with perception in which they have difficulty controlling their position sense and body image. These clients may slump to one side, ignore their left side, or overreach when trying to pick up objects.

Regardless of whether the lesion is in the right or left hemisphere of the brain, the client can benefit from rehabilitation. Members of the rehabilitation team and family members need to be persistent and patient when working with clients with hemianopsia. The person in the early stages of hemianopsia will be anxious, and actions need to be directed to minimizing this anxiety. The individual should be continually oriented to the environment and should always be approached from the unaffected side. When possible, the nurse should position the person so that the unaffected side is toward the door or toward where most of the activity is taking place. Placing the client's personal items such as clock and water glass within view also is helpful.

The client can be taught to scan with the eyes, using horizontal and vertical sweeping motions. This technique can help compensate for loss of peripheral vision on one side, but reinforcement is required when the person is eating, performing self-care activities, and ambulating in the halls. Special visual scanning exercises can be developed to help the client improve scanning abilities.[10] A magnetic spelling board, available at many toy and department stores, is useful because it has large, bright-colored letters and numbers. A board also can be constructed of flannel and felt materials. Initially the letters or numbers can be placed within the client's field of vision and then gradually moved toward the hemianopic side so that the individual is forced to expand the visual field by turning the head. Family members can be encouraged to assist the client with the board game, and in this way they can be involved in the rehabilitation process.

Another exercise that can be used in mastering the scanning technique is asking the person to read using the forefinger as a guide to underscore one line at a time. To help ensure the cooperation of both the client and family, it is important for members of the rehabilitation team to explain the condition of hemianopsia and its effect on vision.

Prisms are other aids that can allow clients to be more aware of objects in their periphery, and these devices can also help the client with severe field restrictions to start scanning more efficiently. The prism is normally placed as close to the center of the client's eyeglass lens as possible. The prism allows the client to make only a small eye movement into the prism, which then displaces objects from the periphery toward the center of the prism. If the central acuity of a client is less than 20/100, then chances of successfully benefiting from a prism diminish.

A bioptic telescope is another device that can expand visual fields. Bioptics are based on the principle of reversed telescopes that minify objects seen by the client. Bioptics are designed so that clients can view through the minification lenses and then look under them with the normal fields. Some states, such as New York and California, allow individuals with diminished visual acuity to drive with a bioptic telescope if it corrects their vision from 20/120 or 20/100 to 20/40.[11]

Newly blind persons: special considerations

How well a newly blind person adapts to the situation depends upon individual personality, attitude, and the attitude of family. To enhance the blind person's ability to communicate, navigate, and take pleasure in the environment, the following guidelines are provided for health professionals and family members:

1. Orient the person to the surroundings and remind visitors to introduce themselves.
2. Maintain personal items such as combs and brushes within easy reach.
3. Do not reorganize the person's life space, for example, bedside stand or chair, without orienting the person verbally and physically.
4. Leave doors completely open or completely closed to prevent injury.
5. When speaking to a newly blind person, use a natural tone of voice and introduce yourself to the person by stating your name and function.
6. Use hand-to-hand contact rather than touching the person on the arm or shoulder, since it allows the person to feel more in control.
7. Allow the individual to be involved in problem solving, because this activity helps set the tone for rehabilitation.
8. Assist the person in organizing his or her

life space, for example, teach how to hang clothes by style or color and how to fold money to aid identification.
9. Provide addresses and telephone numbers of agencies and resources for blind persons.
10. Encourage the person to assume a good posture and to turn directly toward the one to whom speaking.
11. Attach or sew tactile symbols to clothing and personal items to help identify color and contents.
12. Evaluate and train the individual to more effectively use the other senses: auditory, kinesthetic, tactile, olfactory, and gustatory.
13. Assist the person in learning to localize and discriminate sounds.
14. Encourage the individual to become involved as soon as possible in self-care practices and personal decision making
15. Assist the person in learning to detect temperatures and to manipulate objects safely. For example, accurate pouring of a hot beverage can be practiced by placing the palm and fingers of one hand around the cup and hearing and feeling the heat as the hot liquid rises to the desired level.
16. When the person is mastering mealtime activities, such as cutting meat and buttering bread, provide privacy and easily managed foods.
17. Instruct the person to visualize the meal plate as a clock because this can help in communicating about the location of food or other items. For example, the salt shaker is in line with 12 o'clock.
18. When assisting a blind person in walking, walk about a half step ahead of the person, who then grasps the elbow of the guide. The guide's movements can alert the blind person to curbs, turns, and stops.[27]

As stated previously, communication is an important element that requires enhancement for the blind person. Items such as writing guides and check-writing guides are available from the American Foundation for the Blind and may be helpful because they allow the blind person to continue to write by hand. Tape recorders can be used to replace letter writing and can provide privacy for personal correspondence. Rehabilitation team members may want to suggest braille typewriters and braillewriters, depending on the needs of the blind individual. Communication also can be maintained through the use of the telephone by instructing the blind person on memorizing the dial or by using braille or tactile symbols. Mobility is as important a skill as communication. Orientation and mobility specialists can provide training in independent travel. This training takes approximately 180 hours.[27]

Some blind persons may require only short-term rehabilitation, whereas others may require long-term rehabilitation that includes psychological intervention. Finally the rehabilitation team needs to keep in mind the individual's preferences and life-style.

Intraocular implants and prostheses: special considerations

The most popular means used to correct *aprakia* (without lens) has been the implant of an intraocular lens. Intraocular lenses are plastic and are designed to be supported within the anterior or posterior chamber of the eye. In general, the implant is accomplished immediately after the cataract has been removed. Although this procedure is more expensive and increases the complication rate of cataract surgery by 1% to 2%, there are advantages.

One important advantage of an intraocular implant is that it requires no care or maintenance. Also, there is no distortion, magnification, or apparent increase in the size of the image perceived. A client with glaucoma or diabetes is no longer automatically rejected for intraocular implants; each case is individually evaluated.[8,12]

An enucleation, or surgical removal of the eyeball, may for cosmetic reasons require a prosthetic eye. Clients, as well as family members, need to understand that cleaning the artificial eye is important in maintaining comfort and assuring its cosmetic appearance. Some clients, such as those with sinus conditions or allergies, may be more sensitive to the prosthesis. Clients with excessive discharge may have to clean their prosthesis daily, whereas those with less discharge may require cleaning only two or three times each week.

The following steps for cleaning the prosthetic eye should be reviewed with both the client and family members:

1. Remove the prosthetic eye at night and place it in a small container of cleaning solution or warm, soapy water.
2. Allow the prosthetic eye to remain in the solution overnight to help prevent the buildup of secretions on its surface.
3. Remove secretions from the prosthetic eye by using a soft cloth. The eye should be rinsed off with warm water and allowed to remain slightly wet, since this makes insertion easier.

Careful handling of the prosthetic eye is important because of the danger of scratching with the fingernails. At least once each year the prosthesis should be examined by an ophthalmologist who can inspect it for scratches and hardened secretions as well as ensure proper fit.[12]

Referral

Nurses also can be instrumental in referring clients for more extensive assistance. Referrals require thought and a complete awareness of the client's needs and goals. The nurse must be familiar with local and regional resources available for the client with altered vision. The National Eye Institute in Bethesda, Maryland, can provide low vision aids and information on eye disease. (See Appendix E for addresses of additional organizations that can provide help.)

REHABILITATION TEAM INTERVENTIONS

Individuals experiencing more complex visual problems, such as blindness, may benefit from an interdisciplinary team approach. The team may consist of a social worker, occupational therapist, ophthalmologist, rehabilitation nurse, cleric, and family. Together, the team members share expertise and offer options such as braille instruction, guide dogs, white walking canes, and electronic devices to the client. In addition, they aid the client by giving psychological support and relieving anxiety. They aid the family members by assisting them in allowing the client to become as independent as possible.

OUTCOME CRITERIA

To evaluate the success of nursing and rehabilitation team interventions, outcome criteria should be established before the interventions are implemented. The following are some of the outcomes for a client with a visual sensory/perceptual alteration. At the conclusion of contact:

1. The client can explain the basic function of the eye.
2. The client and family can describe reportable symptoms.
3. The client and family can list methods used to compensate for low vision.
4. The client and family can demonstrate proper instillation of eye medications when applicable.
5. The client and family can demonstrate methods for care of glasses and contact lenses.
6. The client and family understand the importance of maintaining appointments with the ophthalmologist.

NORMAL HEARING FUNCTION

At least 1 million Americans are afflicted with a hearing impairment or with total inability to hear sounds.[9] Hearing impairment is a rather benign condition, because overtly there may not be any symptoms. Instead, the affected individual may turn the television set or radio up louder, ask a person to repeat what was said, or ignore the honking of a car while crossing the street. There are many sounds that we take for granted. How would you react if you could never hear the wind blow or the birds chirp? Sounds provide environmental cues, and when they are missing, feelings of frustration and social isolation emerge.

Persons in our society are often impatient with those who are hearing impaired. They may make jokes about them and sometimes assume that the person who cannot hear well must also be mentally deficient. Detection of hearing problems becomes difficult because individuals are embarrassed and feel stigmatized if they have to wear a hearing aid.

Components of the Ear

The ear is a very complex organ located within and protected by the temporal bone. For ease of discussion, the ear can be divided into three parts: external ear, middle ear, and inner ear (Figure 17-5). The *external ear* is composed of the auricle (pinna) and external auditory canal. The *auricle* contains cartilage covered by skin and is the portion of the ear that extends from the side of the

head. The *auditory canal* extends approximately 3 cm (1¼ inches) to provide a passageway by which sound waves reach the tympanic membrane. The temporal bone forms the inner two thirds of the canal. The canal is lined with skin containing cerumen (earwax), sweat glands, and hair follicles. The external ear protects the organ from microorganisms, dust particles, and insects.[12]

The *tympanic membrane* (eardrum) is formed from fibrous tissue and separates the external ear from the middle ear. Normally the tympanic membrane appears pearly gray and semitransparent. When inflammation is present, the membrane may be pink; when pus is present, white; and when there is bleeding, blue. The tympanic membrane is cone shaped and about the size of a pea.

Landmarks on the tympanic membrane include the umbo and the cone of light. The *umbo* is the most retracted part of the membrane. The *cone of light* refers to the reflection seen on the surface of the membrane if a small penlight is shone into the ear.

Directly behind the membrane are three tiny bones called the ossicles: the malleus (hammer), the incus (anvil), and the stapes (stirrup). The *malleus* is the longest bone and is attached directly to the tympanic membrane. The *incus* forms an arm that connects the malleus with the *stapes*, a bone partly embedded in the *fenestra ovalis* (oval window). There is a direct connection between the middle and inner ears. Cranial nerve VII, which controls facial movement, is found within the middle ear. The *chorda tympani*, a branch of this nerve, supplies taste to the anterior two thirds of the tongue.[20]

The *eustachian tube* is another important structure of the middle ear. The eustachian tube opens into the nasopharynx and provides equalization of air pressure between the middle ear and the pharynx. This equalizing mechanism is important when flying at high altitudes or diving under water. The eustachian tube is usually closed but will open when one yawns, swallows, or chews.

The *middle ear* acts as an amplification system. The ossicles form a chain in which the small footplate of the stapes receives vibrations from the tympanic membrane and transmits them to the inner ear.[12,20]

The *inner ear* is a maze formed by a bony labyrinth and a membranous labyrinth. The bony labyrinth is composed of the vestibule, cochlea,

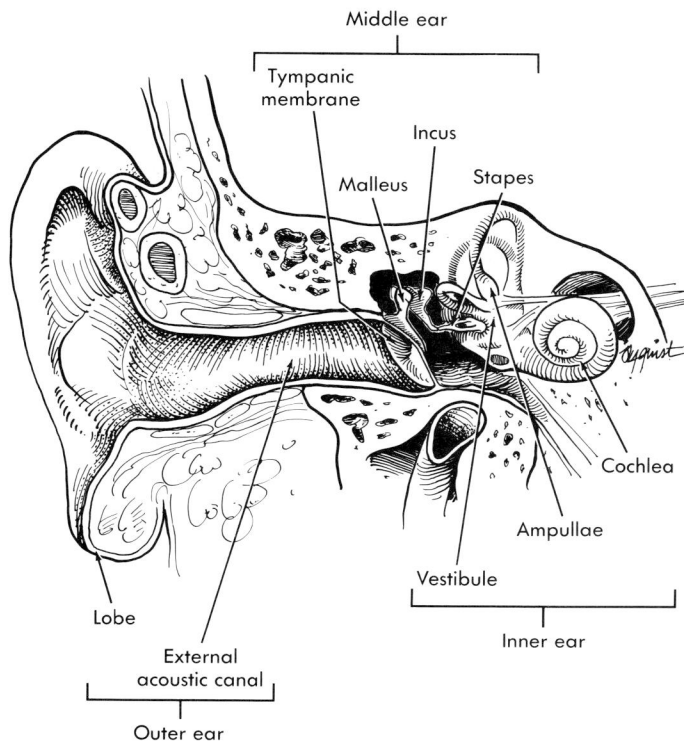

Figure 17-5
Cross section of outer, middle, and inner ear.

and semicircular canals. The *vestibule* makes up the central portion of the bony labyrinth. The fenestra ovalis opens into the vestibule.[12] The *cochlea* houses the organ of Corti, the sense organ of hearing. The cochlea, a tube coiled around several times, has the appearance of a snail and is further divided into three sections, the *scala vestibuli* (the upper section), the *scala media*, and the *scala tympani* (the lower section). Perilymph, a clear fluid, fills both the scala vestibuli and the scala tympani. The *organ of Corti* contains approximately 24,000 hair cells, which become distorted and mechanically bent when sound waves enter the cochlea.[8,21] The hair cells are displaced along the length of the cochlea, and, as they are displaced, they are transformed into neural activity. The neural impulses travel along to the eighth cranial nerve to the brain to produce the sensation of sound. The three *semicircular canals* are at right angles to each other. Within each semicircular canal is a membranous semicircular canal.

Each canal enlarges into an ampulla, which contains receptors from cranial nerve VIII (acoustic nerve).

The membranous labyrinth is composed of the *utricle* and *saccule*. Both the utricle and the saccule are suspended in the vestibule and contain endolymph. A smaller structure, the *macula*, is located in the utricle and saccule. The macula contains hair cells and otoliths (tiny ear stones). The hair cells project into the endolymph and are responsible in part for maintaining balance. When the position of the head is changed, it causes the otoliths to pull on the hair cells.[12] Table 17-3 summarizes the structures of the ear and their functions.

Perception of Sound

The organ of Corti has thousands of tiny hair cells that bend when sound waves enter the cochlea. At this time, sound, which has been a mechanical

TABLE 17-3
Parts of the ear

Structural sections	Component parts	Functional attributes
External ear	Auricle	Passageway for sounds
	Auditory canal	Protects organ from microorganisms
Middle ear	Tympanic membrane ossicles: malleus, incus, stapes	Receives and amplifies sound vibrations
	Eustachian tube	Equalizes air pressure between middle ear and pharynx
	Cranial nerve VII (facial)	Controls facial movement
Inner ear	Bony labyrinth: vestibule, cochlea, semicircular canals	Transmission of sound waves; aids balance
	Membranous labyrinth (inside bony labyrinth): utricle, saccule	Aids balance and equilibrium

force, is converted to an electrochemical impulse. This impulse travels to the temporal cortex of the brain via cranial nerve VIII (the acoustic nerve) and then is interpreted as meaningful sound. The hair cells in the organ of Corti are crucial to hearing. Some of the hair cells are believed to be sensitive to different pitch, whereas others respond to louder sounds.[21]

IMPAIRED HEARING FUNCTION

Most of the time, the ear functions very efficiently in collecting and conducting sound waves. With age, there is a decreased overall sensitivity to sound. Other conditions can create barriers to normal hearing. The following section provides a brief overview of the more common ear alterations (trauma, infection, otosclerosis, and Meniere's disease) and four major classifications of hearing loss.

Trauma and Infection

Trauma can occur from exposure to prolonged intense noise, penetration from a foreign body, a hand slap, rapid deceleration from a nonpressurized aircraft, or a skull fracture. Trauma can result in a perforation of the tympanic membrane. The client may complain of sudden pain, deafness in the affected ear, and perhaps bleeding. In some skull fractures, cerebrospinal fluid may leak through the perforation. An internal ear examination by an otologist (ear specialist) is necessary to determine the extent of the perforation. Small

perforations generally heal by themselves. The ear should be kept clean and dry, and often the client is given a prophylactic antibiotic to prevent infection. If the perforation is large, an operation referred to as a *myringoplasty* may be required to close the membrane. A myringoplasty prevents an infection from entering the middle ear.

Infections of the middle ear can be either acute or chronic. Infection can occur secondary to an upper respiratory tract infection or sinusitis. *Acute otitis media* is most commonly caused by streptococci and pneumococci. The eustachian tube may become inflamed, leading to sealing and blockage of the tube. The client may complain of muffled hearing, pain (earache), and fever. Pus may form and create pressure against the tympanic membrane.

Today antibiotics can be prescribed to reduce the purulent formation. At times, however, it may be necessary to surgically incise the tympanic membrane to release the pus and relieve the pressure. This procedure is called a *myringotomy*. Usually no anesthesia is required. After the myringotomy, when the pus has drained, the client's hearing returns to normal. The client should be instructed to insert new pieces of sterile cotton into the ear canal and should be cautioned to wash the hands, since the drainage is infectious. The client should be instructed not to swim or allow shower water to enter the ear because the tympanic membrane is open, and the infection could become worse.

Although less common, *chronic otitis media* can occur in untreated cases of acute otitis media.

The purulent discharge from the ear may be continuous, and generally more than one type of bacteria can be found in the cultured material. Treatment requires antibiotics and sometimes surgery.

Otosclerosis

Otosclerosis, a hereditary condition caused by progressive overgrowth of bone in the middle ear, generally involves both ears. The footplate of the stapes becomes fixated to the oval window so that sound wave vibrations are prevented from traveling to the inner ear. Women are affected more than men. Surgery can often correct otosclerosis by removing the excess bone and replacing all or part of the stapes with a prosthesis hooked around the incus. This surgical procedure, a *stapedectomy*, is usually done with the client under local anesthesia. The hospital stay is short, but the client should be instructed to change the external dressing, inform the physician if dizziness develops, continue the prescribed antibiotic, and avoid blowing the nose for a week so that the prosthesis does not loosen.[18,20]

Meniere's Disease

The exact cause of *Meniere's disease* is unknown. It seems that the blood vessels supplying the inner ear become constricted. The client may experience vertigo, tinnitus (ringing in the ears), and unilateral hearing loss sometimes accompanied by nausea and vomiting. Between the attacks of dizziness, the client is able to perform activities of daily living normally.

Hearing loss associated with Meniere's disease is usually not incapacitating because the client is still able to hear normally in one ear. Bilateral hearing loss, however, may occur in 10% of those affected. Many forms of treatment have been tried, but no particular one is more effective than another. Reducing fluid intake sometimes helps. Vasodilator drugs or small doses of sedatives also may help. Regardless of the treatment used, the nurse should provide reassurance, because the client may believe that other worse diseases such as a brain tumor are present. In severe cases when the tinnitus is creating a great deal of distress, a *labyrinthectomy* may be performed. This operation is used only as a last resort because it destroys the membranous labyrinth and thereby any hearing sensation remaining in the ear.[16,20]

Major Types of Hearing Loss

Conductive hearing loss, sensorineural hearing loss, mixed hearing loss, and functional hearing impairment can affect communication. Each of these problems and their causes will be examined separately.

Conductive hearing loss occurs when there is damage to the external auditory canal, eardrum, middle ear, or eustachian tube. The damage prevents effective conduction of sound waves to the inner ear. Causes include cerumen buildup, foreign objects, otitis media, trauma (particularly a perforated eardrum), and otosclerosis. Often these clients speak softly because their own voices sound loud to them. Individuals with conductive hearing loss can usually benefit most from a hearing aid because what they principally require is simple amplification.

Sensorineural hearing loss, sometimes called "nerve deafness," is caused by damage to the inner ear or to cranial nerve VIII (acoustic nerve). Prolonged exposure to intense noise, direct head trauma, infections, Meniere's disease, and drugs can cause this type of hearing loss. Drugs such as aspirin, antibiotics (streptomycin, neomycin), certain diuretics, and certain anticancer drugs can damage hair cells. *Presbycusis*, a progressive degeneration of the sensory hair cells and higher auditory pathways, is a special type of sensorineural hearing loss that occurs among older adults.[22] Older men are more frequently affected than older women. This loss is characterized by difficulty in understanding speech versus overall loss of hearing.

Mixed hearing loss, as the name implies, is any combination of conductive and sensorineural hearing loss. Usually the client has reduced speech discrimination, somewhat reduced bone conduction, and unilateral hearing loss.

There is no organic basis for the apparent hearing loss found in *functional hearing loss*. It is believed that this form of hearing loss is caused by emotional factors such as neurotic anxiety.[18,20,23]

NURSING ASSESSMENT

As with visual status, subjective information about hearing status is needed by the nurse so that potential hearing damage can be prevented and appropriate referrals made when hearing problems

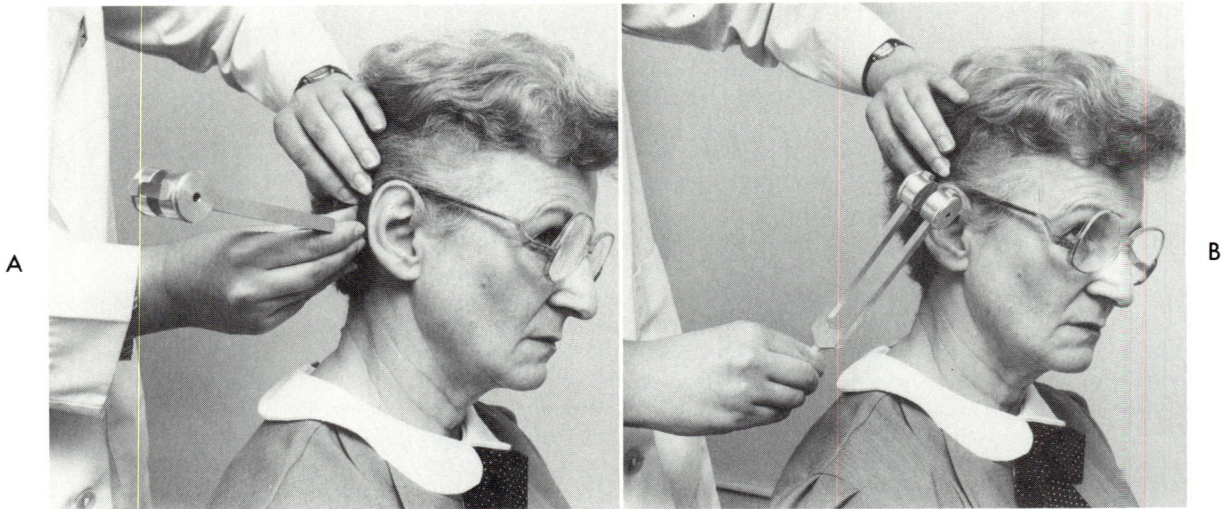

Figure 17-6
A, Rinne test is conducted by placing vibrating tuning fork on mastoid process. **B,** Rinne test continued in which tuning fork is placed by outside of external auditory canal.

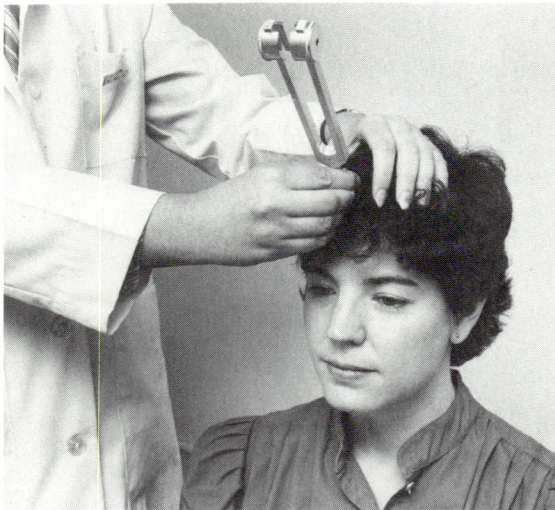

Figure 17-7
Weber test in which vibrating tuning fork is placed on midline of skull.

become apparent. The following questions provide a framework for a more in-depth investigation:

1. Do you now or have you in the past used a hearing aid? If so, what has been your response to the aid?
2. Do you have pain or discharge from your ears?
3. Have you noticed any change in your ability to hear face-to-face conversation, the television, or telephone conversation?
4. If you have noticed an alteration in your hearing, has this affected your activities at home or work?
5. Have you had recent problems with dizziness or ringing in your ears?
6. Have you ever been treated for an ear infection?
7. When was the last time you had a hearing evaluation, and by whom was it done?

Objective data can be obtained by observing the external ear. The nurse should note the size and shape of the auricle. In general, the ears lie in close proximity to the head. The surface of the auricle should be smooth. A variation from normal would include a lesion, a mass, or a *tophus*, which is a white, hard nodule. The nurse also should

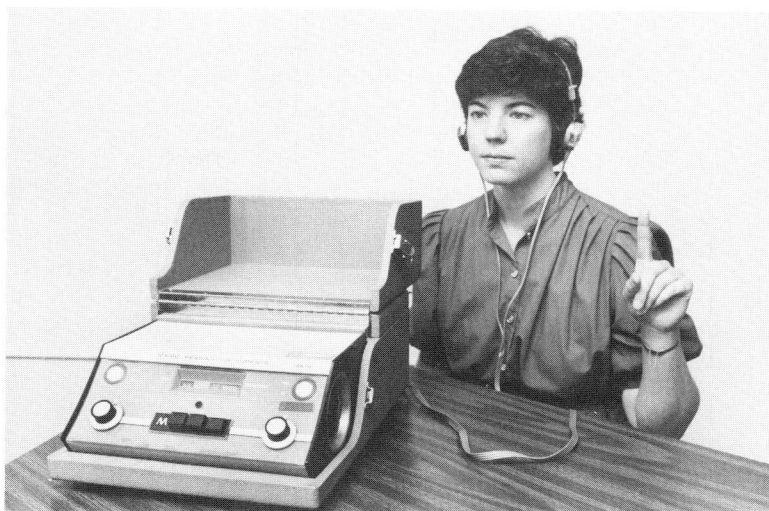

Figure 17-8
Client responding to audiometric test.

inspect the skin color of the external auditory canal and its patency. The color should be similar to the client's skin color. Redness of the canal may signify an inflammation such as external otitis media. The canal should be patent with varying amounts of cerumen. Impacted cerumen, blood, pus, or a foreign object may obstruct the canal.

Some nonelectrical methods can be used to grossly determine hearing ability. One method is *masking speech,* in which the client is prevented from using one ear by having noise produced near that ear. Noise can be produced by crackling paper while at the same time the nurse speaks in a whisper. The client is asked to repeat the word or phrase whispered. If the whispered voice is not heard, a normal conversational voice should be used to elicit a response. Normally a whispered voice is heard at a distance of 18 feet and a conversational voice at 40 feet. Masking speech may localize hearing impairment to one ear.[21]

The *watch tick test* is similar to masking speech. A wristwatch produces a high frequency sound above the range needed to hear speech. This test is easy to administer because it can be done in the client's home. Since loss of hearing often begins with a loss of sensitivity for high frequencies, a defect may be found earlier with this test than with masking.

Tuning forks are designed to produce fre-

quencies that correspond to the musical C scale when they are vibrated. There are two tests that require a tuning fork—the Rinne and the Weber.

The *Rinne test* is designed to compare the client's hearing by air conduction and by bone conduction.[23] The base of the vibrating tuning fork is placed on the bone behind the ear (mastoid process). The client is asked to indicate when a tone is heard and when it dissipates. When the tone dissipates, the vibrating tuning fork is brought close to the external auditory canal. Again the client is asked to indicate when a tone is heard and when it disappears. With normal function, the tone should be heard about twice as long by air as by bone conduction. The client with a conductive hearing loss will hear the tone longer behind the ear than at the canal opening, since the problem involves the outer or middle ear mechanism.

In the *Weber test* the stem of the vibrating tuning fork is placed on the midline of the skull.[23] The client is then asked to indicate in which ear the sound is loudest. Normally the tone is heard equally in both ears. If the tone is lateralized to the poorer ear, then a conductive hearing loss is suspected. In a sensorineural hearing loss, the tone is heard louder in the better ear. Figures 17-6 and 17-7 demonstrate the positions of the forks in the Rinne and Weber tests.

The otologist may refer the client to an audiologist for an audiometric hearing test. The *audiometer* is an electrical instrument calibrated so that what is recorded is not the ability to hear but rather hearing loss in the frequencies tested (Figure 17-8). An *audiogram* is simply a written record of a person's hearing level measured with certain pure tones. The pure tones commonly used to assess hearing sensitivity are the frequencies 250, 500, 1,000, 2,000, 3,000, 4,000, 6,000, and 8,000 Hz/sec. Frequency refers to the number of sound waves emanating from a source per second and is expressed in hertz (Hz). Hearing is most sensitive for frequencies between 500 and 4,000 Hz. Tones are presented through earphones to each ear. Hearing loss can be defined as the number of decibels (db) reached before the client hears the sound for each specific frequency. Zero loudness is calibrated for the sound barely heard by the person with normal hearing. A range of 0- to 20-db loss for a tested frequency is considered normal, whereas a person with a 70- to 89-db loss for a tested frequency is considered to have a profound loss. Persons with a hearing loss of 30 db, even though categorized as having a mild loss, will have considerable difficulty in everyday conversation and will be candidates for hearing aids.

NURSING DIAGNOSES

Three nursing diagnoses are common for clients with hearing impairments.[7] First, the *potential for auditory sensory/perceptual alterations* exists. Increased noise levels in both work and home environments place each of us at risk for noise damage. Normal conversation occurs at about 60 db. A power saw has a sound level of 110 db, and working near a jet plane taking off can expose a person to close to 140 db and can create pain. Lifelong exposure to city noises and loud music can increase the likelihood of hearing impairment in later years.[9]

Second, *social isolation* can easily occur when a person has a hearing impairment. Conductive hearing loss generally signifies that the client can understand speech but has difficulty with reduced background auditory sensation. In comparison, the client with sensorineural loss can hear speech, but often cannot understand it. When a person cannot take part in conversation because of hearing loss, it is only natural to withdraw into one's own world to avoid embarrassment or frustration

when words in sentences are not grasped. Hearing impaired persons may even become suspicious, feeling that others are laughing or talking about them. Suspiciousness can lead to paranoia and even greater social isolation.

Third, the hearing impaired client who must wear a hearing aid may suffer from a *body image disturbance*. An external hearing aid draws attention to the impairment. From a personal perspective, the client may feel that the hearing aid is a signal to others for different treatment and that he or she is not a fully functioning person.

GOALS

The following are some goals that are derived from the previously mentioned nursing diagnoses:
1. To instruct the client about ways to conserve present hearing in the home and work environment
2. To teach the client methods to enhance communication style
3. To assist the client in resolving feelings about the hearing impairment through verbalizations
4. To promote understanding of the communication problem among family members
5. To teach the family methods of communicating with the client

REHABILITATION NURSING INTERVENTIONS

One of the most common procedures the nurse is likely to be involved in is an ear irrigation to remove cerumen, a foreign body, or purulent discharge. Cerumen can be responsible for a profound hearing loss. Clients may attempt to remove hardened wax from the ear by using sharp objects such as a hairpin or a fingernail. Therefore they need to be taught that such a practice not only may push the wax in further but also can injure the canal. A foreign object in the ear is probably the most common ear emergency. Irrigations are the best method of removing hard material. Irrigations should not be used to remove cereal grains, since water causes the grains to swell. When an insect enters the ear, it should be killed before it has the opportunity to sting. This can be accomplished by placing a few drops of oil or alcohol into the ear and then irrigating. When irrigating the ear canal to remove cerumen, the nurse should use tap water or a prescribed solution at body temperature. If the solution is cold, it could stimulate vertigo. The client should be seated with clothing properly protected. A kidney basin held below the ear is used to collect the solution. The auricle should be pulled upward and then backward before injecting the solution along the upper wall of the auditory canal. After the canal has been washed out, it should be dried. If this procedure is not successful in removing the wax, the physician probably will have to use a cerumen spoon.[21,23]

Noise can be an occupational hazard that leads to permanent hearing impairment. It is the nurse's responsibility to teach persons working with noisy machinery ways to protect themselves. There are three basic types of hearing protection: (1) properly fitted earplugs to reduce noise levels up to 30 db, (2) canal caps to close off the auditory canals at the openings, and (3) earmuffs to seal out noise by covering the whole ear. Earmuffs can reduce noise levels by 15 to 30 db. The nurse should encourage persons who work in noise-filled environments to have an annual audiometric test.[28]

The nurse is often in the unique position of providing reassurance to the client and family. The family is a significant support system, but family members need help in learning how to communicate effectively with the client.

Following are some suggestions that can be used by both the nurse and the family to enhance communication with the hearing impaired client[14]:

1. Obtain the client's attention before speaking by calling the client's name or touching the arm.
2. Use a normal tone of voice. Shouting does not help, since sounds of the higher frequencies are the first ones lost.
3. Face the client directly so your lips can be seen in case the client can lip-read. For the same reason, do not cover your face with your hand. Wearing bright lipstick may make it easier for the client to observe lip movement.
4. Remember that facial expressions and body language take on even greater significance and provide cues to the person with a hearing impairment.
5. Reduce distracting noise in the environment when attempting conversation.
6. If you know the client hears better in one ear, speak to that ear.
7. Speak clearly and not too quickly. If the client appears to be confused, rephrase the statement using different words.
8. Use supplemental ways of communicating such as gestures and pen and paper.
9. If the client wears a hearing aid, check to see if the batteries are functioning, that it is not plugged with wax, and that it has been correctly placed in the ear.
10. Recommend a telephone amplifier attached to the receiver if it would be of assistance. Other telephone attachments are available such as the teletypewriter (TTY), which has a keyboard and a readable display. Telephone companies also have various devices available, such as the Signalman, which causes any lamp plugged into the unit to flash on and off when the phone is ringing.
11. Avoid the trap of directing conversation to the family and not including the client. The client who is excluded from conversation loses adult status.
12. Obtain feedback from the client to determine if he or she is following the conversation.

REHABILITATION TEAM INTERVENTIONS

The rehabilitation team may be involved in evaluating the extent of the client's hearing impairment and suggesting the best methods of intervention. Referrals to more specialized health professionals may be warranted based on the client's needs. Can the client be assisted with a hearing aid? If so, what type? Are there financial constraints in selecting a device? What are the client's capabilities? For example, a client with arthritic hands would not be able to handle a small hearing plug that fits into the ear. Would learning to lip-read be the best approach? Or would sign language be more appropriate? These are a few of the potential problems that the team may have to address.

Rehabilitation and counseling a client in lip-reading or using a hearing aid have been estimated to take from 3 to 12 weeks.[13] Certainly, a client's motivation will affect the course of rehabilitation. The client must understand the benefits and limitations of assistive devices. Hearing aids can be of great benefit to some persons. These devices are available in a variety of styles but are not perfect instruments. Hearing aids pick up all sounds in the environment but do not increase the clarity of sound. The rehabilitation team can encourage the client with a hearing aid to become familiar with it. Both the client and family must undergo an orientation phase and be willing to experiment. Often much money goes into purchasing a hearing aid that remains in the client's top drawer. The team therefore should be sure that the client understands the purpose of the aid, the correct method of using it, and how to maintain it.

OUTCOME CRITERIA

To evaluate the success of nursing and rehabilitation team interventions, criteria must be established before a plan is instituted. The following are some examples of outcomes for a client with a hearing impairment. At the conclusion of contact:
1. The client can explain the basic function of the ear.
2. The client can conserve the present level of hearing.
3. The client can demonstrate the application and care of assistive devices when applicable.
4. The client and family can use specific methods to enhance communication.
5. The client can function optimally with assistive devices.

SUMMARY

The responsibility for effective communication does not rest solely with the client who has impaired vision or hearing. The nurse and other team members, including the family, share this responsibility. The impact on a client who has a vision or hearing loss is physical and psychosocial. The nurse must be aware of the function of the eyes and ears and be able to assess function of these organs. The nurse also has to be sensitive to the meaning of an alteration in vision or hearing to the client and family.

TEST QUESTIONS

1. Which of the following statements is *true* regarding the layers of the eye?
   a. The transparent structure covering the iris and pupil is called the sclera.
   b. The middle layer, or uvea, is composed of the choroid, ciliary body, and iris.
   c. The innermost layer is called the sclera and contains a neuronal layer.
   d. The outermost layer, or nutritional layer, of the eyeball is called the retina.
2. A treatment for open-angle glaucoma may be:
   a. Miotic eye drops to constrict the pupil and the ciliary muscle
   b. An iridectomy to remove a section of the cornea
   c. Eyedrops to cure the disease and return previous vision
   d. Eyedrops to dilate the pupil and allow aqueous outflow
3. Of the following statements, which one is *true* regarding the surgical removal of a cataract?
   a. The intracapsular approach involves removing the lens intact.
   b. An iridectomy approach permits lens removal through the anterior chamber.
   c. Retinal extraction is the surgical approach of choice for lens removal.
   d. The extracapsular approach permits lens removal through a corneal incision.
4. A treatment for proliferative retinopathy is:
   a. Good diabetic control, which negates further need for surgical intervention
   b. Fluorescein angiography to reduce microaneurysms and retinal edema
   c. Laser therapy to burn minute openings on the retinal surface for vessel coagulation
   d. Phacoemulsification to break up occluded capillaries and restore vision
5. A retinal detachment may be treated by all of the following methods *except:*
   a. Indenting the retina so that it comes in contact with the choroid
   b. Bonding the choroid and retina together by inducing inflammation
   c. Performing a vitrectomy to prevent pulling of the retina from the choroid
   d. Sealing the retina to the choroid through the use of miotics
6. Optic neuritis may cause visual disturbances in the client with multiple sclerosis. A symptom of optic neuritis is:
   a. Retinal pain
   b. Blurred vision
   c. Crusting of the eyelids
   d. Tearing on the eyes

7. Which statement is *true* regarding hemi-anopsias?
   a. Homonymous hemianopsia refers to loss of vision in the temporal fields of both eyes.
   b. Defective vision or blindness in half of the visual field.
   c. Bitemporal hemianopsia is usually produced by rapidly growing tumors with total vision loss.
   d. Attitudinal hemianopsia affects both eyes and is generally caused by trauma.

8. In collecting subjective data to determine a client's visual status, the nurse is aware that:
   a. A yellowed or reddened sclera is considered a normal finding.
   b. The Snellen chart measures both peripheral and central vision.
   c. Pupil size varies with the color of the iris and with age.
   d. The upper eyelid normally covers all of the iris and pupil.

9. A nursing intervention for the client with visual alteration may be eyedrop administration. The nurse:
   a. Asks the client to tilt the head backward and look downward
   b. Pulls on the client's upper lid to form a small pocket
   c. Places an eyedrop on the surface of the sclera for dispersion
   d. Washes the hands before and after performing eyedrop instillation

10. When instructing the client or family in eye care, the nurse teaches about:
   a. Cleaning contact lenses with a special solution, since mucus may harden and interfere with vision
   b. Making good use of white against white since this combination can be seen more clearly
   c. Glaucoma and hypertension being closely associated since both are characterized by increasing pressure
   d. Saving eyesight for clients with low vision by not engaging in sewing or other close work

11. A nursing intervention for the client with visual field loss as in hemianopsias includes:
   a. Orienting to the environment and approaching from the affected side
   b. Teaching to scan with the eyes using horizontal and vertical sweeping motions
   c. Using prisms that displace central vision objects toward the center of the prism
   d. Positioning so that the affected side faces toward the door

12. A rehabilitation nursing intervention for a newly blind person is to:
   a. Reorganize the person's life space to promote independence
   b. Keep doors slightly open so the person may discriminate among sounds
   c. Walk about one-half step ahead of the person who then grasps the nurse's elbow
   d. Touch the person on the arm or shoulder before initiating conversation

13. Which of the following statements is *true* concerning parts of the ear?
   a. The tympanic membrane separates the middle from the inner ears.
   b. The auditory canal is approximately 6.25 cm (2½ inches) long and provides a passageway to the eardrum.
   c. The inner ear contains the cochlea, which houses the organ of Corti, the sense organ of hearing.
   d. The ossicles are located in the external ear and transmit sound waves to the cochlea.

14. The transmission of sound normally occurs by:
   a. Converting air molecules into electrical energy
   b. Preventing the ossicles from vibrating and disturbing the perilymph
   c. Converting electrical energy to mechanical energy in the semicircular canals
   d. Transmitting energy from the stapes to the oval window

15. In comparing conductive versus sensorineural hearing loss, the nurse knows that sensorineural loss:
   a. Results from prolonged exposure to intense noise or damage to cranial nerve VIII
   b. Is usually treated with use of a hearing aid to provide amplification
   c. Results from damage to the external auditory canal or the middle ear
   d. Has no organic basis and is usually caused by emotional factors

16. In collecting objective data to assess a client's hearing status, the nurse knows:

a. The Rinne test is used to differentiate between a conductive and a sensorineural hearing loss.
b. The color of the external auditory canal normally ranges from light pink to bright red.
c. The watch tick test produces a sound above the range needed to hear speech.
d. The Weber test is designed to compare hearing by air and bone conduction.

17. A nursing intervention that may be ordered to enhance the client's communication is an ear irrigation. In performing this procedure the nurse:
    a. Uses an irrigation solution at room temperature
    b. Injects the solution down the center of the external auditory canal
    c. Removes impacted grains to prevent infection
    d. Pulls the auricle upward and backward for an adult

18. To enhance communication with the hearing impaired client, the nurse instructs the family to:
    a. Exclude the client from noisy conversations to avoid embarrassment
    b. Shout in a loud voice to capitalize on the client's residual hearing
    c. Obtain attention before speaking by calling the client by name
    d. Increase distracting environmental noise when attempting conversation

Answers: 1. b, 2. a, 3. a, 4. c, 5. d, 6. b, 7. b, 8. c, 9. d, 10. a, 11. b, 12. c, 13. c, 14. d, 15. a, 16. c, 17. d, 18. c.

LEARNING ACTIVITIES

1. Place cotton or earplugs in your ears and attempt to listen to your favorite radio station or a special television program. Discuss or record how you felt during that time. How long were you able to tolerate impaired hearing?
2. Ask a colleague or fellow student to blindfold you, and then with assistance, attempt to perform an everyday activity such as going to a cafeteria for lunch. How did others respond to you? How did this make you feel? What was the most difficult obstacle you had to overcome?
3. Arrange to visit a local community agency that assists persons who have visual or hearing impairments. Investigate the services provided and criteria for qualifying for these services.

REFERENCES

1. Anthony CP and Thibodeau GA: Textbook of anatomy and physiology, ed 11, St Louis, 1983, The CV Mosby Co.
2. Bates B: A guide to physical examination, ed 4, Philadelphia, 1987, JB Lippincott Co.
3. Davson H: Physiology of the eye, ed 4, New York, 1980, Academic Press, Inc.
4. Fonda GE: Management of low vision, New York, 1981, Thieme-Statton, Inc.
5. Freese AS: Glaucoma—diagnosis, treatment, prevention. Pub no 568, New York, 1979, Public Affairs Committee.
6. Gaston H and Elkington AR: Ophthalmology for nurses, Dover, NH, 1986, Croom Helm.
7. Gordon M: Nursing diagnosis: process and application, ed 2, New York, 1987, McGraw-Hill Book Co.
8. Havener WH: Synopsis of ophthalmology, ed 6, St Louis, 1984, The CV Mosby Co.
9. Hearing loss: hope through research. Pub no 82-157, Bethesda, Md, 1982, National Institutes of Health.
10. Johnson JJ and Cryan M: Homonymous hemianopsia: assessment and nursing management, Am J Nurs 79:2132, 1979.
11. Jose RT: Understanding low vision, New York, 1983, American Foundation for the Blind.
12. Kapperud MJ: The aging eye: a guide for nurses, Minneapolis, 1983, The Minnesota Society for the Prevention of Blindness and Preservation of Hearing.
13. McCartney JH and Nader G: How to help your patient cope with hearing loss, Geriatrics 34:69, March 1979.
14. McNamee C: Communicating, The Canadian Nurse 74:29, March 1978.
15. Mellor CM: Aids for the 80s—what they are and what they do, New York, 1981, American Foundation for the Blind.
16. Meyerhoff WL and others: Diagnosis and management of hearing loss, Philadelphia, 1984, WB Saunders Co.
17. Miller D: Ophthalmology: the essentials, Boston, 1979, Houghton Mifflin Professional Publishers.
18. Monk HB: Examining the external eye, Nurs. '80 10:58, May 1980.
19. Price SA and Wilson LC: Pathophysiology: clinical concepts of disease processes, ed 3, New York, 1986, McGraw-Hill Book Co.
20. Reinecke RD: Loss of vision: eye pain. In Blacklow RS, editor: MacBryde's signs and symptoms. New York, 1983, JB Lippincott Co.

21. Riley MA: Nursing care of the client with ear, nose, and throat disorders, New York, 1987, Springer Publishing Co.
22. Ryan WJ: The nurse and the communicatively impaired adult, New York, 1982, Springer Publishing Co.
23. Saunders WH and others: Nursing care in eye, ear, nose, and throat disorders, ed 4, St Louis, 1979, The CV Mosby Co.
24. Smith JF and Nachazel DP: Ophthalmologic nursing, Boston, 1980, Little, Brown & Co.
25. Stern EJ: Helping the person with low vision, Am J Nurs 80:1788, 1980.
26. Trevor-Roper PD: The eye and its disorders, ed 2, Boston, 1984, Blackwell Scientific Publications.
27. Wade AS: Occupational therapy for problems with special senses: blindness and deafness. In Hopkins HL and Smith HD, editors: Willard and Spockman's occupational therapy, Philadelphia, 1978, JB Lippincott Co.
28. What you should know about on-the-job hearing conservation. A scriptographic booklet, South Deerfield, Mass, 1983, Channing L Bete, Co, Inc.

ADDITIONAL READINGS

DiPietro L: Deaf patients: special needs, special responses, Washington, DC, 1979, The National Academy, Gallaudet College.

McKenzie GJ and others: The special senses, ed 2, New York, 1986, Churchill Livingstone, Inc.

Pesci BR: When patient's problem is really poor vision, RN 86:22, Oct 1986.

Schein JD and Miller MH: Rehabilitation and management of auditory disorders. In Kottke FJ, Stillwell GK, and Lehmann JF, editors: Krusen's handbook of physical medicine and rehabilitation, ed 3, Philadelphia, 1982, WB Saunders Co.

You and your deaf patients, Washington, DC, 1978, Gallaudet College.

CHAPTER 18

Movement

Margaret Kraszewski Umhauer

OBJECTIVES

After completing Chapter 18, the reader will be able to:

1. Describe the structure and function of bones, muscles, joints and nerves in relation to the production of movement.

2. Assess a client's physical movement.

3. Formulate nursing diagnoses related to physical mobility.

4. Develop goals with the client and family that foster optimum physical movement.

5. Prevent the complications associated with immobilization.

6. Describe correct body alignment in various positions in and out of bed.

7. Discuss positioning aids available to support the client.

8. List types of mechanical beds available for the client with impaired physical mobility.

9. Describe the benefits of various exercise programs designed for the client with impaired physical mobility.

10. Determine methods for moving dependent and partially dependent clients in bed.

11. Describe methods for transferring dependent clients out of bed.

12. Identify transfer technique modifications for clients able to assist in a transfer.

13. Discuss the components of a preambulation program.

14. Describe gait training methods and various types of equipment used to assist walking.

15. Identify concerns unique to clients with lower limb bracing.

16. Identify concerns unique to clients with lower limb prostheses.

17. Discuss wheelchairs as an alternative mode of mobility.

18. Identify health teaching required for clients experiencing impaired physical mobility and their families.

19. Describe the role of other rehabilitation team members in relation to working with the client with impaired physical mobility.

20. List outcome criteria appropriate for the client with impaired physical mobility.

The ability to move about in our own environment is the key to performing activities of daily living independently. Activities of daily living facilitated by physical movement range from self-care activities such as bathing and dressing to fulfilling social roles such as homemaker by performing household tasks. Movement occurs in increasing complexity when sliding from one side of a bed to the other, transferring from the bed to a chair, ambulating from one room to another, or traveling from home to work. The capacity for movement provides an avenue for communication in addition to language. Movement of facial muscles to create a smile communicates pleasure or delight. A rigid posture may indicate a well-controlled, tense feeling. Love or affection can be demonstrated through touching hands or a hug. A person's walk or gait can express a variety of emotions, ranging from dejection to euphoria to anger.

NORMAL PHYSIOLOGY OF MOVEMENT

Movement consists of the action of muscles upon bones and joints. It may involve an involuntary, reflex process or a process of conscious, deliberate choice. The review of anatomy in this chapter focuses on bones, muscles, joints, and nerve pathways for producing voluntary and involuntary motions.

Skeletal Structure and Function

The skeleton, or underlying bony framework of the body, serves multiple purposes. Since it is rigid, it provides humans with form and shape. It also protects vital organs such as the brain encased in the rigid skull and the heart and lungs surrounded by ribs and vertebrae. The skeleton functions as the hemoregulatory system by producing red blood cells with the marrow of the long bones. Movement occurs when the various muscles contract upon the bones. The bones also provide a storage area for salts and minerals.

The human skeleton consists of 206 bones of various shapes and sizes. It can be divided into the axial skeleton and the appendicular skeleton. The axial skeleton comprises the skull, spinal vertebrae, ribs, sternum, and hyoid bones. The appendicular skeleton consists of the other bony structures of the upper and lower extremities.

Bone is a porous rather than a solid substance. The pores contain living cells and blood vessels necessary for maintaining the integrity of the system. The degree of porosity determines whether a bone is categorized as spongy or compact. Spongy bone, also referred to as cancellous bone, contains many large spaces filled with marrow. Compact, or dense, bone contains few spaces and is generally deposited in a thin layer over the spongy bone.

Spongy bone consists of an irregular network of thin plates of bone called trabeculae. The spaces between the trabeculae are filled with red marrow, which is responsible for producing new blood cells (hematopoiesis). Osteocytes, mature bone cells that can no longer produce new bony growth, are contained within the trabeculae. Examples of spongy bone include the sternum and other flat bones of the skeleton.

Compact bone consists of a series of concentric rings and differs markedly in structure from spongy bone. Blood vessels and nerves from the periosteum, the dense, white fibrous covering of the bone, penetrate the compact bone through a structure known as Volkmann's canals. The blood vessels of these canals connect with blood vessels and nerves of the medullary, or marrow cavity, and those of the haversian canals.

The haversian canals run lengthwise throughout the bone and are surrounded by lamillae, which are rings of hard, calcified material. The osteocytes are found in small spaces called lacunae, which are located between the lamillae. The lacunae are connected with each other and with the haversian canals by very minute channels called canaliculi. Each haversian canal with the surrounding lamillae, lacunae, osteocytes, and canaliculi is called a haversian system, or osteon. Within the osteon, bone tissue is constantly created and reabsorbed. New bone is produced by osteoblasts through the process of ossification. The exact mechanism by which ossification occurs is not known. It does, however, involve deposition of mineral salts, principally calcium, within a bone matrix. Osteoblasts are multinuclear cells involved in bone destruction, resorption, and remodeling.

Bone formation and resorption are kept in balance through the regulation of several factors, including local stress, vitamin D, parathyroid hormone, and calcitonin. Local stress or weight-bearing stimulates local bone resorption and formation and also may result in extensive remodeling. Weight-bearing bones are the thickest and strongest in the skeleton. Deformities may be improved through weight-bearing activities. Loss of weight-bearing or stress through immobilization or bed rest results in the loss of calcium from the bone. Vitamin D increases the amount of circulating calcium by enhancing absorption of calcium from the gastrointestinal tract and by mobilizing calcium from the bone.

Parathyroid hormone and calcitonin are the primary hormonal regulators of calcium balance. Calcitonin increases the production of bone. Parathyroid regulates the concentration of serum calcium in part by promoting movement of calcium from the bone.

Bones can be classified according to shape. The five major classifications are long, short, flat, irregular, and sesamoid. The long bones consist of a shaft known as the diaphysis and two extremities known as epiphyses. The diaphysis consists of compact bone that flares at either end into the metaphysis. The metaphysis consists of spongy bone. The femur and the radius are examples of long bones.

Short bones, such as the carpals and tarsals, consist of spongy tissue covered by a thin layer of compact bone. The flat bones, such as the skull and scapula, consist of spongy bone encased in two flat plates of compact bone. The flat bones protect soft body parts and serve as large surfaces for muscle attachment. The vertebrae and ossicles of the ear are examples of irregular bones. The sesamoid bones, such as the patella, are located adjacent to joints and are encased in tendons and muscle fascia. These bones increase the lever capacity of muscles.

The junction between two bones is known as an articulation, or joint. Joints may be fixed or vary in degrees of mobility. The major types of joints are synarthroses, amphiarthroses, and diarthroses. The synarthroses are fixed joints, such as the skull. Amphiarthroses permit slight movement at the articulation. An example is the symphysis pubis. Joints that are freely movable and permit the widest range of position change and motion are the diarthroses or synovial joints. Most of the joints in the body are freely movable.

The diarthroses consist of an articular cavity enclosed by a capsule of fibrous articular cartilage. The cavity is lined with synovial fluid for joint lubrication and for cartilage nourishment. Ligaments reinforce the articular capsule and help to limit motion. Cartilage covers the ends of opposing bones, providing a smooth surface so that bone ends can glide over one another. Some joints are protected by disks located between articular cartilage. Muscles are important stabilizers and maintain the firm contact of articular surfaces.

The synovial joints may be classified according to the shape of the articulating surfaces of the bones: pivot, hinge, saddle, condyloid, gliding, and ball-and-socket joints. The pivot joint consists of rounded, pointed, or concave surfaces that fit into a shallow depression. The movement at pivot joints is rotation. Examples of the pivot joint are the atlantoaxial and radioulnar joints.

The hinge joint consists of a spool-like surface that fits into a concave surface and permits flexion and extension movements. Examples include the elbow, knee, ankle, and interphalangeal joints.

The saddle joint consists of opposing concave and convex surfaces. The joint is capable of flexion and extension, as well as abduction and adduction movements. The carpometacarpal joint of the thumb is a saddle joint.

A condyloid joint is composed of an oval-shaped condyle that fits into an elliptical cavity. The radiocarpal joint at the wrist is a condyloid, or ellipsoidal, joint. It is capable of flexion and extension, as well as abduction and adduction movements.

Gliding joints such as the intercarpal and intertarsal joints in the hand and foot consist of flat articulating surfaces. These joints produce motions of flexion, extension, abduction, and adduction.

The ball-and-socket joint is the most movable joint. It consists of a ball-like head that fits into a cuplike depression. Ball-and-socket joints are located at the shoulder and at the hip. Movements of flexion, extension, abduction, adduction, and rotation occur at ball-and-socket joints. A summary of the major joints of the body, their classification, and range of movement is presented in Table 18-1.

Muscle Structure and Function

Muscle tissue constitutes 40% to 50% of total body weight. Muscle tissue is characterized by irritability, contractility, extensibility, and elasticity. In other words, muscle tissue is capable of responding to stimuli, of shortening and thickening, and of stretching and returning to its original shape after being stimulated. Muscles produce motion, maintain posture, and produce heat through contraction. The three types of muscle tissue are skeletel, visceral, and cardiac. The focus of this chapter is skeletal, or striated, muscle.

Skeletal muscles are attached to bones, connective tissue, other muscles, soft tissue, or skin by tendons or aponeuroses. Tendons are cords of fibrous connective tissue; aponeuroses are broad, flat sheets of connective tissue.

The muscles are composed of parallel groups

TABLE 18-1 _____
Classification of joints and movements

Name	Type	Movements
Atlantoaxial	Pivot	Pivoting or partial rotation of head
Shoulder	Ball and socket	Flexion, extension, abduction, adduction, rotation, circumduction
Elbow	Hinge	Flexion, extension
Radioulnar	Pivot	Supination, pronation
Wrist	Condyloid	Flexion, extension, abduction (ulnar deviation), adduction (radial deviation)
Carpal	Gliding	Gliding
Hand		
Metacarpals	Hinge	Flexion, extension, abduction, adduction
Thumb	Saddle	Flexion, extension, abduction, adduction, rotation, circumduction, opposition
Hip	Ball and socket	Flexion, extension, abduction, adduction, rotation, circumduction
Knee	Hinge	Flexion, extension
Ankle	Hinge	Dorsiflexion, plantar flexion
Foot		
Between tarsals	Gliding	Inversion, eversion
Between metatarsals, phalanges	Hinge	Flexion, extension, abduction, adduction

of muscle cells referred to as fasciculi and are encased in fascia, which is a fibrous tissue. Muscles may consist of both red and white muscle fibers. Red muscle fibers contain a large amount of myoglobin, a hemoglobin-like protein pigment that transports oxygen from the blood capillaries to the muscle cells for metabolism. White muscle fiber contains little myoglobin and is characterized by quick extended periods of contraction.

A sarcomere is the contractile unit of a muscle. When a nerve impulse reaches the motor endplate located in a sarcomere, the neuron releases acetylcholine, causing an electrical charge in the sarcolemma of the muscle fiber. This charge travels over the sarcolemma and is eventually conveyed to the sarcoplasmic reticulum. When the impulse reaches the sarcoplasmic reticulum, calcium ions are released from storage into the surrounding sarcoplasm. The calcium ions move to myosin cross bridges and activate the myosin. Myosin catalyzes the breakdown of adenosine triphosphate (ATP) into adenosine phosphate and phosphate (ADP and P). The calcium ions also permit the tropomyosin-troponin complex to split from the thin myofilament so that the free receptor site of action is permitted to attach to the myosin cross bridge. The energy released from

the breakdown of ATP is used for the attachment and movement of the myosin cross bridges and thus the sliding of myofilaments. As the thin myofilaments slide past the thick myofilaments, they are drawn toward each other, causing the sarcomere to shorten and the muscle to contract. When the calcium concentration in the sarcomere falls at the end of the nerve impulse, the myosin and actin filaments no longer interact, and the sarcomere returns to its original resting state.

ATP is synthesized by skeletal muscle from oxidation of glucose to water and carbon dioxide during low levels of activity. During high levels of activity, sufficient oxygen may not be available, and the glucose is metabolized primarily to lactic acid, as well as some ATP. Therefore, during high levels of activity, increasingly large amounts of glucose are required and must be supplied by glycogen stored in the muscle. Muscle fatigue may occur from the rapid rate of work of the muscle, resulting in depletion of glycogen and energy and in the accumulation of lactic acid. Creatinine phosphate stored in the muscle cell also may be converted to ATP when necessary.

At any one time, some cells in a muscle are contracted while others are relaxed, resulting in muscle tone. Tone is a requirement for maintaining normal posture. If there is less than normal muscle tone, the muscles are characterized as flaccid or flabby and floppy. If the flaccid tone continues over a long period of time, muscle atrophy may occur with consequent loss of muscle mass. Such conditions may result from neurological or muscular disorders or from prolonged inactivity, including bed rest. Spasticity occurs when the muscle tone is greater than normal and causes dysfunctional posture and positioning. Again, neurological disorders or muscle diseases may be responsible. Contracture formation is a serious consequence of spasticity.

Muscle fibers can produce either isotonic or isometric movement of the muscle. In isotonic contraction the muscle shortens, with no increase in tension within the muscle. In isometric contraction the length of the muscle remains constant, but the tension or force generated by the muscles is increased. Isometric contractions do not result in body movement, whereas isotonic contractions do produce movement.

In every movement, there is a prime mover, or agonist, causing a particular movement. Muscles assisting the prime mover are known as synergists. Muscles opposing a prime mover are known as antagonists. The antagonist relaxes while the prime mover contracts.

In flexion of the forearm the biceps is the prime mover, or agonist, and contracts. The antagonist in this case, the triceps, relaxes while the synergists, the deltoid and the greater pectoral, hold the arm and shoulder in a position suitable for flexing the forearm by also contracting. Synergists assume a special importance in the paralyzed individual who may be able to retrain synergists to perform the function of a weakened primary mover.

Skeletal muscles derive their names in several ways. These muscles may be named according to the action produced (flexor), location (femoral), or point of insertion or attachment (sternocleidomastoid). The name of the muscle also may indicate the shape of the muscle body (trapezius), the number of muscle divisions (biceps and triceps), and the direction of the muscle fibers (rectus or transversus).

Nervous System Structure and Function

Voluntary motor activity involves the cerebral cortex, the descending pathways of the spinal cord, and the anterior horn of the spinal cord. Voluntary motor impulses originate in the motor strip just before the central sulcus of the brain. The impulses travel through the hemispheres to merge in the internal capsule and then continue downward through the brainstem. When the pyramidal or upper motor neuron fibers reach the medulla oblongata, the majority decussate, or cross to the opposite side, to descend through the spinal cord in the lateral white column known as the lateral corticospinal tract. In this way, the motor cortex of the right side of the brain controls muscles on the left side of the body and vice versa. On reaching the spinal cord, the impulses synapse with association neurons, which then synapse with neurons in the anterior gray horn known as the lower motor neurons of the cord. The lower motor neurons exit at all levels of the cord to terminate in skeletal muscle (Figure 18-1).

About 15% of the upper motor neurons do not cross at the medulla but descend on the same side to the anterior white column, becoming part of the direct, or uncrossed, corticospinal tract. The fibers of upper motor neurons cross at the spinal cord level to the side opposite the origin of their pathway before synapsing with lower motor neurons. The anterior corticospinal tract provides skeletal muscle impulses primarily for muscles that control the neck and part of the trunk.

The upper motor neuron therefore is the only path between the cerebral cortex and cranial nerve nuclei and the spinal cord. The lower motor neuron is the neuron that actually terminates in a skeletal muscle. Since it is the final common pathway, loss of function of the lower motor neuron through disease or trauma results in flaccid paralysis or loss of both reflex and voluntary movement. If injury or disease occurs in the upper motor neuron pathway, the result is continued muscle contraction evidenced by spastic tone and exaggerated reflexes.

Clients who experience a cerebrovascular accident may become hemiplegic as a result of upper motor neuron damage. Hemiplegia is loss of function of the arm and leg on one side of the body. Clients who have experienced poliomyelitis develop a lower motor neuron flaccid paralysis because the anterior spinal cord is affected. Both upper and lower motor paralyses may occur in spinal cord injury in which both the descending pathways and anterior horn cells are disrupted. When both legs are paralyzed, the resulting condition is referred to as paraplegia; when both arms and both legs are paralyzed, the condition is referred to as quadriplegia.

The extrapyramidal system provides input from the cerebellum and basal ganglia to the muscles, resulting in smooth, accurate, and coordi-

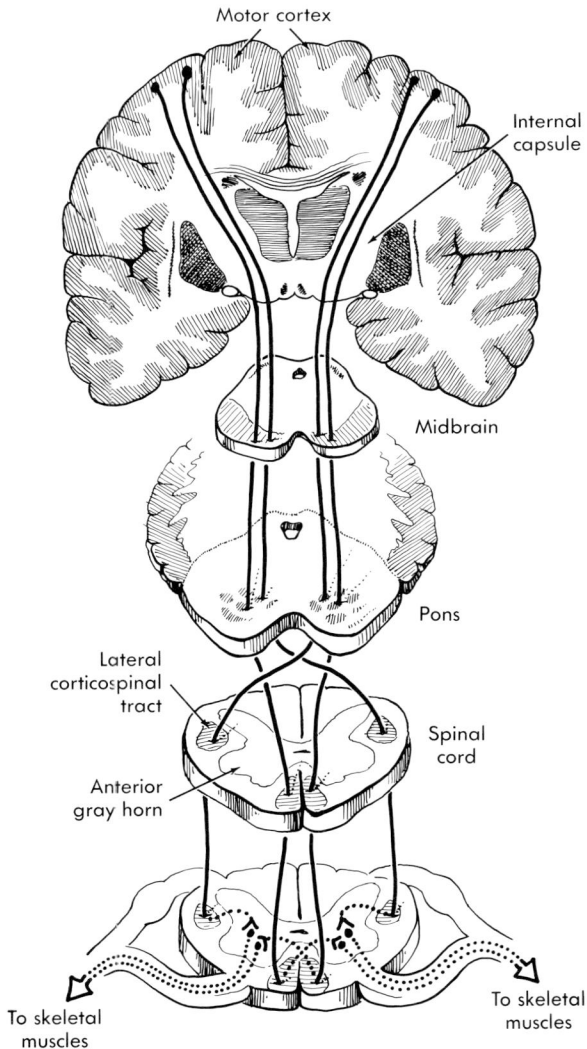

Figure 18-1
Voluntary motor impulses from cortex to skeletal muscles. Impulses arising in cortex descend directly through anterior corticospinal tract or cross at level of medulla and descend through lateral corticospinal tract to anterior horn cells.

nated muscular activity. Impulses that arise in the cerebellum and basal ganglia are transmitted downward through the white matter of the spinal cord. The principal extrapyramidal tracts include the rubrospinal, tectospinal, and vestibulospinal tracts. Dysfunction in the cerebellum or in the extrapyramidal tracts may result in loss of coordinated, controlled voluntary movements. Activities may become disjointed and choppy. Coarse tremor may appear. Gait may be ataxic, staggering, and wide based.

Dysfunction in the basal ganglia or extrapyramidal pathways associated with the basal ganglia results in disturbances of posture and movement and marked muscular rigidity. Coarse tremor may occur. Other involuntary movements, such as athetosis or chorea also may develop. Athetosis is characterized by slow, writhing, twisting motions, and chorea is manifested by spasmodic, grotesque motions of the trunk and extremities with facial grimacing.

NURSING ASSESSMENT

The nurse takes a history and performs a physical examination to obtain data and formulate nursing diagnoses. The specific assessment for the musculoskeletal system is illustrated by using a case study.

History

Mrs. A.K., a 58-year-old white female, is interviewed by the rehabilitation nurse. Her chief complaint is joint pain in the right elbow. She describes the pain as a grinding, stretching sensation that varies from moderate to severe intensity. The pain has been periodic over the last 10 years and increases in severity at night, in cold weather, and during periods of dampness. Mrs. A.K. notes that the joint pain occurs more frequently when she is under emotional stress. To alleviate the pain, she takes two Tylenol tablets and applies a wintergreen-based ointment and a warm flannel. She sometimes experiences similar joint pains in the wrist and fingers of the left arm and in the right hip. When she has right elbow joint pain, Mrs. A.K. also has a sensation of swelling or fullness in the forearm and complains that her skin in that area "feels too tight."

In answering questions during the personal history, Mrs. A.K. reveals that she has been married for 40 years and that her spouse is alive and in good health. Their present income is restricted to Social Security payments.

Her mother complained of similar joint pains throughout her later life, and Mrs. A.K. has two first cousins who have joint disease. One is wheelchair bound following a total hip replacement; the other walks only with assistance of a walker. Her two sisters do not experience joint pain or discomfort of any type. Mrs. A.K. lives in western New York and is exposed to cold, damp winters and springs, as well as muggy summers.

Mrs. A.K. does not smoke and drinks only socially. The only medications she takes are acetaminophen (Tylenol) for joint pain and an occasional headache. She complains of difficulty falling asleep and awakening with joint pain once or twice each night when experiencing a flare-up. During a flare-up of right elbow joint pain, Mrs. A.K. sometimes needs assistance with dressing and other daily activities such as meal preparation and housekeeping. Since her primary occupation for the last 40 years has been homemaker, Mrs. A.K. finds this dependence very frustrating.

Mrs. A.K. lives with her husband in a one-level, rented flat. They have a washing machine but no dryer. Wet laundry must be dried on clotheslines outside or in the laundromat down the street. Mrs. A.K. is very active in church and family activities. She enjoys reading and crocheting and would like to learn to bowl.

In determining the client's previous experiences with illness, immunization status, allergies, and injuries, it is noted that Mrs. A.K. has had an unremarkable childhood history. She suffers occasionally from hay fever, but has no other allergies. She has had the usual childhood diseases of mumps, measles, rubella, and chickenpox. Her immunizations are complete and current. She has experienced three pregnancies resulting in three live births. Her children are a 39-year-old son, and 35- and 38-year-old daughters. Mrs. A.K. underwent gallbladder surgery 3 years ago. She has no recall of any trauma or injury, no fractures or sprains.

The review of systems is begun with questions regarding general health and proceeds to specific questions regarding each body system. Specific questions included in the musculoskeletal system review relate to muscle pain, swelling, lameness, weakness, joint discomfort, leg cramps, arthritis,

fracture, sprains, or dislocations. Information regarding orthopedic appliances and treatment of congenital conditions or trauma also is gathered. Questions related to the neurological system include inquiries about any episodes of unconsciousness, difficulty in walking, decreasing strength in arms or legs, weakness or paralysis, tremors or convulsions, and pain or numbness. The nurse also asks the client if episodes of anxiety, nervousness, confusion, forgetfulness, or nightmares have occurred. The nurse finds that Mrs. A.K.'s review of systems is mostly unremarkable. She does complain, however, of swelling in the lower extremities during the summer and intermittent leg cramps at night.

Physical Assessment

The nurse's physical assessment includes general impression, range of joint motion, muscle tone and strength, deep tendon reflexes, proprioception and position sense, balance and coordination, and gait assessment.

General impression

During the initial interview, the nurse assesses the client's outward appearance. The client's posture is noted. Stooped shoulders, asymmetry, unevenness of length of extremities, absence of digits, and abnormalities of the hands, feet, arms, or legs can affect mobility. Swelling of extremities, asymmetry of facial expression, and involuntary movements or tremors are also noted, as well as weakness of extremities during activities of walking, sitting, rising, writing, or dressing. The nurse is sensitive to clues that some or all of these movements may precipitate pain. After obtaining a general impression, the nurse begins the physical assessment, using the skills of inspection and palpation.

Range of joint motion

Each joint has a specific range of motion that can be described as normal, full, limited, or severely limited and measured in degrees using an instrument called a goniometer. The goniometer resembles a protractor but is specifically designed to measure range of joint motion (Figure 18-2). Several types of goniometers are available; at present, however, there is some discussion about the intertester reliability of goniometric mea-

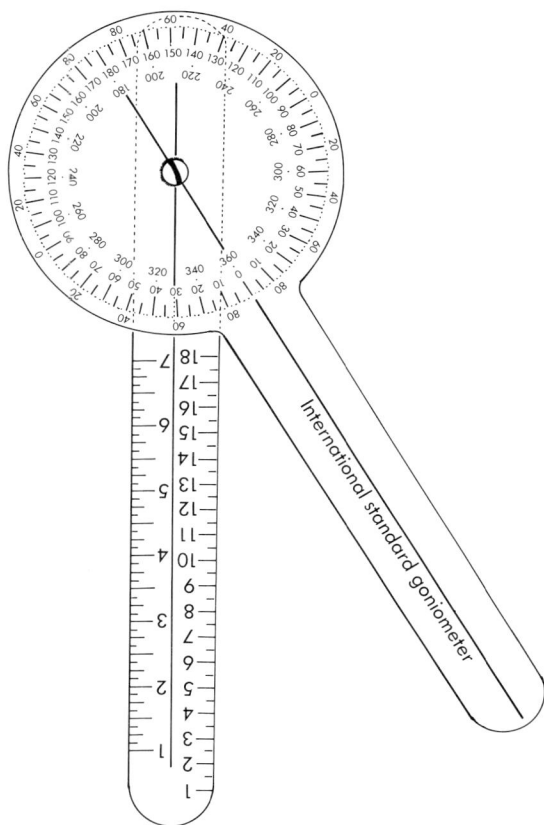

Figure 18-2
Goniometer is used to measure range of joint motion.

surements.[24, 33] Within a given institution, protocols should be established to increase the reliability between testers.

While assessing range of motion, the nurse notes any deviation or limitation of normal range, including joint instability (dislocation or subluxation), or joint stiffness or fixation (ankylosis). Swelling, heat, or tenderness of the joints is noted. Bogginess and bony enlargement are assessed. The nurse palpates for crepitus or a grating sensation while taking an extremity through the range of motion, as well as notes muscle tone and strength, and condition of skin, subcutaneous tissue, and muscle size and shape.

When assessing range of joint motion, the nurse proceeds from head to toe. The jaw or temporomandibular joint is palpated for tenderness or swelling. The client is asked to open her mouth, and the range of movement is observed. Mrs. A.K.'s neck is inspected for deformity or abnormal posture. The muscles of the cervical spine and the trapezius are carefully palpated for tenderness. She is asked to move the neck through the range of motion. Normal range of motion is 45 degrees of forward flexion, 55 degrees of extension, 40 degrees of lateral flexion, and 70 degrees of rotation. Forward flexion is tested by asking the client to touch her chin to her chest; extension by putting her head back; lateral flexion by touching her ear to the corresponding shoulder, and rotation by turning her head to the left and then to the right.

The trunk of the body is commonly inspected while the client is standing. For the posterior inspection, the nurse observes the spine for lateral curvatures such as scoliosis. The trunk is inspected from the side to detect kyphosis and lordosis. Kyphosis is an exaggerated curvature of the thoracic spine commonly referred to as hunchback. Lordosis is an exaggerated curvature of the lumbar spine commonly referred to as swayback. Scoliosis is an exaggerated lateral curvature creating a C or S shape on the client's back. The nurse also notes any differences in the height of the shoulders and iliac crests. The paravertebral muscles are palpated for tenderness and pain. Normal range of motion of the spine consists of 75 to 90 degrees of forward flexion, 30 degrees of extension, 35 degrees of lateral flexion, and 30 degrees of rotation.

To assess the range of forward flexion, the nurse asks Mrs. A.K. to touch her toes while bending from the waist. Symmetry of movement and the distance of the fingers from the toes is noted. If the client has normal range of forward flexion, the rounding of the lumbar concavity is noted. To assess the range of spinal extension, the nurse stands in back of the client and asks her to lean back from the pelvis. Lateral flexion is tested by instructing her to lean to each side, rotation by asking her to turn her shoulders to the right and then to the left while keeping the rest of the body straight. In examining the extremities, all joints are inspected from anterior and posterior aspects, right is always compared to left, and proximal is compared to distal to determine asymmetry and weakness.

The shoulder girdle and joint are inspected for swelling, deformity, or atrophy. The sternoclavicular joint, the acromioclavicular joint, and the shoulder joint itself are palpated for tenderness. Normal range of motion for the shoulder is 50 degrees of extension, 180 degrees of forward flexion, 90 degrees of internal and external rotation, 50 degrees of adduction, and 180 degrees of abduction.

To test shoulder extension, the nurse asks Mrs. A.K. to swing both arms behind as if reaching back for something. To test shoulder flexion, she is asked to raise both arms above the head. The nurse assesses external rotation at the shoulder by asking the client to place her hands behind the neck with elbows out to the side. The nurse assesses internal rotation at the shoulder by asking the client to place her hands behind the waist in the small of the back. The client's ability to adduct the shoulder is tested by asking her to touch the right hand to the left hand while crossing extended arms in front of the body. The process is reversed to determine adduction of the left shoulder. To test shoulder abduction, the client is asked to bring her arms away from the body as far as possible. The elbow is inspected and palpated while flexed at 70 degrees. The nurse supports the client's elbow with one hand while palpating with the other. The olecranon process and grooves and the lateral epicondyle are palpated for tenderness, swelling, or nodules. The normal range of motion at the elbow is 0 degrees of extension to 160 degrees of forward flexion. Elbow range is tested by asking the client to bend and straighten the arms at the elbow. The radioulnar joint also may be tested at this time. The nurse asks the client to keep both arms at the sides with the elbows flexed. The client then turns the palms up (supination) and down (pronation). Normally supination and pronation each have a range of 90 degrees.

The bones of the hands and wrists are inspected for swelling, redness, nodules, deformity, atrophy, or fasciculations. Fasciculations are involuntary twitchings of isolated bundles of muscles fibers. The joints of the wrist and hand, including fingers, are palpated for tenderness, swelling, bogginess, or enlargement. The normal range of motion at the wrist includes 70 degrees of extension, 90 degrees of flexion, 20 degrees of radial deviation, and 55 degrees of ulnar deviation.

At the metacarpophalangeal joint of the hand, 30 degrees of hyperextension and 90 degrees of flexion are possible. The proximal interphalangeal joints are in the neutral position at 0 degrees when extended and 120 degrees when flexed. The distal interphalangeal joint also is in the neutral position at 0 degrees when extended but flexes for a maximum of 80 degrees. The hands and fingers can be tested at the same time. To assess the range of the joints of the hands and digits, the nurse instructs the client to extend and spread the fingers of each hand and to make a fist with the thumbs across the knuckles. The client is instructed to bend the wrist downward and upward and then to move it toward midline (radial deviation) and away from midline (ulnar deviation).

Next the hips are inspected while the client is in the standing position described previously. Observations are made for deformity or asymmetry at the iliac crest. Palpation over the joint can determine the presence of crepitus, nodules, or atrophy. The normal range of motion at the hip is 90 degrees of flexion with the knee straight and 15 degrees of hyperextension. If the knee is flexed, flexion of the hip increases to 120 degrees. The hip adducts to 30 degrees and abducts 45 degrees. The normal range for internal rotation at the hip is 40 degrees; for external rotation, it is 45 degrees. To assess range of motion at the hip, the client is placed in the supine position. The nurse instructs the client to raise each leg separately with the knee straight and then with the knee bent. To assess hip hyperextension, the client is placed in the prone position and asked to lift each leg separately off the surface of the bed. Adduction can be tested by asking the client to cross right leg over left and vice versa. To determine the degree of abduction, the nurse asks the client to slide the leg toward the outer edge of the bed or cot. Rotation may be ascertained as the client bends at knee and hip. As the nurse gently pulls the knee laterally, the hip will rotate externally. The hip rotates internally by pushing the knee medially.

The knees are frequently affected by injury and disease and deserve careful inspection and palpation. Inspection of the knees involves noting deformity, atrophy of the quadriceps muscle around the knee, or loss of normal hollows around the patella. The suprapatellar pouch on each side of the patella and over the tibiofemoral joint space is palpated for thickening, bogginess, tenderness, or fluid. The popliteal space also is palpated.

Specific methods of palpation at the knee include eliciting the bulge sign for small amounts of fluid and ballottement for a floating patella. To test for the bulge sign, the nurse uses the ball of the hand to milk the medial aspect of the knee firmly upward two or three times and displace any fluid. The nurse then taps the knee just behind the lateral margin of the patella and watches for a bulge of returning fluid in the hollow medial to the patella. Normally none is seen. To ballotte a floating patella, the nurse grasps the thigh above the patella with one hand, forcing fluid out of the suprapatellar pouch into the space between the patella and femur. With the fingers of the other hand, the nurse pushes the patella sharply back against the femur and feels for a tap. The tap is not felt in the absence of fluid because the patella is already snug against the femur. Ballottement is a less sensitive test than testing for the bulge sign, but it can be useful when a large amount of fluid is present.[3]

The normal range of motion at the knee is 15 degrees of hyperextension and 130 degrees of flexion. The client is able to demonstrate the degree of flexion most easily when the hip is also flexed while lifting the lower leg off the surface of the bed or cot. The degree of flexion and hyperextension also can be measured in the prone position. The nurse asks the client to bend back the knee and then straighten it as much as possible.

The ankles and feet are inspected for deformity, swelling, nodules, corns, calluses, or bunions. The nurse palpates over the Achilles tendon, the anterior surface of the ankle, and the metatarsophalangeal joints on the anterior and dorsal surfaces. Notes are made of swelling, tenderness, bogginess, or nodules. The normal range of motion at the ankle is 20 degrees of dorsiflexion and 45 degrees of plantar flexion. The foot is capable of 30 degrees of inversion and 20 degrees of eversion at the subtalar and transverse tarsal joints. The toes have a limited range at the metatarsophalangeal joints. To evaluate the range of motion of the ankle and foot, the client is asked to point the toes of each foot up toward the nurse's face (dorsiflexion) and then away (plantar flexion). The nurse then stabilizes the ankle with one hand and uses the other hand to invert (turn the sole inward) and then to evert (turn the sole outward)

the foot at the transverse tarsal joint. By asking the client to clench or ball up the toes and then release them, the nurse is able to determine the range of motion at the metatarsophalangeal joints.

Muscle tone and strength

During the assessment of range of motion, the nurse observes Mrs. A. K.'s muscle tone. Muscle tone is described as normal; flaccid, which is weak and flabby having decreased tone; spastic, which is increased tone usually accompanied by decreased range; or rigid, which is characterized by the inability to relax either flexor or extensor muscle groups and is frequently accompanied by cogwheeling.

Individuals of normal strength can overcome some degree of resistance to movement. The normal individual has equal strength in all areas of the body—on both sides and in proximal and distal positions. To assess the client's relative strength, the nurse examiner applies resistance to the client's movement. For instance, with the nurse's left arm over the client's left shoulder, the client is instructed to flex the left elbow and place the left hand into the nurse's right hand. The nurse then asks the client to straighten her left arm against the resistance of the nurse's right hand. This maneuver indicates the strength of the triceps, the primary muscle in elbow extension.

To test upper extremity strength, the nurse may ask the client to raise both arms and to hold them palms up at shoulder level for 30 seconds. The nurse observes for drifting downward or outward of either arm, which might indicate a muscle weakness. Tremor also may be observed during this "drift" test.

In assessing the strength of the arms and hands, a client is often instructed to grasp and squeeze the examiner's hands. While doing so, care should be taken that neither the nurse nor the client is made uncomfortable. Therefore any large rings should be removed. Facing the client, the nurse crosses her or his own arms so that the client can grasp the index and middle finger of the nurse's right hand in her right hand and the nurse's left hand in her left hand. Crossing the nurse's arms facilitates recall of which, if either, of the client's extremities is weaker.

Grading of muscle strength can be based on a

TABLE 18-2
Scales for grading muscle strength

Letter scale	Percentage scale (%)	Number scale	Interpretation power
Normal (N)	100	5	Normal
Good (G)	75	4	Muscle can make full normal movement but not against resistance
Fair (F)	50	3	Muscle cannot move against resistance or make full normal movement against gravity
Poor (P)	25	2	Full muscle movement possible with force of gravity eliminated
Trace (T)	10	1	No movement of limb or joint, but contraction is visible or palpable
Zero (Z)	0	0	Total paralysis

From Grimes J and Iannopollo E: Health assessment in nursing practice, Monterey, Calif, 1982, Wadsworth Publishing Co.

letter, percentage, or numerical scale. Grimes and Iannopollo[14] have summarized the scales as shown in Table 18-2.

Deep tendon reflexes

The nurse includes testing deep tendon reflexes when the history and other physical findings indicate it is appropriate. Testing should be done during an admission assessment, after severe trauma such as spinal shock, and during reassessments to monitor or detect changes in condition. In testing the deep tendon reflexes, the nurse positions the client comfortably so that the muscle to be tested is mildly stretched. Using a reflex hammer, the nurse strikes the tendon briskly, which in turn produces a sudden additional tendon stretch.

The major reflexes tested are the biceps, triceps, brachioradial, patellar, and Achilles reflexes. The biceps reflex indicates cervical spine function between C5 and C6. Striking the biceps tendon results in elbow flexion. The triceps reflex is innervated by cervical spine segments C6-8. Striking the triceps tendon causes contraction of the triceps and elbow extension. The brachioradial reflex is tested at the styloid process of the radius. Pronation of the forearm and hand is generated in this reflex, which reflects cervical cord function at levels C5-6. The patellar tendon reflex is mediated by L2-4 of the lumbar cord and results in knee extension. The Achilles tendon reflex produces plantar flexion of the foot as a result of stimulation of segments S1 and S2 of the sacral cord.

Grading of reflexes usually ranges from 0 to 4 +. Reflexes are usually compared between sides and between upper and lower extremities. Table 18-3 shows one scale for rating reflexes. In general, hyperactive reflexes are associated with spastic muscle tone, hypoactive reflexes with flaccid muscle tone.

Facilitating an absent or weak reflex may be accomplished through reinforcement. If reinforcement is used, it is documented as such in client records. Reinforcement involves the isometric contraction of another set of muscles, which may increase reflex activity. For example, clenching the jaws may increase upper extremity tendon reflexes, whereas asking the client to lock the fingers and to pull one hand against the other may increase the reflexes in the lower extremities.

Proprioceptive and position sense

Since decisions about motor activities depend in part on sensory feedback about the body's position, the nurse needs to include assessment of position sense. To test position sense, the nurse holds the sides of Mrs. A.K.'s thumb between his or her own thumb and index finger. The client's thumb is then moved up and down. If the client is unable to correctly identify the position of the thumb, then the other joints of the upper extremity should be tested in turn (wrist, elbow, shoulder). In the lower extremity, position sense is determined first in the great toe. If the toe is impaired, the ankle, knee, and hip should be checked in turn.

TABLE 18-3
Grading of reflexes

Reflex response	Grade
Very brisk, hyperactive; may be associated with clonus: often pathological	4+
Brisker than average, possibly pathological	3+
Normal	2+
Diminished, low normal	1+
No response	0

Balance coordination

If Mrs. A.K. were hospitalized, in bed, and indicated some problems in balance or coordination, the nurse would assess for ability to perform independent or assisted movements out of bed and before transfer and ambulation activities. The nurse would assess the client's sitting and standing balance. Sitting balance is first assessed with the client in bed. The bed is raised to a high Fowler's position and the nurse observes whether the client is able to maintain a midline position or if she slumps to the right or the left. If the client can sit upright, the nurse lowers the head of the bed slightly, checking again for slumping toward the side and falling back toward the mattress. If the client successfully sits upright in bed, the nurse assesses the ability to sit on the edge of the bed without supports at the side or back. Swaying, slumping, or falling backward indicates impaired sitting balance.

Standing balance is assessed by assisting the client to a standing position. The nurse carefully "guards" the client as she stands independently. Swaying, reeling, or taking backward steps indicates a deficit in standing balance. The Romberg test also may be used by the nurse to assess balance. In the Romberg test, the client is asked to stand with her feet together, arms stretched out in front together, and eyes closed. A minimum amount of swaying is considered normal. The individual who has profound cerebellar disease falls toward the affected side. During this test, the nurse remains close to the client to prevent injury from falls.

Other tests for coordination include the finger-to-nose test, heel-to-shin test, and various types of rapidly alternating movements, such as touching the thumb rapidly to each finger and pronating and supinating the hands rapidly. Impaired performance in these tests may require modifications in the client's performance of activities of daily living.

Gait

The nurse concludes movement assessment by evaluating gait. The client is instructed to ambulate normally while the nurse observes balance, arm swings, ability to negotiate turns, and actual gait pattern. In normal gait, the client can initiate and terminate ambulation with no difficulty. The movements are smooth and coordinated. The arms swing in opposition to the advancement of the foot. Physical therapists can provide additional information about the client's gait based on determination of the step and stride widths, step and stride lengths, velocity, and cadence, as well as foot angles.[6, 7]

Certain gait patterns are associated with various types of disorders. The client with hemiplegia typically walks with a stiff gait. Knee flexion is diminished on the affected side. The hip is swung out in a wide circle with toes scraping the floor. The affected arm does not swing forward as the opposite foot is advanced. The client who has Parkinson's disease is described as having a festinating gait. Rhythmic arm swinging is diminished, there is hesitation on initiation of ambulation, and steps are small and shuffling. Ataxic gaits reflect damage to the cerebellum or posterior columns of the spinal cord. Clients with ataxic gaits have a broad-based stance with staggering, unsteady steps. Their difficulty is compounded when turning. Bilateral spastic paralysis of the legs observed in some clients with multiple sclerosis results in a scissor gait. This gait is typified by slow steps. The legs cross forward on each other at the thighs, so that the client appears to be walking through water. The steppage gait, associated with lower motor neuron disease, makes the client look as if he or she were walking upstairs. The steppage gait is characterized by lifting the foot up high with the knee flexed and then slapping the foot down. A waddling gait is sometimes observed in clients with muscular degenerative disease.

NURSING DIAGNOSES

Nursing diagnoses that may be made for a client with a mobility deficit include the following[12]:

1. *Impaired physical mobility of the upper ex-*

tremities related to muscle weakness, paralysis, joint swelling or pain, degeneration of bone and muscle, involuntary movement, or absence of an extremity

2. *Impaired physical mobility of the lower extremities* related to insufficient knowledge about the prosthesis, noncompliance with the care plan, lack of support by a family member, insufficient funds to attend therapy, or lack of transportation to therapy

3. *Impaired balance and coordination* related to truncal instability, muscle weakness, paralysis, prolonged bed rest, and loss of or diminished vision

4. *Dysfunctional gait pattern* related to muscle weakness, paralysis, incoordination, involuntary movements, fracture of an extremity, lack of knowledge, fear, and dependence

GOALS

After developing nursing diagnoses that are validated by the client and family, the nurse establishes goals with the client. Goals are based on the client's entire situation. Goals established with each client are unique and specific. The following are potential goals established with the client who has impaired mobility:

1. Prevent complications associated with decreased or absent movement.
2. Increase muscle strength and mobility.
3. Maintain and increase independence in activities requiring motor performance.
4. Prevent injury during activity.
5. Use assistive devices correctly and consistently if appropriate.
6. Adapt to altered mobility.
7. Participate in social and occupational activities.
8. Understand specific interventions related to impaired physical mobility.

REHABILITATION NURSING INTERVENTIONS

When a client is immobilized or bed-bound, the nurse has a responsibility to maintain the client's potential for eventual mobilization. The complications of immobility and an overview of the nursing interventions used to prevent these complications are described.

Rehabilitation nursing interventions to assist the client in maximizing potential for mobilization include a wide range of therapies, such as positioning, use of positioning devices, exercise programs, transfer activities, preambulation and ambulation programs, and wheelchair activities. Maintaining mobility capabilities involves supporting the body in anatomically correct, functional positions; turning the client according to a predetermined schedule; using positioning and mechanical devices when and where appropriate; and maintaining muscle tone and joint mobility through exercise.

While implementing interventions, the nurse frequently seeks input from the client and family and begins to transfer responsibility to them in a gradual, consistent manner. The nurse works closely with other members of the rehabilitation team, including physical and occupational therapists, biomedical engineers, the orthotist, the prosthetist, and the physiatrist, to meet the client's ultimate goals.

Prevention of Complications Associated with Immobilization

Although bed rest was once the most common form of treatment for most diseases and conditions, it is no longer recognized as the panacea for all ills. It is, however, still used to prevent further damage to the body when normal demands exceed the body's ability to respond, such as when the heart cannot provide the volume or force needed for the body to carry out usual daily activities (myocardial infarction) or when the alveoli cannot diffuse adequate oxygen to meet the normal demands of the body cells (pneumonia). Bed rest is also used for short periods for the treatment of many musculoskeletal problems, such as trauma, degenerative disorders, rheumatological diseases, infection, and congenital deformities.[2]

When a person is unable to move part or all of the body because of disease, injury, or treatment method, a number of complications can occur in a short period of time. Olson,[30] in a classic article, described the effects of immobility on every system in the body and noted the nursing interventions that can prevent the hazards of immobility. More recently, Rubin[34] described the physiology and effects of bed rest. After only 3 days of bed rest, plasma and calcium are lost, less gastric juice is secreted, less blood flows through the calves, and glucose tolerance is impaired.[13]

Changes in the cardiovascular system that have been ascribed to immobility include orthostatic hypotension, increased work load of the heart, and thrombus formation.[30] To prevent these complications, passive and active range of joint motion exercises, isometric exercises, and self-care activities should be implemented. One of the most effective measures to change the intravascular pressure and provide a stimulus to the neural reflexes of the blood vessels is to change the client from a horizontal to vertical position by either raising the head of the bed or positioning the person upright in a chair if permissible. Immobilized persons should be taught to avoid holding their breath when moving in bed. To decrease the work load of the heart, attention should be given to preventing constipation and supporting the client in a sitting or squatting position for defecation.[30]

Immobility results in decreased respiratory movement, decreased movement of secretions, and disturbed oxygen–carbon dioxide balance. The nurse should constantly observe the respiratory function of immobilized clients, noting the rate, quality, depth, moisture, work, use of abdominal or neck muscles, and any neurological signs such as restlessness or forgetfulness. The client should be routinely turned and encouraged to cough and sigh. Expelling secretions by coughing helps facilitate adequate oxygen–carbon dioxide exchange. Chest clapping and postural drainage may be needed to help loosen secretions. The nurse should teach the client to use abdominal muscles, the diaphragm, and intercostal muscles and encourage regular deep breathing and coughing exercises.[30]

Immobilization accelerates catabolic activity, resulting in a rapid breakdown of cells and a protein deficiency. The consequent negative nitrogen balance can lead to anorexia, further contributing to existing malnutrition and significantly prolonging the disease process. Therefore attention should be given to discovering the client's food likes and dislikes and providing small, frequent feedings, which are usually more appealing. Supplemental protein may be required. In addition, the stress of bed rest may lead to continued stimulation of the parasympathetic nervous system, producing such symptoms as dyspepsia, gastric stasis, distention, anorexia, diarrhea, or consti-

pation. Through use of tension-reducing interventions, the nurse may be able to help alleviate these symptoms. Attention should be given to the prevention of constipation through the use of stool softeners and the use of exercises to strengthen weak abdominal muscles.[30]

Bed rest also can result in osteoporosis, contractures, and pressure ulcers. Exercises and close attention to body position and alignment, skin condition, diet supplemented as necessary to meet nutritional needs, and client and family education can help prevent these complications.[30]

Immobility also can lead to urinary tract stones and foster urinary tract infection. Prevention of stone formation and urinary tract infection are discussed in Chapter 10.

The nurse should be aware of changes that occur in the production of hormones, sleeping patterns, the immune system, and psychosocial equilibrium. Consequently, no client should be allowed to remain immobile any longer than absolutely necessary. Although it is still not known how often turning is required to prevent some of these complications, it is known that the 2-hour rule of thumb may not be enough for some clients.[34]

Therapeutic Positioning

The bed-bound client benefits from careful positioning by the nurse. The frequency of position change depends on a number of variables, including comfort, amount of spontaneous movement, edema, loss of sensation, overall physical and mental status, and time. Clients may experience discomfort after 30 to 60 minutes of lying prone and need to be repositioned. Clients who can shift weight and move independently may not need to change position more frequently than every 2 to 4 hours. Loss of sensation, paralysis, coma, and edema are indications for position changes every 2 hours or more frequently, since the client is unable to inform the nurse of discomfort or pain and since edematous, paralyzed tissue is more sensitive to pressure than normal tissue. Persons with progressive diseases who are immobilized also may require more frequent position changes to prevent pressure sores. (See Chapter 13 for more information about pressure sores.)

The time of day also may affect the frequency of repositioning. If the client's overall condition permits, a change to every 4 hours during the night is desirable to promote a more normal and restful sleep. To reinforce client and family teaching, a turning and positioning schedule is posted at the bedside. The client and family can then take initiative for position changes and receive feedback from the nurse. (See box below.)

While positioning and turning the client, the nurse is in an excellent position to teach the individual and family about positioning, to have them demonstrate procedures, and to eventually have them share the responsibility in preparing for discharge. The basic positions include supine (back-lying), lateral (side-lying), prone (abdomen-lying) (Figure 18-3), and semi-prone.[39]

Supine

To position the client correctly in the supine position, the nurse assists the client to lay on his or her back (Figure 18-3, A) and provides a small flat pillow to support the head, neck, and upper shoulders. The arms are positioned along the client's sides in a neutral position, with elbows extended and palms downward. The position of the upper extremity is varied by abducting the

---

Positioning and Turning Schedule

Client _____ Room no. _____

Special considerations
Left hemiplegia
Left homonymous hemianopsia

Special equipment
Footboard
Trochanter roll
Three extra pillows
Hand cone (left hand): Remove cone every 2 hours and perform range of motion exercises

Special instructions for supine position
Supine A: Abduct slightly at shoulder, slight flexion at elbows, wrist in neutral position
Supine B: Abduct shoulders, flex arms at elbows above head
Supine C: Elevate arms on pillows

Time	Position	Check when in position
7-9 AM	Supine A	
9-11 AM	Right lateral	
11 AM-Noon	Left lateral	
Noon-1 PM	Supine B	
1-3 PM	Right lateral	
3-4 PM	Prone	
4-6 PM	Supine C	
6-7 PM	Left lateral	
7-9 PM	Supine A	
9-10 PM	Right lateral	
10 PM-Midnight	Left lateral	
Midnight-2 AM	Supine B*	
2-4 AM	Right lateral	
4-5 AM	Prone	
5-7 AM	Supine C	

*When the client builds up skin tolerance, turn every 4 hours at night.

shoulder slightly with a small pillow or pad and by elevating the forearm and hand. Other upper extremity positions include full abduction of the shoulder with extension of the elbow and wrist or full abduction of the shoulder with a 90-degree elbow flexion and the arm and hand positioned upward or downward. The hips are extended and may be supported in place by a trochanter roll. The knees are extended or slightly flexed. Caution is taken to avoid placing pressure on the back of the legs because damage to the blood vessels and a consequent phlebitis could result. Too great a degree of flexion at the knee may result in flexion contracture with impairment of posture and gait. The feet are positioned so that a right angle is formed between the foot and the leg. To prevent contracture formation, resulting in foot-drop, it is best to use some type of device to maintain the desired angle of flexion. Devices include adjustable footboards, firmly folded blankets or pillows, and resting leg splints with footplates or high-top sneakers. For precautions to be taken in using

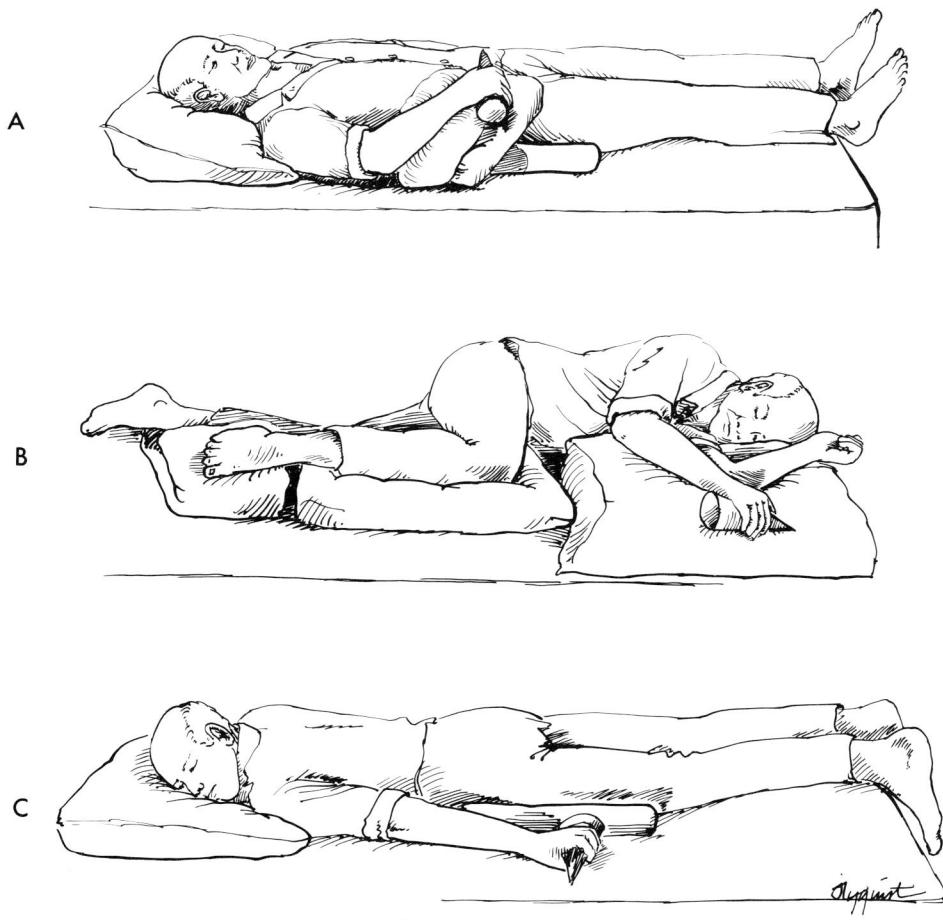

Figure 18-3
A, Supine position with trochanter roll to prevent external rotation of hips. **B,** Lateral position with hand cone to prevent flexion contracture of hand. **C,** Prone position with trochanter roll and hand cone.

these devices, refer to the section on positioning aids.

Lateral position

To place the client in the lateral position, the nurse assists the client to lay on his or her side (Figure 18-3, *B*) and provides a firm pillow to support the head and neck. The lower arm is positioned at the side. The uppermost arm is supported by a pillow to prevent pressure on the chest. The upper leg is flexed at the hip and knee and positioned on a pillow in front of the lower leg to minimize pressure on the lower leg. Another pillow may be used behind the back to maintain the position.

The side-lying position for the individual affected by a stroke incorporates Bobath's approaches and promotes lying on the affected side as much as the client can tolerate. In this position, the client begins to establish weight-bearing and lengthens the trunk, which later helps to counteract abnormal posture in the sitting and standing positions. Positioning on the affected side may stimulate improved muscle tone through weight-bearing and prepare the individual for the bilateral weight-bearing necessary to move up in bed, move on and off the bedpan, and stand. Normally, when lying in bed, a person places the bottom shoulder slightly ahead of the rest of the body and places the hip, knee, and shoulder in some degree of flexion. When positioning the individual who has had a stroke in the side-lying position on the affected side, the head should be placed in a neutral position, the lower shoulder brought forward with the arm extended and the palm facing up, and the hips and knees flexed. When positioned on the unaffected side, the shoulder should be positioned away from the typical spastic pattern observed in hemiplegic posture and a towel or small pillow placed under the trunk at waist level to help elongate the affected side.[31]

Prone position

Before placing the client in a prone position, the nurse reviews the record and assesses the client for any possible contraindications, such as increasing intracranial pressure or cardiopulmonary distress. To position in the prone position, the nurse assists the client to lay on his or her abdomen (Figure 18-3, *C*). The client's head is turned to one side to facilitate breathing and drainage of oral secretions. A small pillow may be placed under the head for comfort, and another pillow may be placed between the chest and the umbilicus to relieve pressure on the chest or breasts. Hips and knees are extended and supported on pillows. The feet and toes are supported by another pillow or are positioned between the edge of the mattress and the bed frame to prevent pressure areas. In the prone position, the client may feel most comfortable with arms flexed over the head or extended along the body in a neutral position

Semiprone

The client is in the semiprone position when resting on the side with the uppermost arm and leg placed farther forward. In the semiprone position, more of the buttocks and back are off of the mattress.

Sitting

All clients should have their feet placed flat on the floor and the hips well back in the seat. Weight should be distributed evenly over both hips. The depth, width, and height of the chair should foster correct sitting position and help the client avoid leaning to one or the other sides of the chair. Pillows can be used if the chair seat is too wide or too deep to allow the hip and knees to be placed at right angles. If the height of the chair seat does not allow the client to place the feet flat on the floor, a stool can be used. When clients affected by a stroke sit up in bed or in a chair, the nurse should instruct them to avoid positions that encourage the development of spastic patterns. The affected shoulder should be placed forward with a pillow for support if needed. The affected arm also could be placed on a table at a comfortable height to achieve this position.[30]

Positioning Aids

To maintain correct body alignment, the use of various positioning aids is sometimes necessary. In general, positioning aids may be developed from materials on the nursing unit or from the client's home, or purchased from hospital supply companies. Other aids such as splints may be prescribed by the physiatrist and designed and fitted by the orthotist or occupational therapist. Even the most customized piece of equipment can cause pressure areas or can impair circulation if not applied correctly, however. To prevent pressure or development of ischemic areas, the nurse checks and removes the equipment every 2 to 4 hours unless ordered otherwise by the physician.

Pillows

Pillows can be used to position, stabilize, and support or provide a bridge beneath a pressure area. Alternatives to pillows include rolled or folded towels, bath blankets, and foam squares covered with washable material.

Trochanter rolls

A bath blanket or flannel sheet blanket can be used to make a trochanter roll. This roll is used to prevent outward rotation of the hip when the client is placed in a supine position. The blanket should be folded lengthwise into thirds and positioned beneath the client's hips from the top of the iliac crest to approximately 6 inches above the knee. It should be rolled under toward the client so that a roll is formed along the outer aspect of the thigh.

Foot supports

The alternatives to a footboard mentioned previously include blanket-covered boxes, resting leg splints, or high-top sneakers. With each of these aids, the nurse checks for pressure areas and ischemia. The nurse also exercises the feet according to the client's capabilities to maintain muscle tone, muscle strength, and joint range. If the legs and feet are spastic, positioning against a footboard may produce an undesirable increase in the tendency of the feet to plantarflex. High-top tennis shoes stimulate the top of the foot as well as the sole and assist in achieving a more beneficial outcome.

Hand rolls

One of nursing's time-honored treatments for positioning the hand in a slightly flexed position was the rolled washcloth or soft rubber ball. If the client has normal muscle tone and voluntary movement, no harm will come of this practice. In the person with a spastic hand, however, overstimulation of the palmar surface can increase flexion synergy, resulting in flexion contracture of the hand and wrist. Rood suggested the use of a firm cone, maintained in position by a strip of elastic over the dorsal aspect of the hand. The cone is believed to provide constant pressure over the

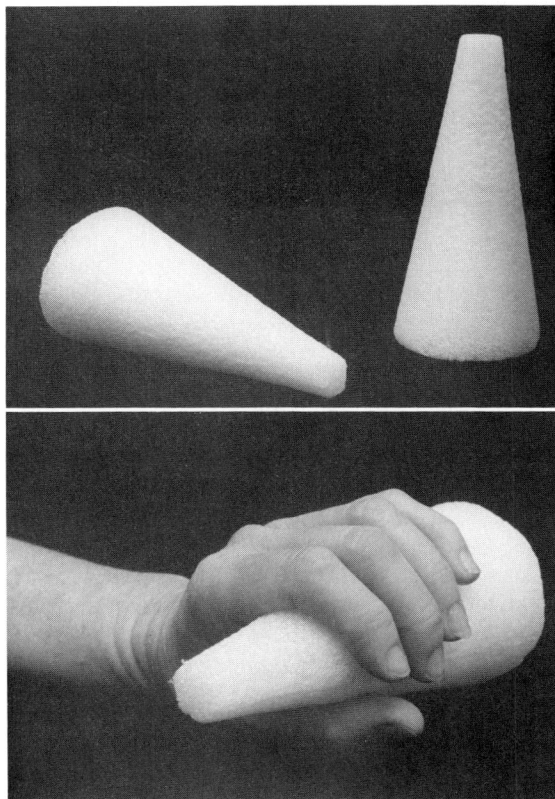

Figure 18-4
Hand cones prevent hand flexion contracture.

entire flexor surface of the fingers and to put pressure on the insertions of the spastic wrist and finger flexors. Pressure on these areas is believed to have an inhibitory effect on the long flexors of the hand (Figure 18-4).[23]

Jamieson and Dayhoff[16] studied the use of a hard cone on eleven individuals with hemiplegia and flexor hypertonicity of the upper extremity. All measurements (composite extension of the finger, opposition of the finger to the thumb, pinch strength, grip strength) were taken with the wrist in the neutral and flexed position. They found that flexor hypertonicity of the fingers and wrist decreased significantly after the hard cone was used for 4 weeks, although only slight changes in function occurred. Their findings were similar to the findings of an earlier study conducted by Dayhoff. She studied three adults with hemiplegia and found the greatest improvement after 6 weeks, when the wrist was placed in a flexed position only.[10]

Splints

Disagreement exists regarding whether splinting spastic extremities facilitates or inhibits spasticity. Many occupational therapists splint only those persons who have moderate to severe spasticity. A study by Mathiowetz, Boding, and Trombly[23] addressed the immediate effects of positioning devices on the normal and spastic hand. They studied the use of the volar resting splint (Figure 18-5), a foam finger spreader (based on Bobath's belief that abduction facilitates extension of the fingers and reduces flexor spasticity of the whole arm), a firm cone, and no device on the normal and spastic hand as measured by electromyography. Their sample was small (eight normal subjects and four with hemiplegia). Their findings suggest a need to further examine these devices, however. In the hemiplegic subjects, the electrical activity of the muscles before and after grasp was not significantly reduced while wearing the volar splint, finger spreader, or hand cone, suggesting that a decrease in spasticity does not necessarily occur when these devices are used. In addition, the volar splint appeared to increase electrical activity during application of the splint and during the grasping period. If an increase in electrical activity is undesirable in a spastic hand, then use of a volar splint would be contraindicated when grasping or performing a comparable activity.[23] The results did not contraindicate the use of a volar splint while the client was resting.

Mills[28] examined the use of bivalve splints to control postural defects caused by spasticity in eight subjects with spastic extremities (ankle, wrist, or elbow flexion contracture). She concluded that no significant change occurred in the spastic muscles as measured by electromyography during splinted and nonsplinted periods. She reported that some individuals experienced an increase in electrical activity while splinted.

A consistent approach by the rehabilitation team is necessary in the use of positioning devices for the spastic hand and arm. Individual response to the device, as well as further research findings, provide the nurse and other team members with the information necessary to determine the best possible approach.

Mechanical Beds

To facilitate changes in position for clients with severe trauma, various types of turning frames and mechanized beds have been developed. These devices, when properly used, enable a minimum of nursing personnel to safely and efficiently provide position changes. Among these devices are Stryker Wedge Frames, CircOlectric beds, Roto Rest,* and air-fluidized beds.

Stryker Wedge Frame

The Stryker Wedge Frame provides for prone and supine positioning. The client is in a lateral position only during the act of turning; therefore variation in positioning is reduced. The Stryker frame has been used with clients who have had spinal cord injuries, plastic surgery, and pressure sores. Individuals who weigh more than 200 pounds cannot be accommodated on the frame. Other limitations of the Stryker frame include limited visibility (the client either stares up at the ceiling or down at the floor), fear or apprehension related to the mechanical turning device itself, and the possibility of human error resulting in injury due to failure to secure frames, straps, or nuts and bolts adequately (Figure 18-6).

CircOlectric Bed

The CircOlectric Bed provides a greater variation of positions from supine to prone, allowing for standing, sitting, and Trendelenburg's positions. Again, acceptability by the client is sometimes a difficulty, since the frame is large and has a number of accessories such as arm support brackets, restraining straps, an overbed table, a mirror assembly, an anterior armsling, a head halter-collar combination, and a spreader bar. The turning procedure from supine to prone or vice versa involves placing the client upright so that weight-bearing is experienced, as well as postural changes. Although both weight-bearing and postural changes can be desirable in preventing osteoporosis and hypotension, the CircOlectric Bed may not be suitable for the individual who should not bear weight or who responds poorly to changes from flat to erect positions, such as the client with a high cervical cord injury. Persons who may benefit from the CircOlectric Bed include those who

---

*Oscillating hospital bed, Kinetic Concepts, Inc., San Antonio, Tex.

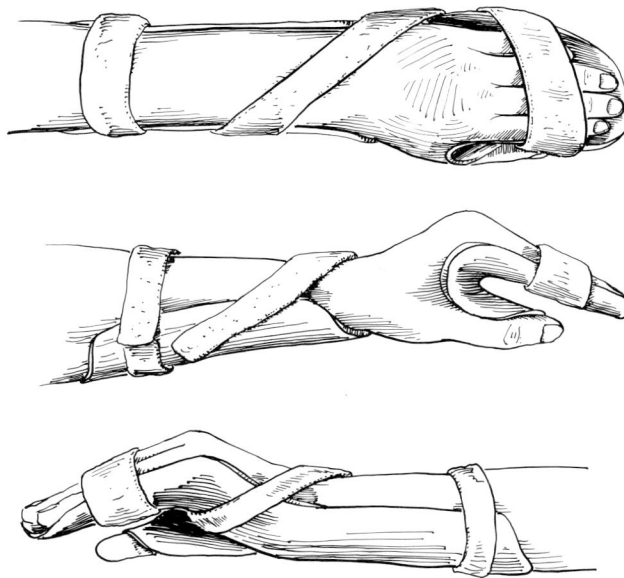

Figure 18-5
Volar resting splint provides support to wrist, thumb, and fingers, maintaining them in position of extension.

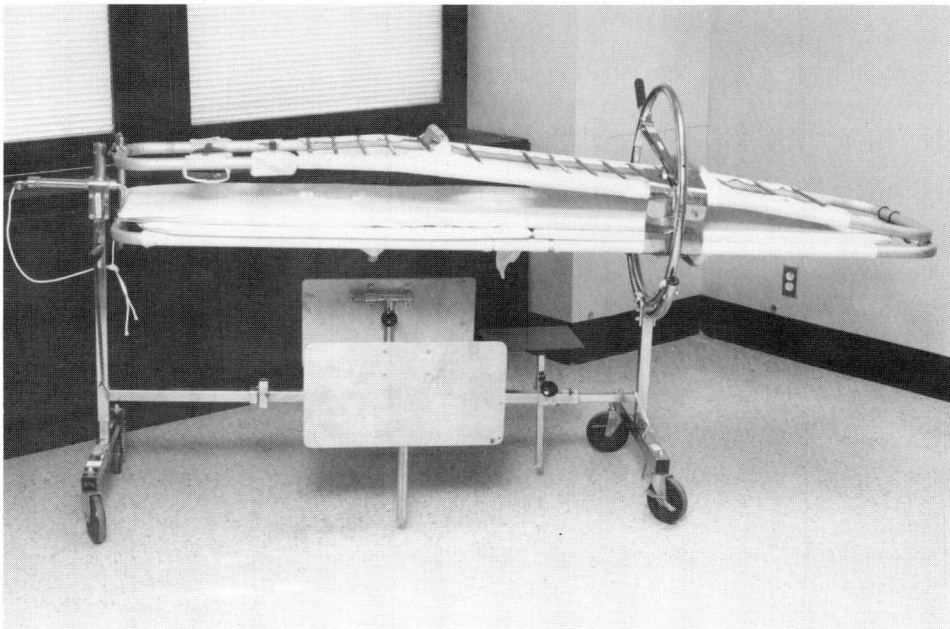

Figure 18-6
Stryker Wedge Frame provides efficient, safe turning for individual with spinal cord injury and for other clients who must be immobilized.

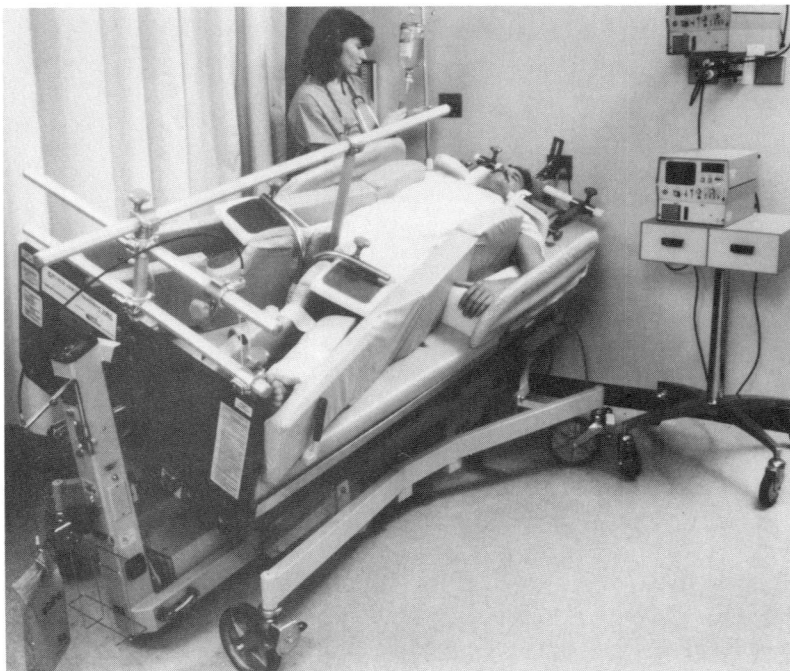

Figure 18-7
Roto Rest model Mark I turns client every 3½ minutes over range of 124 degrees. (*Courtesy Kinetic Concepts, San Antonio, Tex.*)

have experienced multiple trauma, burns, and reconstructive surgery. The nurse is responsible for assuring safe operation of the frame during and after turning.

Roto Rest

The most recent mechanical adjunct to positioning is kinetic therapy developed by Dr. F.X. Keane. The Roto Rest is used to deliver kinetic therapy. This oscillating bed turns the client every 3½ minutes over a range of 124 degrees. The turning is continuous; however, it is so gradual that the individual does not experience dizziness or discomfort. The table can be stopped at any point for nursing or medical care. It conforms to the client with the use of knee and shoulder braces and close-fitting pads placed against the body and extremities. It also minimizes the complications of immobility, such as hypostatic pneumonia, pulmonary emboli, constipation, and pressure ulcers. The table has been used successfully with

clients who have experienced multiple trauma, respiratory disorders, severe burns, paralysis, coma, and pressure areas. Some persons may experience claustrophobia as a result of the pads and braces. If pain is experienced, positioning of the client should be checked (Figure 18-7).[27]

Air-fluidized bed

Air-fluidized beds such as the Clinitron and Kinair* are designed specifically for support while reducing pressure on the skin and permitting unimpeded blood flow. The nurse is responsible for repositioning the client every 3 to 4 hours. The Clinitron bed consists of a loosely fitting polyester filter sheet that covers a tank of 1,500 pounds of tiny, sterile glass beads. Warm pressurized air from a blower lifts the beads, so that the client floats on a dry, fluid medium. Body exudates pass

*Kinetic Concepts, Inc., San Antonio, Tex.

through the filter sheet and fall to the bottom. Since the glass beads are silicone-coated soda lime, an environment with a high pH is created and decreases the potential for bacterial growth.

The Kinair bed supports the client comfortably on a fabric cushion. Compared to standard hospital beds, this air-fluidized bed decreases pressure against the heel by 60 mm Hg, the sacrum by 19 mm Hg, the scapula by 14 mm Hg, the trochanter by 47 mm Hg, and the occiput by 39 mm Hg.

The major potential problems with air-fluidized beds are dehydration related to increased fluid loss from the skin and the respiratory tract; pulmonary congestion, since coughing is ineffective unless the fluidization is turned off; and skin irritation if microsphere leakage occurs through a tear in the sheet.[35] The air-fluidized bed also decreases pain and amount of pain medication while increasing comfort and rest.

Therapeutic Exercise

Regular exercise in an important intervention for the person with impaired physical mobility. Before the client is considered sufficiently stable medically to begin an active physical or occupational therapy program, the nurse implements a program of exercise based upon the client's overall condition. This program is designed to prevent deformity and maintain normal muscle tone and function.

Exercise may take the form of isotonic contractions, producing movement of joint and muscle, or isometric contractions, consisting of shortening of muscle fibers without apparent movement of the limb or joint. The nurse explains the exercise program to the client and family and encourages their active participation. After demonstrating the exercise program, the nurse then teaches through demonstration, encouraging the client and family to practice and redemonstrate. Furthermore, the nurse increases client and family responsibility for the exercise program by sharing responsibility and ultimately by delegating responsibility for the exercise program to the client and family as they prepare for discharge.

Range of joint motion

The most commonly used form of isotonic exercise is range of joint motion exercises. These exercises can be active, active-assistive, passive, or resistive. Range of joint motion exercises are usually performed three or four times a day, with each movement performed on the average of five times. The exercises are considered active if the client performs them, passive if the nurse or family performs them, assistive if some support is used to enable the client to perform them, and resistive if the client performs the motion against a force such as a weight.

In performing range of joint motion, the nurse supports the joint distal to the one moved. The exercises are performed as smoothly and gently as possible. Performing the exercises in a consistent pattern assures thoroughness and facilitates client and family learning. The nurse assesses the client during exercises for pain or resistance and fatigue. Unless otherwise specified, the joint is not moved past the point of resistance or pain.

The type of movement possible at a joint depends upon the type of joint. Hinge joints such as the knee are limited to flexion and extension, whereas ball-and-socket joints such as the hip and shoulder possess a full range of flexion, extension, abduction, adduction, and rotation.

Passive exercise in the supine position. To perform range of motion passively, the nurse explains the purpose of the exercise to the client and family. The client is placed in the correct anatomical position. Privacy is provided for by appropriate screening and bed covers. The first set of exercises is performed in the supine position, and each movement is repeated five times. The nurse supports the client's head with both hands and flexes the neck forward until the chin touches the chest or to the client's tolerance. The client's head is returned to the neutral position. With the head supported, the pillow is removed, permitting extension of the neck back toward the surface of the bed. The nurse then flexes the neck laterally by sliding the client's right ear toward his or her right shoulder and vice versa. Again, while supporting the client's head, the nurse rotates the neck from the right shoulder to the left and vice versa.

Shoulder. The nurse supports the client's elbow and wrist and flexes the shoulder by moving the arm forward, up, and over the client's head. The nurse adducts the shoulder crossing the midline of the body and then abducts the shoulder away from the body. While in the abducted position, with the elbow flexed, the nurse internally rotates the shoulder by turning the arm downward and

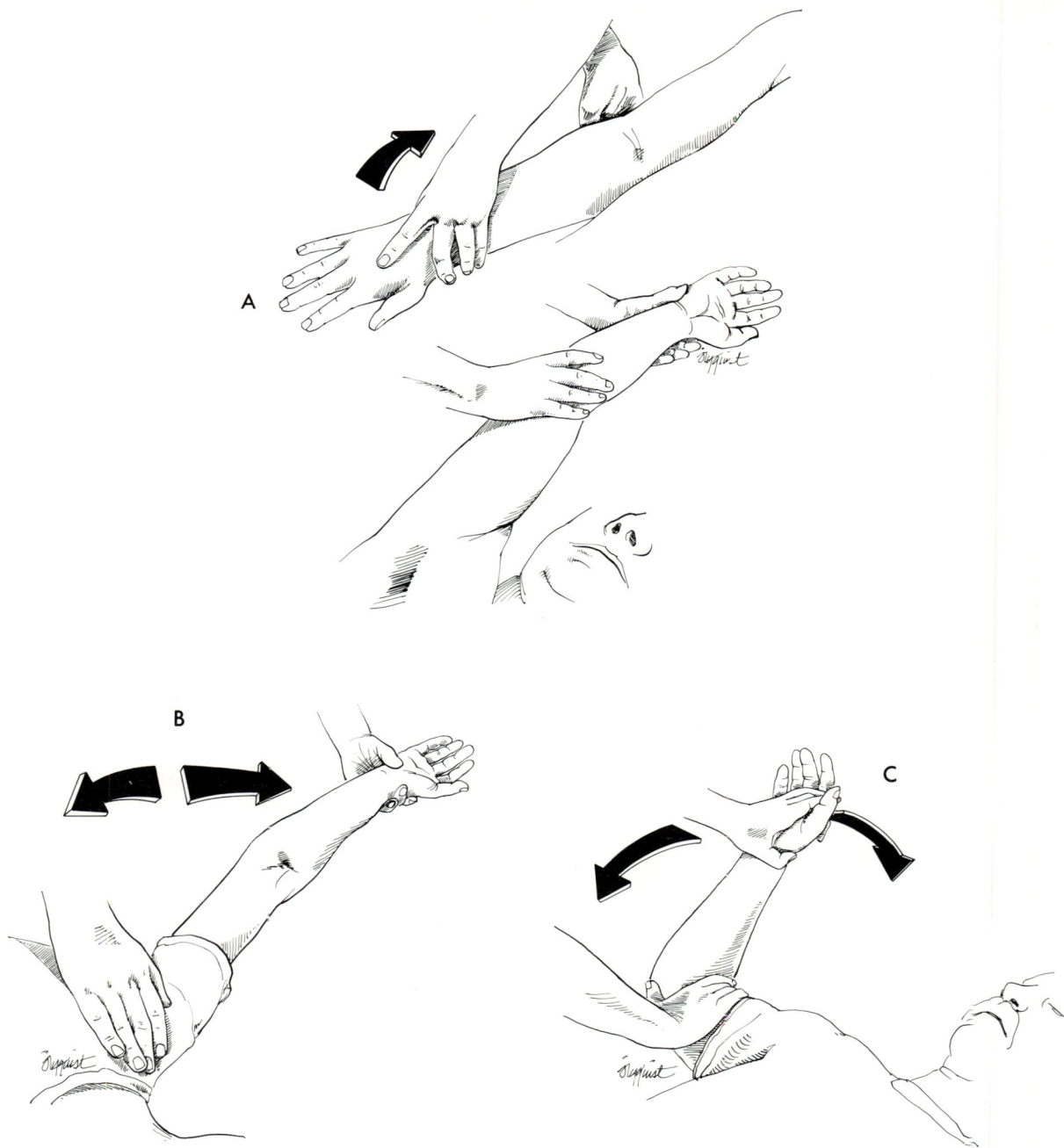

Figure 18-8
A, Shoulder in extended position. Flexion occurs as arm is lifted up and back. **B,** Sliding arm toward body produces shoulder adduction. Sliding arm away from body produces abduction. **C,** As forearm is brought down, internal rotation occurs at shoulder joint. As forearm is brought up and back, external rotation occurs.

externally rotates the shoulder by turning the arm upward (Figure 18-8).

Elbow. With the client's arm in the abducted position, supporting the wrist and stabilizing the arm above the elbow, the nurse extends and flexes the elbow joint (Figure 18-9).

Wrist. The client's arm is flexed at the elbow and abducted at the shoulder. The nurse supports the forearm and hand, flexes the wrist forward, and extends it back. The wrist is moved laterally toward the thumb (radial deviation) and then toward the little finger (ulnar deviation) (Figure 18-10).

Fingers. The nurse continues to support the client's wrist with one hand. With the other hand, the fingers are separated (abducted) and brought together (adducted). The nurse covers the client's fingers with her or his own, flexing them into a fist and extending them. This action moves the metacarpophalangeal joints and the proximal and distal interphalangeal joints through their ranges of motion. While supporting the hand, the nurse moves the thumb through its range of joint motion by flexing and extending the thumb at the interphalangeal joint and at the carpometacarpal joint,

abducting it away from the other fingers and then adducting it back toward the fingers. The nurse then touches the thumb to the base of each finger, returning after each digit to the starting or neutral position. When the fifth digit is reached, full opposition of the thumb has occurred (Figure 18-11).

The final movement of the upper extremity is pronation and supination at the radioulnar articulation. The nurse positions the client's arm, extending the shoulder and elbow. Slipping her or his hand into the client's hand, the nurse supinates the forearm, turning it palm upward, and pronates the forearm, turning it palm downward (Figure 18-12).

Hip. With the client lying in the supine position, the nurse supports the leg below and at the knee. Most persons are more comfortable during hip flexion when the knee is also flexed. The nurse can then combine knee and hip flexion and ex-

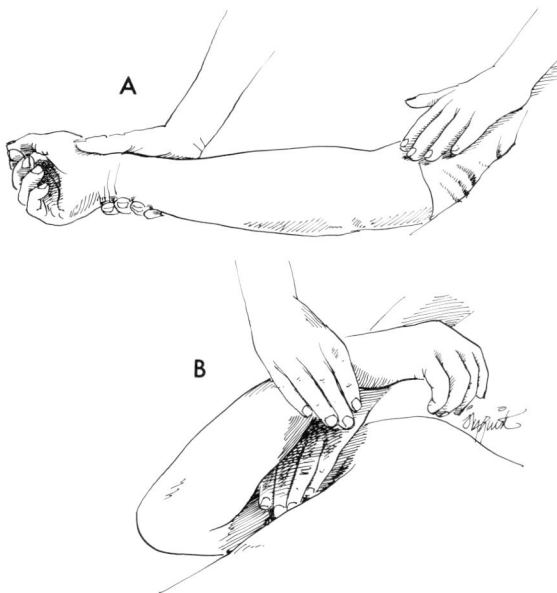

Figure 18-9
A, Elbow extension. **B,** Elbow flexion.

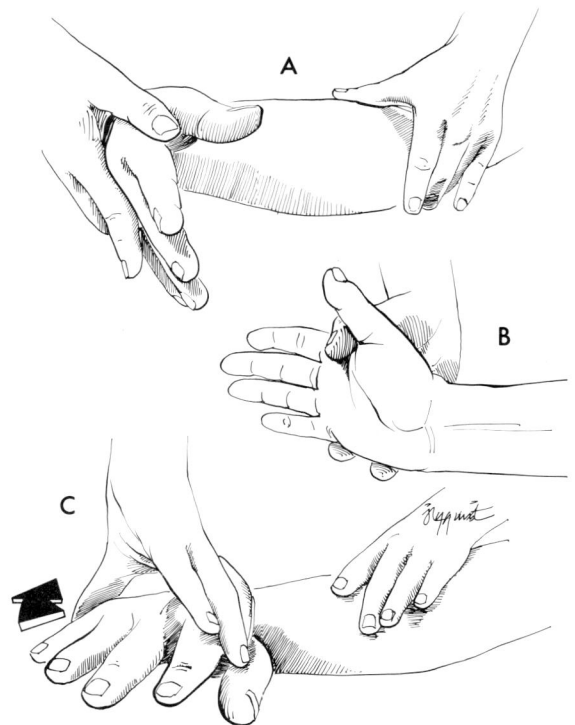

Figure 18-10
A, Flexed wrist. **B,** Extended wrist. **C,** Lateral movement of wrist produces radial and ulnar deviation.

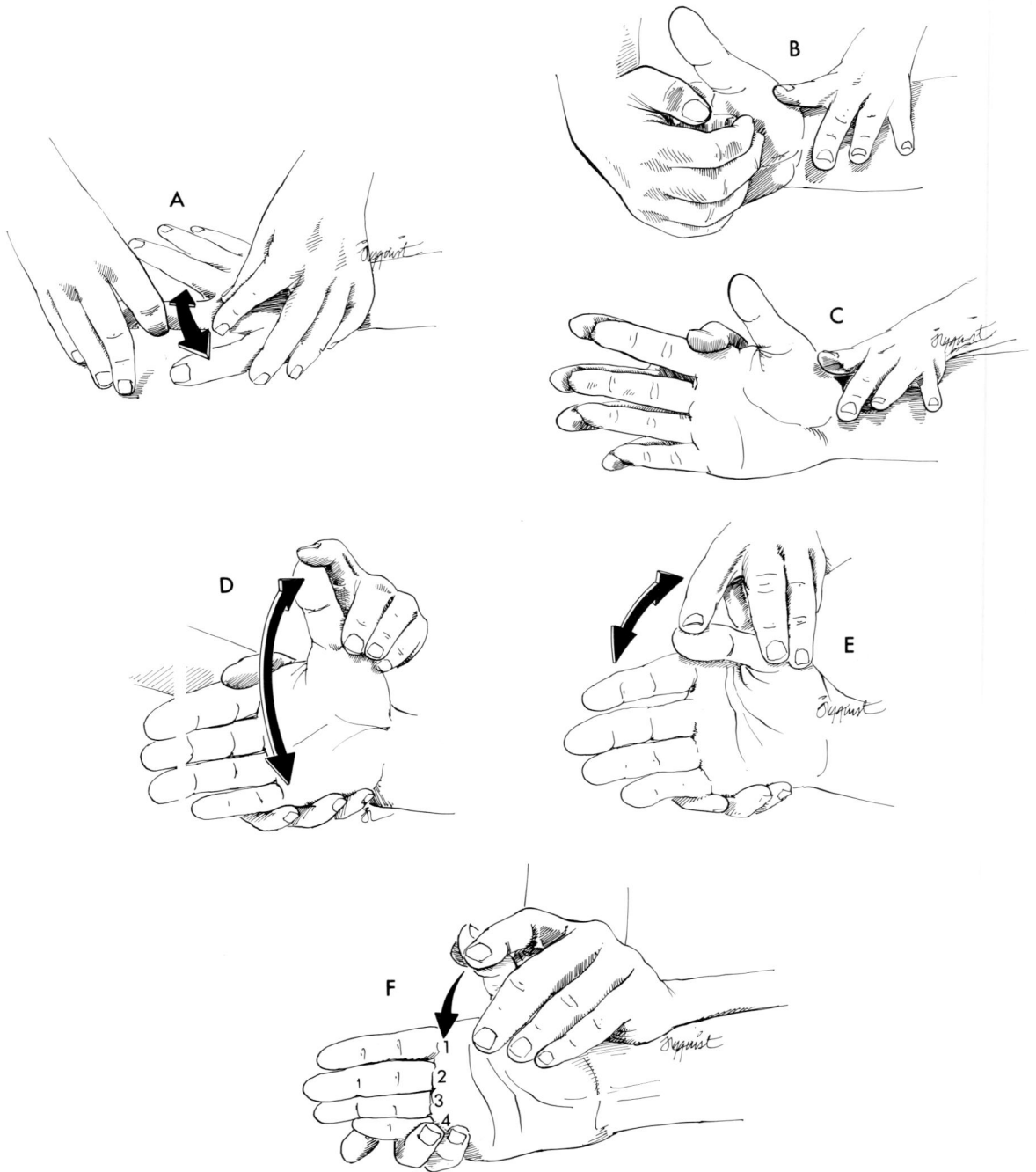

Figure 18-11
A, Fingers abducted away from midline and adducted toward midline (of hand). **B,** Fingers flexed as group into closed fist. **C,** Finger extension is described as open fist. **D,** Thumb flexed toward and extended away from fourth digit. **E,** Thumb abducted and adducted in relation to other fingers. **F,** Thumb moved in opposition to base of each of other four digits.

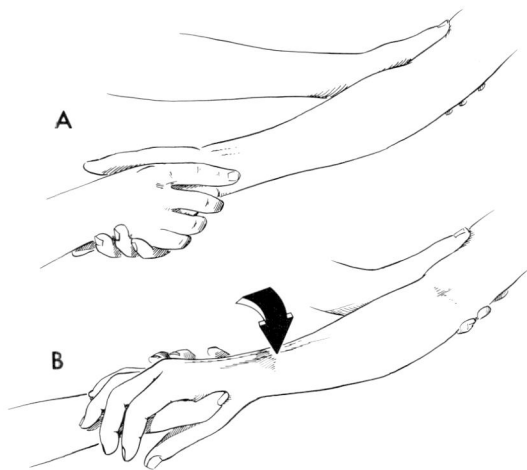

Figure 18-12
A, Forearm in supination. **B,** Rolling forearm downward places it in pronation.

tension in one movement. The client's leg is moved toward the abdomen and then stretched out toward the foot of the bed. The leg is abducted by extending it and then sliding it away from the midline; sliding the leg back to the midline and crossing over it accomplishes hip adduction. To internally rotate the hip, the nurse rolls the client's leg inward; to externally rotate the hip, the nurse rotates the client's leg outward. An alternate method of hip rotation is accomplished by flexing the leg at the hip and knee. The nurse supports the leg at the knee and then moves the knee laterally, causing the hip to rotate externally; by moving the knee medially, internal hip rotation is accomplished (Figure 18-13).

Knee. If the knee is to be put through range of motion separately from the hip, the client is placed in the supine position. The nurse supports the client's leg beneath the knee and beneath the ankle. The knee is bent upward toward the abdomen to provide flexion and is then straightened to provide for extension (Figure 18-14). Hyperflexion of the knee is performed in the prone position and is described later in this chapter.

Ankle. The ankle is moved through range of motion with the leg in full extension. Supporting the leg above the ankle and on the sole of the foot, the nurse points the foot toward the client's

head while dorsiflexing and then points the foot away from the head while plantar flexing. Ankle inversion is accomplished when the nurse moves the sole of the foot inward. Ankle eversion is accomplished when the nurse turns the sole of the foot outward (Figure 18-15). The nurse then moves toes in groups of two away from and toward the midline (abduction and adduction). With the hand over the dorsal surface of the foot, covering the client's toes, the nurse bends and straightens the toes to flex and extend them.

Heel cord stretching. Heel cord stretching is included in range of motion exercises to the ankle to prevent shortening of the muscles that plantar and dorsiflex the foot. Such shortening may occur as a consequence of immobilization, resulting in impaired ability to ambulate. Heel cord stretching is performed with the client in the supine position. The nurse supports the leg with one hand beneath the knee; the other hand cups the heel with the client's foot resting on the nurse's forearm. The nurse maintains a firm grasp on the heel while using the forearm to dorsiflex the foot, thereby stretching the muscles of the heel cord (Figure 18-16).

Passive exercise in the prone position. When the nurse has completed range of motion exercises for the right and left upper and lower extremities, she or he may assist the client to the prone position. In the prone position, the nurse can hyperextend the client's shoulder, hyperextend the hip, and hyperflex the knee. In each action, the nurse supports the limb and moves it away from the bed, monitoring carefully for any client discomfort.

Trunk. For some individuals exercising the spinal joints may be appropriate. With the client in a semi-Fowler's position, the nurse supports the shoulders under the arms and moves the upper torso to the right and to the left to accomplish lateral flexion of the spine. To rotate the spine the nurse supports and lifts the shoulders off the bed and turns the upper torso to the right and to the left. The nurse flexes the spine forward by bending the upper torso forward while supporting under the arms and shoulders.

Although passive range of motion has been a cornerstone of nursing care, recent research questions its widespread application. Clough and Maurin[8] initiated a study based on the premise that range of motion exercises increase spasticity and flexion contractures in clients with upper motor neuron damage by facilitating flexor ac-

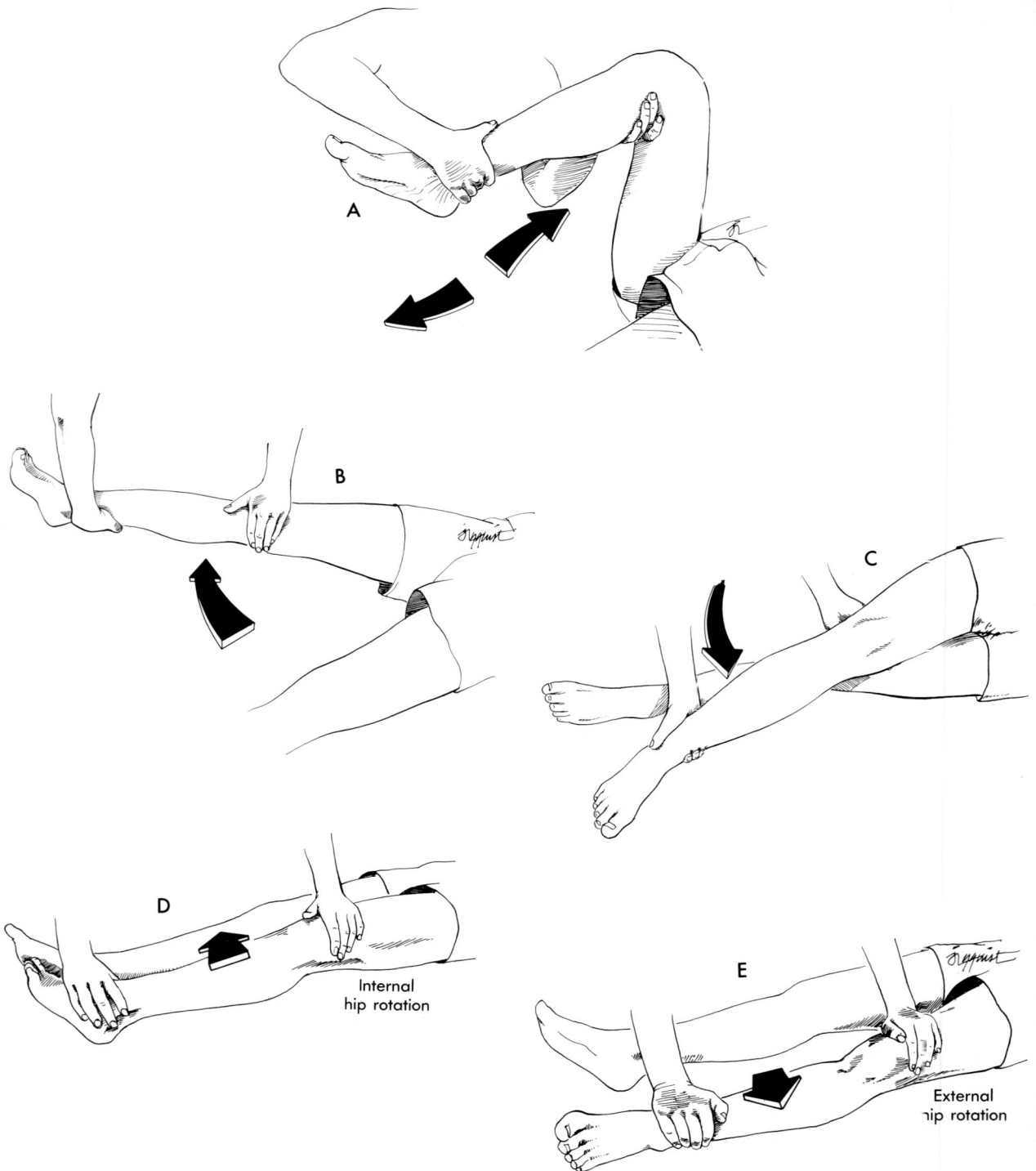

Figure 18-13
A, Caregiver can move hip in flexion by sliding leg back. Extension can be produced by sliding leg forward. **B,** Moving leg away from midline of body abducts hip. **C,** Moving leg toward midline of body and crossing over it adducts hip. **D,** Rolling leg inward causes hip joint to rotate internally. **E,** Rolling leg outward causes hip joint to rotate externally.

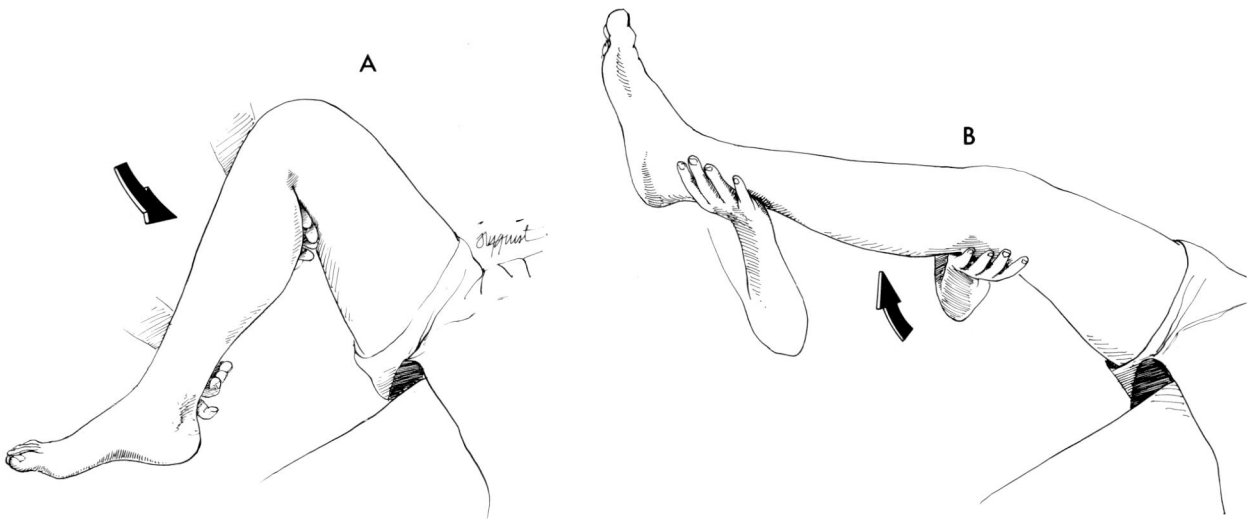

Figure 18-14
A, Knee and hip in position of flexion. **B,** Movement of lower leg upward produces knee extension. Hip also in extension.

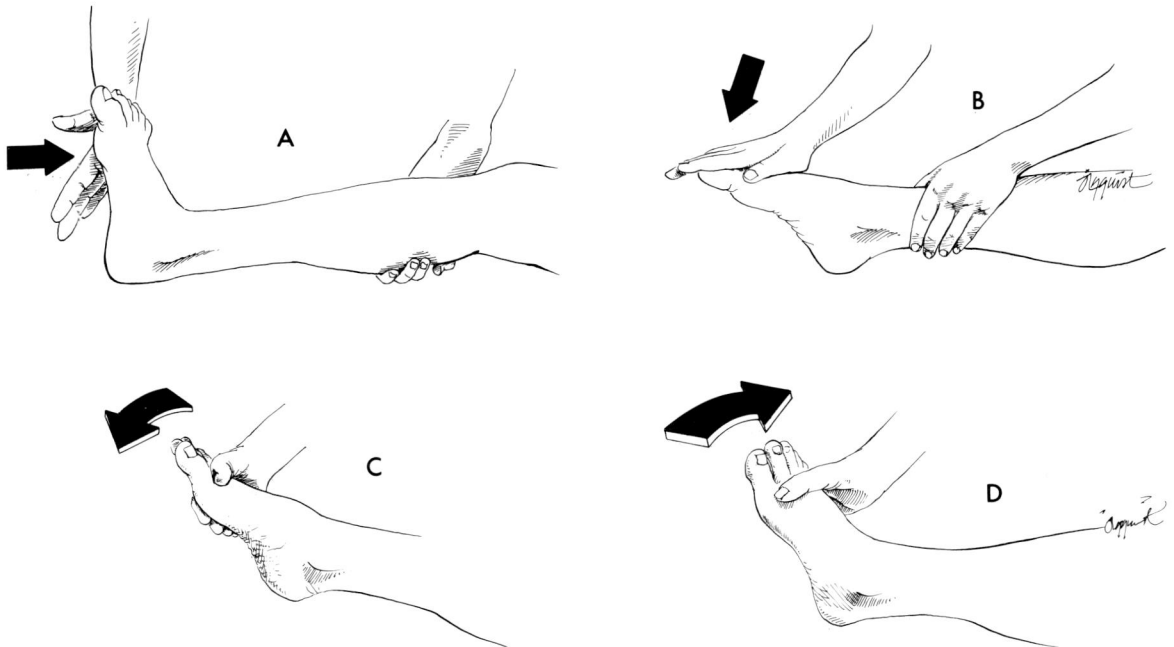

Figure 18-15
A, Pressure with palm of hand against ball of foot causes ankle dorsiflexion. **B,** Pressure against top of foot causes ankle plantar flexion. **C,** Turning foot inward produces ankle inversion. **D,** Turning foot outward produces ankle eversion.

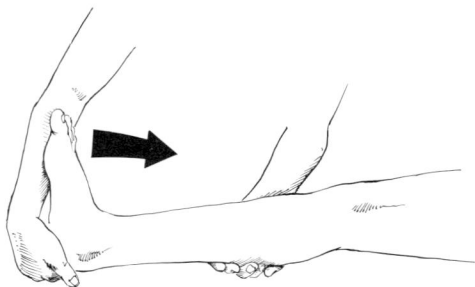

Figure 18-16
Heel cord stretching involves downward pull on heel cord and dorsiflexion of ankle.

tivity when muscle fibers are quickly stretched and maintained in the maximum range. In lieu of range of motion exercises, they used vibration of extensor muscle groups. Vibration reportedly facilitates extensor muscle contraction while inhibiting contraction of the flexor muscle. Results indicated that vibration plus other methods of neurophysiological treatment significantly increased range of motion at the fingers and wrist, decreasing contractures in clients with cerebrovascular accidents. An unexpected finding was that range of motion exercises appeared more effective in decreasing contractures of the shoulder.[8]

Active exercise. In teaching the client to perform active range of motion to extremities affected by disability, the nurse takes into account the general principles of teaching and learning, including motivation, readiness, attention span, and educational level. In general, the client will find the exercises easier to learn if they are demonstrated and if a written form with diagrams is provided. Redemonstration of the exercise to the nurse helps assure accuracy and effectiveness. As with other forms of exercise, a group approach may be helpful. Those persons with similar disabilities may be grouped together during the day for "range" exercises, or the client and an interested family member may exercise together.

Another avenue for the creative nurse to explore would be the hospital television station. A videotape of range of motion and other simple bed exercises could encourage and stimulate the participation of room-bound clients in a daily exercise program.

Modifications in range of motion exercise may have to be made for clients with specific disabilities such as hemiplegia or paraplegia. These individuals need to incorporate methods of moving the paralyzed extremities with the unaffected extremities. For example, many of the upper extremity exercises may be accomplished for the affected arm if the client laces the fingers of the unaffected hand through those of the affected hand, thereby supporting the affected arm, and then proceeds to perform the exercise. In this way, raising the unaffected arm above the shoulder also raises the affected arm. Flexing and extending the unaffected arm at the elbow also flexes and extends the affected arm. To move the legs through range of motion, the client may use a combination of both the unaffected arm and leg, depending on strength and balance. The client with paraplegia may find exercising the legs and feet easier while sitting in bed. The bed assists in maintaining balance and supports the legs and feet. Instruction in active range of motion techniques includes precautions to guard against joint damage, especially if sensation to the extremity has been impaired.

Isometric exercises

Isometric exercises consist of shortening muscle fibers without movement of limbs or joints. Isometric exercises require voluntary participation. The nurse teaches the client how to perform the activity and monitors and evaluates the results of the exercise. Isometric exercises are sometimes referred to as muscle-setting exercises. The most common are abdominal-setting, quadriceps-setting, and gluteal-setting exercises. To teach the client how to perform abdominal-setting exercises, the nurse places one hand on the client's abdomen while asking the client to tense the abdominal muscle. Once contraction is achieved, the client is told to hold it for 10 seconds and then to release the contraction. The client is taught to maintain a normal respiratory pattern during the exercise. Holding the breath may produce undesirable side effects, especially in clients who have had myocardial infarctions or brain injuries. Quadriceps setting consists of contracting the long muscles in the thighs. Gluteal setting is accomplished by tensing the buttocks. Telling the client to pinch the buttocks together may help to explain the desired effect. Other muscles such as the perineal, biceps, and triceps muscles also may be contracted isometrically.

Another type of isometric exercise is achieved by contracting a muscle group against an object. A common example of this type of exercise is pushing or plantar flexing the feet against a footboard to prevent circulatory stasis. In this instance, the isometric exercise is resistive, since the footboard provides resistance to the activity of the muscles of the legs and feet. To maintain normal cardiovascular function, the exercise should be limited to contractions of less than 10 seconds' duration.[1]

Energy expenditure may be a consideration in choosing an exercise program for a particular client. Hathaway and Geden[15] compared subjects' energy expenditure in three types of leg exercise programs (active, passive, and isometric) with energy expenditure in a control group (rest). They found that oxygen consumption and heart rate were comparable and significantly more demanding in isometric and active programs than either passive exercise or rest.

Adjunctive therapies to maintain or increase muscle strength and tone might also include biofeedback and electrical stimulation. Research in normal, healthy subjects suggests that transcutaneous electrical stimulation alone can strengthen skeletal muscle and may have applicability to immobilized or paralyzed clients.[18] Other research indicates that combining biofeedback with isometric exercise produces greater gains in muscle strength than isometric exercise alone.[20] The physical therapist can assess the client to determine whether benefits can be derived from electrical stimulation or biofeedback.

Activities in Bed

The individual who is completely or totally bed-bound should reposition himself or herself or be repositioned by the nursing staff or family. Activities in bed can be divided into turning and moving up and down. If the client is totally dependent, then the nursing staff or family members have to perform the work of moving. If the client is partially able to help, then some assistance or adaptive equipment should be provided. The client with no physical limitations is encouraged to move independently in bed.

To move the dependent client in bed, knowledge of good body mechanics is a must. If possible, the bed is raised to a comfortable working height at approximately hip level. This height coincides with the nurse's center of gravity. The nurse stands with knees slightly flexed and legs positioned apart to provide a wide base of support. The large muscles of the legs and buttocks rather than the small muscles of the back are used to effect the desired position change. Weight is transferred from one leg to the other in producing the motion or movement.

Turning

In turning the client to the side, the nurse stands on the side of the bed toward which the individual is to be turned. The client's arms are positioned on the abdomen. The farther leg is crossed over the near leg at the ankle. The nurse places one leg forward and one leg back. One hand is positioned beneath the client's far shoulder and one hand beneath the hips on the far side. Using a smooth rolling motion, the nurse transfers weight from the forward leg to the back leg, thereby positioning the client on his or her side.

To help the client affected by a stroke learn to bridge with the hips, a movement used to get on a bedpan, the nurse bends the client's knees, instructs the client to place the unaffected foot over the affected one to stabilize it, places a hand on top of the client's affected knee and pulls it down toward the feet, and places the other hand under the affected hip to direct the lifting movement of the hips.[4] Pressure exerted over the client's knee causes the hip to rise automatically.

Moving up in bed

In moving the dependent client toward the top or bottom of the bed, two caregivers are more energy efficient than a single person. The method of moving may depend on the client's weight and breadth.

For a person within the average weight range, two nursing staff members can efficiently effect the move. Using the hands as levers, with elbows bent, one caregiver slides her or his arms under the client's upper back. One arm is positioned under the shoulders, the other arm under the waist. The other caregiver supports the client's lower back, positioning one arm at waist level, the other below the client's hips. The two caregivers coordinate their activities by counting, so that at a given number, weight is shifted from one leg to the other in line with the desired direction of movement. The client is then moved upward or downward in bed.

Alternatively, the caregivers may use the Swedish lift. In this lift each caregiver stands on one side of the bed with feet spread to give a wide base of support. They flex their arms at the elbows and insert them under the client's back, approximately at waist level. Each caregiver's left hand is grasping his or her own right wrist. Beneath the client's back, each caregiver's right hand grasps onto the other caregiver's left wrist, forming a square of locked hands. The two caregivers then lean forward and press against each other's forehead. At a previously chosen count, weight is transferred from one leg to the other in the direction of the desired movement. The caregivers' foreheads must remain pressed together until the move is completed or the mechanical advantage is lost.

For larger clients or those with pain or fragile skin, a bath blanket or sheet folded in half may be used as a lift sheet. The lift sheet should extend from the client's hips to the shoulders. It is rolled under on each side close to the client's body. One caregiver is positioned on either side of the client. Using coordinated movements, weight is transferred from one leg to the other, again in the direction of the desired movement, moving the client up or down in bed. Clients should never be moved up in bed by pulling under their arms. Such pressure exerted under the axilla may damage the brachial plexus nerve, resulting in paralysis in the arm and hand.

To assist the client with a stroke in moving up in bed, the nurse can incorporate Bobath's approaches. The nurse helps the client bridge with the hips and instructs the client to clasp hands, reach forward, and lift the head. The nurse then places his or her hands under the client's affected scapula. By repeating these two movements with support of the nurse under the affected scapula, the client can gradually move up in bed.[4]

Moving to the side of the bed

To move the dependent client to the side of the bed, the caregivers may use the turn sheet, substituting a pushing-pulling motion for the sliding motion used in moving the person up in bed. If a turn sheet is not used, then the two caregivers

may stand at the same side of the bed. Using their arms as levers, they "divide" the client into two halves. One caregiver supports the client under the shoulders and under the waist; the other supports under the waist and at the hips. Each caregiver stands with knees slightly flexed and one foot forward. At the given count, weight is transferred from the forward to the back leg, and the client is moved to the edge of the bed. A single caregiver can follow the same principles. It may be easier, however, to move the client in "thirds," a section at a time, before the movement is completed. The caregiver would first slide head and shoulders over, then waist and hips, and finally legs and feet.

The client affected by stroke can be assisted to the side of the bed by using Bobath's approaches. The client is instructed to clasp hands and stretch them forward, bend the knees, turn the head and look in the direction of the turn, swing the extended arms to the side of the turn, and let the knees follow to complete the turn.[4]

Encouraging participation

When the client is able to assist in activities in bed, the nurse encourages participation and provides instruction. In turning to the side of the bed, the client is taught to use the siderail, pulling with either upper extremity. If an arm is immobilized, the client is taught to position the arm on the abdomen so that it is not left behind during the turn or to position the arm carefully when turning onto the paralyzed side. The affected leg is positioned over the unaffected ankle to make the task of turning simpler and so that the leg is not malpositioned. If one or both legs are mobile, then the client can facilitate the act of turning by pushing in the direction of the turn with the sole of the foot. The nurse emphasizes that the sole of the foot, rather than the heel, is used to prevent pressure area formation. If siderails are not available, then the edge of the mattress can be used as a support.

To move up toward the head of the bed, the client grasps the siderails and pulls up with the arms at the same time, pushing up with the soles of both feet. The head of the bed or a trapeze suspended on a Balkan or overbed frame also can be used to pull up on. The trapeze is useful for the client to pull up on for bedpan positioning or when the bed is being made. The physical therapist can assess the client for use of a trapeze and can teach bed exercises to strengthen the upper extremities.

Activities Out of Bed

Activity out of bed may be a nursing prescription for completely dependent clients, as well as for those who require some assistance. Generally the client is moved out of bed to a chair or wheelchair to provide a change in physical position and minimize the effects of immobility, as well as for a change in surroundings. Before sitting in a chair, the client spends time sitting in Fowler's position with the head of the bed elevated 90 degrees and also dangles the legs on the edge of the bed while supervised by nursing staff members. These activities help the client to adjust to a sitting posture. Readiness to sit in a chair is assessed by monitoring vital signs and comfort level while the client is sitting in a high Fowler's position or dangling. Circulation to lower extremities is assessed with the legs dangling, since venous pooling in the legs and feet when sitting can have serious consequences. If venous stasis occurs, application of antiembolism stockings or elastic bandages before activity out of bed may be indicated. Elevating the legs and feet on a stool also may be helpful.

Transferring a dependent client

Transferring a dependent client to a chair may be accomplished by mechanical devices or by nursing personnel. Nursing personnel can use lift transfers and pivot transfers to assist the client. Sitting posture and weight shifts are monitored when the client is sitting in a chair.

Mechanical devices. The most commonly used mechanical device is the pneumatic lift. The Hoyer lift is an example of such a device. The client is positioned on a one- or two-piece sling connected by chains to a crossbar on the lift. As the hydraulic pump is jacked up, the client is lifted off the bed in a sitting position. A broad base of support that is sometimes adjustable makes it possible to wheel the suspended client from the bed to a chair. As the pressure is released

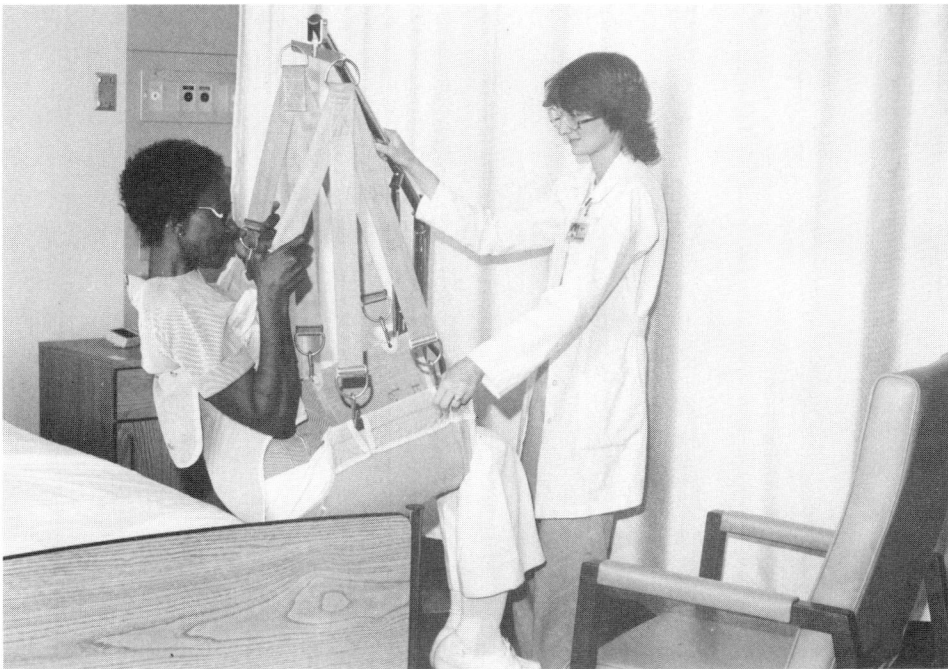

Figure 18-17
Hoyer lift provides safe and practical transfer for totally dependent client.

slowly from the hydraulic pump, the client descends into the chair. Depending on the client's size and disability, one, two, or three caregivers may be required to safely transfer the client to a chair. The slings may be left in place until it is time for the client to return to bed or may be removed for use with another client. Hooks on the slings should be turned away from the client to prevent injury (Figure 18-17).

Lift transfer. Two nurses or caregivers can transfer clients of average weight from the bed to a chair. The bed surface is elevated slightly higher than the chair. One nurse stands at the head of the bed and reaches under the client's arms with both arms. She or he grasps the client's wrists with opposite hands. The other nurse supports the client's legs and feet. While using good body mechanics and on the predetermined count, the client is lifted out of bed and slid into the chair (Figure 18-18).

For a heavier-than-average client, a sturdy lift sheet may be used with four caregivers, one at each of the client's shoulders and one at each of the client's knees. At the predetermined count, the caregivers slide the client over the surface of the bed with the lift sheet and into the chair.

Pivot transfer. If weight-bearing is not contraindicated, a dependent client can be pivot transferred to the chair. In a pivot transfer the client is first brought to a sitting position on the side of the bed. The nurse positions the client's arms around her or his neck. The nurse's arms pass under the client's arms to support the lower back. The nurse then flexes the knees and thighs and rocks back and forth with the client to gain momentum. When the client and nurse are ready,

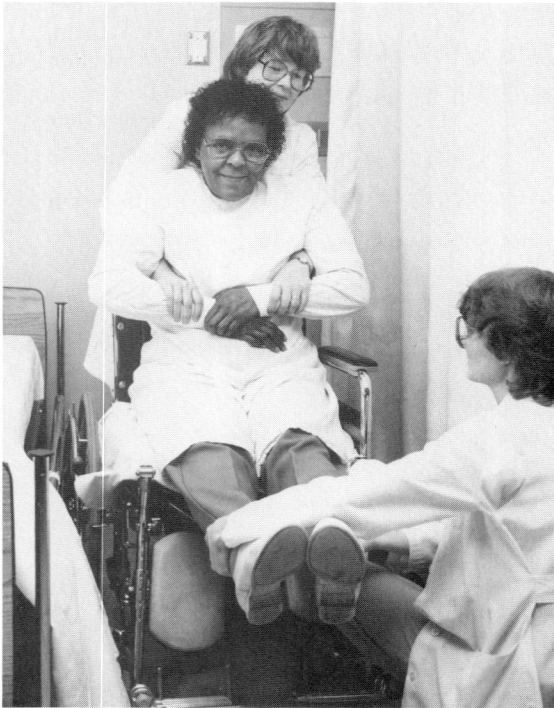

Figure 18-18
Dependent client is transferred from bed to chair by two caregivers.

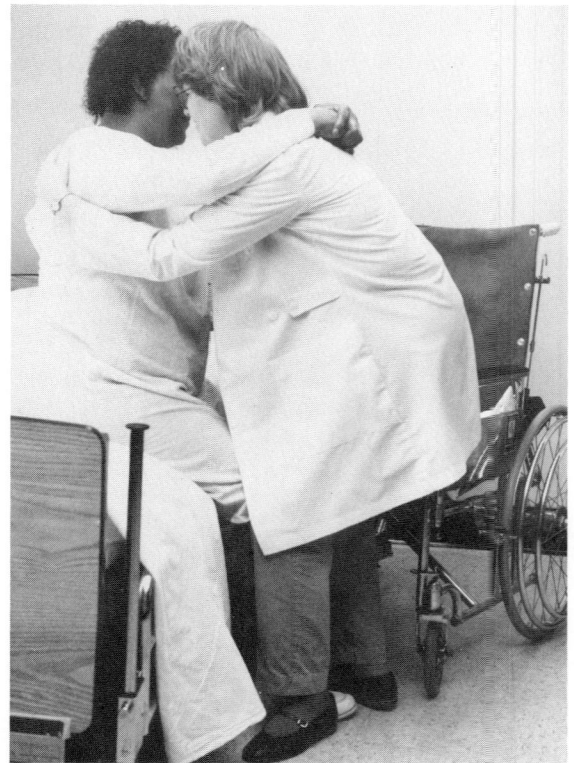

Figure 18-19
Dependent client is transferred from bed to chair by one caregiver using pivot transfer.

the nurse shifts weight from the forward to back leg, lifting the client off the bed and turning the client toward the chair. The nurse shifts weight from the back leg to the forward leg, bending at the hip and knee as the client is lowered into the chair (Figure 18-19).

Positioning in the chair. Once the client reaches the chair, the nurse checks the posture and corrects any problems. The best sitting posture for most clients is with a straight, slightly relaxed back, hips and knees flexed at 90 degrees, and feet flat on the floor. The nurse adjusts the physical characteristics of the chair to meet the client's requirements. If the chair is too high, a footstool is provided to maintain good posture. Pillows may be positioned on each side of the client to prevent leaning toward one side or the other if a chair is too wide. A pillow also may be used at the back to prevent slumping if a chair is too deep. When a chair is too low, the hips and knees are flexed more acutely than is desirable, predisposing to the development of contractures. A foam pad or pillow should be placed under the client before transfer to the chair.

The client and family are taught that position change is important even when sitting in a chair. Two or three times an hour the client's weight should be shifted by leaning forward, to the right, or to the left. Depending on the client and family's ability and motivation, this activity can be shared by the nurse and the client and family and can be transferred gradually to the client and family before discharge.

Assisting the client to transfer

Partially dependent clients can increase their independence by using several other transfer techniques. Included are a technique used by persons who are paraplegic, use of a transfer board, and a technique used by persons who are hemiplegic. The nurse encourages participation, is available for assistance, and breaks the transfer procedure down into steps while instructing the client in each of these transfer techniques.

Paraplegic transfer. The client who is paraplegic or who has limited mobility from the waist down can use the following transfer. The chair is placed perpendicular to the bed at the middle of the bed. The wheels on the bed are locked. If a wheelchair is used, the wheelchair is locked and footrests are removed. The client raises to a sitting

position. Using the upper extremities, the trunk and legs are turned to line up with the chair. With the client's back nearest the seat of the chair, the client reaches back with both arms to grasp the armrests and slides the hips and legs from the bed back into the chair. The chair is then moved back from the bed, and the client lowers the legs carefully (Figure 18-20).

Transfer board. A transfer board can be used for the client with limited use of the lower extremities. The wheelchair or chair is placed alongside the bed. Brakes are locked, and armrests are removed if possible. The transfer or sliding board is placed between the chair and the bed. The client is assisted to position a portion of the transfer board under the buttocks. Using the upper extremities, the client pulls himself or herself toward the far armrest of the chair, thereby causing the hips and lower extremities to slide along the board and into the chair. The transfer board also may be used in transfer activities between the chair and tub, the chair and toilet, the chair and car, and so forth. Generally the physical therapy department initiates upper extremity strengthening and the training necessary for the client to begin to use this method of transfer. The nurse reinforces instruction received in physical therapy and provides encouragement as this type of transfer is integrated into daily activities.

Hemiplegic transfer. The client with less muscle strength on one side of the body, such as the person with hemiplegia, can be instructed to transfer independently in many situations. Most sources advocate that the chair or locked wheelchair be placed at a slight angle to the bed on the client's unaffected side. The client comes to a sitting position on the side of the bed by using the unaffected hand to position the affected hand across the abdomen. The unaffected foot is slid under the affected ankle; both legs are moved over the side of the bed on the client's unaffected side. The client grasps the edge of the mattress and pushes with elbow and forearm against the bed, coming to a half-sitting position. After moving one hand to the rear, the client pushes to a full sitting position. The client is now ready to transfer to the chair. Keeping the feet beneath the body and leaning forward, the client places the unaffected arm near the edge of the bed and pushes to a standing position. The client then steadies himself or herself. The unaffected hand

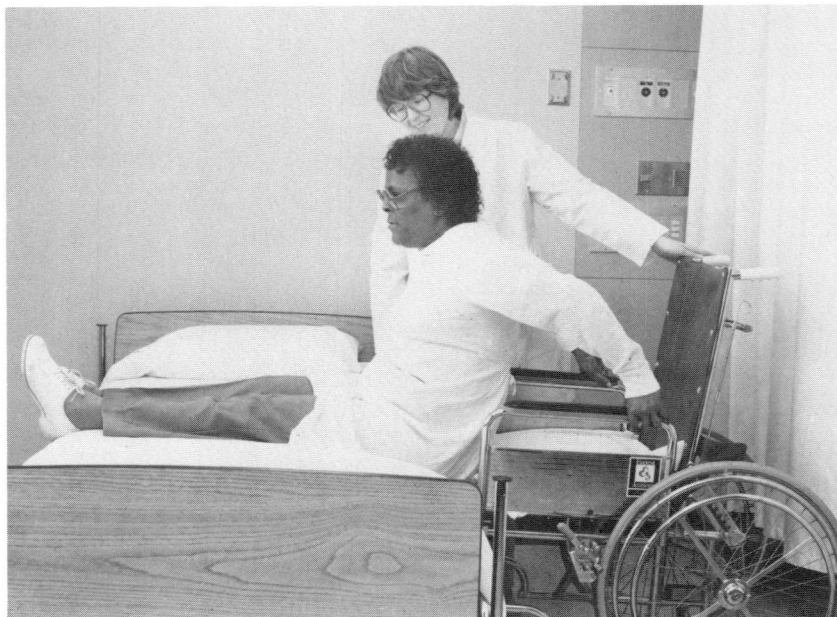

Figure 18-20
Paraplegic transfer enables client with good balance and upper extremity muscle strength to transfer independently.

is then moved to the farther armrest of the chair. The client turns on the unaffected foot toward the chair and lowers to a sitting position.

When incorporating Bobath's approaches, the chair is placed at an angle to the bed on the client's affected side. The chair is locked and the armrest closest to the bed removed. The client is assisted to the side of the bed, and the feet are positioned flat on the floor with the heels under or slightly behind the knees. The client is helped to clasp the hands and extend the arms, leaning forward until the head and trunk are in position over the feet. The nurse then leans over the client's back and assists the client in moving the hips. The nurse rocks back, shifting the weight to the back foot, and pivots the client's hips toward the chair, affected side first. The client is then gently lowered to the chair or other transfer surface.[4]

Ambulation/Gait Training

To assist the client in achieving a goal of functional ambulation, the rehabilitation team members work together. Generally the physical therapist

establishes a plan reinforced through activities on the nursing unit and in occupational therapy. The plan includes isometric and other exercises designed to prepare the muscles used in walking, practice in maintaining sitting and standing balance, passive standing using specialized equipment, and finally selection of adaptive equipment and assistive devices used with specific gait training techniques.

Preambulation exercises

The exercise program to prepare muscles for standing and walking is initiated while the client is still bed-bound. The purposes of the exercises are to strengthen muscles of the lower extremities; muscles of the trunk, including the gluteal and abdominal muscles; and muscles of the upper extremities. Isometric exercises such as those described earlier in this chapter are implemented. The nurse reinforces instruction from physical therapy and encourages client compliance with the program. Involvement of family members in the exercise program is encouraged as well. Other exercises that are performed in bed preparatory to walking are modified sit-ups in the supine position and modified push-ups in the prone position. The nurse monitors the client's cardiovascular response to these and other exercise programs.

Sitting balance

Sitting balance is developed by assisting the client to a sitting position on the side of the bed. The client's feet are resting on the floor or are firmly supported by a footstool. The nurse or therapist guards the client while the client is instructed to raise the arms left, right, forward, and upward. Demonstrating the ability to perform these maneuvers without a loss of balance indicates readiness to progress in the ambulation program. If walking with crutches is the eventual goal of the ambulation program, the client is taught to perform sitting push-ups using both upper extremities to support the entire body weight while sitting in a locked wheelchair or very sturdy armchair.

Standing balance

The client is taught to come to a standing position and practices this activity until it is performed safely. Basically the client is reminded to slide to the edge of the sitting surface, keeping the feet back under the body. He or she is taught to push down with the legs and arms while leaning the trunk forward to come to a standing position. Some clients require the assistance of rehabilitation personnel to achieve a standing position and are then trained to use assistive equipment to compensate for weakness or disability. The client practices standing next to a stable support until an erect position and trunk balance can be maintained while moving the extremities. During these activities, care is taken to guard the client against injury from falls. Research is needed with the elderly whose balance is often impaired because of loss of arm movement, abnormal gait patterns, and increased body sway. Activities such as passive rocking in a rocking chair have been suggested as possible methods to increase vestibular stimulation, thereby improving balance.[32]

Passive standing activities

Passive standing activities may precede transfer activities and standing activities. Passive standing is prescribed to prepare the cardiovascular system

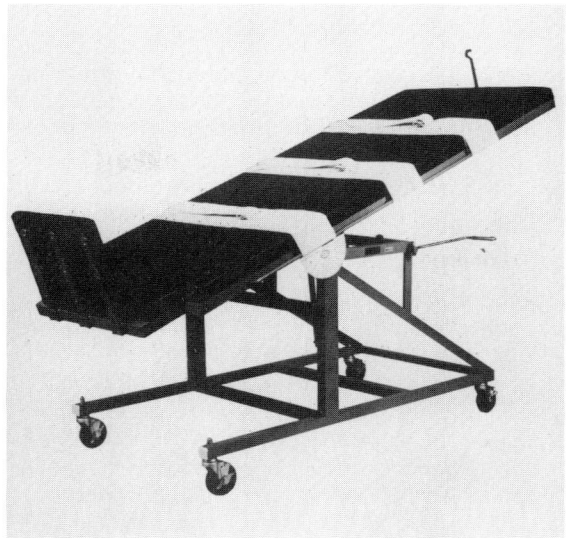

Figure 18-21
Tilt table adjusts to erect position. (*Courtesy LaBerne Manufacturing Co, Inc, Columbia, SC*)

to adjust to the change in circulatory demands between the recumbent and erect positions.

Tilt table. Most commonly the tilt table is used to passively stand the client (Figure 18-21). The tilt table is generally located in the physical therapy department. The client is transferred to the table in the supine position and then secured with safety straps. The feet rest on a support. A baseline blood pressure and pulse are obtained. The tilt table is elevated initially at a 15- to 20-degree angle. Thereafter the degree of tilt is increased by 5- to 10-degree increments until a standing position is tolerated for 10 to 30 minutes. During tilt table activities, the blood pressure and pulse are checked for abnormalities, the feet and legs are monitored for dependent edema and mottling, and the client is asked to indicate if faintness, dizziness, or headache occur. If the client has been bed-bound for a prolonged period before beginning passive standing or has a poor cardiovascular response, the legs may be wrapped with elastic bandages and an abdominal binder applied in preparation for tilt table activities. Squires[38] found the following advantages in using electrically powered tilt tables with the elderly: relief of gluteal pressure, maintenance of postural reflexes, enhanced bladder and bowel function, un-impeded chest expansion, and psychological motivation to participate in an ambulation program.

Standing frame. A standing frame or table also may be used to passively stand the client. When using standing frames or tables, the client adjusts to transfer from a sitting position to immediate upright standing. There is no gradual increase in degree of erect position as with the tilt table. Standing frames or tables generally have stabilizers that may be padded supports at the knees and abdomen or actual counters or tabletop surfaces. The posterior stabilizers may include heel cups, knee stabilizers, and pelvic or gluteal supports. The use of the standing frame or table permits the client to enjoy the physiological and psychological rewards of an erect position, while increasing standing balance and freeing the individual to use the upper extremities for occupational therapy exercises or diversional activities.

The physical therapist assesses the client for ability to ambulate in a functional manner, prescribes assistive equipment most appropriate for the specific disability and most acceptable to self-image, and initiates teaching and training of the client and family to accomplish the desired goal.

Use of assistive equipment

The type of assistive equipment selected often depends on the client's physical limitations. Crutches are appropriate for clients with full use of upper extremities who have limitations in lower extremity function because of amputation, fracture, or paraparesis or paraplegia. Broad-based canes or tripod or quad canes are appropriate for clients who have weakness or paralysis of one side of the body, including those who have had strokes. Walkers are chosen for those persons who have generalized weakness in both upper and lower extremities and are used with the aged who have generalized arthritis, hip fracture, and neuromuscular diseases.

The physical therapist measures the client so that the assistive equipment is tailored to height, weight, and specific needs. For this reason, assistive equipment such as crutches, canes, and walkers should not be shared among clients. In teaching the client to ambulate with any assistive equipment, the following points are covered: care of the device, coming to a standing position, actual gait training, maneuvering stairs or curbs, re-turning to a sitting position, and coming to a sitting or erect position after a fall.

Crutch walking. The physical therapist measures the client for crutches that allow the elbow to flex at 30 degrees to hold the handgrips. The length of the crutch is the measurement of the distance from 2 inches below the axilla to a mark placed 2 inches out and 6 inches ahead of the tip of the shoe. The nurse and therapist stress and reinforce the fact that weight is supported on the handgrips, never under the axillae.

Depending on the client's abilities, the physical therapist prescribes a four-point alternate, two-point, or swing gait. The four-point alternate gait is commonly used for clients with muscle weakness or lack of balance. It is a very stable and safe gait pattern; however, it also is a slow method of ambulation. The client starts in a crutch stance with slightly flexed elbows and with crutches held 6 inches out and 6 inches away from the shoe tips. The axillary bar is 2 inches below the axilla and is pressed against the chest for lateral stability. The gait pattern is left crutch, right leg, right crutch, left leg, repeated until the desired distance is reached.

The two-point gait most closely resembles the normal gait pattern. It is more rapid, but requires better balance, since there are only two points of contact with the floor at any given time. The client begins in the usual crutch stance and then shifts weight to advance the right leg and left crutch at the same time, following through with the left leg and right crutch and so on.

Swing gaits are used for clients with a non-weight bearing lower extremity caused by hip or leg fracture or by single amputation. Swing gaits are broken down to the slower but more stable swing-to or step-to gait and the more rapid, but more complex swing-through gait.

In the step-to-gait, the client starts in the usual crutch stance with no weight-bearing on the affected extremity. Both crutches are moved ahead as a unit while the client bears weight on the unaffected extremity and shifts weight onto the crutches, stepping up to the crutches, and then repeating the process. In the step-through or swing-through gait, the client begins in a crutch stance. Again, both crutches are moved 4 to 6 inches ahead as a single unit as the client supports weight on the unaffected extremity. The client then shifts weight onto the crutches, advancing the unaffected leg so that the foot lands ahead of the crutches. The process is repeated until the client ambulates the required distance.

Ambulation with a cane. In selecting a cane, the rehabilitation team can choose from a straight cane, which has a single point of contact with the floor, or from quad or tripod canes, which have broader bases of support, but are bulkier to handle (Figure 18-22). The length of the cane is mea-

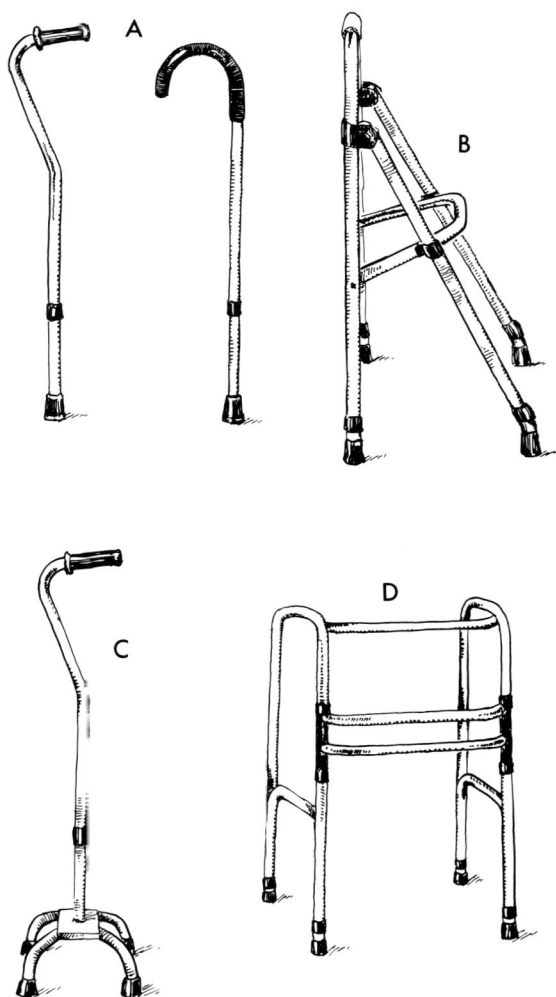

Figure 18-22
Assistive devices for ambulation. **A,** Straight canes. **B,** Pickup walker. **C,** Quad cane. **D,** Standard walker.

sured by determining the distance between the greater trochanter and the floor. When the proper length of cane is selected, it enables the client to stand with elbows slightly flexed while the cane is about 6 inches to the side of the foot. To walk with a cane, the client stands with weight on both feet and the hand on cane. The cane is advanced approximately 4 to 6 inches. The weaker leg is moved up to the cane, then the unaffected leg is moved past the cane; this process is repeated for the desired distance.

For a client with hemiplegia, bracing of the affected lower extremity may be necessary. A short leg brace may be prescribed by the physiatrist. This brace is attached to the shoe and extends to just below the knee. The brace assists the client in raising the toes off the floor when walking, in striking the heel of the affected leg back to the floor, and in preventing the ankle from turning inward during ambulation. In addition, the standing balance and ambulation activities of clients with hemiplegia may be more successful if a sling is used on the affected arm. A sling keeps the weight of the affected arm close to the body, improving balance and preventing accidental injury and dislocation of the affected arm. Slings are often prescribed and tailored to meet client needs by the occupational therapist.

The construction of the sling varies, but most consist of a one- or two-piece support for the affected arm, supported by straps or webbing to distribute the weight of the affected arm to both sides of the upper trunk. More recently, dynamic slings fashioned of elastic, denture dam, or tourniquet hosing have been suggested. Dynamic slings are designed to give resistance to the triceps as it contracts and to provide a quick stretch to the triceps as the arm snaps back up because of the sling's elasticity.[23] In addition to providing support, such a sling increases range at the shoulder.

Ambulation with a walker. Walkers vary according to structure and purpose. Lightweight, adjustable, pickup walkers are available for clients able to lift the walker and maintain balance; reciprocal walkers are suitable for persons who might lose their balance backward when lifting a regular walker. Rolling walkers are available with and without seats, permitting energy-efficient ambulation. The instability of rolling walkers, however, makes their use impossible for some persons. Measurement for the walker is the same as for the cane described previously. The gait pattern with the pickup walker consists of advancing the walker, and then stepping with each leg, keeping steps equal. An alternate gait with this type of walker is to advance the walker, step with the right foot, advance the walker, step with the left foot and so on. The client is reminded not to step or walk while the walker is off the floor (Figure 18-22).

Lower limb bracing. The client with paraplegia may be a candidate for functional ambulation based on multiple factors. Among the devices used to achieve this goal include long leg braces with crutches or a walker, and the Orlau Swivel Walker. Electrical stimulation also is used to promote functional ambulation.

Long leg braces, or knee-ankle-foot orthoses, provide stabilizers at the knee, ankle, and foot, making ambulation possible with the assistance of crutches or a walker (Figure 18-23). Research indicates, however, that persons with paraplegia with knee-ankle-foot orthoses expend five to almost thirteen times as much energy during ambulation as the able bodied.[26]

The Orlau Swivel Walker (Orthotic Research and Locomotor Assessment Unit) consists of a rigid, stable steel frame. The wearer is held upright in the frame by a thoracic band, sacral band, and knee clamp. The footplates are sloped upward and outward. The client shifts weight from one side to the other causing the walker to move forward. The Orlau Swivel Walker has advantages of increased stability and easy mobility, without de-

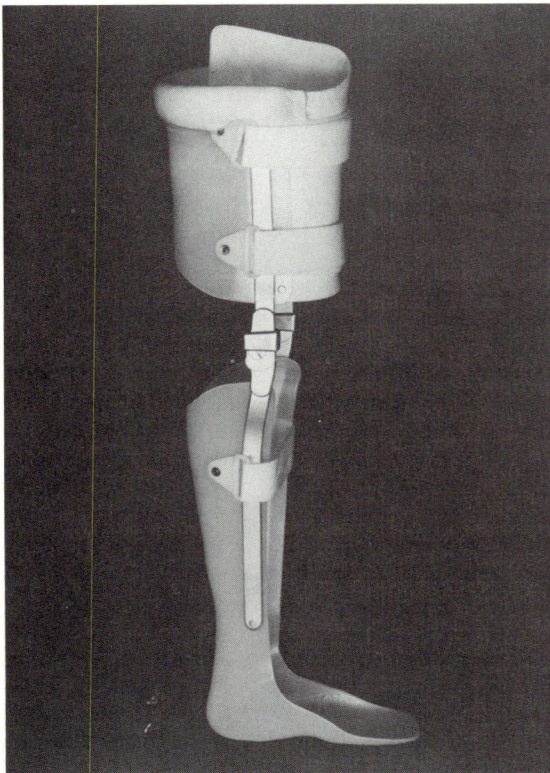

Figure 18-23
Foot-knee-ankle orthoses, also known as long leg braces, provide stabilizers at client's knee, ankle, and foot.

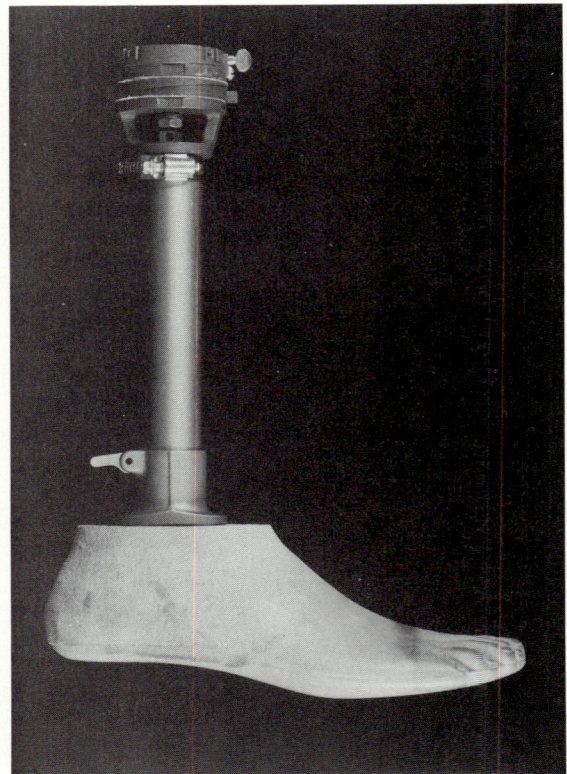

Figure 18-24
Immediate postsurgical fitting pylon before application of plaster dressing.

pending on the upper extremities for support. However, it provides a very slow method of mobility. Research indicates that it is the least efficient metabolically when compared to knee-ankle-foot orthoses and wheelchair mobility.[36]

Most recently research has been conducted with the use of electrical stimulation as an ambulatory aid for paraplegic clients. Such stimulation has been used with limited populations to date. A four-channel stimulator enables the client with paraplegia to sit, stand, and walk. Equipment and procedures need to be streamlined and further developed before the stimulators can be widely used.[5,22]

Lower limb prosthesis. Although the person with an amputation is mobile with a walker or crutches, more stable and acceptable ambulation is possible with a prosthesis. Depending upon the recommendations of the rehabilitation team, a rigid plaster dressing and pylon may be applied immediately after the amputation. Such an immediate postsurgical fitting permits the person to participate in transfer and ambulation activities very soon after surgery (Figure 18-24). These clients, as well as those with traditional postoperative treatment, must wait until stump shrinkage subsides before being fitted with a permanent prosthesis.

The prosthesis is tailored to each client through the joint efforts of the physiatrist who provides the prescription and the prosthetist who constructs the limb. Basically the lower limb prosthesis for a person with an above-knee amputation consists of a socket, joints at the hip and knee, a suspension system, and a foot and ankle. Because of the diversity of the components available, the prescription and construction are complicated. The suspension system, for instance, may involve a suction system, pelvic band, waist belt, and leather thigh corset (Figures 18-25 and 18-26).

For clients with above-knee amputations, a prosthesis has been developed that incorporates a hydraulic cylinder to coordinate gait at the hip and knee. This type of prosthesis permits the person to use a wider range of walking speeds and to improve the equality of durations of successive swing and stance phases.[19,29]

The prosthetist designs the leg, taking into account the length and condition of the stump, the general assessment of the client, including age, weight, agility, and endurance. Consideration is given to present financial status and medical in-

surance coverage, as well as social and occupational goals. Individual motivation and family support are important factors in the actual use of the prosthesis on a day-to-day basis.

The prosthetic limb is designed to match the normal limb in length and skin tone; the prosthetic foot corresponds to the size of the normal foot. Care is taken that pelvic tilt is avoided in the standing position and during ambulation. The prosthesis should be functional while appearing as normal as possible.

Once fitted with the prosthesis, the amputee continues gait training using a four-point or swing gait. Eventually the person with an amputation walks with a cane or may be able to maneuver without any assistance except for the prosthesis.

The nurse teaches the client and family to inspect the stump daily for redness, abrasions, or

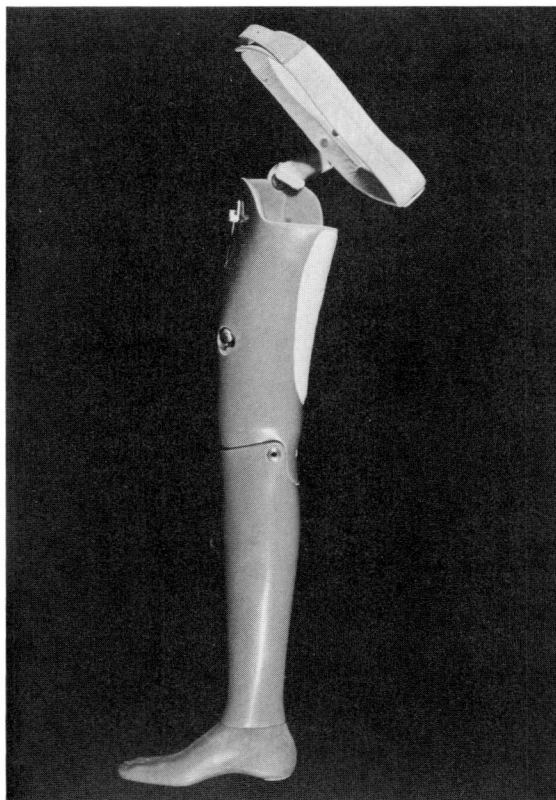

Figure 18-25
Above-knee prosthesis.

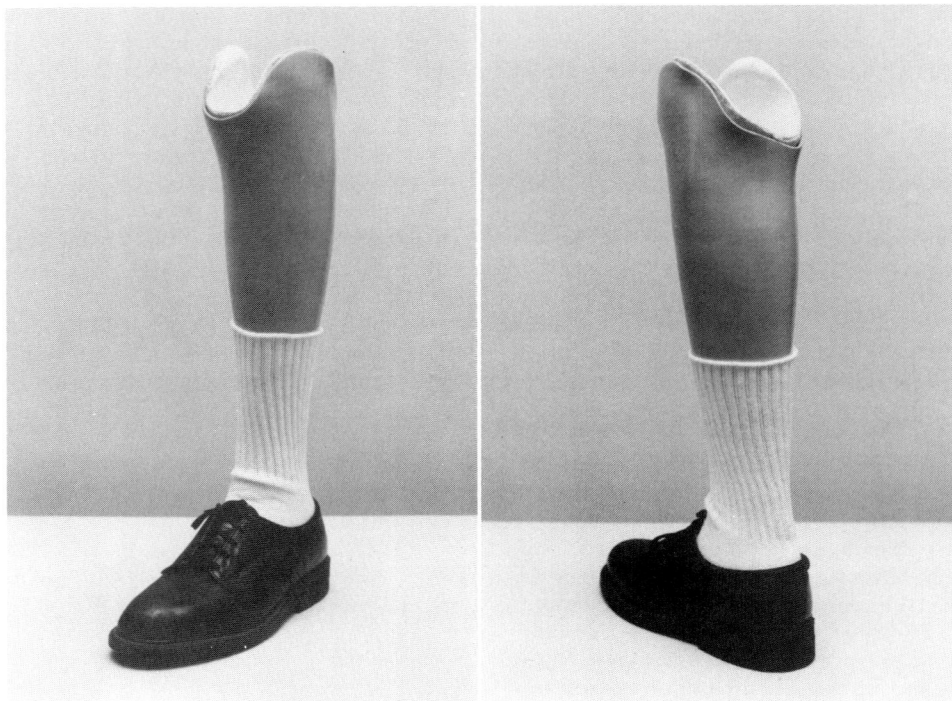

Figure 18-26
Below-knee prosthesis.

irritation and provides instruction about stump hygiene, stressing cleanliness and gentle care. Information is given to the client and family about the care of stump socks, prevention of stump swelling, and care of the prosthetic limb. The client is cautioned that the prosthesis should not be mechanically altered or adjusted, but the prosthetist should be consulted if problems arise and for regular maintenance.

Wheelchair Mobility

The United States Bureau of Vital and Health Statistics revealed in 1977 that 645,000 persons required wheelchairs, translating into an estimated cost of over $550 million.[9] Findings of a West Coast study conducted in 1983 suggested that when used about 9 hours a day, the average life span of a wheelchair was only 25 months and that only 49 to 79 percent of the wheelchairs were used in an optimum manner.[17] The same study recommended further evaluation of wheelchair

usage based on a team approach involving physical and occupational therapists, the rehabilitation engineer, physiatrist, social worker, and psychologist. The study also strongly recommended consulting the consumers of wheelchair products for their evaluations.

Modifications

Wheelchairs are as diverse as the clients who use them. The prescription for a wheelchair is usually a joint effort of the rehabilitation team with specific recommendations for modifications made by physical and occupational therapists. The wheelchair height and width are based on the client's dimensions, so that as normal a sitting posture as possible can be maintained when sitting in the wheelchair. The back and seat of the chair can be modified to accommodate antipressure devices and additional positioning supports. High-backed and reclining-back chairs are available for clients who need head and neck support or who tolerate the erect seated position poorly. In initial transfer activities out of bed, the nurse may make use of a wheelchair that flattens out completely so that a simple sliding transfer can be performed. The chair is then cranked into a sitting position.

Wheelchairs can be constructed to fold so that the chair is transportable from one area to another. Armrests and legrests may be detached to facilitate transfer activities. Generally the more modifications in the wheelchair design, the more the wheelchair costs. Financial circumstances and individual needs and goals are considered when choosing a wheelchair. The weight of the chair and the size and type of tires can facilitate traveling within or outside the home. Generally, heavier chairs with tires of more durable construction are better suited to the outdoors. Wheelchairs consisting of lightweight frames, high-quality bearings, and tubular tires can be specifically designed for racing. Manual hand controls of differing types, as well as electronic touch and breath control, can be used for propulsion of the wheelchair. Research into more energy-efficient methods of manual propulsion has examined the use of arm cranks, as well as handrims.[37] Efforts are made to use hand controls even when the client is quadriplegic; it is believed that self-image is improved if the client is able to use the hands, rather than the chin for propulsion. Persons who are quadriplegic appear to develop better balance when hand controls are used, since a manually operated chair does not require a control box. Some clients use the control box to lean upon for support.[25]

Psychological aspects

Although dependency on a wheelchair for mobility may be a threat to self-esteem, the energy saved makes possible the performance of more diverse activities within a day and may outweigh the psychological need to ambulate. A study involving elderly clients with bilateral below-knee amputations concluded that wheelchair mobility was preferable to ambulation on prostheses, since oxygen use and heart rate during ambulation were significantly higher during ambulation.[11] Competitive sports such as wheelchair racing promote physical, emotional, and social rehabilitation of persons who are paraplegic.[21]

Prescription criteria

Criteria that help determine the prescription of the wheelchair as the primary mode of mobility include energy cost, physiological factors, cosmetic and psychosocial factors, and occupational and educational goals. The nurse and other rehabilitation team members teach the client and family how to transfer to and from the wheelchair, checking dependent body areas for signs of pressure; change position in the wheelchair, including push-ups; maintain the wheelchair; and propel the wheelchair.

As the client is prepared to leave the facility, the rehabilitation team focuses on accessibility of the wheelchair. Doorways and room dimensions are measured to determine if the wheelchair can be accommodated. Exits and entrances are evaluated for ramp placement; adaptations in living arrangements may be necessary if the living unit is located on multiple levels or has "step-down" areas. Consideration is given to the method of transportation to and from the living quarters. Feasibility of transfer to a traditional motor vehicle is assessed and compared to that of vans or other vehicles modified to accommodate persons in wheelchairs as passengers or operators.

OUTCOME CRITERIA

Outcome criteria for the client with impaired physical mobility depend upon the client's individual situation. The following criteria can be adapted for a person's specific problems in mobility:

1. The client is free of secondary complications of immobility.
2. The client participates in all activities planned to increase mobility as demonstrated by:
   a. Participation in exercise and positioning programs on the nursing units.
   b. Participation in activities in the physical and occupational therapy departments.
   c. Explanation and demonstration of specific exercises and positioning programs prescribed to maintain and increase function.
   d. Communication with health team members regarding personal needs and goals.
3. The client functions safely at an optimum level of independence as demonstrated by:
   a. Safe levels of function in activities in bed, transfer activities, and ambulation/wheelchair activities.

b. The realization of need for and acceptance of assistance from others.

4. The client successfully adjusts to the psychological impact of impaired physical mobility as evidenced by:
   a. Compliance with exercise and activity programs.
   b. Use of prescribed prostheses, braces, ambulatory aids, and wheelchairs.
   c. Continued interaction with family, friends, and rehabilitation team members.

5. The family provides effective support for the client as demonstrated by the ability to:
   a. Explain the importance of correct body alignment.
   b. Explain and demonstrate therapeutic positioning with and without supportive equipment.
   c. Explain and demonstrate how to move the client in bed.
   d. Explain and demonstrate safe transfer methods for the client.
   e. Explain and demonstrate safe ambulation methods for the client.
   f. Explain and demonstrate modifications needed for wheelchair mobility.
   g. Accept need for adaptive equipment, including braces, prostheses, crutches, canes, walkers, and wheelchairs.
   h. Identify potential problems arising from the use of such equipment (such as pressure areas).
   i. Realize the importance of the need to be as independent as possible.
   j. Understand reasons for consulting the rehabilitation team (such as equipment dysfunction, change in status).

SUMMARY

Working with clients who have impaired physical mobility requires that the nurse possess a knowledge of the structure and function of muscles, joints, bones, and nerves. A complete assessment of the musculoskeletal and nervous systems enables the nurse to formulate nursing diagnoses and set goals with and unique to specific clients. Nursing interventions complement the interventions of other members of the rehabilitation team. Educating the client and family about reasons for and methods of optimizing mobility increase the chances of compliance and successful adjustment.

TEST QUESTIONS

1. Voluntary motor activity impulses originate in:
   a. The pyramidal tract of the cerebral cortex
   b. Gray matter of the anterior horn of the spinal cord
   c. White matter of the lateral spinal cord
   d. Basal ganglia and cerebellum

2. The nurse knows that movements at ball-and-socket joints such as the hip include:
   a. Flexion and extension
   b. Abduction and adduction
   c. Internal and external rotation
   d. All of the above

3. In assessing a client's mobility, the nurse:
   a. Assesses range of motion of joints
   b. Determines relative strength of muscle groups
   c. Checks deep tendon reflexes
   d. All of the above

4. A nursing intervention(s) to prevent contractures is (are):
   a. Range of joint motion exercises
   b. Frequent turning and positioning
   c. Use of hard hand cones
   d. All of the above

5. A nursing intervention to promote correct body alignment in the supine position includes all of the following except:
   a. Placing a trochanter roll at the hips
   b. Elevating the foot of the bed 30 degrees
   c. Using a footboard
   d. Placing a flat pillow to support the shoulders and head

6. When using Bobath's approaches to positioning, the nurse positions the client with a stroke on the affected side and places the:
   a. Affected shoulder behind the unaffected shoulder with the affected arm flexed
   b. Affected shoulder forward with the arm extended
   c. Affected shoulder forward with the arm flexed
   d. None of the above

7. According to recent nursing research, the best nursing intervention for placing a spastic hand in a functional position is to use
   a. A soft rubber ball
   b. A rolled washcloth
   c. A firm cone
   d. No device, best left unsupported

8. A nursing intervention used to prevent the hazards of immobility and that turns a person every 3½ minutes over a range of 124 degrees on a continuous basis is the:
   a. CircOlectric Bed
   b. Stryker Wedge Frame
   c. Clinitron
   d. Roto Rest
9. In transferring a client who is hemiplegic, the nurse is aware that:
   a. Independent transfer activity is improbable.
   b. The client's feet should be positioned flat on the floor with the heels under or slightly behind the knees.
   c. The client always transfers toward the unaffected side.
   d. The wheelchair is always turned toward the foot of the bed.
10. The client using a four-point gait exhibits the following pattern:
    a. Right crutch, left foot, left crutch, right foot
    b. right crutch, right foot, left crutch, left foot
    c. Right crutch and foot, left crutch and foot
    d. Right and left crutch, right and left foot
11. The nurse assists the client in mastering the following activity(ies) before ambulation:
    a. Isometric exercises
    b. Sitting balance
    c. Standing balance
    d. All of the above
12. When collaborating with the physical therapist and occupational therapist to prescribe a wheelchair, the nurse knows that wheelchairs:
    a. Are designed only for indoor activities
    b. Provide an alternative to ambulation when ambulation is not energy efficient
    c. Are inexpensive to purchase and maintain
    d. Always require use of upper extremities
13. The nurse teaches the client and family all of the following procedures to care for a stump *except:*
    a. Wash once a week
    b. Inspect for redness, abrasions, or irritation
    c. Elevate of the stump
    d. Wear and clean stump stocks

Answers: 1. a, 2. d, 3. d, 4. d, 5. b, 6. b, 7. c, 8. d, 9. b, 10. a, 11. d, 12. b, 13. a.

LEARNING ACTIVITIES

1. Work in groups of three students or three nurses. One person plays the nurse, one acts as a client, and one acts as an evaluator. The nurse positions the client in the basic bed positions (supine, lateral, prone, and semiprone). Use supportive devices as needed. The evaluator checks the client's alignment and provides feedback to the nurse. Alternate roles. During and after positioning practice, share subjective feelings about relative comfort of each position.
2. Practice turning and moving a fellow colleague in bed. Ask another colleague to check your body mechanics and techniques as you turn your "client," slide him or her to the edge of the mattress, and move him or her up in bed. Consider your colleague's subjective comments about comfort, discomfort, and strain during movement.
3. Demonstrate passive range of motion exercises on another colleague. Watch for verbal and nonverbal indications of discomfort. Measure the range of each joint with a goniometer. Verify your measurements with those made by another colleague.
4. Depending on the availability, practice using the following equipment: CircOlectric Bed, Stryker Wedge Frame, Roto Rest, Hoyer lift, crutches, cane, walker, wheelchair. Take the role of both the client and the caregiver. Discuss your feelings about using the equipment and of being a "client" dependent on such equipment.
5. Practice getting a colleague out of bed using a pivot transfer and a two-person transfer. Role-play teaching the client with paraplegia and the client with hemiplegia how to transfer independently from the bed to chair or wheelchair.
6. Visit a physical therapy and an occupational therapy department in a rehabilitation facility. Observe the roles of the therapists. Consider how the prescribed activities of specific clients can be complemented and reinforced by nursing activities.
7. Take a field trip and visit an orthotist/prosthetist. Observe the construction and fitting of a brace and a limb prosthesis. Compare different models of limbs. Determine the costs involved in obtaining a brace and prosthesis, including

fitting and maintenance. Determine what types of braces and prostheses are fully or partially covered by different medical insurance policies and Medicare.

8. Speak with a group of disabled individuals who have undergone rehabilitation. Ask them about factors that facilitated their use of adaptive and assistive equipment. Try to determine the factors that impeded their progress. Use input in planning care for specific clients.

REFERENCES

1. Ahrens WD, Carter R, and Kinney MR: The effect of antistasis footboard exercises on selected measures of exertion, Heart Lung 14(4):366, 1983.
2. Akeson WH and others: Effects of immobilization upon joints, Clin Orthop 219:28, June 1987.
3. Bates B: A guide to physical examination and history taking, ed 4, Philadelphia, 1987, JB Lippincott Co.
4. Bobath B: Adult hemiplegia: evaluation and treatment, ed 2, London, 1978, Heinemann Medical.
5. Bojd T and others: Use of four channel electrical stimulator as an ambulatory aid for paraplegic patients, Phys Ther 63(7):1116, 1983.
6. Cerny K: A clinical method of quantitative gait analysis, Phys Ther 63(7):1125, 1983.
7. Clarkson B: Absorbent paper method for recording foot placement during gait, Phys Ther 63(3):345, 1983.
8. Clough DH and Maurin JT: ROM versus NRx, J Gerontol Nurs 9(5):278, 1983.
9. Congressional Research Service, Library of Congress: Digest of data on persons with disabilities, Washington, DC, 1984, Mathematica Policy Research, Inc.
10. Dayhoff N: Rethinking stroke: soft or hard devices to position hands? Am J Nurs 75:1142, 1975.
11. Dubow LL and others: Oxygen consumption of elderly persons with bilateral BKA: ambulation versus wheelchair propulsion, Arch Phys Med Rehabil 64(6):255, 1983.
12. Gordon M: Nursing diagnosis: process and application, ed 2, New York, 1987, McGraw-Hill Book Co.
13. Greenleaf JE and Koslowski S: Physiological consequences of reduced physical activity during bed rest, Exerc Sport Sci Rev 10:84, 1982.
14. Grimes J and Iannopollo E: Health assessment in nursing practice, Monterey, Calif, 1982, Wadsworth Publishing Co.
15. Hathaway D and Geden EA: Energy expenditure during leg exercise programs, Nurs Res 32(3):147, 1983.
16. Jamieson S and Dayhoff N: A hard hand-positioning device to decrease wrist and finger hypertonicity: a sensorimotor approach for the patient with nonprogressive brain damage, Nurs Res 29:285, 1980.
17. Kohn J and others: Provisions of assistive equipment for the handicapped, Arch Phys Med Rehabil 65(8):378, 1983.
18. Laughman RK and others: Strength changes in the normal quadriceps femoris muscle as a result of electrical stimulation, Phys Ther 63(4):494, 1983.
19. Lehneis HR: Using prosthetics to aid in independence, Patient Care 17(1):45, 1983.
20. Lucca JA and Recchiuti SJ: Effect of biofeedback on an isometric strengthening program, Phys Ther 63(2):100, 1983.
21. Madorsky JGB and Madorsky A: Wheelchair racing: an important modality in acute rehabilitation after paraplegia, Arch Phys Med Rehabil 64(4):186, 1983.
22. Marsolais EB and Kobetic R: Functional walking in paralyzed patients by means of electrical stimulation, Clin Orthop 5(175):30, 1983.
23. Mathiowetz V, Bolding DJ, and Trombly CA: Immediate effects of positioning devices on the normal and spastic hand measured by EMG, Am J Occup Ther 27(4):247, 1983.
24. Mayerson NH and Milano RA: Goniometric measurement reliability in physical medicine, Arch Phys Med Rehabil 65(2):92, 1984.
25. McClary I: Electric wheelchair propulsion using a hand control in C4 quadriplegia, Phys Ther 63(2):221, 1983.
26. Merkel KD and others: Energy expenditure of paraplegic patients standing and walking with two knee-ankle-foot orthoses, Arch Phys Med Rehabil 65(3):121, 1984.
27. Milazzo V and Rash C: Kinetic nursing—a new approach to the problems of immobilization, J Neurosurg Nurs 14(3):120, 1982.
28. Mills VM: Electromyelographic results of inhibitory splinting, Phys Ther 64(2):190, 1984.
29. Murray MP and others: Gait patterns in AKA hydraulic swing versus friction, Arch Phys Med Rehabil 64(8):339, 1983.
30. Olson EV: The hazards of immobility, Am J Nurs 4:781, 1967.
31. Passarella P and Gee Z: Starting right after stroke, Am J Nurs 87:802, 1987.
32. Roberts B and Fitzpatrick J: Improved balance: therapy of movement, J Gerontol Nurs 9(3):140, 1983.
33. Rothstein JM, Miller PJ, and Roettger RF: Goniometric reliability . . . in a clinical setting, Phys Ther 63(10):1611, 1983.
34. Rubin M: The physiology of bedrest, Am J Nurs 88:50, 1988.
35. Sanchez DG, Bussey B, and Petorak M: Air fluidized beds, revolutionary skin care, RN 46(6):46, 1983.
36. Seymour RJ and others: Paraplegic use of Orlau Swivel Walker, Arch Phys Med Rehabil 63(10):490, 1982.

37. Smith PA and others: Arm crank versus handrim wheelchair propulsion: Metabolic and cardiopulmonary responses, Arch Phys Med Rehabil 64(6):259, 1983.

38. Squires AJ: Using the tilt table for elderly patients, Physiotherapy 69(5):150, 1983.

39. Up and around—a booklet to aid the stroke patient in activities of daily living, US Public Health Service Pub No 1120, Washington, DC, US Government Printing Office.

ADDITIONAL READINGS

Appell HJ: Skeletal muscle atrophy during immobilization, Int J Sports Med 7(1):1, 1986.

Bergstrom D and Coles CH: Basic positioning procedures, Rehabilitation Publication 701, Minneapolis, 1971, Sister Kenny Institute.

Bohannon RW: Taping and stabilizing ankles of patients with hemiplegia, Phys Ther 63(4):524, 1983.

Bohannon RW, Thorne M, and Mierer AC: Shoulder positioning devices for patients with hemiplegia, Phys Ther 63(1):49, 1983.

Chin PL: Physical techniques in stroke rehabilitation, J R Coll Physicians 16(3):165, 1982.

Creason NS, and others: Validating the nursing diagnosis of impaired physical mobility, Nurs Clinics North Am 20:669, 1985.

Crockett JE: Power grasp aid to rehabilitation, Physiotherapy 68(7):224, 1982.

Davies P and Ryan DW: Stevens-Johnson syndrome managed in the Clinitron bed, Intensive Care Med 9(2):87, 1983.

Getz PA and Blossom BM: Preventing contractures: the little extras that help so much, RN 45(12):44, 1982.

Hale SS and Stephens SE: Neurological treatment, Physiotherapy 69(3):76, 1983.

Hill I: Equipped for the job: mobile hoists, Nurs Times 79(27):24, 1983.

Hoffman D, Kusek N, and Tonjuk AM: Pneumatic lift as an aid to positioning the strength compromised patient, Phys Ther 63(6):979, 1983.

Hultman E and Sjoholm H: B/P and HR response to voluntary and nonvoluntary static exercise in man, Acta Physiol Scand 115(4):499, 1982.

Knapik J and others: Isokinetic torque variations in four muscle groups through a range of joint motion, Phys Ther 63(6):938, 1983.

Konikow NS: Alterations in movement: nursing assessment and implications, J Neurosurg Nurs 17:61, Feb 1985.

Lainey CG, Walmsley RP, and Andrew CM: Effectiveness of exercise alone versus exercise plus electrical stimulation in strengthening the quadriceps muscle, Physiotherapy Can 35(1):5, 1983.

Lowenthal DT, Bharadwaja K, and Oakes WW, editors: Therapeutics through exercise, New York, 1979, Grune & Stratton, Inc.

Malkiewicz J: A pragmatic approach to musculoskeletal assessment, RN 45(11):56, 1982.

McCabe JB and Nolan DJ: Comparison of the effectiveness of different cervical immobilization collars, Ann Emerg Med 15(1):50, Jan 1986.

O'Sullivan SB, Cullen KE, and Schmitz TJ: Physical rehabilitation: evaluation and treatment procedures, Philadelphia, 1981, FA Davis Co.

Passarella PM and Lewis N: Nursing application of Bobath principles in stroke care, J Neurosci Nurs 19(2):106, 1987.

Reddy MP: A guide to early mobilization of bedridden elderly, Geriatrics 41:59, Sept 1986.

Regan TJ: Proper use of wheelchairs, J Am Geriatr Soc 31(2):126, 1983.

Scales JT and Lowthian PT: Vapern patient-support system: a new general purpose hospital mattress, Lancet 2(8308):1150, 1982.

Selkurt EE, editor: Basic physiology for the health sciences, Boston, 1982, Little, Brown & Co.

Siegel IM and Silverman M: Contoured seating for the wheelchair bound patient with neuromuscular disease, Phys Ther 63(10):1625, 1983.

Siegler S, Selektar R, and Hyman W: Simulation of human gait with the aid of a mechanical model, J Biomech 15(6):415, 1982.

Shelton ME and Guise EP: Variation on pylon for BKA, Phys Ther 62(11):1601, 1982.

Soderberg GL and Cook TM: Electromyographic analysis of quadriceps femoris muscle setting and straight leg raising, Phys Ther 63(9):1434, 1983.

Sorenson L and Ulrich PG: Ambulation guide for nurses, Rehabilitation Publication 707, Minneapolis, 1974, Sister Kenny Institute.

Stanton KM and others: Wheelchair transfer training for right cerebral dysfunctions: an interdisciplinary approach, Arch Phys Med Rehabil 64(6):276, 1983.

Stephens TE and Lattimore J: Prescriptive checklist for positioning multihandicapped residential clients, Phys Ther 63(7):1113, 1983.

Stern RB and Walley M: Functional comparison of upper extremity amputees using myoelectric and conventional prostheses, Arch Phys Med Rehabil 64(6):243, 1983.

Sullivan PE, Markos PD, and Minor MAD: An integrated approach to therapeutic exercise theory and clinical applications, Reston, Va, 1982, Reston Publishing Co.

Tiller J and others: Treatment of functional chronic stooped posture using a training device and behavior therapy, Phys Ther 62(11):1597, 1982.

Toth L: Spasticity management in spinal cord injury, Rehabil Nurs 8(1):14, 1983.

Walker J: Modified strapping of roll sling, Am J Occup Ther 37(2):110, 1983.

Walker J and others: Active mobility of the extremities in older subjects, Phys Ther 64(6):919, 1984.

Warren ML: A comparative study on the presence of the asymmetrical tonic neck reflex in adult hemiplegia, Am J Occup Ther 38(6):386, 1984.

Wevers HW: Wheelchair and occupant restraint system for transportation of handicapped passengers, Arch Phys Med Rehabil 64(8):374, 1983.

Weiss PL and St. Pierre D: Upper and lower extremity EMG correlations during normal gait, Arch Phys Med Rehabil 64(1):11, 1983.

Wilder PA and Sykes J: Using an isokinetic exercise machine to improve the gait pattern in a hemiplegic patient, Phys Ther 62(9):1291, 1982.

Winter DA: Knee flexion during stance as a determinant of inefficient walking, Phys Ther 63(3):331, 1983.

Woodburne R, editor: Essentials of human anatomy, ed 7, New York, 1983, Oxford University Press.

CHAPTER 19

Sexuality and Sexual Function

Joyce Santora

OBJECTIVES

After completing Chapter 19, the reader will be able to:

1. Describe sexuality as a component of optimum health.
2. Explain the physiology of sexual response in able-bodied males and females.
3. Describe the psychosocial factors affecting quality of sexual response.
4. Discuss physical and psychosocial alterations in ability to function as a sexual being.
5. Assess a client's physical and psychosocial abilities and limitations as a sexual being.
6. Formulate nursing diagnoses associated with alterations in sexuality and sexual function.
7. Develop goals with the client and partner that foster maximum satisfaction as a sexual being and with sexual function.
8. Determine nursing interventions to assist the client in maintaining and restoring concept of self as a sexual being.
9. Identify other rehabilitation members who assist the client in maintaining and restoring concept of self as a sexual being.
10. List outcome criteria used to evaluate the effectiveness of planned intervention to maintain and restore concept of self as a sexual being.

Human sexuality is a broad concept that includes how one thinks, feels, and acts as a sexual being. Each person is capable of a wide range of feelings and actions that help to define oneself as a male or female. Definition of oneself as a sexual being with needs and drives is important for most individuals. Intimate involvement with another person is desirable for both able-bodied and disabled persons. The involvement may vary in intensity according to the role played, personal interactions, and the context in which those interactions take place.

With the spread of acquired immunodeficiency syndrome (AIDS) and the concurrent rise in incidence of other sexually transmitted diseases, a climate fostering liberal sexual expression has been tempered by caution. Despite the supposed availability of knowledge about sexuality, the need for this knowledge and sexual dysfunction problems continue to exist among able-bodied and disabled people. Persons who are disabled, however, face additional problems such as fatigue, body-image disturbances, fear, general debility, and lack of opportunity.

Members of society frequently regard disabled persons as asexual beings. Myths and misconceptions are perpetuated by the lack of discussion by health care professionals about sexual needs and behaviors. Sexuality remains one of the most difficult topics for rehabilitation team members to discuss. Thus the disabled individual faces attitudes based on misinformation about a disease or disability, misconceptions about the sexual partner's expectations, unrealistic goals for sexual performance, and lack of open communication about the topic from those most able to help with sexual readjustment.

The rehabilitation nurse's effectiveness in assisting a disabled person to meet sexual needs depends upon knowledge about sexuality and sexual function, comfort with one's own sexuality, comfort in discussing sexual function with disabled clients, comfort with the client's sexual preferences and practices, and awareness and respect for a client's desire not to discuss this aspect of life. This chapter presents information about sexuality and sexual function, effects of disability upon sexual function, potential problems of clients in resuming former sexual activities, and ways in which the nurse and other rehabilitation team members can provide information and counseling about sexual options to a client with a disability.

SEXUALITY: A COMPONENT OF OPTIMUM HEALTH

Maslow[38] identified the sexual drive as a basic human need that must be satisfied before higher needs could emerge. The ability and desire to function as a sexual being depend upon an individual's culture, position in the life cycle, current life status, state of physical and emotional well-being, and availability of opportunities.

The sexual needs of an individual must be recognized if the nurse is to deliver holistic care. Studies conducted in the early 1970s demonstrated that despite the trend in educating health professionals about sexuality, registered nurses scored lower on sexual knowledge and had more conservative attitudes than nursing students, medical students, and other graduate students.[33] Later studies showed that although sexual knowledge did not differ from other groups, graduate nursing students generally had more conservative sexual attitudes than students in other disciplines.[32]

Sexuality refers to a person's capability of having sexual feelings and capacity. In a broad sense, it includes any subjective and objective activities of an individual. More specifically, it includes an erotic component, in the form of arousal with or without concurrent physiological changes, and interpersonal, emotional, and nongenital aspects of eroticism.[27] Sex or gender role refers to a set of societal expectations about the way an individual should act in a given situation. Sexual identity refers to the objective and subjective private responses of an individual.[34,42] Sexual response is the physiological ability to experience genital sensations, erection, ejaculation, vaginal lubrication, pelvic thrusting, and other responses to stimulation.[53]

The ability to function as a sexual being may be altered by physical disability. Although a person's opportunities may decrease and ability to perform and respond to sexual acts may be altered, an individual may compensate for these changes and with the assistance of rehabilitation team members, achieve sexual health.

The World Health Organization defined sexual health as "an integration of somatic, emotional, intellectual, and social aspects of sexual being, in ways that are positive, enriching, and that enhance personality, communication, and love."[52] Included in this definition are three basic elements: (1) ability of a person to enjoy sexual and reproductive behavior in accordance with personal and social ethics, (2) freedom from fear, guilt, shame, and false information that impair a sexual relationship and inhibit sexual response, and (3) freedom from organic diseases and disabilities that present barriers to sexual and reproductive functions.[52]

Maddock[35] adds that to judge sexual health there must be (1) congruency between one's gender identity and comfort with a range of sex role behaviors; (2) effective interpersonal relationships with both sexes, including the potential for love and commitment; (3) capacity to respond to erotic stimulation so as to experience sexual activity as positive and stimulating; and (4) a high correlation between one's sexual behavior and value system.

PHYSIOLOGICAL ASPECTS OF SEXUAL RESPONSE

The ability to perform sexual acts depends upon stimuli that initiate a reaction, nerve tracts to carry stimuli to various centers in the nervous system, nerve tracts to return messages to appropriate body parts, and sexual organs that react to the messages carried. In addition to a physiological response to sexual stimulation, a psychological desire also must be present for successful sexual performance.

A sexual response may be elicited either by mental stimuli, such as pictures in books and magazines, movies, or sexual thoughts and dreams, or by touch stimuli applied to erotic zones of the body. Rhythmic rubbing of the genitalia is usually the most effective means of stimulating sexual response in a person with intact neurological pathways. When carried on for periods of time, this action may lead to a full sexual response. It is believed that direct touch stimulation is carried to the S2-4 segments of the spinal cord by the pudendal nerve. Messages are then conducted to the brain through the lateral spinothalamic tracts.[53] Messages are conducted down through the pyramidal tracts to T11-12 and S2-4, resulting in erection in men and vaginal lubrication in women. "Mental" erections are not possible when there is a lesion at or above T10 to L1 but may be possible when the lesion exists in the area of the L2 to to S1 segments. Touch erections are possible when a lesion exists at or above T10 to S1 segments but are not possible when the S2-4 segments are destroyed and the genital-sacral reflex is lost. Ejaculation does not occur when there is a complete lesion at or above T10 to S4 spinal cord segments. Individuals with complete interruption of the neurological pathways in the central nervous system cannot experience orgasm when touch is applied to erogenous areas.[53]

Whether sexual acts are performed as part of masturbation or homosexual or heterosexual activity, the physiological response of the body is the same. Many years ago, Masters and Johnson[40] described the changes that occur during sexual responses as (1) excitement, (2) plateau, (3) orgasm, and (4) resolution. Body changes occur during the sexual response in able-bodied males and able-bodied females.

Sexual Response in the Able-Bodied Male

Sexual response in the able-bodied male is characterized by erection, ejaculation, and orgasm. Following initial and prolonged tactile or visual stimulation, changes in the body begin to appear.

There is a systemic increase in circulation and the appearance of a penile erection. Erections of psychogenic origin require an intact spinal cord and parasympathetic nervous system. The stimulus message originates in the brain and travels to the psychogenic erection centers located in T11-12 segments of the spinal cord and then, via the parasympathetic fibers, from S2-4 segments to the penis. Reflex erections require an intact sacral spinal cord and sacral nerve roots S2-4. Light touch or friction applied to the penis elicits this type of erection.[53] The term "spontaneous erection" is sometimes used when the erection is caused by some internal body event. Because of the involuntary control of this type of response, the erections are not useful for sexual intercourse.

Two processes occur during ejaculation: seminal emission and true ejaculation. Seminal emission occurs as a result of peristalsis of the smooth muscles of the vas deferens, seminal vesicles, and prostate. A bolus is formed by the combination of seminal fluid and sperm. This bolus is pushed into the posterior urethra by the contraction of smooth muscle. Clonic contractions of the urethra, penis, and lower pelvis result in expulsion of the ejaculate. The skeletal muscles and somatic nervous system are responsible for this latter phase of ejaculation. When a spinal cord injury is complete at any level, communication between the brain and genitalia is lost and ejaculation (from genital stimulation) is not possible.

Orgasm is a sensation coinciding with seminal emission and ejaculation. Rhythmic rubbing of the breasts, neck, inner thigh, perineum, or perianal areas may lead to orgasm. Again, orgasm does not occur with complete spinal cord lesions due to loss of the brain-genitalia connection.

Body changes during the male sexual response

Within the first 3 to 8 seconds of the excitement phase, a penile erection takes place. As the phase is prolonged, there is a thickening, flattening, and elevation of the scrotal sac as well as an increase in size of the testes. In approximately 30% of the male population, there is nipple erection and skin flushing.[28]

An increase in the penile coronal circumference occurs during the plateau phase. In some males, a purple hue appears below the corona. The testes become swollen and fully elevated in the scrotum. A slight mucoid secretion exudes from Cowper's glands. This phase is characterized by a generalized skeletal muscle tension, hyperventilation, increased blood pressure, and an increased heart rate ranging from 100 to 160 beats/minute.[28]

The orgasmic phase consists of a series of contractions resulting in ejaculation of semen through the urethral duct of the penis.[21] At the time of orgasm, the male's body movement consists of plunging into the vagina and holding this position.

In the resolution phase the male begins a refractory period where ejaculation is not possible although erection may be maintained. There is a rapid loss of pelvic vasocongestion. Loss of penile erection occurs in primary (rapid) and secondary (slow) stages.

Sexual Response in the Able-Bodied Female

Sexual response in the able-bodied female results when touch is applied to the erogenous zones (breast, neck, inner thighs, perianal areas, vulva, clitoris), thus leading to sexual arousal. Messages are carried via the pudendal nerves to S2-4 spinal cord segments and then via the lateral spinothalamic tracts to the brain. Messages are sent down to the T11-12 and S2-4 spinal cord segments, resulting in vaginal lubrication.[53]

Complete cord lesions at any level allow touch lubrication but preclude orgasm from genital stimulation. Also, orgasm is not possible as a result of genital stimulation when there is a complete lesion at L2 to S1 spinal cord segments.

Body changes during the female sexual response

Changes in the clitoris, vagina, cervix, and skin occur during the excitement phase. When stimulated, the clitoris becomes engorged with blood.

The walls of the vagina excrete a lubricant, thicken, and expand. The labia and lips of the vagina become swollen with blood. Other changes include elevation of the cervix and uterus, tumescence of the clitoris, consistent nipple erection, and often skin flush.[16]

These physiological changes continue and intensify during the plateau phase. There is marked discoloration in the engorged labia minora and withdrawal of the clitoris. Full expansion of the outer two thirds of the vagina occurs with a swelling of the outermost third. The uterus enlarges and contracts rapidly and irregularly. The breasts reach full expansion, and a more pronounced "sex flush" than in males is observed. Bartholin's glands release a mucoid substance. As in the male response, the female response is characterized by a generalized skeletal muscle tension, hyperventilation, increased blood pressure, and an increased heart rate ranging from 110 to 160 beats/minute.[28] If stimulation ceases at this point, an orgasm does not take place.

During the orgasmic phase, the female experiences a series of contractions that vary in intensity and number. These contractions may be accompanied by an expulsion of clear fluid at the time of orgasm. Orgasm may result from stimulation of the clitoris or vagina and may be felt in the genital area.[1] In their early studies, Masters and Johnson[40] found that orgasm resulting from rubbing of the clitoris could not be distinguished from a physiological standpoint from orgasm resulting from intercourse alone. However, this does not mean that all orgasms feel the same. Feeling and intensity are matters of perception, and many psychosocial factors may influence satisfaction.[41]

Female response in the resolution phase consists of a loss of clitoral tumescence and a return to normal position. Initially, the sex flush disappears and then the pelvic vasocongestion. Nipple erection is lost, and the muscles of the body relax. Heart rate, blood pressure, pulse, and respirations return to normal. Women are capable of repeat orgasms if stimulation continues.[28]

PSYCHOSOCIAL FACTORS AFFECTING QUALITY OF SEXUAL RELATIONSHIPS AND RESPONSE

A number of psychosocial factors affect the quality of sexual relationships and responses in males and females. These factors include communication, surroundings, timing and mood, and sensory stimulation.

Communication

Communication between partners is the key to initiation and satisfaction with sexual experiences. Telling a partner what is pleasant does a great deal to enhance sexual relationships and sexual acts. Being honest with another person helps each partner enjoy the other as a whole person. Thoughts, feelings, and concerns, when shared openly and without embarrassment, contribute to the quality of the sexual relationship.[8] "Love talk" is helpful in creating the mood for and subsequently assisting in sexual arousal.

Wolf[51] describes the importance of letting a partner know when there is fatigue, discomfort, or frustration. Saying no when a person is too tired for sexual activities does not mean that an individual will not want to engage in these activities an hour later or at another time. It helps to tell this to a partner. He states that "partners of men with erectile problems often fear they are at fault. It is reassuring to tell her that you still love her and are still turned on by her, but the signals are not getting through to your penis."[51] She may still think you are wonderful, and then it becomes a problem that can be worked on together.

When there is sensory loss, it is particularly helpful to tell your partner what feels good and that touching in some areas may be painful. Also, the person with a disability may want to tell a partner that there is a chance of bladder incontinence even after voiding before sexual activities.[51]

Sometimes a sexual relationship is improved if times are set aside for conversation with no physical contact except for holding if desired. Talking about feelings and experiences helps persons know and understand each other better. By allowing this time, some surprises about the other person may occur that help to enhance physical contact and the sexual relationship.[51]

Masters and Johnson[39] developed a technique that they call "sensate focus" and that is used by some sex counselors. In this technique, the partners decide beforehand to explore different parts of each other's body and not to let the exploration lead to intercourse or orgasm. The person explored concentrates completely on the touches and lets the partner know what feels good and what does not. The genitalia are considered as only one part of the body, and attention is given to pleasurable feelings when the rest of the body is touched.

Surroundings

The surroundings in which sexual activity takes place are limited only by one's imagination. Any setting that is comfortable and affords a chance for preparation, relaxation, and enjoyment is appropriate. Mirrors can help in observing what a partner is doing even when no sensation is present. Water beds facilitate some positions and allow for a temperature-controlled environment.

Variations in surroundings may add to the sexual experience. New settings such as the floor, chair, or bathtub can be used to enhance the sexual act. Most persons prefer a setting where safety and privacy can be assured.

Timing and Mood

Certain times of the day may be more comfortable for engaging in sexual activities. Some persons prefer sex only at night in a dark room, whereas others prefer sex with soft lighting or during the daylight hours. The best time is when persons feel rested and relaxed. Morning hours and weekends may be better for some people than nights during the week after working hard all day.[8] Candlelight, music, and a drink of wine in a romantic setting may heighten sexual arousal.

Some couples prefer to plan sexual activities when both know they will not be fatigued. At other times, one partner may be fatigued and let the other person take over while the tired person relaxes and enjoys, expecting to repay the favor at some point.

Sensory Stimulation

Added sensory touches can enhance the psychological desire for sexual activity. Among the added sensory touches are the use of scented oils, creams, or lotions for body massage; engaging in foreplay for extended periods; and sharing fantasies with a real or imagined partner.

Certain smells may serve to relax a partner and lead to sexual arousal. A wide range of products can be purchased to decrease noxious body odors and give off pleasurable body scents. Natural body scents, known as pheromones, are believed to stimulate sexual desire.[1] The reaction to smell is highly individualized. A scent pleasant to one individual may be a "turnoff" to another.

Foreplay is an important aspect of arousing psychological desire for sexual activity. It includes lightly touching genitalia, breasts, neck, ears, lips, thighs, back, buttocks, anus, palms, and feet. Kissing and licking these erogenous zones also are a part of foreplay. Males become more quickly aroused than females, so these activities may have to be stopped to forestall male orgasm and started again if the enjoyment of foreplay is to be prolonged. Disabled individuals also may require more time and stimulation for arousal. The longer the foreplay, the greater is the likelihood that the female will achieve orgasm. Foreplay can be enhanced by using hot and cold sensations, applying objects such as vibrators, and rubbing the partner with textured materials.

Fantasy as a form of sexual arousal consists of thoughts of lovemaking with a real or imagined partner. Thoughts may be purposefully stimulated by erotic material including sexually explicit magazines and films, or they may occur spontaneously during everyday activities. Many people have sexual fantasies in their dreams. Fantasies are often associated with masturbation (individual sexual activity) and intercourse. These images can be used to stimulate sexual arousal, heighten pleasure, assist in remembering feelings in previous sexual encounters, and provide a release of sexual tension.

ALTERATIONS IN SEXUAL FUNCTION

Shrey and associates[47] identify individuals with altered sexual function as those with chronic disease or disability who are significantly inconvenienced because of sensory limitations or disorders involving one or more of the body's systems, for example, musculoskeletal, respiratory, cardiovascular, or digestive. Disease and disability may affect sexual function whether or not the sex organs are affected. Not only is the sexual function of the ill or disabled person altered but also the partner's ability to participate in sexual activities is affected. A frequent concern of the disabled person and partner is the fear that engaging in sexual activity may accelerate the disease process or adversely affect the disabled individual. This

section therefore briefly discusses functional problems that may occur as a result of a disease or disability and alter the individual's ability to function as a sexual being.

Physiological Alterations

Physiological alterations that interfere with sexual activities include impaired physical mobility, lack of or limited sensation, pain, lack of bladder and bowel control, and fatigue.

Impaired physical mobility

A freely movable body is an asset in expressing oneself as a sexual being. When small joints are affected by disease, the individual may have difficulty in communicating with sensitive touching and caressing motions. When knees, hips and vertebral joints are affected, the person may have difficulty assuming comfortable positions. In addition, management of personal hygiene, insertion or application of birth control devices and ability to relax may pose difficulties.

Paralyzed persons may have obvious mechanical difficulties and often may experience spasticity.[10] Little is known scientifically about specific sexual dysfunctions related to stroke. Some researchers have found little change in sexual desire after stroke, particularly in individuals under 60 years old.[7,15] Impaired physical mobility for these individuals results in obvious mechanical difficulties, but psychological factors may have a greater impact on sexual relationships.[13]

Altered sensation

When sensation is altered, the pleasure derived from stimulation may no longer be possible in some erogenous zones of the body. The higher the level of a neurological lesion, the less skin surface is available for stimulation. With decreased sensation during sexual activities, the affected partner remains relatively passive. However, the potential for giving genuine pleasure to another through physical and emotional contact still exists.

Pain

Pain contributes to perceived sexual dysfunction. In a number of chronic diseases, pain is constant and can create real barriers to one's own perception of sexuality and physical attractiveness.[26] Pain also can cause difficulty in assuming positions required for sexual activities. Continued pain often results in depression, which may decrease the sexual desire. Pain has been identified as a greater barrier to sexual intimacy than deformity.[10]

Bladder and bowel incontinence

Both men and women worry about offensive perineal odors and bladder and bowel accidents during sexual activities. These accidents are more likely when sexual activity occurs spontaneously because the individual has not taken time to tend to personal hygiene. Women may have more problems with bowel accidents than men because the penis inside the vagina presumably activates bowel reflexes.[53] These problems, to a lesser degree, also can be concerns of able-bodied men and women. Thus attention is given by males and females to preparation for sexual intimacy, use of powders, deodorants and perfumes, and perineal hygiene.

Concern about the possibility of an accident often inhibits the enjoyment of sex. The person with a disability should be as knowledgeable as possible about bowel and bladder management. Some able-bodied partners can assist the partner with a disability with bladder and bowel care; however, many persons have difficulty switching from the role of sexual partner to that of care giver.

Fatigue

Valleroy and Kraft[48] report that the most common complaint of women with multiple sclerosis is fatigue. Men also reported this problem although to a lesser degree. Fatigue can be a symptom of depression. Persons whose daily living activities require a great expenditure of energy may have little energy left to engage in sexual activities.

Psychosocial Alterations

Psychosocial alterations occurring concurrently with disability and chronic illness include lack of knowledge about fertility and safe birth control, difficulty in meeting persons of the opposite sex, negative self-concept, and concerns about engaging in sexual acts other than intercourse.

Lack of knowledge about fertility

Often the disabled individual and society assume that a disability leads to infertility. Fertility is profoundly affected for the male with a spinal cord injury, although no specific predictions can be made without a thorough fertility workup.[12] Walbroehl[49] recommends that sperm be obtained as soon as possible after spinal cord injury because spermatogenesis ceases shortly after interruption of spinal tracts. When sperm is not banked within several weeks of injury, the chances of obtaining viable sperm are significantly reduced.

A young woman's fertility is usually not altered by any disability, although there may be some contraindications to pregnancy such as thrombophlebitis and significant renal insufficiency. The typical orgasm is not present in women with complete cord lesions, although tactile stimulation above the level of the lesion will result in heightened arousal.[21] Women with spinal cord injury cease to menstruate for a brief period after injury, but within 6 to 12 months menses return to normal, and they are able to conceive and deliver with no more difficulty than able-bodied women.[18] They are, however, prone to complications of autonomic dysreflexia, urinary tract infection, and premature labor. Women who do not wish to bear children should be counseled about methods of contraception.

Lack of knowledge about birth control is common among able-bodied and disabled persons. The person with a disability may face added physical and psychosocial problems if an unplanned and unwanted pregnancy takes place.

Difficulty in meeting persons of the opposite sex

Disabled individuals may find it more difficult to meet persons of the opposite sex if circumstances limit social contact. When relationships are established, it may be more difficult to communicate a willingness to engage in sexual activity based on their own and others' reactions to disease and disability. Persons who are wheelchair bound, for example, need to become adept at making others feel at ease despite the presence of the wheelchair.

Self-concept

Self-concept includes all the beliefs people hold in regard to themselves. This includes beliefs about the body, beliefs about the value of self or self-esteem, and the internal feelings one has about the body parts and the body's physical appearance.[30] External factors such as makeup, clothes, and jewelry also contribute to one's self-concept.

Self-concept is closely allied with the concept

of body image. Throughout the life span, persons develop positive or negative views of self as they interact with others.[22] Acceptance by others, warm and loving relationships, and positive interactions contribute to a positive self-concept; lack of acceptance by others, poor relationships, and negative interactions contribute to a negative self-concept.

The disabled person may be forced to abdicate usual social roles for brief or extensive periods of time. To be productive as a family member and financially responsible may not be feasible. The ability to adapt to and accept these changes varies among individuals, but almost always, there is some loss of body image and self-concept.[24]

Disabled persons who have had a positive body image before disability will accept body changes more readily than individuals who viewed themselves negatively before the disability. Those who are able to engage in self-care tasks and resume social roles are more likely to adapt to body changes positively and to possess a positive self-concept.

Concerns about engaging in sexual acts other than intercourse

For many persons, sexual activity means traditional intercourse: the female beneath and the male above with the erect penis inside the vagina. Other options such as oral-genital stimulation of the woman's genitalia (cunnilingus) and of the man's genitalia (fellatio) are viewed as "preliminary acts" that lead to the "real thing." Some persons regard these acts as perverse. Cultural and social mores also may preclude masturbation. Masturbation is a normal sexual option that allows for relief of sexual tension and allows an individual to become better acquainted with the body and its pleasurable function.[25] Unfortunately, myths and misconceptions regarding this activity may lead to guilt, shame, and anxiety.[11]

NURSING ASSESSMENT

Sexuality and sexual response may not be priorities early in the rehabilitation process. However, as rehabilitation progresses, this function may become a major consideration for the client and the sexual partner if one is involved. The nurse's response to the client's concerns about maintaining or restoring sexual function can greatly influence the client's sexual adjustment and total rehabilitation.

Nurses should possess the knowledge, experience, and interviewing skills to provide sexual adjustment counseling, but it is not realistic to assume that all nurses feel comfortable in discussing this area in detail. One of the unfounded assumptions of health professionals is that a client will be able to ask questions about sex. In most situations, it is the nurse's responsibility to ask about needs in this area.

All too often, nurses have not been adequately prepared in their educational programs to feel comfortable discussing human sexuality. Until the 1970s, schools of nursing did not include human sexuality in the curriculum nor was there substantial information on sexuality in the nursing literature. Lack of knowledge in this area or discomfort in discussing this topic should alert the nurse to the need to refer the client and sexual partner to another member of the rehabilitation team. According to Hott,[26] sexual counseling is not the exclusive province of any given discipline. Golden and Golden[17] found that clients desire direction and support as they reestablish sexual function and relationships. They suggest that health care providers should be comfortable in discussing sexual issues, be knowledgeable about sources of referral if they are in conflict with the client's cultural and religious beliefs, and introduce discussion of the client's sexual concerns at various stages of the rehabilitation process, but in particular when the diagnosis is made, when planning for treatment occurs, during early convalescence, and when on the road to recovery.

An adequate sexual assessment includes preparing the client for the questions, obtaining a sexual history, identifying physical and psychosocial strengths and limitations, determining the client's sexual values, and assisting with or performing diagnostic tests.

Client Preparation for the Sexual History

Preparing the client for the sexual history involves a number of techniques to make the client feel more comfortable in answering the questions posed. Initially the nurse tells the client that questions will be asked in order to plan care. The client should be informed that some of these questions will be personal but will help identify areas where assistance may be needed. The client can refuse to answer any questions and should be so informed at the outset of the interview. Sociocultural orientation may dictate sex as a taboo topic among certain ethnic groups. Age and gender also may be barriers between the nurse and client in discussing sexual concerns.

Questions should proceed from the less to the more sensitive areas. A matter-of-fact and objective approach should be taken. For instance, the nurse can make a general statement about masturbation as a normal form of sexual release and then ask the client's opinion about this practice. Sometimes it is helpful to ask about the ideal rather than the real to facilitate communication. For example, the client could be asked how a sexual relationship differs from what was expected.[31] After establishing rapport with the client and giving information about the nature of some of the questions, the nurse who feels knowledgeable and comfortable in this area can proceed with the sexual history.

The Sexual History

The nurse obtains a sexual history by asking the client questions in three general areas: (1) physiological strengths and limitations, (2) psychosocial strengths and limitations, and (3) sexual values and attitudes.[47] Areas and issues addressed are listed in the box. Additional information regarding level of fertility; hormonal changes; hereditary and genetic factors; residual functional capacity, including cardiovascular status, perceptual difficulties, and communication disorders; and physiological deficits and assets should be obtained from the physician and other professionals. Since the long-term use of certain recreational and prescribed drugs, such as antihypertensives, antipsychotics, and antidepressants, also may contribute to sexual difficulties, the nurse should review the client's current medications.[5]

Open-ended questions can be asked to help the client talk about sexual concerns. For example, the nurse may state that "many persons with your condition have concerns about their sexual functioning. Do you have any concerns in this area?"[37] The interviewer should proceed from the least taboo to the most taboo topics and toward the end of the interview move to closed-ended questions that require "yes" or "no" answers. A summary of the interview allows the client to disagree, add, or delete information.[37]

Areas to Assess During Sexual History

Physiological assets and deficits
1. Physical mobility
2. Sensations, such as hot, cold, touch, pain
3. Degree of spasticity, if applicable
4. Levels and areas of pain
5. Bladder and bowel continence, including use of appliances
6. Difficulties with vision and hearing
7. Endurance
8. Balance
9. Medications used and reactions to these medications
10. Genital and extragenital sexual response, that is, capacity for lubrication, erection, ejaculation, orgasm

Psychosocial deficits and assets
1. Client's motivation and commitment to explore psychosocial deficits and assets
2. Client's level of psychosocial adjustment to disability
3. Client's premorbid and present coping mechanisms and skills
4. Client's interpersonal skills and behavior
5. Significant others in client's world
6. Attitudes of significant others in client's world
7. Client's body image
8. Client's level of satisfaction or dissatisfaction with current relationships (interpersonal and sexual)

Sexual values
1. Religious beliefs and attitudes on, for example, birth control, premarital sexual relationships
2. Priorities of sexual relationships
3. Cultural beliefs and attitudes
4. Marriage and family priorities and value
5. Preferences in sexual activities, for example, masturbation, oral-genital sex, manual stimulation, fantasy, sexual positions, gender of partner
6. Use of physical stimulation appliances, such as vibrators
7. Values regarding flexibility of male-female roles
8. Sexual preferences: heterosexual or homosexual
9. Physical appearance of other and self
10. Preferred areas or locations (environmental) to initiate interpersonal and sexual relationships

Modified from Shrey DE, Kiefer JS, and Anthony WA: J Rehabil 45:28, April/May/June 1979.

Language substitutions are sometimes required to coincide with the client's use of sexual terms. "Making love" may have to be substituted for sexual intercourse or "coming" for ejaculation or orgasm. Any signs of shock or disapproval at what the client says should be avoided.

Although the sexual history is only one part of the comprehensive nursing assessment, continual assessment of this function takes place throughout the rehabilitation process. In addition to the sexual history, the nurse may perform or assist with diagnostic tests that indicate capacity for sexual performance in the client who has an interruption in neural pathways.

Diagnostic Tests

Two tests can be performed to determine if orgasm might occur in males and females with neurological lesions. These are a test of pain or temperature sensation and a test of voluntary contraction of the anus. The first test is used to establish intact voluntary pathways between the genitalia and the brain and gives information about the lateral spinothalamic tracts. The client should respond either to a pinprick or be able to correctly identify hot and cold objects applied to the penis or vulva.[53] The latter test is used to provide information about the motor tracts traveling to the genitalia from the brain. If the client correctly perceives pain and temperature and voluntarily contracts the anus, the neurological pathways for sensation and orgasm are intact. If either one of these tests is negative, the client will not be able to experience orgasm or ejaculation because there is injury somewhere along the pathways for sensation and orgasm. The male may, however, be able to have a reflex touch or mental erection depending upon the level of the injury.

Three reflexes used to assess the male client's physical abilities to engage in sexual activities are (1) the bulbocavernosus reflex, (2) the anal tone reflex, and (3) the testicular reflex. The bulbocavernosus reflex and anal tone reflex have been previously described (Chapter 11). Presence of the bulbocavernosus reflex indicates that the sacral segments of the spinal cord are open and reflex touch erections are likely to occur. Ability to contract the internal anal muscles indicates that the sacral and lumbar segments of the cord are intact. When both of these reflexes are present, the reflex touch erection can be expected to be strong because the lesion is probably higher up in the cord. The significance of these reflexes for assessment of sexual function in women is still not understood.

To find out whether the injury is above or below the T9 spinal cord segment, the testes should be squeezed until pain is experienced. Since the sensory fibers from the testes enter the spinal cord at the T9 level, it can be assumed that the client who cannot feel any pain has a lesion at or above this level. Mental erections do not occur in this instance, since the fibers necessary for this type of erection exit around the T11-12 segments of the spinal cord. If there is acute testicular discomfort, the lesion is most likely located below the T11-12 area and mental erections will probably occur.[53]

It is rare for a neurological lesion to occur below the L1 level. When a lesion does occur in this area, the bulbocavernosus, anal tone and testicular reflexes can be elicited, but there is no perception of pain in the genitalia, no anal tone, and no voluntary ability to contract the anus. Although mental and touch reflex erections can be expected, these will be of poor quality. Orgasm and ejaculation will not be possible.[53]

NURSING DIAGNOSES

Nursing diagnoses related to sexuality that are accepted by the North American Nursing Diagnosis Association include the following[20]:

1. *Sexual dysfunction, altered sexuality patterns:* Lack of or compromised ability to respond to those activities or behaviors associated with stimulation of the erogenous zones. Planning is directed toward designing interventions to meet sexual adjustment goals that are realistic and attainable.

2. *Body image disturbance, personal identity disturbance, self-esteem disturbance:* Lowered self-concept possibly caused by impaired motor or sensory function, pain, fatigue, disfigurement, or depression. Planning is directed toward facilitating the process of adequate sexual adjustment while focusing on improving body image through attention to personal hygiene, dress, and mannerisms; assisting the client to resume social roles and change prevailing attitudes regarding male and female sexual roles; reestablishing personal identity; and improving self-esteem as former activities and roles are resumed in the usual or adapted ways.

3. *Social isolation:* Lack of or limited ability for social interaction because of impaired motor or sensory function or self-imposed isolation. Planning should focus on the identification of acceptable social interactions, recreational opportunities, and transportation options.

4. *Knowledge deficits:* Lack of knowledge regarding alternative ways to achieve sexual functioning, lack of knowledge regarding birth control. The client may not be aware of alternatives to traditional sexual activities, and the disabling condition may result in motor or sensory impairments that interfere with the ability to perform sexual activities in the usual manner. The client may not be aware of ability or lack of ability to produce children. Planning should be directed toward teaching the client about options to facilitate satisfaction of sexual drives and birth control methods.

GOALS

Realistic goals, mutually established with the client and partner, should include the following:
1. To maintain or restore the client's function as a sexual being
2. To facilitate the sexual adjustment goals of the client and partner
3. To offer the client and partner information about sexual options
4. To teach the client and partner about nontraditional positions for sexual intercourse
5. To decrease pain during sexual activities, if applicable
6. To teach the client with bowel and bladder problems how to avoid accidents and manage appliances
7. To maintain or restore positive self-concept, including improving body image when necessary
8. To offer the client and partner information about birth control
9. To refer the client and partner to knowledgeable and skillful members of the rehabilitation team when necessary

REHABILITATION NURSING INTERVENTIONS

If holistic care is to be delivered to disabled clients, the rehabilitation nurse must intervene when problems are discovered, observed, or expressed in the area of sexual function. The disabled client should be offered information and services related to sexual function.

Frequently, health care providers are uncomfortable with their own sexuality. A first step before intervening with a client is becoming comfortable in this area. According to Griffith and Trieschmann,[21] counseling is one approach that can be used in uncomplicated cases by any rehabilitation team member who is "(1) comfortable with his or her own sexuality, (2) knowledgeable about the psychosocial and learned components of sexuality, (3) aware of the various religious and cultural prohibitions of certain sex acts, and (4) familiar with the relevant medical-physical factors of the individual care." Giving information is another intervention strategy, although information alone has not proved to be an effective way of changing behavior.[3] When referral is made to a sexual therapist or another rehabilitation team member, it is essential that the physical-medical and psychosocial status of the individual receiving treatment be known by the therapist.

Counseling

When the client's medical condition stabilizes, sexual concerns may become more evident. Over a period of time, the nurse has the opportunity to establish a good rapport and a trusting relationship with the client. Thus it may be the rehabilitation nurse who is first approached with these concerns or who can initiate discussion with the client regarding sexuality and sexual function. A review of the sexual history at this time may suggest approaches to the topic.

Aside from the presentation of basic facts related to sexuality and the effects of disability on sexual function, the role of the rehabilitation nurse encompasses counseling. Effective counseling begins with a willing listener, and the nurse should be available to listen to the client express needs as a sexual being. Involvement and responsibility of both partners, the expression of their feelings, the importance of learning, and the creation of a nurturing, caring environment can be facilitated by the rehabilitation nurse.[6]

Techniques of counseling

Kerfoot and Buckwalter[29] outline several techniques that the nurse can use in sexual counseling. They include using empathic and active listening, giving information to significant others, allowing a client to express anger and grief over loss of function, identifying strengths, using humor when appropriate, providing reassurance and permission, and anticipating and preparing for certain surgeries and procedures that may threaten self-esteem.

Listening is probably one of the nursing skills most undervalued by nurses. By simply being there and actively listening to what the client has to say, the nurse can guide the client through the steps of problem solving, thus helping the client to become more comfortable in discussing sexuality and specific needs in relation to self and family members. The nurse also may assist the family through empathic and active listening.[29]

Counseling family members involves giving information. Knowing how to react to changes in body image, being prepared for what can happen during sexual intercourse, and understanding the effects of medications and certain disabilities on sexual function can help alleviate the partner's anxiety about engaging in sexual acts.[29]

The client often experiences a change in self-perception as a sexual being as a result of developmental processes, divorce, medications, surgeries, procedures, specific disabilities, and many other experiences. Nurses can help restore body image by listening to these clients express grief and anger and introducing them, when they are ready, to other clients who have successfully coped with similar situations. Both the client and partner may need help in dispelling myths and misconceptions about alternate sexual options and overcoming changes in body image.[29]

The use of past successful coping strategies often will help a client place events in proper perspective. Nurses and family members can assist the client in identifying strengths and previous successes. The client who can adopt the attitude that things have changed but will not necessarily be worse than before has a better chance of success in coping with alterations in sexual ability.[29]

Humor may be used when appropriate to help a client cope. All too often in western culture, sexual acts are taken too seriously. Humor can be used, according to Kerfoot and Buckwalter,[29] "to release anxiety, to help clients anticipate potentially embarrassing moments, and can teach the client to help people laugh with him or her as a way of relieving tension associated with changes in sexual functioning."

The nurse also can provide reassurance and support to experiment with alternative forms of sexual expression. The nurse can act as a validator to confirm that a particular sexual practice is acceptable and will not be harmful. Response to clients must be geared to their sexual lifestyles and needs.

Nurses can be much more effective as counselors if they can anticipate what the reactions of clients may be to certain surgeries, procedures, and disabilities. By supplying information before surgeries and procedures, they can help alleviate threats to self-esteem related to lack of knowledge and loss of control. Experience with numbers of clients with similar disabilities, knowledge of the comprehensive health assessment, and experience with successful interventions for individuals of like developmental level and cultural, religious, and ethnic values can be helpful to the nurse in counseling clients.

The PLISSIT model

If the rehabilitation nurse is uncomfortable counseling clients about sexual needs, the PLISSIT model may be helpful.[2] The PLISSIT model, developed by Annon and Robinson,[2] can be easily adapted to sexual counseling. PLISSIT is an acronym for permission, limited information, specific suggestions, and intensive therapy. Using four levels of involvement, the health professional engages in counseling at his or her level of comfort. As comfort and experience increase, the nurse may employ more complex levels but continues to be free to make referrals at any time.[2]

The levels in the PLISSIT model are as follows:

Level I: Permission is given to the client by the nurse to discuss concerns and problems related to sexuality. The willingness of the nurse to discuss any area will help relieve anxiety and tension on the part of the client. The nurse can give permission and reassurance that the current sexual practices of the client are appropriate and healthy. Permission also can be given to experiment with new forms of sexual expression. The nurse remains nonjudgmental while encouraging discussion. Many clients involved in the rehabilitation process may feel uncomfortable discussing sexual function unless the topic is initiated by the nurse or other rehabilitation team member. The nurse can inform the client that to worry about sexual function is normal.

Level II: Limited information is given to the client. The information is usually quite basic but provides the client with specific information. The information given to enhance understanding about a specific concern should be limited, since it is difficult to remember complex information beyond the scope of the client's immediate concern. Behavior change may or may not result.

Level III: Specific suggestions may be offered by the nurse to address specific concerns. These involve direct problem-oriented strategies or referral for specific medical interventions. The suggestions may help the client to rethink the problem and make changes to alleviate the concern. Griffith and Trieschmann[21] recommend that opportunity to practice new behaviors be provided and reports obtained on progress and problems.

Level IV: Intensive therapy is the mechanism used to meet the needs of the client whose problems cannot be solved using levels I, II, or III. It is desirable to refer the client for intensive therapy with professional counselors at this point. This level of intervention is required by only a few clients involved in the rehabilitation process but is appropriate for persons with significant psychosocial sexual dysfunctions.[21]

Rehabilitation nurses who are uncomfortable with any of these levels should refer the client to knowledgeable and skillful members of the rehabilitation team for further counseling and education. Other team members who may be skilled in sexual counseling include the psychologist, social worker, rehabilitation counselor, gynecologist, urologist, and sex therapist.

Client and Partner Education

Client and partner education is designed to provide information about sexual options, positions for sexual activities, relief of pain, control of bladder and bowel accidents, psychosocial aspects of human sexuality, effects of medications on sexual function, and birth control methods. The information preferably should be presented to both the client and the partner. Another way of presenting information would be to schedule a session on human sexuality as part of ongoing, regularly scheduled client education programs. Information should be tailored to individual, partner, or group needs and abilities. Groups can be composed of individuals who have new changes in sexuality and individuals who have previously experienced the same alterations but have successfully coped. Groups also can be composed of clients who are at similar stages in the adjustment process.[29]

Sexual options

Masturbation, the self-manipulation of the genitalia, is a normal sexual option allowing for release of sexual tension for clients with normal sensation or limited loss of sensory function. In some disease processes, such as myocardial infarction, masturbation is considered the first step back to sexual activity.[50] This option may be appropriate for any client with intact sensory perception.

Manual sexual stimulation and oral-genital sexual stimulation are other options for some disabled individuals. Two types of oral-genital activity are possible, depending upon the sex of the person receiving the stimulation. Cunnilingus is very pleasurable for some women. For women who are pregnant, however, this activity is not without hazard, because air forcibly blown into the enlarged uterine veins may result in a fetal embolism. However, if air is not blown into the vagina, this activity can be continued.[41] Fellatio can provide pleasurable sensations and orgasm with or without ingestion of the ejaculated semen by the partner. A client with loss of sensation may perform manual and oral-genital sexual stimulation on the partner and gain a sense of fulfillment from pleasing another person.

When the male is unable to have or sustain an erection, the partner may choose to use the "stuffing technique" where the female "stuffs" the semisoft penis into the vagina, contracts the vaginal (pubococcygeal) muscles, and holds the penis in the vagina.[22] A thrusting or circular motion may be carried out by the woman when she is in the dominant position. This technique may be particularly useful for the partner of an impotent client, regardless of the underlying pathophysiology.

Penile implants are another option for some males who are impotent as a result of spinal cord injury, diabetes, arterial ischemia, extensive pelvic surgery, or long-term use of certain drugs such as antihypertensives. Implantation of these devices may diminish ability to achieve partial erection. If sensations during intercourse were present before surgery, they will remain afterward. Also, presurgical sperm count will not be affected. As with any surgical procedure, complications can occur. Malfunction of the hydraulic mechanism, kinks in the tubing, and fluid leaks are some of the complications. (See Chapter 10 for an explanation of the mechanics of penile implants.) Usually these problems can be corrected to the client's satisfaction. Although some physicians limit implantation to clients with organic impotence, some will now perform this procedure for clients with functional or psychogenic impotence considered refractory to current forms of sex therapy.[19] Clients who cannot tolerate or do not wish penile implant surgery may want to use an artificial penis. This device is strapped onto the groin and simulates a natural erection. Another penile option is a stiff-walled condom into which the man places his penis.[49] Clients who do not have partners and those who are too weak to have intercourse or to control hands may wish to use a vibrator.[49]

Some clients will not accept any of these options because of socioculturally based attitudes or a partner unwilling to experiment and try new approaches. An understanding and nonjudgmental nurse or rehabilitation team member can be helpful in counseling the couple about sexual options.

Positioning

Many positions may be used to enhance comfort and facilitate sexual activities; however, not all clients and their partners are aware of these. Nurses should encourage clients to experiment with positions that are comfortable and appropriate for them for the chosen activities. Information about alternate positions, as well as encouragement to experiment, are often welcomed by the disabled individual and sexual partner.

Clients who have difficulties with mobility may need equipment such as side rails or bed loops to increase ease and safety in changing positions.[44] Some clients may not be able to assume "on top" positions and may need encouragement and support to try new positions. Loss of motion in the joints, particularly in the hips, may limit movements during sexual activity. Consideration should be given to helping clients and their partners select positions that will place the least stress on involved parts of the client's body, thus causing the least pain and allowing for the most sexual pleasure.

Individuals who experience spasticity may have difficulty remaining in any position. Involuntary movements may be a source of embarrassment, as well as a matter of inconvenience during sexual activity. Medication taken before sexual activity may provide relief from or reduce the spasticity.[44] Individuals should be informed that antispasmodic medications such as diazepam (Valium) may decrease libido but are necessary if spasms are to be relieved.

Disabled persons may use variations in the four basic positions. These positions include face-to-face contact with the man on top, face-to-face contact with the woman on top, face-to-face in a side-lying position, and a rear-entry position. These positions provide access for genital-genital contact, cunnilingus, and fellatio.[1,25] The advantages and disadvantages of these positions are described briefly.

1. *Face-to-face, man-above position:* This position, often referred as the "missionary position," provides the opportunity for the partners to engage in continued kissing and hand touching of the body. The male is in control and may have a psychological advantage. Good sensation is possible, since there is opportunity for deep penile penetration. Pillows placed under the back and buttocks of the woman allow for deeper penetration. This position may be helpful if impregnation is desired, because the semen is pooled in the vagina. Sexual activity may be difficult if the man is overweight or if the woman is pregnant. There are at least four disadvantages to this position: (1) a woman may feel "pinned" underneath the weight of her partner, making it more difficult to engage in pelvic movement; (2) a woman has little control over the depth of penetration; (3) a man may find it tiring to support his weight on his elbows and knees; and (4) a man may have less control over ejaculation than he does in other positions.[41]

2. *Face-to-face, woman-above position:* This position allows for increased control by the female both from a psychological and mechanical viewpoint. Both partners may engage in kissing and touching of the body.[46] Some men do not feel comfortable emotionally with the control exercised by the woman in this position.

3. *Face-to-face, side-lying position:* This position provides for freedom of movement for both partners. It allows for kissing, touching, and exploration. Since neither partner is supporting the weight of the other, it can be less tiring and more relaxing over an extended period of time. Pillows may be used to support various areas such as the back and legs and to provide for increased comfort and decreased strain on muscles and joints. Penetration in the side-lying position is not as deep

as in those positions where the male or female is dominant.[23]

4. *Rear-entry position:* Rear entry is possible from a side-lying or sitting position or when the woman is kneeling or lying prone. Hand stimulation is possible for both partners, and penetration into the vagina may be regulated. Variations in this position are possible because multiple approaches using pillows as supports can be used. Persons who feel that face-to-face contact is important during intercourse may not find this position acceptable.[46]

Specific disabilities may preclude certain positions. For example, clients who have cardiac problems should avoid positions that place undue stress on the arms for sustained periods. In this circumstance, the client may find the supine position less stressful as long as breathing is not restricted. Often, the side-by-side position and the face-to-face position create less worry about compromising cardiac function.

Efforts to avoid complications and provide a comfortable means of sexual activity should be the goal in experimenting with positions. Persons with arthritis, for example, should select positions that place the least stress on the involved joints. Loss of motion in joints will limit movement during sexual activity, and the client and partner may need to experiment with several positions before finding one that permits comfort and flexibility.

Those with multiple sclerosis who experience fatigue and spasticity may need to consider positioning that is the most comfortable and least tiring. Similarly, persons with spinal cord injuries should be encouraged to experiment with various positions to enhance sexual activity. The male may assume the bottom position, thus enabling easy placement of the penis by the sexual partner. Clients may find it easier to roll from side to side from this position. Females often find the missionary position the most comfortable, especially with the strategic placement of pillows. The female also may wish to experiment with the prone and side-lying positions.

Other diseases and disabilities require specific knowledge on the part of the nurse or other team members involved in the sexual counseling of the client and partner.

Alleviation of pain

Malek and Brower[36] suggest several techniques that can be used to alleviate the pain of rheumatoid arthritis when engaging in sexual activi-

ties. They stress the necessity to avoid fatigue and engage in anticipatory planning and activity management. These suggestions also would be helpful to clients with other conditions involving painful muscles and joints and include:

1. Practice muscle relaxation techniques and mental imagery to promote comfort and tranquility.
2. Practice range-of-motion exercises without resistance to promote comfortable movement.
3. Apply moist heat to painful joints 10 to 15 minutes before sexual activities to reduce swelling and promote increased range of motion. This may be in the form of compresses, a warm bath, or a shower.
4. Rest after completion of bathing and grooming activities.
5. Position pillows under affected, painful limbs for support. Always remember to remove these pillows after sexual activity to prevent contractures.
6. Schedule pain medications, and arrange for sexual activities around the periods of maximum drug effectiveness. This, of course, is not always possible or appropriate for each client.
7. Explore alternative styles of sexual expression to convey caring, concern, and love.[36]

Aging women and women with spinal cord injuries may experience discomfort because of decreased lubrication and should be advised to use a water-soluble lubricant, such as KY Jelly, to promote comfort. Petroleum jelly should not be used because it does not dissolve in water and may increase the chances of vaginal infection.[4]

Clients with spinal cord injuries above the T6 spinal cord segment may become uncomfortable if autonomic hyperreflexia occurs during sexual activity and should be advised of the symptoms and treatment for this condition (Chapter 10).

Management of bowel and bladder problems

Persons with bowel and bladder problems are anxious about the possibility of urinating or defecating during sexual activity. When these problems exist, the partner should be so advised in order to prevent embarrassing surprises. Disabled individuals should empty their bladders before sexual activity and reduce or avoid drinking for a few hours beforehand. Maintaining a consistent bowel program will help prevent accidents.

The need to use urinary drainage appliances

routinely also may be a major concern. If a man prefers to leave an indwelling catheter in place, it should be taped to the penis or sheathed in a condom. Females should be advised to tape an indwelling catheter to the abdomen. If the client has difficulty accepting the presence of the catheter during sexual activity, it should be removed and replaced. Suprapubic or ileoloop appliances need not be removed but should be taped to the abdomen. Foley catheters, suprapubic tubes, and ileoloops should not be kinked off for any period of time.

Psychosocial factors

The self-concept may be adversely affected by altered sexual abilities. To help maintain or restore self-concept, the client should be advised gently and tactfully about ways in which appearance can be improved. The nurses may need to discuss good genital hygiene with the client and sexual partner. Applying cosmetics, using toiletries, and dressing in attractive clothing can help in maintaining self-concept. Applying braces when ordered helps keep the limbs in alignment and improves appearance. If role changes are necessary for sexual activities, the nurse should be available to provide support and encouragement.

Males may be extremely anxious about sexual problems and may voice concern about their ability to provide satisfaction for their partners. Men with spinal cord injuries may worry about a decrease in the length of the penis. However, most men can be taught to increase the length by applying pressure to the perineum. If erection is affected by the disability, manual stimulation of the genital organs, dildos (devices that simulate a penis), and vibrators may be used to help the sexual partner achieve sexual satisfaction.

The ability to father children is frequently a very sensitive subject for males whose neurological pathways have been interrupted. When a male is unable to father children, the reasons for this problem should be shared with both him and his partner, including the rationale for inability to maintain an erection, inability to ejaculate, decreased sperm motility, and any altered thermoregulation of the body affecting sperm production.[45]

Open communication between partners and a positive attitude toward experimentation can help to create more satisfying sexual experiences for both persons. Efforts should be made by the nurse

to encourage clients and their partners to realize that satisfaction may be achieved through a variety of methods and that learning about each other's body reactions to various stimuli may provide enjoyment not previously experienced.

Nurses should be acutely aware that the client whose self-concept is threatened may avoid contact with others and become socially isolated. Involving the client in social interactions, complimenting efforts to appear attractive, allowing the individual to discuss sexual concerns, and accepting this expression matter-of-factly may help the client maintain or restore self-concept. The nurse's positive attitude and nonjudgmental approach early in the rehabilitation process can help alleviate client concerns and provide a climate for adaptation to the disability by the individual and partner.

Birth control

Nurses need to develop a good rapport and a trusting relationship with clients to obtain information regarding the client's needs and desire for birth control information. This need is particularly prominent among adolescents. Often society and the client assume that disability results in infertility, and thus no precautions are taken.

The nurse should provide information to clients of all ages about available methods of contraception. Ideally, the sexual partner should be included in the discussion. Verbal and nonverbal interactions between the partners will give the nurse clues about the acceptance or nonacceptance of specific methods.

Instruction of the client and partner should include a visual demonstration of sexual organs, the physiology of contraception, and birth control devices. The nurse should evaluate how well the information was received by obtaining feedback after the presentation of information. Partial grasp of the knowledge could result in unwanted pregnancy.

A brief discussion of several methods of birth control, focusing on effectiveness, availability, advantages, and disadvantages of each, is presented. The nurse must be aware of both basic information and changing information regarding the various methods. Failure to present this information to the disabled client who has the ability to impregnate or become pregnant may result in future physical, social, emotional, vocational, and spiritual problems for the client and partner.

The pill. The pill is an oral contraceptive composed of synthetic hormones similar to those that naturally regulate a woman's menstrual cycle. Birth control pills are obtained by prescription after the woman has had a thorough physical examination by a physician. This method is 99% effective when the schedule for administration is followed. Among the advantages of the pill are effectiveness, uninterrupted protection, reduced fear of pregnancy, increased sexual enjoyment, and lack of mechanical preparation before or after intercourse. The side effects may include weight gain, headache, spotting, nausea, vomiting, and sore breasts. Some emotional side effects attributed to the pill are diminished sexual interest and depression.[43] Severe headaches, loss of vision, or sudden chest or leg pains should be reported immediately to a physician.

Oral contraceptives containing estrogen present thromboembolic hazards; thus this method may not be an appropriate birth control option for a woman who must spend a large part of the day in a wheelchair. Oral contraceptives containing progesterone may cause weight gain and depression, thus decreasing levels of function for a woman with a disability.

The intrauterine device. The intrauterine device (IUD) is a plastic device with strings attached that is inserted into the uterus by a physician or nurse. For reasons not completely understood, it prevents pregnancy 97% of the time, provided it is properly inserted and checked for proper placement after each menstrual cycle.[1] Advantages include effectiveness and continual placement. Side effects or problems associated with the IUD include cramping, bleeding, spotting, and an increased risk of endometritis. IUDs also can cause pain, discharge, and odors that interfere with sexual satisfaction. Not all women can use this device because of uterine rejection The client should consult a physician for symptoms of pain, bleeding, fever, or discharge.[14]

The diaphragm. The diaphragm, a shallow rubber cup, when combined with spermicidal cream, is 97% effective if used correctly and consistently. The rubber cup fits inside the vagina, forming a seal or barrier between the uterus and sperm. The correct size is determined and prescribed by a physician or nurse following a pelvic examination.[1] Advantages include effectiveness and safety. One of the side effects is vaginal irritation.[14] Another brand of cream may be tried if this

becomes a problem. Other problems with this method are that some women may find it messy or difficult to insert or may be unable, because of cultural taboos, to touch their own genitalia.

A woman lacking fine finger movement and finger strength will have difficulty inserting a diaphragm. Trunk balance and flexibility also are required for placement of the device. Frequently the sexual partner can be taught and will choose to insert the diaphragm.

Spermicidal foam, jelly, or cream. Spermicidal jellies and creams may be obtained in tubes; foams are packaged in aerosol cans or are available in individual applications. These substances contain a chemical that kills sperm and provides a barrier between sperm and the uterus when inserted into the vagina.[14] This method is 90% to 97% effective if used correctly and consistently.[12] The chosen substance is inserted into the vagina within 30 minutes before intercourse and inserted again before intercourse is repeated.

Condom. The condom, or "rubber," is a sheath designed to fit over the erect penis to prevent sperm from entering the vagina during intercourse. If used correctly and consistently, it is 97% effective.[14] Advantages are safety, effectiveness, and protection against sexually transmitted diseases. These appliances are conveniently purchased without a prescription at drugstores.[1] Difficulties arise when condoms are sporadically used: the sheath breaks or is defective, or allergic reactions to the rubber occur. In the latter instance, rubber-free condoms, called skins, can be purchased.[15] Some persons object to this method of contraception, because it interrupts foreplay and following ejaculation, the penis must be immediately removed from the vagina. Application of the condom also requires fine finger movement, but it may be applied by the partner.

Condom and foam. The use of a condom and foam in combination provides 100% effectiveness if used correctly each time intercourse occurs. Foam must be inserted within 30 minutes before intercourse, and the condom must be placed on the erect penis before contact with the vagina.[14] The advantages and disadvantages are the same as those discussed in relation to spermicidal foams, jellies, and creams and condoms.

Rhythm. The rhythm method requires the woman to determine the fertile days of each menstrual cycle (ovulation time) and avoid intercourse at those times. There are three methods of determining the fertile time of a woman's cycle: (1) calendar, (2) basal body temperature, and (3) vaginal secretion methods. With the basal body method, the temperature is taken daily. Slight increases in temperature indicate the time of ovulation. With the vaginal secretion method, observations are made of times when secretion increases, indicating ovulation. These methods will be 90% to 97% effective if followed consistently, and if the woman has a fairly regular menstrual cycle.[14] One method may be used in combination with another to increase effectiveness. No adverse side effects occur with this type of birth control. However, the woman must be willing to keep accurate records and avoid intercourse for a significant part of the cycle. The sexual partner also must be willing to adhere to this schedule.

Sterilization. Sterilization procedures (vasectomies for males and tubal ligations for females) consist of tying and cutting the reproductive ducts, thus preventing sperm from reaching the egg. These procedures are usually considered the most effective in preventing pregnancy. Surgical procedures carry with them some degree of risk but generally result in few complications. Occasionally, there may be a regrowth of the tubes. With the fear of pregnancy virtually removed, sexual relations may improve following surgery.[14] These procedures seldom are reversible and should not be performed should a couple desire to have children.

Other considerations. In addition to effectiveness, availability, side effects, and cost, there are other considerations for choosing or not choosing a method of contraception. Persons may need to consider the broad financial aspects of their lives, their desire to have or not have children, their current health status, the presence of a disability, the prognosis of a chronic disability, the religious and moral overtones of each method, their mental and emotional stability, and willingness and ability to follow through with a method of birth control. The nurse has a responsibility to inform clients who are able to bear children of these options.

Discharge Planning and Follow-Up

Although much adjustment work to illness occurs after hospitalization, the rehabilitation nurse is instrumental in identifying problems that will re-

quire early intervention for discharge planning and follow-up. When the client is discharged home, problems can become more acute if not given attention during hospitalization. The nurse can create an environment on a hospital unit that allows privacy for the client to experiment alone or with a partner. All staff members should be encouraged to knock on a client's closed door and wait for permission to enter. Weekend passes planned with the client and partner while the client is still hospitalized can be helpful in providing opportunities to try out new sexual options in the privacy of their own surroundings. Time should be planned to discuss the experiences at home with them.

Rehabilitation nurses also need to know the community in which they work well enough to provide appropriate referral sources for individuals who require continuing therapy. These arrangements should be part of the team plan. Follow-up appointments with a member of the rehabilitation team may be scheduled to deal with sexual difficulties related to the disability. Other individuals may require intensive therapy. Two professional organizations, the Society for Sex Therapy and Research (New York) and the American Association of Sex Educators, Counselors, and Therapists (Washington, DC), publish national directories of qualified sex therapists. Local medical societies, psychological associations, and other nurses working in rehabilitation centers or as members of a sexual management team also may be helpful in identifying qualified sex therapists.

REHABILITATION TEAM INTERVENTIONS

Expert sex therapists and researchers agree that the sexual concerns of the client with a disability and the partner can best be managed by an integrated rehabilitation team approach.[9,4-53] Although the nurse may be able to listen to the client's concerns, give permission to talk about problems, offer limited information, and specific suggestions at the client's level of comfort, the integrated team approach offers the client opportunities for individual or group counseling and the resources of a number of health care professionals. Learning of the successes and failures of others who are coping with sexual problems associated with disability is helpful in the adjustment process. Didactic and informational sessions led by members of the interdisciplinary team, although not sufficient to lead to behavioral change or resolution of sexual problems, provide a forum for discussion.[21]

Many rehabilitation facilities have begun sexual treatment programs by first educating members of the designated sexual management team. Opportunities are provided for health care professionals to desensitize themselves through programs such as the Sexual Attitude Reassessment (SAR) workshops, in which both able-bodied and disabled persons are presented with a number and variety of sexual stimuli in an intense program. Opportunities are then provided for discussion and consideration of personal feelings and beliefs about sexual behavior for themselves and others.[9] Rehabilitation team members must be presented with information about normal sexual anatomy and physiology and changes associated with various physical disabilities before they can comfortably assess, intervene, and evaluate problems related to sexual function.

The PLISSIT model enables interdisciplinary rehabilitation team members to address the sexual needs and problems of the disabled client and partner at a comfortable level. Most team members are comfortable at levels I and II. Working together, a urologist, gynecologist, sex therapist, rehabilitation nurse, social worker, rehabilitation counselor, psychologist, physiatrist, and other members of the team may help the client and partner achieve desirable outcomes.

OUTCOME CRITERIA

Outcome criteria associated with satisfying sexual function for the client and partner are:
1. The client and partner assume responsibility for setting realistic sexual adjustment goals.
2. Sexual activity of the client and partner is maintained and restored.
3. The client and partner understand:
   a. Their sexual options
   b. Changes that may be necessary in male and female sexual roles
   c. Methods of birth control and ways to use them correctly and consistently if desired

4. If applicable, the client deals with specific problems by:
   a. Minimizing bladder and bowel accidents
   b. Practicing methods for pain control
5. In relation to self-concept:
   a. The client demonstrates a positive self-concept.
   b. The client and partner understand the relationship between self-concept and sexual function.
   c. The client understands the importance of physical appearance, good genital and personal hygiene practices, and neat and attractive dress.
   d. The client asks for assistance from rehabilitation team members when help is needed in maintaining a positive self-concept.
6. In the area of discharge planning and follow-up:
   a. The client and partner use community resources appropriately.
   b. The client and partner call for assistance if problems arise and return for follow-up appointments if scheduled.

SUMMARY

The ability to function as a sexual being is a basic need of all persons and can no longer be ignored if rehabilitation is to be addressed holistically. Sexual concerns sometimes become a major focus for persons who are chronically ill and disabled. In most cases, sexual concerns are tremendously complex. Consequently, no simple behavioral or medical approach will suffice to assess or treat individual sexual problems. Ideally a sexual management team whose members are comfortable with their own sexuality, knowledgeable about human sexuality, and willing to commit a considerable amount of time is required to plan and implement a team approach for the individual with sexual problems.

Rehabilitation nurses frequently deal with these problems at their level of comfort, refer to other team members if unable to address the problems expressed, and participate as members of a sexual management team. It is a responsibility of the rehabilitation nurse to give the client permission to discuss sexual concerns and then to deal with any expressed difficulties appropriately.

TEST QUESTIONS

1. The term *sexuality* encompasses what aspects of eroticism?
   a. Interpersonal
   b. Emotional
   c. Nongenital
   d. All of the above
2. Of the following statements, which statement is *true* regarding the normal female sexual response?
   a. Messages sent down to the T2-4 and L2-4 spinal cord segments result in vaginal lubrication.
   b. Complete lesions at T10 to L2 spinal cord segments preclude touch lubrication from genital stimulation.
   c. Complete lesions at T10 to L2 spinal cord segments allow orgasm from genital stimulation.
   d. Complete lesions at L2 to S1 spinal cord segments preclude orgasm from genital stimulation.
3. Of the following statements, which one is *true* of the normal male sexual response?
   a. The term *spontaneous erection* is commonly used to describe clonic contractions of the urethra and expulsion of ejaculate.
   b. Reflex erections require an intact sacral spinal cord and sacral nerve roots S2-4.
   c. Complete lesions of the T10 to L2 spinal cord segments result in the ability to ejaculate from genital stimulation.
   d. The psychogenic erection centers are located in the T2-10 segments of the spinal cord.
4. One of the most important psychosocial factors in enhancing the quality of a sexual relationship is communication. The couple should be aware that:
   a. Telling a partner what is pleasant is quite embarrassing and inhibits communication.
   b. Being honest by giving information helps persons to enjoy each other.
   c. Saying no to sexual activity makes the partner feel positive.
   d. Conversation with no physical contact inhibits sexual relationships.
5. A person with impaired physical mobility:
   a. Should no longer engage in sexual activities
   b. Has no difficulty with engaging in sexual activities
   c. Has no desire for sex
   d. Often must explore options if he or she wishes to begin or continue sexual activities
6. A person who becomes physically disabled:
   a. Can always perform social roles
   b. Has no difficulty in meeting persons of the desired sexual identity
   c. Has no difficulty in engaging in a variety of sex acts
   d. Often must make changes in social relationships
7. When performing a sexual assessment, the nurse:
   a. Judges the client's sexual values
   b. Discourages the client from engaging in deviant or abnormal sexual behavior
   c. Identifies the client's physical and psychosocial strengths and limitations
   d. Concentrates on the client's limitations when setting goals for sexual health
8. When assessing the client, the nurse knows that:
   a. Tests of pain or heat and cold sensation provide information about motor tracts traveling from the genitalia to the brain.
   b. The bulbocavernosus reflex in males indicates that the sacral segments of the spinal cord are open and reflex "touch" erections are likely to occur.
   c. Contraction of the internal anal muscles demonstrates that the thoracic segment of the cord is intact and erections are likely to occur.
   d. Voluntary contraction of the anus establishes that there are intact voluntary pathways between the genitalia and the brain.
9. Following the PLISSIT model, the nurse, at his or her level of comfort, intervenes to promote sexual health with a person who is physically disabled by giving:
   a. Permission
   b. Limited information
   c. Specific suggestions
   d. All of the above
10. The nurse who is instructing a couple on the side effects of the pill informs them that all

of the side effects listed below *except* _____ might occur.
  a. Infection
  b. Headache
  c. Loss of vision
  d. Spotting
11. The nurse instructs clients who have difficulty with pain when engaging in sexual activities to:
  a. Engage in activities after completion of bathing and grooming activities
  b. Practice range-of-motion exercises without resistance to promote comfortable movement
  c. Take pain medication after sexual activity
  d. Leave pillows under affected limbs for support after sexual activity

Answers: 1. d, 2. d, 3. b, 4. b, 5. d, 6. d, 7. c, 8. b, 9. d, 10. a, 11. b.

LEARNING ACTIVITIES

1. Assess your feelings regarding masturbation and oral-genital sex. Determine your willingness to discuss these topics with clients and their sexual partners.
2. Form a discussion group with fellow students or staff members, and share your feelings with each other about masturbation and oral-genital sex.
3. Role play the following situation with a colleague: You are a man with a spinal cord injury at T10 and have received a weekend pass from the hospital. You and your partner have received sexual counseling and information about your sexual abilities. What situations occur to you on this pass? How do you and your partner handle these situations?
4. Visit an adult bookstore and investigate available materials and devices used to substitute for or enhance sexual activities.
5. Contact or visit your local planned parenthood organization and obtain information and pamphlets about birth control and family planning.
6. Identify resources in your community that offer counseling services to persons with sexual problems.
7. Attend lectures addressing sexual problems presented by other health professionals such as urologists, counselors, and gynecologists.

REFERENCES

1. Allgeier AR and Allgeier ER: Sexual interactions, Lexington, Mass, 1984, DC Heath & Co.
2. Annon J and Robinson C: Behavioral treatment of sexual dysfunctions. In Sha'Ked A, editor: Human sexuality and rehabilitation medicine: sexual functioning following spinal cord injury, Baltimore, 1981, The Williams & Wilkins Co.
3. Bandura A: Principles of behavior modification, New York, 1969, Holt, Rinehart & Winston.
4. Barbach L: For each other: sharing sexual intimacy, New York, 1982, Doubleday & Co, Inc.
5. Bianchine JR and Lubbers JR: Drugs and sexual dysfunction. In Pariser SF, Levine SB, and Gardner ML, editors: Clinical sexuality, New York, 1983, Marcel Dekker, Inc.
6. Blanchard MG: Sex education for spinal cord injured patients and their nurses. In Krueger DW: Rehabilitation psychology, Rockville, Md, 1984, Aspen Systems Corp.
7. Bray GP, DeFrank RS, and Wolfe TL: Sexual functioning in stroke survivors, Arch Phys Med Rehabil 62:286, 1981.
8. Bregman S: Sexuality and the spinal cord injured woman, Minneapolis, 1976, Sister Kenny Institute.
9. Cole T and Cole S: A guide for trainers: sexuality and physical disability, Minneapolis, 1976, University of Minnesota Medical School, Multi-Resource Center, Inc.
10. Conine TA and Evans JH: Sexual reactivation of chronically ill and disabled adults, J Allied Health 11:261, 1982.
11. Dagon EM: Aging and sexuality. In Nadelson CC and Marcotte CB, editors: Treatment interventions in human sexuality, New York, 1983, Plenum Press.
12. Doherty M and Prato SA: Cardiac impairment. In Martin N, Holt NB, and Hicks D, editors: Comprehensive rehabilitation nursing, New York, 1981, McGraw-Hill Book Co.
13. Fairburn CG, Dickerson MG, and Greenwood J: Sexual problems and their management, New York, 1983, Churchill Livingstone, Inc.
14. Family planning methods of contraception. DHEW publication HSA 78:5646, Rockville, Md, 1973, US Dept of Health, Education and Welfare, Health Services Administration.
15. Ford AB and Orfiren AP: Sexual behavior and the chronically ill patient, Med Asp Hum Behav 8:10, 1976.
16. Geiger RC: Neurophysiology of sexual response in spinal cord injury, ARN J 5:16, Nov/Dec 1980.
17. Golden JS and Golden M: Cancer and sex, Front Radiat Ther Oncol 14:59, 1980.
18. Goller H, and Paeslack V: Pregnancy damage and birth complications in children of paraplegic women, Paraplegia 10:213, 1972.

19. Googe MCS and Mook TM: The inflatable penile prosthesis: new developments, Am J Nurs 83:1044, July 1983.
20. Gordon M: Nursing diagnosis: process and application, ed 2, New York, 1987, McGraw-Hill Book Co.
21. Griffith ER and Trieschmann RB: Sexual dysfunctions in the physically ill and disabled. In Nadelson CC and Marcotte DB, editors: Treatment interventions in human sexuality, New York, 1983, Plenum Press.
22. Griggs W: Sexuality. In Martin N, Holt NB, and Hicks D, editors: Comprehensive rehabilitation nursing, New York, 1981, McGraw-Hill Book Co.
23. Harmatz MG and Novak MA: Human sexuality, New York, 1983, Harper & Row Publishers, Inc.
24. Herbst SH: Impairment as a result of cancer. In Martin N, Holt NB, and Hicks D, editors: Comprehensive rehabilitation nursing, New York, 1981, McGraw-Hill Book Co.
25. Hogan RM: Human sexuality, a nursing perspective, Norwalk, Conn, 1980, Appleton-Century-Crofts.
26. Hott JR: Sex and the heart patient, Topics Clin Nurs 1(4):81, 1980.
27. Katchadourian H: Human sexuality, Berkeley, Calif, 1979, University of California Press.
28. Katchadourian HA and Lunde DT: Fundamentals of human sexuality, ed 2, New York, 1975, Holt, Rinehart & Winston.
29. Kerfoot KM and Buckwalter KC: Sexual counseling. In Bulechek GM and McCloskey JC, editors: Nursing interventions: treatments for nursing diagnoses, Philadelphia, 1985, WB Saunders Co.
30. Kozier B and Erb G: Fundamentals of nursing, ed 2, Menlo Park, Calif, 1983, Addison-Wesley Publishing Co, Inc.
31. Krozy R: Becoming comfortable with sexual assessment, Am J Nurs 78:1036, 1978.
32. Kuczynski HJ: Nursing and medical students' sexual attitudes and knowledge, JOGN Nurs 9:339, 1980.
33. Lief HI and Payne T: Sexuality—knowledge and attitudes, Am J Nurs 75:2026, 1975.
34. Lubkin IM: Chronic illness: impact and interventions, Monterey, Calif, 1986, Jones & Bartlett Publishers, Inc.
35. Maddock JW: Sexual health and health care, Postgrad Med 58:52, July 1975.
36. Malek CJ and Brower SA: Rheumatoid arthritis: how does it influence sexuality? Rehabil Nurs 9:26, Nov/Dec 1984.
37. Marcotte DB: Sexual history taking. In Nadelson CC and Marcotte DB, editors: Treatment interventions in human sexuality, New York, 1983, Plenum Press.
38. Maslow A: Motivation and personality, New York, 1954, Harper & Row Publishers, Inc.
39. Masters W and Johnson VE: Human sexual inadequacy, Boston, 1970, Little, Brown, & Co.
40. Masters W and Johnson VE: Human sexual response, Boston, 1966, Little, Brown & Co.
41. Masters W, Johnson VE, and Kolodny RC: Human sexuality, ed 2, Boston, 1984, Little, Brown & Co.
42. Money J and Ehrhardt A: Man and woman, boy and girl, Baltimore, 1972, Johns Hopkins University Press.
43. Notman MT: Fertility, infertility, and sexuality. In Nadelson CC and Marcotte DB, editors: Treatment interventions in human sexuality, New York, 1983, Plenum Press.
44. Robinault IP: Sex, society and the disabled, New York, 1978, Harper & Row Publishers, Inc.
45. Sandowski C: Sexuality and the paraplegic, Rehabil Lit 37:11, Nov/Dec 1976.
46. Schulz DA: Human sexuality, ed 2, Englewood Cliffs, NJ, 1984, Prentice-Hall, Inc.
47. Shrey DE, Kiefer JS, and Anthony WA: Sexual adjustment counseling for persons with severe disabilities: a skill-based approach for rehabilitation professionals, J Rehabil 45:28, April/May/June, 1979.
48. Valleroy ML and Kraft GH: Sexual dysfunction in multiple sclerosis, Arch Phys Med Rehabil 65:125 March 1984.
49. Walbroehl GS: Sexuality in the handicapped, Am Fam Phys 36:129, July 1987.
50. Watts RJ: Dimensions of sexual health, Am J Nurs 79:1568, 1979.
51. Wolf J: Mastering multiple sclerosis: a guide to management, ed 2, Rutland, Vt, 1987, Academy Books.
52. World Health Organization: Education and treatment in human sexuality: the training of health professionals. WHO Technical Report Series No. 572, Geneva, 1975, World Health Organization.
53. Zejdlik CM: Management of spinal cord injury, Monterey, Calif, 1983, Wadsworth Health Sciences Division.

ADDITIONAL READINGS

Barbach L: For yourself: the fulfillment of female sexuality, New York, 1975, Signet.
Barrett M: Sexuality and multiple sclerosis, New York, 1982, National Multiple Sclerosis Society.
Becker E: Female sexuality following spinal cord injury, Bloomington, Ill, 1978, Cheever Publishing, Inc.
Brecher E and the editors of Consumer Reports: Love, sex, and aging, Boston, 1984, Little, Brown & Co.
Burdette JA: The routine sexual history, Am Fam Phys 18:145, Oct 1978.
Comfort A: More joy, New York, 1975, Simon & Schuster, Inc.
Comfort A: The joy of sex, New York, 1974, Simon & Schuster, Inc.

Dickerson J: Oral contraceptives: another look, Am J Nurs 83:1392, 1983.

McCormick GP, Riffer DJ, and Thompson MM: Coital positioning for stroke afflicted couples, Rehabil Nurs 11:17, March/April, 1986.

Mooney TO, and others: Sexual options for paraplegics and quadriplegics, Boston, 1975, Little, Brown & Co.

White EJ: Appraising the need for altered sexuality information, Rehabil Nurs 11:6, May/June 1986.

Who cares? A handbook on sex education and counseling services for disabled people, Washington, DC, 1979, Sex & Disability Project, George Washington University.

Yoshino S and Uchida S: Sexual problems of women with rheumatoid arthritis, Arch Phys Med Rehabil 62:122, March 1981.

CHAPTER 20

Work and Recreation

Dorothy P. Byers

OBJECTIVES

After completing Chapter 20, the reader will be able to:

1. Define the functions of work and recreational activities in daily living.

2. Identify ways in which chronic illness and physical disability may affect a client's work and recreational activities.

3. Explain the methods used and data collected when performing a nursing assessment of work and recreational activities.

4. Formulate nursing diagnoses associated with a client's alteration in work and recreational activities.

5. Develop goals collaboratively with the disabled client for work and recreational activities.

6. Determine nursing interventions appropriate for the client with alteration in work and recreational activities.

7. Identify the interventions of rehabilitation team members related to the ability of a client to engage in work and recreational activities.

8. List outcome criteria used to evaluate the success of rehabilitation in work and recreational activities.

To be human is to want to be active, and work and recreational activities for many disabled clients represent a central point in successful rehabilitation. Sir William Osler, in an address to medical students stated, "Though a little one, the master word (work) looms large in meaning. It is the open sesame to every portal, the great equalizer in the world, the true philosopher's stone which transmutes all the base metal of humanity into gold."[5] Comparing Frankl's description[6] of the apathy that can envelop the life of a concentration camp prisoner to the life of a person with a disability, the person with a disability also can be rendered unable to feel normal emotion able only to numbly sense the advantage of being alive. A life without a purpose, without a true goal, leads an individual to believe that everything that had meaning is gone, and as Frankl notes, there will be retreat to the inner life or life of the mind. Those who cultivate a rich inner life will realize the importance of love (of another person, humankind), the value of simple appreciation of art and nature (beauty), and most important, the ability to choose one's attitude. This inner decision helps determine the rehabilitation outcome and can make life meaningful and purposeful. Even if a creative or active life is not possible for the person with a disability, the inner life can give purpose to existence. Survival may well depend on the ability of the person to test inner strength.[6] The contemplation of work and the meaning it has for the client can be a great resource in building a sturdy inner life.

When working with a disabled client, the nurse is in a position to assess with the individual the various aspects of work and recreation that may in time be meshed into the fabric of a strong inner life. This chapter focuses on the role of the rehabilitation nurse in this process and on interventions that will help prepare the client to achieve goals for work and recreation.

FUNCTIONS OF WORK AND RECREATIONAL ACTIVITIES

Webster defined work as toil, employment, task, job, deed, or achievement; something produced by mental or physical effort or physical labor. It also means to exert oneself physically or mentally and to perform work regularly for wages. The normal function of work relates to activity, either mental or physical, that results in wages or remuneration. The wages thus acquired allow the individual to purchase basic necessities such as food, clothing, and shelter.

Recreation or having fun is defined differently by each individual. Some clients will plan carefully for highly structured "play" activities; others may rarely take time for recreation, and still others will seek out fun as a way of life. Recreational or play activities can be defined as a refreshing of strength, diversion, or relaxation. The person with a disability will have to seek a balance among work, recreation, and rest, defining each of these activities to fit a particular life-style. Some individuals will choose to do nothing during leisure time.

During work or recreation, the individual, perhaps without conscious effort, expends physical and mental energy. Walking, running, lifting, bending, sitting, jumping, climbing, and fine motor activities, such as writing and assembling, may be involved. Planning, organizing, solving problems, following instructions, and communicating are mental activities that may be required for both work and recreation. Not to be overlooked is the expenditure of emotional energy in relating to coworkers and others in the course of a day.

The functions of work and recreation, however, go beyond these primary concerns. Work may be a means of socialization, a chance for power and prestige, a way of providing for others, a source of self-fulfillment, or an opportunity to amass a fortune, and an individual may assess personal worth in relation to the work role. Others may judge an individual in the same way. Recreational pursuits also help to define the person.

Historically work and recreation have had different meanings. Greco-Romans thought of work as a curse to be avoided. Early Hebrews considered idleness to be offensive and thought even lowly jobs provided dignity. In biblical times, Jesus' teachings advised giving away worldly wealth to gain Heaven. Early Christian doctrine recognized work as a means to a worthy end, but it was given no intrinsic value. In early Catholicism, the religious and intellectual efforts of those in the monastery were highly valued, whereas manual labor was left to lay people. Worldly concerns were overshadowed by concerns for gaining the hereafter.[16]

Martin Luther removed the distinction between everyday work and service to God by teaching that all activity was divine and that each person should be satisfied with his or her own work. Calvinism held it was God's will that all must work but shun wealth, possessions, and "soft" living. Puritanism arose from Calvinism and encouraged the greatest possible gain from work so those gains could benefit needy people. For the first time, the pursuit of wealth was justified. This belief was the predecessor to the modern age, where work is valued for its own sake. However, rest and pleasure were abhorred.[16]

The machine age made it possible for humans to mold, control, and manipulate the environment, and the work necessary to achieve this became important in and of itself. As machines increased productivity of goods, consumerism developed to keep the system going. As hard physical labor lessened, the prominence of sports as a substitute increased, and the tie of work to religious belief waned.[16]

The industrial society of the past has been replaced by an information society, meaning that many heavy and light industrial jobs no longer exist. The change began in the mid-1950s when fewer people were producing goods and more people produced services. Currently, 65% of employed persons work with information directly, whereas others hold information jobs within manufacturing companies. Service jobs account for 11% to 12% of the work force, whereas only 12% of workers are engaged directly in manufacturing. Naisbitt, a futurist, states that:

Professional workers are almost all information workers—lawyers, teachers, engineers, computer programmers, systems analysts, doctors, architects, accountants, librarians, newspaper reporters, social workers, nurses and clergy. . . . Everyone needs some kind of knowledge to do a job. Industrial workers, machinists, welders, jig makers . . . are very knowledgeable about the tasks they perform. The difference is that for professional and clerical workers, the creation, processing and distribution of information *is* the job.*

As we near the twenty-first century, a rapidly changing world will alter the normal function of work for many people. Adler[1] mentions six activity areas: (1) sleeping or all biological acts that must be performed by a living person; (2) toiling, or monotonous repetitive acts that teach us nothing; (3) leisuring, or learning, playing, or activities engaged in for their own sake; (4) play, or amusement for pleasure; (5) idling, or killing time; and (6) resting . . . "which is worshipping for those who believe in religion, or the appreciation of art for those who do not believe in religion."

Until the early part of this century, most people spent their lives in a combination of sleeping and toiling, but by the year 2100, many people will work only 25 hours per week and will devote the remainder to recreational activities. Mechanical or toiling tasks will be performed by computers, lasers, and robots, thus freeing people to lead four- or five-part lives. According to Adler, "There is nothing good about toil. The sooner we get rid of that, the better."[1]

*From Naisbitt J: Megatrends, New York, 1984, Warner Books.

The implications for the nurse and the disabled client are many. First, the variety of jobs in the information society opens new doors for training and retraining, even for a client with many limitations. Second, clients whose work was in industry may be disadvantaged if they are unable or unwilling to accept changes in the workplace. Last, the nurse as a therapist will need comprehensive knowledge of current and future vocational trends and recreational resources to interact effectively and plan work alternatives and recreational options with a disabled client.

IMPAIRED ABILITY TO ENGAGE IN WORK AND RECREATIONAL ACTIVITIES

Some kind of activity, whether physical, social, mental, or emotional, is involved in work and recreation. A disabling condition that restricts the client's function in any of these activities will alter employment potential and the ability to engage in recreational pursuits. The degree of restriction will depend upon the severity of functional loss measured against the requirements of the desired activity.

A secondary effect of impaired ability to engage in work and recreational activities may be loss of the provider role and loss of sources of socialization in the workplace. The client to whom power and prestige were the primary work satisfactions may lose the position of power because of disablement. As with any major loss or change in life-style, self-image and feelings of worth may be altered. Along with financial uncertainty, a grieving process may ensue, further adding to client problems. Reversal of roles within the family unit can be a negative or positive development for the client.

Some families, when faced with these losses, grow stronger; others are weakened, overwhelmed by myriad changes and problems. Loss of family support may interfere with the client's motivation to cope with the disability and hinder rehabilitation efforts aimed toward returning the client to the workplace.

The client who has a disability needs careful nursing assessment of remaining abilities. Although a medical diagnosis is helpful, assumptions made on that basis alone may be faulty. For example, a client who has had a mild stroke may have no functional loss and will probably be able to resume desired activities. Conversely, a sudden trauma, such as a severe head injury, may leave the client with impaired physical, social, emotional, and mental function. The recovery period may be lengthy and costly, limiting work and leisure options. In another example, a sudden spinal cord injury may leave a young, active client wheelchair-bound and in need of continuous care. Education or a beginning career may be suddenly interrupted; emancipation from the family may be reversed; and the customary life-styles of the family may be altered significantly.

A condition with more gradual onset, such as multiple sclerosis, commonly results in problems with mobility, weakness, urinary incontinence, spasticity, and numbness. Speech, vision, and intellect also may be affected. Often, the condition is progressive, and predicting the extent of functional limitation is difficult. Persons between 20 and 40 years of age are affected at a time in their lives when they are active in terms of career and family life. Since at present there is no cure for multiple sclerosis, the treatment is symptomatic and directed toward preventing severe disability. The uncertainty of occurrence and extent of signs and symptoms adds to the difficulty of planning for both work and recreation.

Other chronic medical conditions can result in functional disabilities affecting work and recreation. For example, the client with chronic obstructive pulmonary disease may find the energy needed to work is increasingly taken up by the effort used for breathing. As the condition progresses, anxiety produced by chronic shortness of breath can interfere with ability to concentrate on work or recreational activities. Similarly, individuals with chronic renal failure, in addition to dealing with reduced physical strength, must make time for dialysis treatments and may have other medical problems. Planning with certainty for work and recreation must center around a treatment program.

Oncological conditions can alter the individual's ability to work and play in several ways. Physical appearance after major head and neck surgery distorts body image and, if a laryngectomy is performed, speech patterns are altered. The client with a colostomy often has difficulties with body image. Treatment modalities such as chemotherapy may be time consuming and produce side effects such as nausea and hair loss, in addition to interfering with the client's usual patterns of work and leisure activities. In many instances, the uncertainty of prognosis makes planning for a future vocation and for recreation difficult.

Various acute and chronic disabling conditions alter the client's physical, emotional, mental, and social functioning. The nurse working in a rehabilitation setting must be prepared to assess clients in these areas to formulate a care plan that returns the client to an optimum level of function in preparation for future roles in work and recreation.

NURSING ASSESSMENT

The nurse has many opportunities to interact with the client during the daily rehabilitation program. In discussing the role of work, recreation, and the future of both with the client, emphasis should be placed on the client's abilities, not limitations, and what physical, mental, and emotional abilities are required to participate in work and recreational activities. The assessment process should be ongoing and should lead to a picture of the abilities needed by the client to work before the disability compared to current or expected function. The nurse, through the assessment, determines the meaning of work for the client. Is the provider role important, or does the workplace provide socialization for the client? What recreational pursuits does the client enjoy?

A suggested framework for documenting information gained from the client is found in the book *Rehabilitation Client Assessment*.[12] Referred to as the initial order roster, this framework can be used to establish a baseline. Because it is open ended, it can be amended as more facts are obtained. (See box on p. 434.) The categories serve as a guideline for questioning the client in areas pertinent to work and recreation.

The roster consolidates much pertinent information and is useful to an interdisciplinary team, as well as to a nurse working in a small institution or in the community. Whatever the method of gathering data, it is important to realize that the answers lie within the client, and the more skillful the nurse's interviewing techniques, the more useful the information gathered.

Interaction with the client in all rehabilitation settings allows the nurse to discuss work and recreational concerns. With knowledge of the client's functional abilities, the nurse can begin to construct a picture of future possibilities in these areas with the client. The assessment process is

---

Initial Order Roster

Personal-social information

1. Physical appearance, age, nationality, speech
2. Mannerisms, reactions, statements during interview
3. Method of thinking about problems, peculiar class habits
4. Family and home situation: Married? Number of children? Living with parents?
5. Statements about relations with others, comments from others about personal adjustments, quirks, interactive behaviors

Vocational-educational information

1. Years of schooling, success in school
2. Number of jobs, level of jobs, skills learned
3. Test material and client statements about job interests, training, aspirations

Medical-environmental information

1. Client's disability, prognosis, possible restorative procedures
2. Miscellaneous data on environment: How well does client know present area? Client owns and operates a car, owns home?

From Miller L: Everybody's system for interpreting client information like a vocational counselor. In Bolton B and Cook DW: Rehabilitation client assessment, Baltimore, 1980, Baltimore University Press.

---

ongoing and can be accomplished during casual conversation. The nurse, along with other rehabilitation team members, encourages the client to begin to realize what will be possible and impossible. In this manner, the client is assisted in establishing some of the structure for developing "inner strength." The initial conversations in relation to work and recreation can be painful for both the nurse and client. A quiet, empathic acceptance of whatever is expressed by clients will help to bring conflicting feelings out, open the door to future communication, and help clients realize that others can appreciate their plight. To be a good listener is part of the therapeutic use of self.

In the assessment it is important to look closely at recreational interests, especially if full-time work seems to be unlikely. Do the recreational interests involve physical exertion such as in active sports or manual dexterity such as in crafts or woodworking? Are there new untried recreational activities that interest the client and might be possible with adaptive devices? Recreational activities can provide a healthy new outlet for the client and allow use of remaining abilities.

An interview guide for nursing assessment of recreational activities follows:

1. What did you do during your leisure time before your disability (for example, watch television, read, engage in sports, go out for dinner, engage in arts and crafts, go to the theater, play musical instruments, play cards or other table games, continue work activities, sew, cook, visit with friends)?
2. Did you prefer to engage in recreational activities with others or by yourself?
3. What do you do now for recreation?
4. Do you prefer to spend your leisure time with others now or by yourself?
5. What would you like to do now for recreation?
6. What do you think you can do now?
7. What are your goals for use of your leisure time in the future?
8. Do you prefer to spend your leisure time with others or by yourself in the future?
9. How do you plan to accomplish your goals for leisure time in the future?

NURSING DIAGNOSES

Impaired physical, mental, or emotional function affects the ability of the individual to engage in work and recreational activities. The disabled person needs to establish a balance of activities in life. Too much emphasis on one area will mean sacrifices in other areas. If the individual is spending great amounts of energy in the work role (and the energy expenditure can be tremendous), there may be no energy left for fun. The individual who wants and values performance like a "normal" person in the work role may become exhausted in the attempt. The benefits of play and diversional activities are the same for everyone. These activities serve to free the spirit, restore balance, and restock the storehouse of pleasant memories.

Alteration in the ability to function physically, mentally, or emotionally affects the ability of the individual to work and enjoy recreation. Pronounced deficits in any of these areas contribute to the nursing diagnoses of *change in vocational potential* and *diversional activity deficit.* Other nursing diagnoses that relate to a person's ability to perform work and recreational activities are listed below.

Physical Limitations

1. *Impaired physical mobility:* Affected clients may have partial or total loss of the use of arms or legs (impaired fine motor skills with arthritic changes in the hands), or gross motor control (spasticity found in multiple sclerosis) may be lost. The client has a loss or decrease in motor control that interferes with the ability to move from place to place independently, as in quadriplegia.

2. *Activity intolerance:* The client tires easily with even minimum exertion, as in emphysema.

3. *Impaired verbal communication:* The client has difficulty in expressing thoughts verbally or understanding the speech of others. For example, the individual may experience aphasia after a cerebrovascular accident.

Intellectual Limitations

1. *Altered thought processes:* The client has difficulty in forming concepts, memory problems, and a short attention span. Also, the client may have difficulties with judgment and be unable to check and control behavior and correct errors.

2. *Sensory-perceptual alteration:* The client has impaired sensation or perception. There may be difficulty with visual or auditory perception. There also may be kinesthetic, gustatory, tactile, and olfactory impairments.

A client who has central nervous system damage after a head injury or a cerebrovascular accident has some of these deficits, which directly affect work and recreational activities.

Emotional Limitations

1. *Body image disturbance, self-esteem disturbance:* The client has a problem accepting altered appearance or activity. Disturbances in self-concept may occur as a result of the physical or mental changes. The individual may devalue self or lack feelings of self-worth.

2. *Altered role performance, personal identity disturbance:* In this instance, the client may see his or her role assumed by others or may no longer be able to make a meaningful contribution to society through work. Feelings of loss may be experienced when the client can no longer function

as provider, homemaker, student, or parent. When a client achieves personal identity primarily through a work role and is no longer able to work, personal identity may be difficult to define.

3. *Anticipatory or dysfunctional grieving:* In this instance, the client may not be able to participate in rehabilitation therapies because of not adjusting to the disability.

4. *Ineffective individual coping:* The client may cry without an immediate stimulus and be unable to control emotions.

GOALS

Goals are established with the client and relate to the nursing diagnoses. Goodkin and Catlin state, "The goal of rehabilitation is maximum independence, and the role of the rehabilitation professional nurse, doctor, or therapist is to foster and encourage this independence in all areas to ensure that the disabled individual is able to make decisions and to control his own life."[7]

Short-term goals for work and recreation involve facilitating the client's participation in various therapies designed to maximize physical function. The nurse can reinforce programs in physical and occupational therapies by encouraging the client to practice therapeutic activities until these become integrated into activities of daily living. The act of buttoning a shirt can improve a client's fine motor skills and provide a sense of satisfaction, and the nurse must allow time for these activities.

If the client expresses a desire to resume a former job, this decision must be evaluated in terms of the physical and mental activities that the job requires. Like any other job seeker, the disabled client needs to explore the qualifications for the position. When working with the client, the available options are examined. The nurse avoids passing judgment. "To be effective and productive, counseling must allow for latitude, change of mind, trial and error, and the choice to do nothing; above all, it must allow for failure. All of these, although negative in their superficial context, are positive means for self-exploration vis-à-vis the world of work and should be encouraged rather than discouraged."[19]

Trieschmann[17] cites studies of spinal cord–injured clients which show that employability is related to vocational responsibilities before injury, work-related interests before injury, and acceptance of responsibility for predisability educational planning. Goals often can be based on predisability orientation to work.

Goal setting in collaboration with the client provides a continuum of activities leading to an attainable outcome. If the client's goal is too global, for example, "returning to work," the nurse can assist by helping the client break down the large goal into a series of smaller goals that, as achieved, may led to the larger goal.

If the goal of returning to work seems unrealistic, a substitute goal that also is satisfying needs to be established. If poor self-image or lingering in the grief process occurs, the nurse may assist the client in exploring feelings about self, with a goal of helping the client accept the losses while emphasizing remaining strengths and abilities.

REHABILITATION NURSING INTERVENTIONS

The role of the nurse varies depending upon the setting. In an institution with a rehabilitation unit or in a rehabilitation agency, the nurse functions as a member of an interdisciplinary team. Many disciplines are involved in rehabilitation therapy, and the nurse contributes to the care plan in a cooperative effort with other members of the rehabilitation team. The nurse working in community health or home care may have a more direct role in therapies or referral to community resources. For example, a community health nurse may refer a client to the local office for vocational rehabilitation or may facilitate mobility by locating a firm to supply adaptive equipment for a car.

Nurses who work for insurance companies and evaluate the progress of workers undergoing rehabilitation can refer clients to a work-hardening program. In this work-oriented treatment program, the outcomes for the client are measured in terms of increased productivity until the client achieves a level that will be acceptable in the competitive labor market. This type of program was developed in the late 1970s at Rancho Los Amigos Medical Center in Los Angeles and is proving to be very successful in determining which individuals will succeed in the competitive job market.[11]

The client with a speech impairment needs encouragement and time to practice outside of therapy sessions. The nurse can assist the family

in learning what is being done in therapy so that they can help the client in learning to use speech and language skills outside the therapy milieu.

The nurse's role in promoting health maintenance activities cannot be overemphasized. The client who is wheelchair bound after a spinal cord injury, for example, must be taught the importance of skin care and bowel and bladder programs to avoid the complications of skin breakdown and urinary tract infections. The nurse must have a knowledge of the equipment and techniques available to assist the disabled client in avoiding these secondary complications. Intermittent self-catheterization, for example, can be taught to some individuals and make possible a life free of an indwelling catheter. Decreasing the chance of infection contributes to better health status.

An individual who has had a stroke and who needs temporary bed rest can be assisted in maintaining maximum range of motion, assisted in frequent position changes, and taught bed mobility. These efforts will help prevent contractures, muscle atrophy, and skin breakdown. The nurse prepares the client for transfer activity and facilitates ambulation when appropriate. Knowledge of wheelchair management and the proper use of prostheses and orthoses enables the client to receive maximum benefit from these devices.

Psychosocial Interventions

A major alteration in life-style such as a change of role, employment, or ability to move about freely can be stressful to any individual. By anticipating the possibility of a stress reaction, the nurse can be alert for stress-related behaviors such as undue fatigue, difficulty in sleeping or withdrawing by too much sleep, decrease in interaction with others, or irritability. If these behaviors are not typical for the client and begin to interfere with progress toward vocational goals, the nurse can tactfully make the client aware of the observed behavioral changes. A way to begin dialogue with the client might be: "I've noticed you don't seem to come to the lounge with your buddies in the evening, John, for the usual poker game. And you're in bed so early and asleep right away. This is a change for you, and I wonder if you can tell me why?" If the nurse's tone is non-threatening, the client has the freedom to express personal feelings.

If the client reacts with anger, the underlying

reasons can be elicited and discussed. A client who has tried very hard to meet goal expectations may react with relief that the nurse has noticed his or her plight. Or a client may express fear— fear of leaving the program and the shelter of the hospital. These feelings are not abnormal. It is helpful to ask the client to recall possibly experiencing similar feelings before the disability in a period of stress. The checklist below can be used as a guide when intervening in problems related to stress:

1. Identify behavioral change.
2. Look for a pattern, not an isolated occurrence.
3. Decide if the behavioral change is interfering with progress toward goals.
4. Share observations and allow the client to express feelings about the situation.
5. Identify possible sources of stress with the client.
6. Decide with the client what steps to take to change the situation.
7. Monitor progress and supply feedback to the client.

Difficulties with role change, body image, and sense of personal worth may be problems for some disabled individuals. If the work role has been a strong integrating factor, the client may experience an unfavorable reaction to change. Kohl states, "Full-time employment, volunteer work, or full time family are alternatives that require exploration without any judgmental response that only return to paid employment is the mark of successful rehabilitation."[10]

The nurse can anticipate problems in these areas and offer therapeutic assistance to clients and families. The full impact of problems with body image, personal identity, and role change may not be evident in the rehabilitation program setting. A programmed exercise called *Human Interaction and Physical Differences* presents eight attitudinal dimensions commonly expressed toward disabled persons. Although the exercises are designed to be used by two people, the material can be adapted for use by families, staff, and others.[18] The reality of possible negative reactions can be discussed and the strength of the disabled individual enhanced.

Acceptance of changed body image can be facilitated by contact with individuals who have successfully made a transition to community life. For example, ostomy societies and stroke clubs exist in many communities, and the nurse can arrange for representatives to talk to clients and families. These individuals can serve as role models for the client attempting to reenter the community and as such are helpful to some clients.

Reentry into social situations can be facilitated by role-playing sessions. Clients can have an opportunity to enact strategies that will be used in going to a social function, shopping, keeping an interview for a job, or going to a movie. The nurse can be the pivotal person in arranging this activity and is supported by other rehabilitation team members.

A distorted self-image is a problem of some individuals who continue to anguish over altered appearance and ability. Small revisions in goals may be made, such as changing a goal of walking without a limp to doing things despite a limp.[15]

Client and Family Education

Much of the progress toward integrating disabled individuals into the community is the result of the activism and determination of disabled people themselves. Clients and families need to be aware of current legislation that affords opportunities for even those who are severely disabled to be able to obtain and hold a job. The Rehabilitation Act of 1973 established the right of a disabled person to equal consideration for employment and required agencies receiving federal funding to make their facilities accessible to the handicapped. Amendments to the law in 1978 provided for independent living services to more severely disabled persons who may not be able to work.

Knowledge of assistive and adaptive devices for leisure activities helps the nurse to encourage clients to seek play and recreation. Special skis are available for persons who have amputations, as well as "water limbs" for swimming. A sled called the "Sit 'n Ski" is available for downhill skiing, cross-country skiing, and waterskiing. Clients with upper extremity limitations can be supplied with special easels to facilitate writing and artistic activities.

In many areas, special programs have been developed to offer ice-skating and horseback-riding lessons to blind clients. The Colorado Outdoor Education Center for the Handicapped and the Voyageur Outward Bound programs offer challenging experiences for disabled persons. Unique Reservations will arrange for cruises to many destinations for individuals who need dialysis (Dialysis at Sea). Participating in a marathon run has been a positive and possible experience for some persons with ostomies.

Community newspapers and contact with community groups can supply information for the nurse interested in referring clients to sources of recreational activities. Numerous agencies operate to provide support and services for disabled persons, and the nurse may facilitate contacts with these groups even before discharge. For example, the National Paraplegia Foundation is a source of support for clients with spinal cord injuries. (See Appendix E for address.) Self-help organizations such as stroke clubs are a source of information and also socialization. Information regarding accessible recreational facilities can be obtained from a number of agencies, as well as travel publications listing accommodations and services for the disabled. (See Appendices D to F.)

Transportation may be a problem for both work and recreational activities. Automobiles and vans may be adapted and the disabled person taught to drive. At the Veterans' Administration Hospital in Long Beach, California, a driver training program enabled 154 out of 169 eligible candidates to successfully learn to drive. Ages of these disabled persons ranged from 21 to 53 years, and the group included clients with spinal cord injuries, multiple sclerosis, and amputations.[9]

In many areas, coalitions and consortiums have been developed by disabled people to make communities more aware of their presence and their needs. An excellent guideline for this effort is *Planning Effective Advocacy Programs* by Bowe and Williams.[2]

Discharge planning should take place during all stages of rehabilitation and intensifies as the client begins to achieve some of the goals established for maximum independence. Special equipment sources must be located, and if necessary, plans for adapting the client's home to make it accessible need to be implemented. Appropriate referrals to community agencies such as the local office of vocational rehabilitation should be made to determine if the client is employable. Availability of a driver-retraining program and a source of the needed auto adaptations should be found. Liaisons should be established between the rehabilitation nurse and the community health nurse when referrals are made to ensure continuity of the rehabilitation team plan.

Follow-Up

The period of reentry into the community after the initial phase of rehabilitation is vitally important to the disabled client. A significant goal of rehabilitation is for the individual and family to apply the assistive and adaptive techniques in the community after discharge from the rehabilitation facility. Although the rehabilitation facility has been supportive and encouraging, the community at large may be less hospitable or even hostile. Disabled people desire reintegration into the community and have been encouraged by rehabilitation professionals to think that this is possible. "Disabled persons themselves, however, have little or no awareness of the intermediate steps necessary to attain this goal."[4] The nurse should collaborate with the client in planning for possibly difficult or embarrassing social interactions and situations that may occur upon return to the community. For example, the nurse may role play a citizen asking the client about the disability or wheelchair so the client can anticipate this situation and practice responses.

Clients with spinal cord injury have been known to use sequential selection of social settings and associates in coping with reentry to the community. Also, they engage in positional maneuvering. "In essence, what newly disabled people can do is learn how to concentrate the attention of others on their positive characteristics in order to shift attention away from their disability."[4]

Using this knowledge, the nurse may assist the client in role-playing efforts in expected social situations. It may be beneficial to maintain phone contacts at regular intervals with clients to monitor progress and provide support. Another approach would be to offer a meeting place for discharged clients where experiences in the community are shared. Planned liaison with community health nurses who are actively assisting the client is another method of sharing knowledge. The postdischarge period is one that rehabilitation workers know the least about and for which they offer the least assistance and support to those adapting to a new disability.[4]

REHABILITATION TEAM INTERVENTIONS

Achievement of the client's work and recreational goals is the concern of the interdisciplinary team. In a large hospital or rehabilitation agency, the nurse is a member of a large team comprised of many disciplines, and when they work together, roles may blur or overlap. In addition to each discipline asking, "What is our unique role?" Browne suggests asking, "What is the task?" "Who can do what?" and "How should those persons work together?"[3] For example, nurses, occupational therapists, and physical therapists all work with the client to maximize physical strength and endurance. It may be that one particular therapist has the best rapport with an individual client and can best facilitate goal attainment. The social worker, psychologist, and nurse may all be involved in assisting a client to resolve a grief reaction. The psychologist may be the key person in moving the individual toward better emotional health. Once the task at hand is determined, rehabilitation team members with the most appropriate skills are used. This approach necessitates negotiation and compromise.[3]

Outside the institution, the nurse may need to structure a rehabilitation team approach to suit the needs of a particular client. The "team" may be two people and may exist for a short time until a particular goal is achieved. For example, a community health nurse may contact a resource for auto adaptation and supply the initial information regarding the client's abilities. A source of financing should be located, especially if the adaptation will enable the client to work. The nurse then follows through to determine if the needed equipment is in place and if the client is able to use the adaptive devices to travel to the place of employment or recreation.

Roles and functions of other rehabilitation team members in assisting the client to resume work and play activities include the following:

Physiatrist: Responsible for diagnosis; prescribes various treatment modalities for the client, provides follow-up evaluation, and communicates with the client's personal physician.

Occupational therapist: Assists in developing and restoring skills related to self-care, recreation, and vocational interests; assists in increasing muscle strength and coordination; instructs in use of assistive and adaptive devices.

Physical therapist: Develops specific exercise programs to increase muscle strength and facilitate ambulation; instructs in the use of prostheses; instructs in pulmonary function exercises; uses treatment modalities such as diathermy, ultrasound, transcutaneous electrical nerve stimulation, massage, and traction.

Vocational counselor: Evaluates client in terms of vocational aptitudes, abilities, and interests using techniques such as job analysis, psychological testing, work samples, and the situational work approach; assists the client with retraining and education; educates employers about the benefits of hiring disabled persons; serves as an advocate for disabled persons in the workplace.

Social worker: Assists the client with financial concerns; identifies sources of income replacement; works with the client and family on adjusting to the specific disability; identifies community resources appropriate to client needs such as transportation, housing, and recreation; supports the client and family to facilitate discharge.

Recreational therapist: Encourages the client to establish or reestablish recreational and leisure interests; offers the client opportunities for group and individual recreational activities within the institution and the community; helps prepare the client for socialization upon reentry into the community.

Industrial engineer: Serves as a consultant to the interdisciplinary team; identifies potential problems in job demands and environmental accessibility; selects procedures for modifying the workplace and job tasks to accommodate the individual using job analysis and workplace design. (See box on p. 440 for the steps followed in job adaptation.)

OUTCOME CRITERIA

As with any client problem, outcome criteria relate to goal setting and how well the client was able to achieve goals. If the goal was to return to a former job, one needs to consider whether this has been possible for the client. If returning to work was only possible with adaptation of the workplace, has this been achieved? If traveling to and from work was the problem, has the client found transportation? If the client was a homemaker, have the necessary adaptations to the home been made to allow resumption of this role? Does the client have a network of social support to call upon; if not, can the nurse help the client

---

Steps to Effective Adaptation of Jobs

Vocational counseling considerations
1. Determine vocational limitations of the person.
2. Determine vocational interests of the person.
3. Identify local job opportunities consistent with interests.

Job analysis considerations
1. Estimate potential job/person fit in terms of:
   a. Job tasks
   b. Environmental accessibility
2. Isolate potential problem areas in a selected job or jobs.
3. Develop detailed information for job modification.

Workplace design and modification
1. Identify methods to resolve problems.
2. Redesign a job or facility.

Job training
1. Provide training for a job.
2. Measure job performance.

From Priest JW and Roessler RT: Rehabil Lit 44:202, July/Aug 1983.

---

maximize function in all areas. Functions include setting realistic goals with the client and tailoring nursing therapies to meet those goals. Also involved is referral to agencies in the community best equipped to assist the client. Follow-up efforts to encourage the client during community reentry are important.

A vitally important area for all rehabilitation team members is client advocacy, which means encouraging employers to consider hiring disabled persons as well as encouraging communities to face problems of transportation, accessibility, recreational programs, and programs for independent living.

To quote Frankl, "An abnormal reaction to an abnormal situation is normal."[6] In assisting the client with a disability to reorder both the external and internal life, the nurse can be reassured that the client who is struggling to go on with life is "being normal." The nurse, in collaboration with members of the interdisciplinary rehabilitation team, can help give clients tools to adjust their behavior to changed circumstances.

or family identify the beginnings of such a network?

If retraining for new work was necessary, has this been possible for the client? If the client was a student, is the chosen school accessible? If work was not possible, does the client have an adequate income source? Has the client achieved maximum independence in self-care skills in the activities of daily living? If help is needed, how much, what type, and for how long to accomplish what activities?

Finally, have the client and family successfully adjusted to an altered life-style? Are recreational activities pursued successfully? Does the client have easy access to a support system if unrealistic goals must be altered? Do the client and family express satisfaction with the current life situation?

SUMMARY

The rehabilitation nurse's role in assisting the client with work and recreational activities is to

TEST QUESTIONS

1. When assessing the client's potential for work and recreational activities, the nurse:
   a. Focuses on the client's limitations and particular loss of function
   b. Establishes baseline data by asking questions requiring "yes" or "no" responses
   c. Conducts the interview close to the client's discharge date to avoid undue anxiety
   d. Emphasizes physical, mental, and emotional abilities required for future vocational and leisure endeavors
2. All of the following are nursing goals established with the client *except:*
   a. Denying the opportunity to try any activity that the client feels able to accomplish
   b. Providing time to practice therapeutic activities until these become integrated into activities of daily living
   c. Facilitating the client's participation in various therapies designed to maximize physical function
   d. Fostering independence in all areas of rehabilitation to ensure that the client is able to make decisions that affect his or her life

3. The Rehabilitation Act of 1973 established the right of a disabled person to have:
   a. Accessibility to driver-retraining programs
   b. Equal considerations for employment
   c. Accessibility to recreational facilities
   d. Opportunities to establish self-help organizations
4. Which statement is *true* regarding the disabled client and the period of reentry into the community?
   a. Disabled persons have a great awareness of the intermediate steps necessary to attain community reintegration.
   b. Nurses are the rehabilitation team members who structure the client's progress toward reintegration.
   c. The community at large may not accept or may even be hostile toward the disabled client.
   d. Disabled people generally do not desire or aspire toward community reintegration.
5. The role of the rehabilitation counselor as a member of the rehabilitation team is to:
   a. Evaluate the client in terms of vocational aptitudes, abilities, and interests.
   b. Assist in developing and restoring skills in self-care activities.
   c. Instruct in the use of prostheses.
   d. Prescribe various treatment modalities.

Answers: 1. d, 2. a, 3. b, 4. c, 5. a.

LEARNING ACTIVITIES

1. You are a student in a nursing program or a fairly new graduate practicing in a rehabilitation setting. You have just been diagnosed with multiple sclerosis, and because of severe disabilities you are already experiencing, you will not be able to pursue your profession. How would you proceed to restructure the work and recreational activities of your life?
2. Interview a disabled person who has made a successful return to employment. Make a list of the community barriers overcome and ways in which these have been overcome.
3. In your own community, survey recreational facilities, restaurants, auditoriums, churches, and other public places for accessibility. Discuss their accessibility with a disabled person to determine whether you have the same perceptions regarding accessibility to recreational activities.
4. Select a business and make an appointment with the personnel director. Ask questions about hiring disabled workers, for example, philosophy, practice, numbers of disabled workers employed, and work records. If the workplace has been designed and modified for the disabled worker, find out how it was accomplished. Share your findings with colleagues.

REFERENCES

1. Adler M: What we should know about work and leisure, Speech delivered at Daeman College, Buffalo, NY, 1984.
2. Bowe F and Williams J: Planning effective advocacy programs, Washington, DC, 1979, American Coalition of Citizens with Disabilities.
3. Browne JA: Position statements on social work education. In Browne JA, Kirber BA, and Watt S, editors: Rehabilitation services and the social work role: challenge for change, Baltimore, Md, 1981, The Williams & Wilkins Co.
4. Cogswell BE: Socialization after disability: reentry into the community. In Krueger DW, editor: Rehabilitation psychology, Rockville, Md, 1984, Aspen Systems Corp.
5. Cushing H: The life of Sir William Osler, New York, 1925, Oxford University Press.
6. Frankl V: Man's search for meaning, New York, 1963, Pocket Books.
7. Goodkin HF and Catlin JH: Making the world accessible. In Murray R and Kijek JC, editors: Current perspectives in rehabilitation nursing, St Louis, 1979, The CV Mosby Co.
8. Gordon M: Nursing diagnosis: process and application, ed 2, New York, 1987, McGraw-Hill Book Co.
9. Kent H and others: A driver training program for the disabled, Arch Phys Med Rehabil 60:273, 1979.
10. Kohl SJ: Psychosocial stressors in coping with disability. In Krueger DW, editor: Rehabilitation psychology, Rockville, Md, 1984, Aspen Systems Corp.
11. Matheson LN and others: Work hardening: occupational therapy in industrial rehabilitation, Am J Occup Ther 39:5, May 1985.
12. Miller L: Everybody's system for interpreting client information like a vocational counselor. In Bolton B and Cook DW, editors: Rehabilitation client assessment, Baltimore, 1980, Baltimore University Press.
13. Naisbitt J: Megatrends, New York, 1984. Warner Books, Inc.
14. Priest JW and Roessler RT: Job analysis and workplace design: resources for rehabilitation, Rehabil Lit 44:202, July/Aug 1983.

15. Stryker R: Rehabilitative aspects of acute and chronic nursing care, ed 2, Philadelphia, 1977, WB Saunders Co.

16. Tilgher A: Homo faber, San Diego, 1930, Harcourt Brace.

17. Trieschmann RB: Spinal cord injuries: psychological, social and vocational adjustment, New York, 1980, Pergamon Press, Inc.

18. Yerxa EJ: Human interaction and physical differences, Costa Mesa, Calif, 1974, Concept Media.

19. Zuger R: Vocational rehabilitation: its philosophy and practices. In Murray R and Kijek JC, editors: Current perspectives in rehabilitation nursing, St Louis, 1979, The CV Mosby Co.

ADDITIONAL READINGS

Adler M: A vision of the future, New York, 1984, Macmillan Publishing Co, Inc.

Bowe F: Rehabilitating America, New York, 1980, Harper & Row Publishers, Inc.

Commission on Practice: Work hardening guidelines, Am J Occup Ther 40:841, Dec 1986.

Hull K: The rights of physically handicapped people, New York, 1979, Avon Books.

Norback J: Sourcebook of aid for the mentally and physically handicapped, New York, 1983, Van Nostrand Reinhold Co.

Roth W: The handicapped speak, Jefferson, NC, 1981, McFarland & Co, Inc.

CHAPTER 21

Accessing Home and Community

Theresa P. Dulski

OBJECTIVES

After completing Chapter 21, the reader will be able to:

1. Describe an accessible and safe environment in the home and in the community.

2. Identify facilitators to safe access in the client's home and in the community.

3. Give examples of physical considerations in providing for an accessible and safe environment in the home and in the community.

4. Assess a client's physical environment for accessibility and safety.

5. Formulate nursing diagnoses associated with accessing the physical environment.

6. Determine goals with the client and family to maximize accessibility and safety in the home and in the community.

7. Determine nursing interventions that will enable the client to gain access and perform activities of daily living safely in the home and in the community.

8. Identify the interventions of rehabilitation team members in promoting an accessible safe environment for the client.

9. List outcome criteria used to evaluate the effectiveness of planned intervention to achieve accessibility of the client's environment.

Trieschmann defines rehabilitation as the "process of learning to live with one's disabilities in one's own environment."[20] Orem's theory,[18] first published in 1959, focuses on the individual need for self-care and the unique role of the nurse in this process. Before an individual can meet higher level needs, safety and security needs must be met. In Maslow's hierarchy of needs,[13] safety and security needs are placed immediately above physiological needs in importance.

Rehabilitation nursing uses components of Trieschmann's definition and Orem's and Maslow's theories in a philosophy that espouses the uniqueness of the individual, client independence whenever possible, health promotion, and client and family involvement in the rehabilitation process. The client exists on a continuum extending from community to rehabilitation facility and back to community. The purpose of health care in the rehabilitation facility is to prepare the client for independent life after discharge.

The nurse can assist the client in gaining accessibility in the home and in the community. Accessibility refers to the ability to enter, move around in, and exit a residence; move about on streets and sidewalks; enter, move around in, and exit buildings; obtain transportation for work, recreation, and socialization; park; obtain living quarters; attend church; obtain services of choice; and vote.

The rehabilitation nurse is unique in helping the client access the community because interaction with clients and families is constant, daily, and often less formal than that of other rehabilitation team members. The nurse has the opportunity to help the client realize that disabilities need not become handicaps and to establish optimistic, realistic goals with the client and family for achieving and maintaining access in the home and in the community.

FACILITATING ACCESS

Each year millions of dollars are spent helping the individual who is disabled achieve maximum independence. During the total rehabilitation process, the person is prepared physically and emotionally to return to the community. Transition from a supportive institutional environment can be frightening and discouraging. Adjustment to the community environment in a new role can be challenging to some, but overwhelming to others. Self-care to the limit of abilities helps an individual preserve a sense of dignity and personal worth, whereas dependence deprives a person of initiative and self-esteem.

Historically in the United States, persons who are disabled have experienced attitudinal and architectural barriers as they attempt to gain access to community. The presence of an obvious physical deformity often generated prejudice, ignorance, condescension, and anxiety in others. Disabled persons were separated from the rest of the population and either confined to their homes or placed in institutions where custodial services were provided.[7]

After World War II disabled soldiers returning home were rehabilitated and assimilated into the work force and the community. In most instances, rehabilitation was not considered complete until the individual was able to work and become self-sufficient. It became evident that these veterans could learn new skills, adapt to disabilities, and cope with certain aspects of the environment.

Many rehabilitation programs helped bridge the physical and psychological gap between institution and community by giving attention to the needs of disabled persons for housing, transportation, education, employment, recreation, service, and social needs. Yet independent function remained impossible for many of these persons to achieve because of attitudinal and architectural barriers in their environments.

Persons who were disabled became increasingly determined in their quest for personal rights, participation in decisions affecting them, and full participation in community life. As they gained a broader view of independence, they pressed for legislation that would give them access to the entire community. The goal of barrier-free design is autonomy for the disabled. A person with a disability should be able to participate in all everyday activities.

Housing

Studies indicate that disabled people desire to return to their own home rather than move to housing designed solely for them,[5,6] but often adaptive features are needed to maximize functioning in the home. Housing accessibility needs are unique to the user and should be tailored to meet individual needs. Most new residences can be easily and inexpensively adapted to facilitate accessibility and can be planned with adequate parking; ramps; doors wide enough to accommodate wheelchairs, crutches, and walkers; reach considerations in kitchens and bathrooms; and sufficient space to maneuver equipment.

Until recently it was impossible for persons with severe disabilities to live independently. Lack of housing options and support services forced them to live in institutions. Now, however, a variety of living options exist. Congregate housing with or without attendant care has been the most common housing alternative. Some persons live by themselves with attendant care. Lack of available live-in attendant care, however, continues to be a major obstacle to independent living. Independent living centers in a number of communities offer support services that allow persons who are severely disabled to continue living in their own dwellings. Services supplied may include personal care, peer counseling, congregate meals, transportation, and housing.

The U.S. Department of Housing and Urban Development has as its assigned responsibility within the federal government the development and provision of accessible buildings and living facilities for low-income elderly and disabled citizens. This department also provides and maintains subsidized housing for these citizens. Because programs are administered by the states, quality and quantity of service vary. Laws have been passed to help make housing available and accessible to the disabled. Among these laws are the Housing Act of 1959, which provided mortgage loans to finance construction or rehabilitation of housing projects, including housing for the elderly and handicapped persons; the Architectural Barriers Act of 1968, which required that federally funded buildings be accessible to physically disabled persons; Section 504 of the Rehabilitation Act of 1973, which prohibits discrimination based on handicap in the sale or rental of federally subsidized housing; the Housing and Community Development Act of 1974, which provided housing assistance payments to lower income families; and Title VII Comprehensive Services for Independent Living, which provides services to the severely disabled. Title VII is the first law that does not require vocational potential as a requirement for service. Some areas of the country have apartment complexes for the disabled or group housing with shared services such as attendant care.[14]

Transportation

When the disabled do not have adequate access to public transportation because of high steps, narrow doors and aisles, and inadequate signs for information, their world shrinks to the immediate environment.[12] Access to shopping, medical, and other support services is crucial if disabled per-

sons are to continue to maintain function and participate in everyday activities. Access to shopping centers allows purchase of necessary goods such as food, clothing, medical supplies, and toiletries. Access to other medical and support services, such as clinics, churches, and recreational facilities, enables individuals to maintain and promote health.

The Urban Mass Transportation Act of 1964 funded research aimed at encouraging consumer groups across the country to identify basic criteria regarding accessible public transportation for the disabled. Consumer groups are still active in trying to minimize the inequities that deny accessibility to public transportation.

The Urban Mass Transporation Act of 1969 made it a national policy for elderly and disabled persons to have the same rights to use mass transportation as others. Lower floors, shorter steps, wider doors and aisles, ramps or lift systems, and space to accommodate wheelchairs were suggested. After September, 1979, buses were required to use new access specifications.[15]

Today interstate bus companies, the national railroad system, and airlines offer assistance to the elderly or physically disabled traveler. Most travel services are accommodating if alerted to special needs before a trip.

Section 504 of the Rehabilitation Act of 1973 mandated accessibility at terminals and planes that are part of intercity, urban, or suburban systems. Travel outside a person's immediate community requires that airlines, trains, or bus transport companies be contacted in advance to determine services available and accommodations made for disabled passengers. If contacted ahead of a scheduled trip, the Chambers of Commerce in most cities will supply accessibility booklets. The U.S. Department of Transportation will supply guides to national highways and airports.[24]

The current thrust of federal government programs is to provide rehabilitation, job training, recreation, and regulations that assure the disabled equal access to the community.[3] Understanding the need for a barrier-free environment means understanding the needs of people with functional and mobility problems. Their needs vary greatly according to the type and degree of disability; therefore it is impossible to generalize about environments needed. Each person is unique and has individual abilities and needs.

Lack of physical function is influenced by the degree of dysfunction, adaptive skill, training, ability, and attitude of the individual.[11]

Building Accessibility

When the disabled began to reenter the community after World War II, they gained a new prospective of the world from a wheelchair. Curbs and steps presented frustrating barriers. During the civil rights movements of the 1960s, the disabled pressed for legislation to allow them the right to share in the joys and responsibilities of the community. Disabled activists lobbied for legislation to modify building design and for accessibility to employment, education, transportation, and recreation.[1] To make buildings more accessible, persons with disabilities stressed the need for external grading, walkways, parking ramps, doorways, restrooms, lower telephone placement, and location of utilities such as water fountains.

The Rehabilitation Act of 1973 included the Birth Right Act for disabled people. This legislation established the Architectural and Transportation Barrier Compliance Board to monitor discrimination and support affirmative action. The board initially consisted of eleven representatives of federal agencies assisted by a consumer advisory panel appointed by the board. In 1978 an amendment to the Rehabilitation Act added eleven members to the board. These members were appointed by the president. At least five members must be disabled. The board establishes minimum guidelines and requirements for accessible design and ensures accessibility and availability of public conveyances for the disabled. The board coordinates other federal departments and agencies within the Department of Education to develop standards and to provide technical assistance to public or private facilities, persons, and organizations as efforts are made to overcome barriers created by architecture, transportation, and communication. Specifications for making buildings accessible to and usable by the physically handicapped are enforced. Standards for an accessible, barrier-free design that would allow all people—able bodied, disabled, young, or old—to move more freely, independently, and safely in the community address such problems as wheelchair clearance; curb ramps; parking requirements; specifications for lavatories, eleva-

tors, and drinking fountains; telephone accessibility; and tactile warning signs. These standards were developed by the American National Standards Institute and comply with Uniform Federal Accessibility Standards.

Education

Legislation has been enacted that affects the educational programs offered to persons with disabilities and makes any type of program much more available to persons with disabilities. In accordance with Section 504 of the Rehabilitation Act of 1973, all elementary and secondary educational programs receiving federal funds must identify and notify qualified disabled persons that free appropriate education is available. Postsecondary education programs receiving federal funds must not discriminate in admission and recruitment on the basis of handicap. In addition, all school buildings must be accessible. The Education for All Handicapped Children Act of 1975 was passed to emphasize the needs and protect the rights of disabled children and their parents or guardians, give financial assistance to states and their localities, and assess the effectiveness of education for children who are disabled.[14]

Many educational institutions offer services specifically for disabled students, such as special parking, special equipment, mobility assistance, tutors, and wheelchair storage. Talking books, braille books, Kurzweil reading machines, reader services, and textbook recording may be available for blind students. Interpreters and notetakers are often available for hearing impaired students.

The Vocational Education Act mandates that states have boards responsible for vocational education programs. The Rehabilitation Comprehensive Services and Developmental Disabilities Act of 1978 required that states develop and implement a system to protect and advocate for rights of persons with developmental disabilities.[14] In addition, these amendments created the National Institute for Handicapped Research, which was to later become the National Institute for Disability and Rehabilitation Research.

Employment

Access to employment and to the worksite and resources to assist individuals in obtaining this access vary from state to state. State offices of vocational rehabilitation and private rehabilitation companies may provide assessment of the person for the job market; assessment of training facilities, equipment, and transportation; employer development; job modifications; placement and follow-up; supportive employment, including full or part-time coaches; and work-hardening programs.

Several pieces of legislation have influenced employment opportunities available to persons with disabilities. The Fair Labor Standards Act requires that the minimum wage cannot be less than 50% of the wage paid to nonhandicapped workers for the same type of job. Section 503 of the Rehabilitation Act states that any contract with a federal department or agency must include a provision requiring a contractor to take affirmative action to employ and promote qualified individuals who are disabled. Amendments to the Comprehensive Employment and Training Act of 1978 require local sponsors to include affirmative action programs to identify and recruit persons who are disabled.

The Civil Service Reform Act of 1978 mandates that agencies make reasonable accommodations for qualified persons with known physical or mental limitations and prohibits the use of selection criteria that would screen out such persons from employment. In addition, the Tax Reduction and Simplification Act of 1977 allows employers to take limited tax credits for employing disabled persons. As part of the Tax Reform Act of 1984, Congress reenacted the business tax deduction that had lapsed in 1982. This law gives firms a tax deduction of up to $35,000 for providing accessibility to public facilities and transportation.[3]

Voting

The Voting Accessibility Act was enacted in 1984 to improve access to registration and polling places for the elderly and disabled. This act mandates that accessible sites be provided for the elderly and handicapped. Laws governing state and local elections, however, may vary.[14]

NURSING ASSESSMENT

Information the nurse obtains before observing the client function in the environment provides insight into some of the problems the client may experience. Knowledge of physical deficits or alterations in mobility helps the nurse identify the client at risk for injury.

The nurse incorporates findings from the physical assessment to identify any alterations that may affect ability to function in the environment safely. Data from the physical assessment that must be considered are sensory alterations (vision, hearing, thermal/tactile) and mental status. The physical assessment also allows the nurse to learn about the client's mobility and ability to ambulate with or without assistive devices.[2]

An environmental assessment enables the nurse to identify interactions between the client and the environment. The best indication of suitability of the home environment is the ability of the client and family to manage activities of daily living. The established data base assists the nurse in planning individualized intervention.[16] The nurse asks the following general survey questions about the client's home, community, transportation, and support systems before making an environmental assessment:

Questions about the home environment

1. Where do you live?
2. What type of home do you have (apartment, duplex, single home)?
3. Do you rent or own your home? (Important if recommendations are made for modifications.)
4. Do you have concerns about getting into your home?
5. Do you anticipate any difficulty getting around in your home?
6. What safety measures will have to be taken around your home?
7. Who is responsible for cooking? (Response will determine extent of modifications that have to be made in the kitchen.)

Questions about the community environment

8. What buildings in the community do you use regularly (school, place of employment, bank, post office, grocery store, department store, church)?
9. Do you anticipate a problem getting in or around in these buildings?
10. Do you anticipate difficulty functioning in these buildings because of the physical environment (type of desk, high counters, inaccessible toilets)?

Questions about transportation

11. Do you own a car?
12. Do you have a driver's license?
13. Are you able to drive your car? (Information from a physical assessment may make this question inappropriate.)
14. Is there someone who can drive your car or drive you where you want or need to go (family, friend, church member)?
15. Is there public transportation near your home (bus, taxi, van service)?
16. Do you anticipate any problem in using public transportation (cost, difficulty getting in and out of vehicle)?

Questions about support systems

17. Is there anyone living with you who could assist you in getting around in the home and community?
18. Is anyone else willing and able to help you (relatives, friends, church members, civic group members)?

To assess the client's safety and level of independence and to determine any needed modifications, the nurse should have the client demonstrate activities of daily living in the home and community using assistive and adaptive devices if needed and learned skills.

Assessment in the Home

The nurse, often in collaboration with physical and occupational therapists, assesses physical features of the home for obstacles or hazards, accessibility, safety, and the client's level of independence within the environment. The type of dwelling (apartment, private residence), design (one floor, two floors, split level), and floor plan (number and placement of rooms) should be noted. The following areas of the home are assessed in questions answered in relation to accessibility and safety:

Entrance	Distance from transportation? Adequate lighting? Ramp width, slope, railing? Door width? Difficulty opening, closing doors? Threshold height? Adequate space for maneuvering (wheelchair, walker, crutches) on landing?
Stairs	Handrails, height, width, carpeting, lighting, obstacles, (such as clutter)?
Hallways	Width, carpeting, handrails, lighting?
Elevator	Control accessibility? Timing of automatic door? Threshold height?
Kitchen	Location? Space for maneuvering wheelchair, walker, devices? Cupboard height? Ability to open? Countertop height? Work space? Sink height? Opening under sink for wheelchair? Ability to operate faucets? Type of stove (electric, gas, microwave oven)? Safety features? Ability to operate stove safely (attention to placement of clothing when turning on)? Ease of refrigerator opening? Accessibility of contents? Accessibility of appliances and utensils? Ability to use safely?
Bathroom	Location, space for maneuvering wheelchair, walker, devices? Height of toilet? Accessibility of sink, tub, shower? Ability to use safely? Height, threshold, safety of sink, tub shower? Placement of faucets?
Bedroom	Location, space, obstacles? Height of bed? Firmness of mattress? Ability to get in and out of bed safely?
Floors	Type of surface (wood, carpet, linoleum)? Condition (deep-pile, frayed, loose carpeting; slippery linoleum)? Scatter rugs? Obstacles (such as toys)?
Furniture	Type (such as functional)? Arrangement (obstacles)? Ability to use safely?

Assessment in the Community

The nurse, often in collaboration with the social worker, determines accessibility of the places the individual uses for acquiring goods and services, work, worship, and pleasure and recreation. The following areas commonly used by clients in places they frequent may be assessed through client and family interviews and direct observation:

Parking areas	Marked for handicapped and have adequate space to get in and out of vehicle?
Ramps	Height of incline, width?
Sidewalks	Width, incline?
Entrances	Ramp, landing space before and after door adequate for wheelchair, crutches, walker?

Doors	Automatic? Height of door handles, ability to operate? Width?
Hallways	Marked for handicapped route, width, lighting, carpeting, railings (height, security, width for grasping)?
Rooms	Accessibility? Room to maneuver wheelchair, crutches, walker?
Furniture	Sturdiness, height, firmness, ability to use, arrangement so as not to be a hazard?
Function	Can client perform function intended in building (for example, bank, store)? If not, what physical environmental factor prohibits function?
Church	Ramp available? Restrooms available for disabled? Accessibility to drinking fountains? Seating available?
Library	Clear space at card catalogs and reference stacks of at least 35 inches? Clear aisle width in stacks of 42 inches (minimum of 36 inches)? Accessible public areas?

The type of transportation used to travel from the home to the destination in the community also should be assessed. The ability to ambulate in the community, operate a private vehicle, and use public transportation are factors considered. Observations made include the following:

Ambulation	Uses assistive devices? Avoids hazardous behavior, crosses with light, crosses at corner, avoids walking at night or in high-crime areas alone?
Vehicle	Type of vehicle? Able to get in and out? Able to operate safely alone? Uses seat belts? Individual driver operates vehicle safely?
Public transportation	Distance from home? Able to reach pickup area? Able to access? Amount of assistance needed? Can driver assist? Is anyone available to assist? Cost?

NURSING DIAGNOSES

Data obtained from assessment of the client's environment are used in formulating nursing diagnoses. Factors that the nurse identifies as actual or potential hazards to the client's health and safety provide direction for nursing intervention.

Accepted nursing diagnoses from the North American Nursing Diagnosis Association that are related to an accessible environment include the following[8]:

1. *Self-care deficit (specify).* Client cannot be independent in activities of daily living because of barriers in the environment.

2. *Potential for injury (specify).* Information obtained during assessment of the client's ability to engage in activities of daily living in various settings will help the nurse identify physical hazards and unsafe practices. Sensory or motor deficits are identified.

3. *Knowledge deficit (specify).* The client and family members may not be aware of environmental hazards. The nurse identifies hazardous features of the environment and advises the client and family on how to eliminate them.

GOALS

Goals or expected outcomes established with the client and family are aimed at providing a safe, accessible environment. Individual client strengths and limitations are considered in order to help the client establish realistic goals. Short-term goals reflect immediate or less involved steps toward functioning safely in the environment. Long-term or ultimate goals reflect the long-range effect of planning or intervention. The ultimate goal should be the client's safe practice of activities of daily living in an accessible environment.

Actual and potential environmental hazards are identified after the nurse completes an assessment by observing the client perform activities of daily living in his or her own environment. Nursing judgment concerning the client's ability to function safely helps determine the goals established. The client and family members should be involved from the beginning in establishing goals, because they are ultimately responsible for creating a safe and accessible environment.

Examples of goals related to accessibility in the home and in the community follow:

1. To assist the client in gaining safe access when entering, moving about, and exiting from the home
2. To assist the client in performing activities safely as a participating member of the community

3. To assist the client and family in identifying hazards in the home and in the community.

REHABILITATION NURSING INTERVENTIONS

Disabled persons should participate in decision making concerning their own environment. Rehabilitation team members may be concerned about clients' functional potential after discharge and often may be reluctant to support their desire to attempt living in what the rehabilitation team may regard as a less than ideal living arrangement. Clients should be given the chance to test out the living arrangements they choose, however, and support should be given during a trial period.

Home Modification

Every effort should be made to support the client's decision about return to the community. The nurse can help facilitate client independence by making recommendations about the living quarters.

Garage. At least 12 feet in width should be allowed for transferring and maneuvering a wheelchair or hydraulic lift. A remote control should be used to open the garage door either from within the car or by an electric switch that can be reached from the car.[9]

Entrance. When a home has more than one entrance, the one closest to the client's designated parking place or transportation should be chosen. The outside walk should be free of obstacles and should not be broken or cluttered. In addition, the walk should be wide enough to accommodate a walker or wheelchair (36 inches wide). A doorway clearance of 32 inches is needed to accommodate a wheelchair. Entrances to buildings should include at least one entrance accessible to people in wheelchairs. The route to the entrance should be accessible.

Ramp. A ramp should be at least 36 inches wide to accommodate a wheelchair. It should have a low guardrail at the side, handrails on both sides that extend 1 foot beyond the top and bottom of the ramp, and a nonslip, smooth surface. There should be a level area at the top of the ramp before the doorway so the client can manipulate the walker or wheelchair while opening the door. Edges should be protected to prevent slipping

off. Ramps should have a gradient rise no greater than 1 foot in 12 feet.[19] Ramps also should have a 6-foot level clearance at the bottom.[14]

Floor. Highly waxed, slippery floors and scatter rugs should be avoided. Wheelchairs can be propelled easier on an unwaxed linoleum floor or on a rug with short pile and no underpad. Rugs should be secured to the floor and not frayed or worn.

Stairs. Risers on stairs should be slanted or beveled. Handrails at least 32 inches above the step level along steps and hallways act as safety devices to aid balance when walking or propelling a wheelchair.[19] Handrails on both sides of the stairs should extend at least 12 inches beyond the top and at least 19 inches from the bottom step. Tread heights and risers should be uniform. Risers should be no more than 7 inches high.

Halls. A width of 36 inches is needed for wheelchair access. Doors should swing into rooms, not into the hall.[19] Adequate indirect lighting is needed to safely maneuver the chair.

Doorways and doors. Doorways should be widened when necessary and should be at least 32 inches wide. Doors should not require over 5 pounds of pressure to open. Doors can be replaced with sliding or folding doors or curtains or rehung with step-back hinges. Doorknobs may be replaced with levers to facilitate opening when the client is unable to grasp and should be able to be opened in a single effort. Thresholds over ½ inch high should be removed and replaced with an inclined threshold. Floors should be level for at least 5 feet in the direction of the door swing and extend 3 feet in the direction opposite to the door swing. It should takes at least 3 seconds for doors to swing close.[14] For persons with limited hand function, keys may be adapted by attaching a short length of dowel to the key or by screwing a wooden handle to it.[9]

Rooms

Modifications can be made in rooms to promote safety and accessibility. These modifications are of benefit not only to the disabled but to the able bodied as well. Modifications to the kitchen, bedroom, and bathroom are discussed.

Kitchen. The kitchen should have sufficient space for maneuvering a wheelchair. Five feet of floor space is needed to turn a wheelchair 180 degrees.[19] Cupboards should be accessible. Accessibility from a wheelchair or sitting position should be considered and easy-open latches installed according to the client's ability to use fine finger movements and manipulate articles. Items should be stored and arranged to decrease the need for bending and reaching. Some of the most frequently used equipment should be stored within the client's maximum reach.

Pegboards with hooks provide a means of storing frequently used items. A knife rack permits handles to remain upright for easy grasp. A dish rack or divider may help use space and make dishes more accessible. Drawer dividers help organize contents and make them more accessible. Sliding racks and turntables bring items to the front of the cupboard without the need for reaching.[12] Sinks should be no more than 34 inches high and the sink and counter width a maximum of 30 inches. Ranges and cooktops and their controls should be insulated or protected to prevent burns, abrasions, or shocks. Self-cleaning ovens are recommended. A reacher should be available to retrieve articles that have fallen to the floor or to reach articles on high shelves.

Controls placed on the front of the stove allow the client to independently turn on the stove without reaching over the burners. A mirror positioned over the stove helps a person in a wheelchair check the progress of food cooking on top of the stove. Safety around the stove is always a concern. Lighting a gas stove if the automatic pilot has extinguished can best be accomplished with a long wooden fireplace match.[12] The client should be alerted to the fact that liquids or food heated in a microwave oven may be hot while the container stays cool.

Conservation of energy is an important factor when working in the kitchen. Performing tasks in a sitting position should be considered. Dishwashing is a task particularly suited to this position. The cupboard under the sink should be open or recessed for wheelchair accessibility. Hot water pipes should be covered or insulated to prevent burns. For clients with altered sensation, hot water temperature can be regulated to avoid burns. The counter should be large enough so that working space can be efficiently and safely arranged.[10]

Consideration may be given to the Universal Kitchen developed at the Georgia Institute of Technology. This kitchen features a variety of work surfaces, storage units, and appliances that can be easily installed, removed, or rearranged to fit the user's needs. The Universal Kitchen permits builders to fit, remodel, and change a kitchen to accommodate the individual's disability.[4]

A variety of aids enable the disabled person to function more independently in the kitchen. Among these are an easy-to-use peeler, chopper, electric blender, one-handed can opener, and jar opener. Long-handled utensils for reaching and safety around the stove are available.

Bathroom. The doorway should permit wheelchair access to the toilet and bath facilities, with a turning space of 60×60 inches for maneuvering a wheelchair. The area around the toilet should be large enough to accomplish a transfer. A raised toilet seat and grab bars may facilitate use of the toilet. The toilet should be contained in an area that is at least 3 feet wide and 4 feet, 8 inches deep; have a door that is 32 inches wide and swings out; and have a seat 17 to 19 inches high from the stand.

Bedroom. Removing rollers from the bed prevents rolling during transfers. A firm mattress facilitates mobility in the bed. Clutter and obstacles, such as poorly arranged furniture, should be avoided. Three feet of space is needed on one side of the bed for a client in a wheelchair to position himself or herself next to the bed for transfer. Drawer pulls may require adapting, such as using handles rather than knobs. Wheelchair users need closet rods placed at a height of 3 or 4 feet.

Furniture

Sturdy, easily cleaned furniture should be arranged in rooms in such a way that it does not present obstacles. The client should use the furniture safely (for example, not sit on the edge of a chair or bench), equalize weight when transferring in and out of a chair to avoid tipping, and avoid standing on furniture to reach high places. Climbing should be avoided when there is any loss of function in the upper or lower extremities, incoordination, or weakness.

A variety of cleaning devices have been designed to aid the disabled homemaker. Long-handled dusters and dustpans, reachers, lightweight vacuum cleaners, and sit-down ironing boards are only some of the devices available. (See Appendix D for suppliers of assistive/adaptive devices.)

Environmental modification to accommodate for sensory deficits

During the assessment the nurse identifies any decrease in the client's functional ability because of alterations in vision, hearing, and touch. Vision may be improved by using corrective lenses. Hearing may be enhanced with hearing aids and in some cases corrective surgery. Another option, often ignored by health care professionals, that can be used to enhance sensory function is modification of the physical environment.

Vision. Two major problems related to altered vision are reduced color discrimination and inability to tolerate glare. Intervention is directed toward providing variation in color and avoiding glare. This can be accomplished by using red, orange, and yellow colors and avoiding pastels. Monotones make it difficult for the client with decreased discriminatory ability to function. For example, dark furniture on a dark floor or light furniture against a light wall may interfere with the client's ability to distinguish items in a room.

Contrasting colors make it easier for the client to distinguish objects. Dishes with contrasting rims help prevent table accidents. Door frames painted in contrasting colors help distinguish doorways. Bright stripes on the edge of each stair and landing help in distinguishing stairs. Brightly colored nail polish can be used to make a dot on the stove or appliance control knob to indicate the "off" position.

Signs in public buildings should be painted in colors against a black background. Numbers on doors and elevators should be painted in contrasting colors.

A black telephone with white lettering makes it easier to see the letters on the dial. A circular device with large numbers is available from the telephone company and can be fastened around the circular telephone dial.

When the client's eyes are sensitive to bright light, glare should be reduced. Exposed light bulbs and shiny surfaces, such as highly waxed floors, should be avoided. Fluorescent light may be used to prevent indoor glare and sunglasses to prevent outdoor glare. Tinted glass or sheer curtains reduce glare from large windows. Lamps should be located to create a pleasing, safe environment. (See Chapter 17 for further discussion of impaired vision and nursing interventions.)

Hearing. Deterioration in hearing usually progresses slowly and often goes unnoticed until the deficit is severe enough to interfere with functional ability. Changes in the vestibular apparatus of the inner ear may affect equilibrium and cause falls. Diminished ability to distinguish words and locate direction of sounds interferes with a person's participation in conversation. Conversation without visual cues often may be misunderstood, causing the affected person to avoid groups and conversational opportunities.

Radios and televisions can be adjusted so lower tones, which are easier to hear, are more prominent. Background noise, such as the noise of appliances, also may affect ability to hear. Capturing the person's attention, facing the person and speaking distinctly in a slightly lower volume improve communication.

Amplification devices for the telephone can be installed rather inexpensively. A light activated when the telephone rings or when a smoke detector alarm goes off alerts a hearing-impaired individual and promotes safety in the environment. (See Chapter 17 for further discussion of impaired hearing and nursing interventions.)

Touch. When impaired touch sensation accompanies decreased function of the extremities, the affected person is vulnerable to burns. Extra care should be taken when cooking, using hot water and heating pads, and operating appliances such as an iron. Interior arm surfaces and the back of the hand are more sensitive than the palm of the hand and can be used to test the temperature of water and objects.[11]

Decreased sensation in the lower extremities contributes to unsure footing and decreases awareness when bumping into objects. The nurse should advise the client of the resulting safety hazards and focus on teaching techniques to compensate for the sensory deficit. (See Chapter 16 for further discussion of touch.)

Environmental Modifications in the Community

A safe, accessible community includes consideration of buildings, facilities, equipment, and transportation. Attention to safety and accessibility of these areas facilitates mobility for the disabled in the community. Nurses can become involved as advocates for the disabled in establishing a safe, accessible community.

Outside buildings

Community access for people with mobility limitations depends on pedestrian right of way. Right of way should be given attention in loading and unloading zones, rest stops, waiting areas, and parking lots. The international access symbol displayed on public buildings indicates these facilities are accessible for wheelchair users and others with limited mobility. This symbol, displayed in parking lots, indicates areas reserved for persons with disabilities (Figure 21-1). Arrival sites should provide adequate information regarding parking and direction to the accessible entrance.

Designated parking should be as close to the building entrance as possible. The parking space should be at least 12½ feet wide to allow space for loading and unloading a vehicle. This area should have access to an open area or ramp leading to a walkway or route of travel. Curb cuts should be marked to alert visually impaired individuals (Figure 21-2). Ramp length should not exceed 30 feet without a level rest area and should not exceed an 8.33% slope. Walkways should be at least 48 inches wide. The entrance also should display the international symbol of access. Benches situated in areas that require long walks to and from buildings provide rest opportunities (Figure 21-3).

Many public buildings have exterior doors that open outwardly. There must be a level landing of at least 5 square feet connected by a level or ramped approach walkway (Figure 21-4). Entry doorways should be at least 36 inches wide, and doors should be easy to operate. Automatic sliding doors help. Thresholds should not be over ½ inch high, and door kickplates at least 12 inches high should be provided.

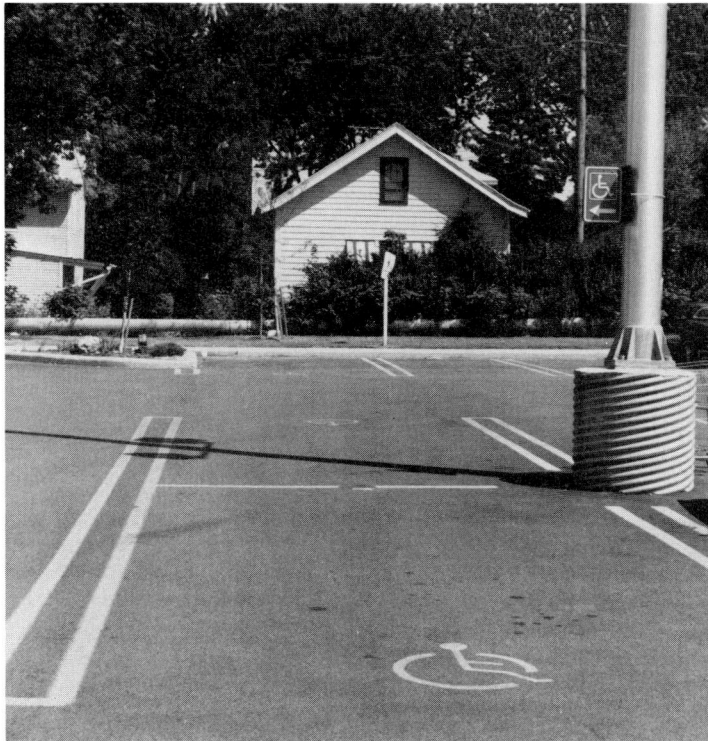

Figure 21-1
International symbol of access.

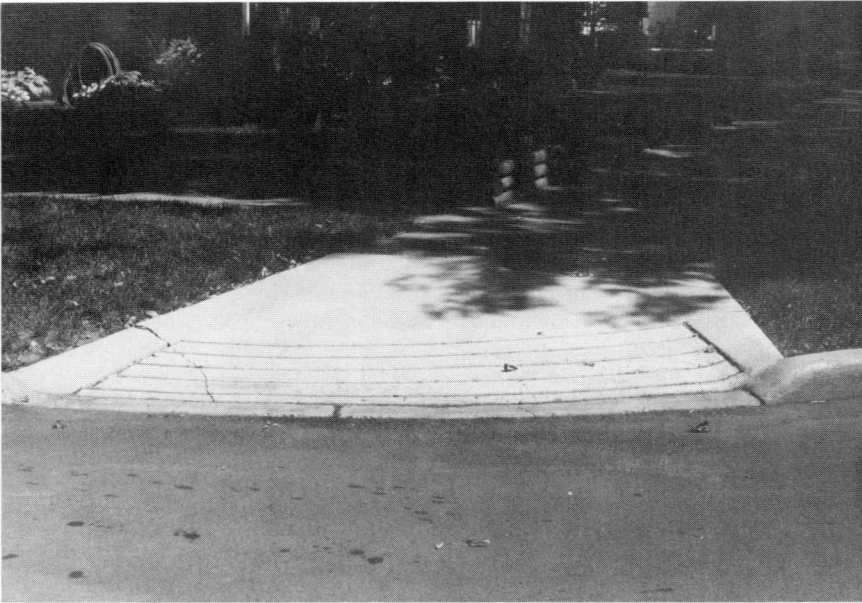

Figure 21-2
Curb cut.

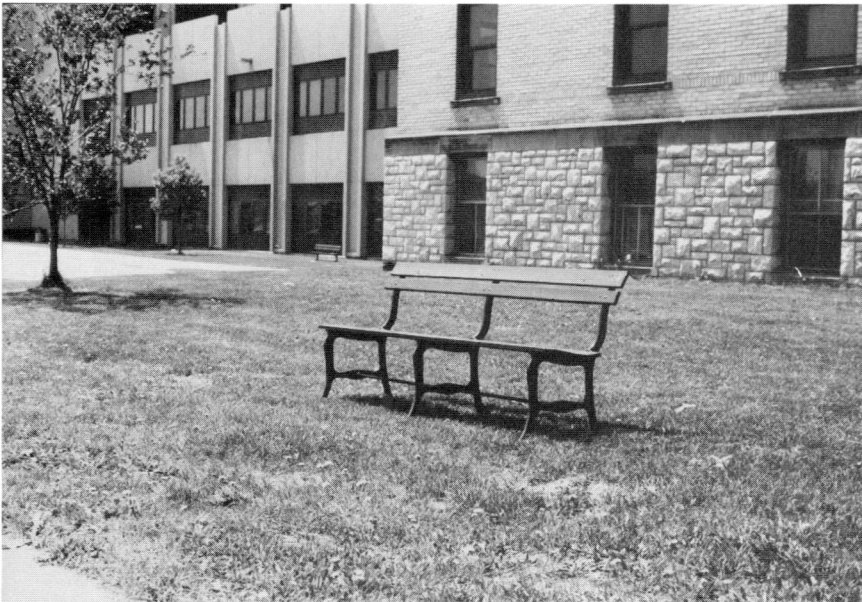

Figure 21-3
Bench provides opportunity for rest on way to health care facility.

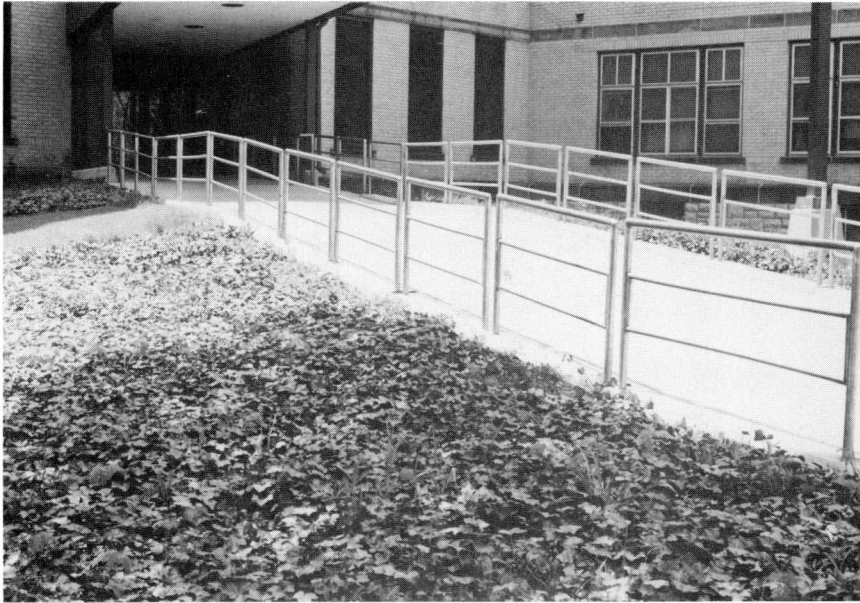

Figure 21-4
Ramp to health care facility.

Inside buildings

Route information from the entrance to areas around the main building should be clearly marked and free of obstacles. Interior doorways should be at least 32 inches wide. Stairways adjacent to the accessible route of travel should not have open risers or overhanging steps. Handrails that are easily grasped should be securely mounted along stairwells (Figure 21-5). Elevator control buttons should be well within reach of a seated person at least 48 inches or less from the floor, and directional signals should be audible and visible. The automatic door opener should be timed to allow the client to step or wheel in and out of the elevator safely and should remain open at least 3 seconds. The cab should be at least 5 feet by 5 feet. A person in a wheelchair facing the rear of the elevator should be able to see the floor numbers by means of a mirror or floor identification at the rear of the elevator. The threshold of the elevator should be flush with the floor.

Public assembly rooms, rest areas, public telephones, and drinking fountains should be accessible with easily manipulated controls and hardware. Levers or controls that operate without precise movements are recommended. The height of the dial on a public telephone and the coin slot should be 48 inches or less from the floor. There should be enough space (30 × 40 inches) to allow a forward or parallel approach to public telephones. Persons in wheelchairs should be able to wheel up to water fountains and use the hand-operated up-front spout and controls.

Public restrooms should have adequate maneuvering space for a wheelchair. Compartment doors should swing out and close automatically with lever-type hardware. Toilet seats should be slightly higher (17 to 19 inches from the floor). Grab bars should be securely installed no more than 18 inches from the middle of the toilet and no more than 34 inches high (Figure 21-6). Toilet tissue dispensers, towel racks, and shelves should be within easy reach. Mirrors should be low enough to use when seated. Wheelchair maneuvering space is needed around and beneath sinks. Hot water pipes should be insulated or otherwise protected to avoid the danger of burns.

Carpeting can be a hindrance unless it has low pile or is unpadded. All carpeting should be glued down or anchored securely.[12] Highly waxed floors should be avoided.

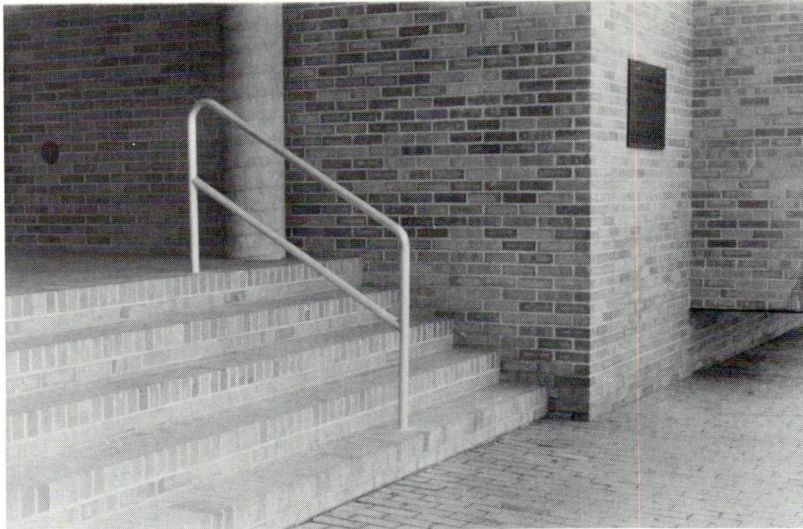

Figure 21-5
Handrails.

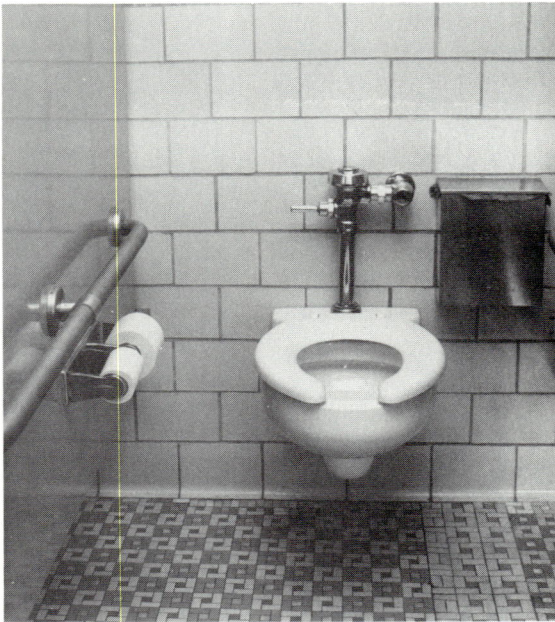

Figure 21-6
Grab bars and high toilet seat in public restroom.

School and employment environments

Although legislation mandates architectural specifications or modifications, buildings still may not be accessible to each individual with a disability. Not all changes can be made to accommodate each disabling condition unless removal of an architectural barrier would make the difference between complete dependence and complete independence.[3]

Employers must be continually sensitized and educated about the capabilities of potential employees with physical limitations. They need to know about systems and devices that permit otherwise limited individuals to function effectively and perform jobs previously believed impossible for them.

If the school or employer is not willing or able to spend additional money needed to make individual modifications or provide specific equipment, other organizations may be a source of this funding. (See Appendix E for listing.)

A team effort, including nursing referral, vocational rehabilitation counseling, direction from occupational and physical therapists, and assistance from social services can assist the employer and employee in discovering accessible school and employment prospects.

Recreational, social, and cultural events

Progress is being made toward participation of the disabled in all life activities. Major breakthroughs in sports and recreational activities are occurring, as evidenced by the ever-increasing number of people with disabilities who are making the most of the world around them. Athletic, recreational, and social events help the disabled improve physical fitness, learn new skills, develop independence, make new friends, relax, and have fun.

With modified equipment and rules, the disabled can participate in a variety of sports and recreational activities. The National Wheelchair Association is the governing body for regional and national competitive meets in track and field events, swimming, table tennis, weight lifting, and archery. A rule and guidebook for sports participation by the disabled is available from this association.

Other organizations promote and coordinate competitive sports such as basketball, bowling, softball, and marathon racing. With adaptive equipment where necessary, proper training, and encouragement, persons with disabilities are now participating in and enjoying most sports, recreational, and social activities.[17] (See Chapter 20 for further discussion.)

Consumerism and public awareness have contributed to the removal of architectural barriers. Access features are now incorporated into the design for parks and buildings where recreational and cultural events are held. The nurse should inform the disabled client about these recreational, social, and cultural opportunities and make referrals to other team members who can assist the client in participating in these events.

Transportation

Transportation is the key element in linking the disabled to shopping, medical, and other support services. Without transportation the world shrinks to one's immediate surroundings.

Private vehicles provide the most independence, but limited financial resources often restrict private transportation for the disabled. Automobiles can be equipped with hand or foot controls to facilitate use of the brake and accelerator. Safety and transfer equipment such as grab bars, retractable running boards, wheelchair loaders, transfer devices, emergency lights, citizen band radios, and automatic garage door openers are some of the options available.

Small vans for personal and group transportation have sliding, wide doors, and ramps for easy access. Motorized wheelchairs, golf carts, and scooters are examples of other vehicles that increase mobility for the disabled.

Vehicles must be adapted to the individual's functional ability. In some instances this may involve costly modifications. The Georgia Institute of Technology is working on development of the Universal Car, which staff members hope can be economically produced.[4]

A need for access to low-cost transportation services exists in the community. Door-to-door small vehicle transportation to serve the disabled is expensive and needs considerable subsidization, but is preferred by many planners as an alternative to incorporating costly changes into existing public transportation. Although some advances have been made, availability and access to public transportation remains a critical problem for the disabled.

Participation in the Political Process

Nurses can act as advocates for the disabled in the community and support legislation and seek appropriations to help make communities more accessible and safer. They also can write letters to congressional representatives supporting proposed legislation and continuation of current legislation that ensures equal rights to community participation for persons who are disabled. In addition, rehabilitation nurses can participate in consumer activist groups and assist them with letter-writing campaigns and transportation to polling places. They can volunteer to work in election campaigns for politicians who support the rights of the disabled. Some nurses are now running for legislative seats where they can cast the vote on bills concerning these issues. The most important contribution that nurses as a group and political force can make in assuring community access and safety is to become more aware of the platforms and voting records of legislators and to vote for those who support the rights of persons who are disabled.

Referrals, Follow-Up, and Maintenance

Many disabled people begin their rehabilitation in a general hospital. They may be transferred to a rehabilitation facility after their condition stabilizes. When the rehabilitation process is successful, the client is discharged back to the community and followed-up by a community nursing agency.

The initial environment in which the client resides has a great deal of influence on the total rehabilitation program. The responsibility for creating this introductory atmosphere is ascribed to the nurse in the general hospital. It is essential for nurses in each rehabilitation agency to understand the total rehabilitation needs of the client and be aware of previous nursing interventions. The better the interagency communication, the better is the continuity of rehabilitation.

Coordinating the client's day, teaching procedures, and reinforcing skills learned in other rehabilitation therapies are some of the responsibilities of the rehabilitation nurse. For the disabled client the unit is "home" after a physically and emotionally fatiguing day. The nurse should provide a relaxed atmosphere and be sensitive to the client's feelings about the day's progress.

After a certain amount of independence has been gained, the client may be given a pass for a weekend visit. Teaching the client and family about equipment, procedures, and medications before the weekend home visit helps the client and family test out ability to manage in the home. A home visit by the rehabilitation team (nurse and therapists) provides the opportunity to evaluate the environment and offer recommendations for improving accessibility and safety.

Family members should be discouraged from making early, expensive alterations in their home until after a home visit is made by the rehabilitation team. Any specific recommendations for changes should be planned and discussed with the client and family because they are the ultimate decision makers. Recommendations geared to adapting what is currently in the home, rather than buying expensive equipment, help avoid undue financial stress.

The community nurse observes and reinforces the efforts initiated during the acute and rehabilitative phases of care. Activities started in these phases of care have no value unless the client is prepared and encouraged to function outside the protected environment. The community nurse must be alert to the entire complex of the client's environment.[1]

Assessment of the client's functional ability in the home environment is continued by the community nurse. The nurse works with the client

and other team members to plan appropriate interventions and accomplish desired outcomes. Periodic evaluation and reassessment of the client's ability to perform activities of daily living are necessary to monitor any changes (either increasing or decreasing levels of independence), and to plan appropriate interventions.

REHABILITATION TEAM INTERVENTIONS

Rehabilitation is a team effort and involves collaboration among team members to assure a safe and accessible environment for the client. A home visit with the physical therapist and occupational therapist present facilitates analysis of the client's functional ability in the home. The team works with the client and family to determine what additional alterations or substitute rehabilitation skills may be needed for the client to accomplish activities of daily living with maximum safety, efficiency, and mobility in the home.

The team analyzes the problems encountered in the home and the community. Recommendations are offered after input is received from the client and family members. Consideration must be given to cost, extent of alterations, and the effect these alterations may have on others living in the home. The final decision concerning home modification is made by the client and family members. Once they make the decision, they should be supported and assisted by rehabilitation team members.

The rehabilitation counselor works with employers and educational institutions in the community to find positions for disabled clients who are returning to work or school. Equipment, transportation, and support needed at work or school are explained to potential employers and teachers and efforts are made to ensure these are available. The social worker and rehabilitation counselor often work together closely to obtain equipment, supplies, and support services in the community.

OUTCOME CRITERIA

Outcome criteria related to safety and accessibility in the home and the community include the following:
1. The client functions at an optimum level in an accessible environment.
   a. The environment is adapted or modified according to the client's abilities.

b. Assistive/adaptive devices and rehabilitation skills are used to encourage maximum independence.

c. The client has mobility in the community and is able to travel to and from work, school, and recreational, social, and cultural activities.

d. The client, family, and community assume responsibility for providing and maintaining an accessible environment.

2. The client functions safely within his or her own environment.

a. The client incorporates safe practices while engaging in activities of daily living in the home and in the community.

b. The family incorporates safe practices while assisting the client in activities of daily living in the home and in the community.

SUMMARY

The relationship between the client and the environment is a major consideration in the rehabilitation process. The client's environment may make the difference between complete dependence or complete independence.

Observation of the client in his or her own environment helps the nurse identify the accessibility of the environment and the client's ability to perform activities of daily living safely. The assessment provides insight into the client's awareness of actual and potential hazards. Rehabilitation nursing interventions focus on working with the client and family to change or adapt restrictive or hazardous barriers in the environment.

TEST QUESTIONS

1. Legislation has facilitated accessibility in the community for disabled individuals. The _____ established the Architectural and Transportation Barrier Compliance Board to monitor discrimination and support affirmative action.
   a. Rehabilitation Act of 1973
   b. Rehabilitation Amendments of 1978
   c. Comprehensive Employment and Training Act of 1978
   d. Urban Mass Transportation Act of 1964

2. Title VII of the 1978 Rehabilitation Amendments was important to the severely disabled because it provided for:

   a. Accessibility in buildings erected with federal funds
   b. Comprehensive services for independent living
   c. Mainstreaming in the schools
   d. Boards responsible for vocational education programs

3. When assessing the home, the nurse should consider _____ and how it (these) will affect the client's ability to move about in the home environment.
   a. Type of dwelling
   b. Design
   c. Floor plan
   d. All of the above

4. When assessing a client's home, the nurse or therapist recommends that:
   a. Doorway width be 42 inches to accommodate a wheelchair.
   b. Ramps should be at least 46 inches wide to accommodate walkers or wheelchairs.
   c. Doorways should be at least 32 inches wide to accommodate wheelchairs.
   d. At least 20 feet should be allowed for transfer and maneuvering of a wheelchair in the garage.

5. During a home assessment the nurse or therapist asks, "Do you own your own home?" What is the best rationale for asking this question?
   a. The answer will help the nurse determine the wealth of the client.
   b. This matter is personal and should not be asked.
   c. The answer will help determine what physical modifications can be made in the home.
   d. The answer will help the nurse decide how attached the client is to his or her home.

6. Another question asked during the home assessment is "Who is responsible for doing the cooking?" The response to this question helps the nurse determine:
   a. If a microwave oven would help the client
   b. To what extent modifications should be made in the kitchen
   c. What new appliances are needed
   d. If the cupboard under the sink must be removed

7. When assessing the home of a client who has difficulty walking, attention should be given to the floors. All of the following statements are true *except:*

a. Clutter should be removed from the right of way.
b. Scatter rugs should be tacked or removed.
c. Floors should be waxed to prevent wear.
d. Deep pile rugs are difficult to walk on and could cause the client to fall.

8. One of the major problems associated with poor vision is the individual's ability to discriminate color. All of the following recommendations of the rehabilitation nurse can be effective in helping the client discriminate color *except:*
   a. Use pastels to avoid glare.
   b. Use red, orange, and yellow.
   c. Use dishes with contrasting rims.
   d. Use light-colored letters on a dark background.
9. Doors in the home can be a problem for a client who is in a wheelchair. All of the following recommendations of the rehabilitation nurse are appropriate interventions *except:*
   a. Replace the door with a sliding door.
   b. Replace the door with a curtain.
   c. Replace the door with a full-length glass door.
   d. Replace the door with a folding door.
10. Nursing interventions that will assist the client in achieving and maintaining access in the home and community are:
    a. Recommendations for home modification
    b. Recommendations for safety procedures in the kitchen
    c. Participation of the nurse in the political process as an advocate for the disabled
    d. All of the above
11. To assure safety in the kitchen, the nurse should recommend that:
    a. Controls be placed on the back of the stove.
    b. Gas stoves should be lit with standard matches.
    c. Frequently used equipment should be stored in upper cupboards.
    d. Controls should be placed on the front of the stove.
12. Rehabilitation nurses can participate in the political process and advocate for the rights of persons who are disabled by:
    a. Supporting legislation that ensures equal rights to community participation
    b. Assisting consumer advocate groups with letter-writing campaigns

c. Volunteering to work in election campaigns of politicians who support the rights of the disabled
d. All of the above

Answers: 1. a, 2. b, 3. d, 4. c, 5. c, 6. b, 7. c, 8. a, 9. c, 10. d, 11. d, 12. d.

LEARNING ACTIVITIES

1. Conduct an assessment of your home and community. Identify potential or actual environmental hazards. Identify barriers to mobility. What modifications would you suggest?
2. Assess the home environment of an adult with a physical disability. Identify actual or potential hazards. Identify barriers to mobility. Plan modifications with the client to make the home environment accessible and safe.
3. Assess the environment of a person with a visual deficit. Identify actual or potential hazards. Plan modifications with the client to make the home environment accessible and safe.
4. Assess the community environment of an adult with a physical disability. Identify actual or potential hazards. Plan modifications with the client to make the client's community environment accessible and safe.

REFERENCES

1. Beland IL and Pasos JY: Clinical nursing: pathophysiological and psychosocial approaches, ed 4, New York, 1981, Macmillan Publishing Co, Inc.
2. Bellack JP and Bamford P: Nursing assessment a multidimensional approach, Monterey, Calif, 1984 Wadsworth, Inc.
3. Burkhauser R and Haveman R: Disability and work—the economics of American policy, Baltimore 1982, Johns Hopkins University Press.
4. Ellis R and Sewell J: Sensible products from a one of a kind technology center, Disabled USA 2:32, 1984.
5. Fenton J: Residential needs of the severely physically handicapped non-retarded children and young adults in New York state, Rehabilitation Monograph No 46, New York University Medical Center, 1972, Institute of Physical Medicine and Rehabilitation.
6. Fogel ML and Columbus D: Survey of disabled persons reveals housing choices, J Rehabil 37:26, March/April 1971.
7. Goldenson R: Disability and rehabilitation handbook, New York, 1978, McGraw-Hill Book Co.

8. Gordon M: Nursing diagnosis: process and application, ed 2, New York, 1987, McGraw-Hill Book Co.

9. Laurie G, editor: Housing and home services for the disabled: guidelines and experiences in independent living, New York, 1977, Harper & Row, Publishers, Inc.

10. Lowman E and Rusk H: Self-help devices, New York University Medical Center, 1965, Institute of Physical Medicine and Rehabilitation.

11. Luckmann J and Sorensen K: Medical-surgical nursing: a psychophysiological approach, ed 3, Philadelphia, 1987, WB Saunders Co.

12. Martin N, Holt NB, and Hicks D, editors: Comprehensive rehabilitation nursing, New York, 1981, McGraw-Hill Book Co.

13. Maslow A: Motivation and personality, New York, 1970, Harper & Row, Publishers, Inc.

14. Mumma CM, editor: Rehabilitation nursing: concepts and practice, a core curriculum, ed 2, Evanston, Ill, 1987, Rehabilitation Nursing Foundation.

15. Murray R and Kijek JC, editors: Current perspectives in rehabilitation nursing, St Louis, 1979, The CV Mosby Co.

16. Murray RB and Zentner JP: Nursing concepts for health promotion, Englewood Cliffs, NJ, 1979, Prentice-Hall, Inc.

17. National Easter Seals Society: The widening world of sports and recreation, Chicago, 1983, The Society.

18. Orem DE: Nursing: concepts of practice, New York, 1980, McGraw-Hill Book Co.

19. Toth LL: The professional nurse's attitude, knowledge and application of the concepts of home modification for the severely disabled adult, master's thesis, Buffalo, NY, 1983, State University of New York.

20. Trieschmann RB: Spinal cord injuries: psychological, social and vocational adjustment, New York, 1980, Pergamon Press, Inc.

ADDITIONAL READINGS

Bachman C and Preston K: Effective rehabilitation: reintegration into the community, Rehabil Nurs 9(1):14, 1984.

Bowe FG: Transportation: a key to independent living, Arch Phys Med Rehabil 60:483, 1979.

Elliott F: Nursing interventions to improve adjustment to aging, Rehabil Nurs 7:2, March/April 1982.

Goldman F: Environmental barriers to sociosexual integration: the insiders' perspective, Rehabil Lit 39:6, June/July 1978.

Hale G, editor: The sourcebook for the disabled, New York, 1979, Paddington Press, Ltd.

Hays A: Caring for the hospitalized elderly, Am J Nurs 82:6, 1982.

Hodgeman K and Warpeka E: Adaptations and techniques for the disabled homemaker, Minneapolis, 1973, Kenny Institute.

May EE, Waggoner NR, and Hotte EB: Independent living for the handicapped and elderly, Boston, 1974, Houghton Mifflin Co.

Moorat D: Accidents to patients, Nurs Times 79:20, May 1983.

O'Brien MT and Pallett PJ: Total care of the stroke patient, Boston, 1978, Little, Brown & Co.

Vash C: Employment services for women with disabilities, Rehabil Lit 43:7, July/Aug 1982.

CHAPTER 22

Coping

Kathy M. Graham

OBJECTIVES

After completing Chapter 22, the reader will be able to:

1. Apply general systems theory when assisting a client and family to cope with the loss of function.

2. Describe the grief responses to loss of function.

3. Explain ways in which loss of function affects the client.

4. Determine ways in which loss of client function affects the family.

5. Assess a client's coping ability.

6. Formulate nursing diagnoses associated with coping ability.

7. Develop goals with the client and family that foster maximum coping abilities.

8. Determine nursing interventions to assist the client in maintaining and restoring coping ability.

9. Identify rehabilitation team interventions to assist the client and family in maintaining and restoring coping abilities.

10. List outcome criteria used to evaluate the effectiveness of the planned intervention to help the client and family maintain and restore coping abilities.

A 13-year-old junior high student practices a newly learned jackknife dive into a neighbor's swimming pond, only to discover the dry weather left only 4 feet of water in the pond. He suffers a fracture of the cervical spine, resulting in quadriplegia.

A 24-year-old newlywed woman drives home from the grocery store, but forgets to fasten her seatbelt and is hit by a drunk driver. Her right femoral artery is severed, resulting in the eventual amputation of her right leg.

A 16-year-old high school student is thrown from a toboggan during a Saturday afternoon winter carnival. She suffers an injury of the thoracic spine, resulting in paraplegia.

During a routine doctor's appointment, young parents are told their two-year-old boy may have cerebral palsy.

Imagine yourself in a typical hospital room and being given one of the diagnoses described above. What is your immediate reaction? Shock? Fear? Anger? Despair? Consider how this injury or disease will change your life-style and future.

More than 50% of the U.S. population suffers from one or more chronic diseases, and approximately 70% of the population will become disabled at some point in their lives.[3] Consequently, health care providers, whether employed in an emergency room, general medical-surgical unit, outpatient clinic, or private practice setting, are caring for and interacting with people who have experienced either abrupt or gradual physical or mental losses, resulting in disability.

Diagnosis of a chronic illness and physical disability is a difficult experience for most individuals. Although grief responses of the terminally ill and bereaved survivors have been studied, research concerning the grief response in the chronically ill and disabled client has been sparse. Most literature reflects the principles of grief and coping that were originally described for terminally ill individuals and their families. Personal accounts, however, indicate that the loss of one's own function may be different from the loss of someone outside of one's self.[49]

Years ago the family had primary responsibility for the care of disabled members. Although some individuals were placed in a custodial institution, often located at a distance from the family, most remained at home. Then, for several decades, our society entered a period in which custodial care for persons with severe impairments was believed the best approach. This practice meant that ties with home and family were often broken and never resumed.[18]

Ryder and Ross[37] contend that a hospital's organizational structure makes care routinized rather than individualized and consequently often unsuitable to the needs of clients and their families. Furthermore, the orientation of the medical profession and hospital personnel toward clients with traumatic injuries and debilitating diseases

has been cure rather than care. To fulfill this expectation, staff members devote their time to helping clients recover. Since chronic illness and disability are characterized most often by a limitation of power over the disease process, those providing care must be driven by commitment to the person rather than the excitement of care.[38]

Integral to the rehabilitation philosophy is the belief in assisting individuals to function with their remaining abilities by using the resources of expert rehabilitation team members. The family is viewed as a major health care resource, and the home environment in most instances is the most appropriate living arrangement. The family is identified as the first line of social support and can serve as a vital link between the client and the larger community.[18] The client can be viewed as part of a family system.

GENERAL SYSTEMS THEORY

A system can be defined as a set of relationships between objects and their properties with bonds that join the system together as a functioning unit.[21] Systems theory is fundamentally a method of viewing systems as a whole composed of related parts that interact together. Every system has an environment that is open or closed to outside influences. Contained in the surrounding environment are sets of objects that affect both the system and the changes that may occur within it.

Putt[35] described several attributes that a true system will possess. All systems must have *structure*, that is, a specific arrangement to component parts. There must be a *process* and *order* to every system. In this manner, a system receives and exchanges energy and information. All systems are arranged into an interlocking hierarchy. Any system can be further divided into subsystems. Although the system is perceived as a whole, a change in one part can affect the total system. A dysfunction in one part would cause an overall system disturbance rather than a single isolated functional loss.

Proper system functioning requires an *exchange of energy*. This exchange may occur at varying rates, with both reversible and irreversible exchanges. Through the intake and output of energy, a system will *change with time*. The change may be either deterioration or maturity toward a higher level of organization. As a system increases in complexity, one part must emerge as the controlling unit. A system's interaction with the environment tends to move it toward more specialization of function.

Every system has some degree of *openness*. Systems are either open or closed to their environment. A closed system has rigid boundaries that prevent interaction with the environmental surroundings, whereas an open system has free exchange of energy between system parts and the environment. An open system may become closed if the exchange of information or energy is temporarily or permanently stopped. Likewise, a closed system may become open if an exchange of energies erupts between the system and its environment.

A system must possess a *feedback mechanism* to provide a means of self-correction. That is, a portion of the system's output is returned as input information to allow the system to adjust to any future output. This feedback mechanism allows the system to maintain some *degree of stability*, or homeostasis.

The Family as a System

Traditionally, health care providers have been trained to focus on the hospitalized person's basic needs, not the emotional needs of visitors and family members.[15,45] Since families play a significant role during the time of illness, their reactions will contribute to the client's response to the initial illness or injury and resultant disability.[25]

The family unit is described as more than a number of people living together; it is a community whose members nurture and teach one another. Hospitalization of one member tends to disrupt the family unit. Consequently, when one member is gone, the family falters and all its members are affected.[45] Because the client is part of a greater unit, total client care infers that the nurse must be effective in supporting the family, as well as the client. Craven and Sharp[9] concur and comment:

> If the nurse expands her concept of the patient from that of an individual in a bed to that of a participating member of a family, then she will expand her role to assist relatives to cope with the patient's illness while simultaneously maintaining the family functions.

Goldberg and Goldberg[17] believe that to understand an individual, we must examine that person's various relationships with other people, particularly those within the family framework. The family is a natural social system with characteristics and attributes all its own. A family is a system that has developed a set of rules, roles, power structures, forms of communication, and styles of problem solving that allow specific tasks to be accomplished effectively.

Putt[35] viewed the family as a group of individuals bonded together by the interests of members. Kandzari and Howard[22] agreed that the family consists of interacting people who are interdependent in sharing goals and meeting each others' needs. Leavitt[26] views the family as an integrated system of interdependent functions, structures, and relationships, a unique and complete entity.

The wholeness of the family unit is reflected in the interdependence and interrelatedness of its members.[31] Although each member has a unique personality, each interacts with others to comprise the larger whole. The welfare of one family member is likely to depend upon the welfare of the other members. It is impossible to assess the needs and strengths of one family member without also assessing how these needs and strengths relate to the total family unit.

Families are rule-oriented systems; members behave in an organized, repetitive pattern of interaction with one another. Unwritten family rules may include division of labor, power, and child-rearing responsibilities.[17] These patterns usually are closely tied to cultural and sex-role beliefs. Family rules often determine patterns of behaviors between members because each person's behavior directly relates to and depends on the behavior of all the other members.

Every family unit has boundaries, or delineations between its own subsystems and the larger outside systems. These boundaries specify who can participate within the system and also to what extent one can interact with members in the system. They also designate the degree to which members will allow input into the system from other systems. Since a family is a living system, it must relate to broader systems of community, country, and universe.[50] Boundaries, therefore, separate the family system and its individual members from the surrounding environment.[31]

Boundaries also help maintain a family's equilibrium and permit the family to gradually adapt to changes and growth. All families develop a set of homeostatic mechanisms that keep the system in balance. This homeostatic mechanism assures proper family functioning, because it regulates the input information according to the family's ability to cope with input from the outside.

It is difficult for families to function efficiently without adequate resources. Family resources come from a variety of areas such as extended family members, knowledge, financial means, and religious affiliations.

All family system characteristics discussed are aimed at one eventual outcome—the optimum functioning of the family unit, that is, the extent to which the family members operate in harmony with one another. In this instance, family communication lines are open and expressed freely, the family members are well-bonded together, and the family reaches decisions and allocates tasks to benefit the whole.[31] When a family no longer interacts between and among its subsystems and the surrounding environment, it becomes dysfunctional. Therefore a healthy family that is functioning optimally, is an open system with members freely exchanging materials and information with each other and with the environment.

GRIEF IN THE DISABLED INDIVIDUAL

Webster defines grief as "the intense emotional suffering caused by a loss or deep sorrow."[48] It is an emotion experienced by every human being and one with which we learn to deal sometime during the life span. Hafen and Frandsen[20] believe experiencing grief is necessary, because without it, healing cannot take place. It is a form of sorting out one's emotions about the loss and eventually continuing on with life.

Charmaz[5] defined grieving as a process that consists of facing the reality of a loss and reorganizing one's life and self-image. The process of grieving usually depends on the nature of the loss. A person may grieve longer and more intensely over a loss that was of greater value and significance than over a loss that held little consequence in one's life.

When individuals experience an illness or injury that affects function, they may experience a profound sense of loss. The obvious inability to use one or more of the extremities coupled with other overt and covert losses such as loss of mobility; impaired communication, bowel and bladder function, and sexual performance; and loss of body image, self-esteem, and independence can result in a feeling of loss of control over one's own life.

There is a predictable end to grief experienced during a terminal illness. Persons who die are not reappearing constantly to reactivate the feelings of loss. According to Werner-Beland, a nurse who suffered a cervical spinal cord injury, the loss of one's own function is ever present. Although feelings of despair may wane with time, events frequently occur that remind the affected person that he or she is "less than perfect."[49]

Any loss or change of sufficient magnitude produces crises that threaten one's psychological equilibrium. A disability presents the affected person with a crisis that calls for an adjustment.[36] Engel[13] showed that psychological and emotional adjustments must be achieved during the grieving process to facilitate eventual acceptance of the loss. Both the client and family must work through the stages of grief.

Stages of Grief

The stages of grief proposed by Engel as necessary to successful grieving include shock and disbelief, developing awareness, restitution, and finally resolution. Although grieving is individualized, almost everyone who grieves exhibits signs of denial, a period of reality awareness, and a gradual culmination of the mourning process. A person's grief responses to illness and disability occur within the context of the person's total environment. If illness, disability, or any threat to wellness is viewed as a dangerous situation, the client's situation and response is easier to understand. Therefore nurses must consider where the person is coming from in terms of natural, cultural, and experiential clues to danger.[49]

Shock and disbelief

The first stage of grief, shock and disbelief, occurs upon learning of the disability. It is difficult for any individual to accept or comprehend this fact. This stage is characterized by a period of stunned numbness in which the person does not emotionally acknowledge the reality. The affected person may try desperately to keep busy with the daily hospital routines and with visitors in an effort to avoid the full emotional impact of the loss. Clients may express their initial feelings as "being a spectator in a bad dream" and tell family members and nurses not to worry because "the doctors have made a mistake." This phase may last a few minutes, hours, or even days.

Awareness

The length of denial and the course that grief takes will depend on each person's coping style, that is, as an individual tries to cope by avoiding stressful events, denial may be prolonged.[4] As the reality of the situation begins to penetrate a person's consciousness and the person feels safe and supported enough to let go of denial, awareness develops. The person realizes the actual pain and anguish of the loss and experiences feelings of emptiness, frustration, anger, and loneliness. Physical symptoms of grief may be exhibited during this time.

Lindemann's early observations[28] of patients during normal grief reactions identified the following symptomatic syndrome: tightness in the throat, choking and shortness of breath, sighing, an empty feeling in the abdomen, lack of muscle power, and tension of mental pain. The duration of this grief reaction seemed to depend upon the success with which a person accomplished the work of mourning identified as separating oneself from the deceased, readjusting to the environment in which the deceased is missing, and forming new relationships.

Engel[13] states that the outward expression of grief, such as crying, is important in the work of mourning. The disabled person who cries receives support and help from peers. Environmental or cultural demands must not cause involuntary suppression of crying, causing the individual to cry inwardly or wait until he or she is unobserved before showing tears.

Restitution

Restitution is the third stage in the work of grieving. During this stage, friends and relatives gather together to mutually share the loss. When a person dies, traditional religious practices of the wake, the funeral, expression of condolences by friends, flowers, mass cards, and contributions help the bereaved through the period with supportive interpersonal interactions.[51] When a person suddenly becomes ill or disabled, friends and relatives gather around initially to lend support. It is during this period that the reality of the disability becomes apparent. Disabled persons are faced with their own helplessness and need to feel control of their own life or death. Once this struggle to control events is resolved, persons do not feel as helpless or despairing.[49]

Resolution

Resolution occurs as disabled persons adjust to their individual loss. They attempt to deal with the empty void and feeling of lost self-wholeness. Something happens during grief resolution that allows disabled individuals to find pleasure in small accomplishments.[49] During this process, disabled individuals begin to respond to rehabilitation therapies. As Werner-Beland describes, "if and when the disabled person can allow himself to look to new experiences, each of these experiences is like an adventure. . . . The person who continues to downgrade every achievement and refuses to let the old self die tends to remain unrehabilitated."[49] After resolution of one's grief, the individual and family feel free to once again plan for the future, explore alternative life-styles, and redirect their desires and goals.[33] Werner-Beland noted that in her experience, the sense of helplessness was worse than the lack of physical sensation in her legs. She described helplessness as the "ultimate in psychic pain" and described herself as being on an uneven keel, struggling with her helplessness for the right of survival. If she won, it equaled elation; if helplessness won, it equaled emotional despair.[49]

Nurses should be attuned to the responses of the client and family and explore the client's values and attitudes to appropriately prepare the client for reintegration within the family and adaptation to altered or new social roles.[14] Also, the disabled person needs help in dealing with the attitudes and reactions of family members and friends. Although rejection or overprotection are quite common, often family and friends wonder why this disability happened to their loved one and sometimes feel guilty about contributing to the occurrence of the disability by not paying attention to some detail. At other times, the disabled person may have to handle comments or facilitate open communication about themselves so that they can teach others to live with them.

Anticipatory Grief

Lindemann's early investigation[28] into the grieving process revealed a syndrome termed *antici-*

patory grief, in which the person involved in a significant loss begins the grieving process before the actual loss occurs. Anticipatory grief is a form of social, psychological, and emotional preparation for the loss when the individual imagines himself or herself at a lower functional level.

Unlike acute illness or trauma, chronic illness and disability require an adjustment period between first diagnosis and eventual loss of function. For example, in degenerative diseases such as arthritis, multiple sclerosis, and amyotrophic lateral sclerosis, the client and family have the chance to begin working through the process of grief. During this time, family members and the individual affected may express feelings of depression and a heightened concern. The process of going through anticipatory grieving may even help clients and their families approach the loss more constructively. A person's resources and strengths may surface and allow them to remain in control of the situation.[43]

Time Period for Accomplishing Grief Work

As the person accomplishes grief work, preoccupation with the loss of function may progressively lessen, allowing the disabled individual to reinvest feelings in other relationships such as family, work, and school. After grieving present and past losses, the person may return to living by reestablishing relationships and assimilating a changed identity and self-image. Chronic illness and disability, however, are constant reminders of the frailty of life, which often can create a state of grieving lasting much longer than that experienced with terminal illness.[27]

EFFECTS OF DISABILITY ON THE INDIVIDUAL

Chronic illness and disability imply an altered health state that cannot be cured by a simple surgical procedure or a short course of medical therapy. The individual usually experiences impaired functioning in more than one body system and the illness-related demands may never be completely resolved.[32]

The grieving process may become a cycle of hopelessness, helplessness, and dependency in which one realizes over and over various limitations in life.[33] Chronic grief may be pictured as waves of repeated grief that "build on previous

grief like bricks placed by the mason creating a wall."[39] These periods of increased grief are associated with exacerbations of the physical condition and require a person to face new limitations or meet new indignities. Every new episode means a renewed struggle through the various stages of grief.[39]

Servoss[39] contends that persistent grief may result in depressive illness or pathological grief. Depressive illness exists when the client exhibits a constant state of sadness or loses enthusiasm for all usual activities. The person appears worried or anxious and gradually becomes apathetic, with occasional outbursts of irritability and hostility. Alterations in appetite and sleep patterns also are usual during this time.

In contrast to depressive illness, pathological grief involves a state of chronic and false hope in which the client continually attempts to regain that which has been lost. The client is unable to become intellectually and emotionally detached from the loss. This prevents one from reinvesting in the possibilities that remain. Denial becomes this person's means of coping. A client suffering from pathological grief may forget to take prescribed medications and to wear braces to clinic appointments or delay the installation of adaptive equipment in the home.

Dell Orto[11] made several pertinent observations about a person coping with the enormity of illness and disability:

- No one is completely prepared for illness or disability.
- Illness brings out the best and worst in people.
- Illness changes a family and challenges its resources.
- Disability can deplete resources, as well as create them.
- Often the only support a patient has is the family.
- All people do not have family they can depend on.
- Not all families are capable of responding to the illness and disability of a family member.
- Coping with a chronic disability is an ongoing developmental process.
- Existing health care resources can help, as well as hinder adjustment to a disability.

Many of the emotional, social, and economic implications of chronic illness have a devastating effect on the individual's life-style and perception of life's goals. Remember the case histories given at the beginning of the chapter. Consider how the 13-year-old with quadriplegia might view himself as financially and socially unacceptable because he doesn't believe he will be able to work, drive a car, rent an apartment, or even date and court a marriage partner. Or the 24-year-old wife, left with only one lower extremity. Will her husband continue to find her physically attractive? Will he be patient with the many doctor visits and needs for expensive prosthetic equipment? Will her potential children understand why she is unable to run as fast as them or teach them to ski?

An individual's emotional state, as well as attitude toward the loss of health and well-being tends to vary.[33] Pereira describes health as a state of personal well-being and integration of life encompassing the physical, social, emotional, and spiritual well-being of the individual, family, and society. For her, being healthy is a matter of being totally comfortable with whatever circumstances in which one finds oneself. Therefore she believes a state of being chronically ill can be a healthful event if the individual can fully comprehend that, in chronic illness, there is some control over life and future activities.

Strain[42] identified several psychological reactions that a person may experience after the diagnosis of a chronic illness:

1. Loss of control over one's body that threatens self-esteem and sense of body wholeness
2. Fear that illness and dependence on others will cause significant others to withdraw love and general approval of the person
3. Loss of independence and loss of control over body functions
4. Anxiety because of separation from loved ones and familiar environment due to hospitalization
5. Fear of the loss of or injury to body parts
6. Guilt and fear of retaliation from family for having incurred the health problem in the first place
7. Fear of pain
8. Fear of strangers providing intimate care

Pertinent to all these reactions is the underlying fear of powerlessness and lack of control over one's fate.

For the person with a spinal cord injury, several factors have been considered when looking at the psychological reactions to paralysis. These include place of the person in the life cycle when the paralysis occurs, the nature of the onset, the role of guilt, the personal meaning associated with the paralyzed part, the antecedent personality structure, and the role of significant associated defects such as skin breakdown and infection.[41]

Developmental disabilities originate before the age of 18 and usually continue indefinitely. Persons with developmental disabilities have established relationships with others while they were disabled. Usually they have not engaged in interpersonal relationships except as a person with a disability. Since "normal" function is not the basis for comparison with others, their self-image often remains intact. These individuals do not have to grieve for what was first there and then lost. People with developmental disabilities, however, do battle with envy of what others have and can do and grieve for what could have been for them.

When a disability occurs further along in the life cycle, it takes on a different significance for the disabled individual. Adolescence is a period of normal uncertainty concerning a person's life-style, independence, career choice, and sexual development. Paralysis superimposes another element of uncertainty because it disrupts peer group membership and affects acceptance by peers, viewed as so vital during this period. Chronic disability also forces the adolescent to prematurely face issues of loss and deterioration normally associated with the elderly.

Middlescense is a period of gradual physical decline exhibited by beginning hair loss, deterioration of strength, and death of close friends and family. This is a time when individuals are open to taking responsibility for wellness.[6] Persons begin to see that they are alone and mortal. They begin to seek internal validation. It is also a time when persons move out of roles defined by others and begin to find their own self-fulfillment.[40] Disability occurring at this stage may amplify a person's preexisting fears about anticipated decline and discourage attempts to achieve high-level wellness.

The time or nature of disability onset is another factor affecting psychological adjustment. Clients often feel remorse if their own actions, such as reckless diving or driving, played a role in causing their dysfunction. The self-recrimination that clients experience can be lifelong, intensifying at the time of the anniversary of the event. Clients may exhibit self-recrimination tendencies by saying "If only I hadn't. . . . " "Why was I so stupid?" Individuals with cerebral palsy or stroke may be angry at "fate" and become bitter against God for their condition.

The significance of the paralyzed body part to the individual also constitutes a powerful determinant of the emotional reactions toward the disability. Spinal cord injuries at the lumbar sacral level affect sexual performance, bowel control, and bladder control. Loss of these functions is associated not only with inconvenience, but also with humiliation, because in our society, children learn at an early age that bowel and bladder control are important for social acceptance. Later in life, loss of voluntary control over these functions reactivates the feelings of shame associated with poor sphincter control as a young child. Impairment of sexual function is associated with loss of male or female identity.

Paralysis of the lower extremities forces a person to depend on a wheelchair for mobility and could create a sense of decreased self-esteem because of the belittling experience of always looking up at other people. Paralysis of upper extremities compromises the individual's ability to perform self-care. Feelings of helplessness and humiliation are generated when one is unable to feed, wash, dress, and groom oneself. The use of the hands is perceived as essential for the demonstration of love and affection. Loss of this ability may render a person psychologically unable to express or receive love and tenderness.

Depression may result from the loss of self-esteem caused by the paralysis, since self-esteem rests on the foundation of feeling strong, loved, and able to return love. Disabled persons must be able to adjust to and make the best use of a body that does not live up to former standards. If they cannot give up the quest for functions no longer possible, constant frustration and depression may result.[41]

Pereira[33] maintains that hope is the key element in achieving gratifying levels of personal fulfillment and self-worth while sustaining optimum levels of physiological, emotional, and psychological functioning. It is important to the emotional survival of the disabled person to keep sight of the essence of inner being harbored within the body. The acquisition of a new self-image, new skills, different ways of performing former skills, and engaging in self-satisfying work and leisure activities are all part of grief resolution for both the newly disabled and the significant others.[49]

EFFECTS OF DISABILITY ON THE FAMILY

Those people most closely associated with the disabled person join in the client's sense of mourning because of the significant impact the loss also has for them. Often disabled clients are forced to not only handle their own burden of grief, but also to handle the brunt of others' grief on their behalf.[49] Not all members of a family work through the stages of grief at the same rate.[23] One griever may be in a state of shock, whereas another may be depressed. As each person goes through an active mental change, the family system as a whole proceeds through intensive change.

Serious and prolonged illness is a common source of stress, posing major problems of adjustment for both the client and family.[23] Severe injury, the diagnosis of chronic illness, and resultant disabilities also can mean catastrophe for the family, as well as the individual family members. It often means living with uncertainty, accompanied by depletion of a family's monetary and psychological resources. The actual illness is probably only one of the many stresses placed on a family.[9] Interpersonal problems occur between family members as important lines of communication break down. Debts begin to rise as the family faces unemployment and often astronomical medical bills. Expenses of medical and rehabilitation care in conjunction with home remodeling for adaptive modifications and purchases of expensive equipment can be a source of economic stress for any family.[46]

All family members are subjected to social and psychological stress and may find themselves undergoing an adjustment process as they respond to changing roles and functions within the family unit.[3] Problems associated with child care and discipline come about as changes in living routines need to be made. Introduction of a disabled family member into an already structured household causes difficulty when sleeping and eating arrangements are upset. Problems associated with the lack of a consistent authority figure arise when older siblings are expected to care for younger brothers and sisters.

The social stigma and economic stress placed on the family often lead to decreased social mobility.[3] An otherwise mobile family might find itself permanently dwelling in one place rather than change areas and loose contact with medical and rehabilitation care providers and social support systems. Likewise, the main financial provider for the family may decline job advancements and opportunities if moves to another location are required. The adult family members may decline social invitations from friends and neighbors rather than deal with architectural barriers and embarrassing questions inflicted on their children.

Family responses to chronic illness and physical disability can be positive and supportive or negative and destructive. A poorly organized family is vulnerable to stress. Their inability to be flexible in reorganization of role sharing in an emergency tends to create problems within the family structure.[44] These families have difficulty in making long-term commitments to the client. Their responses and interactions can lead to overprotection, neglect, avoidance of future planning, denial of the diagnosis, and excessive and inappropriate demands on the client and the nursing staff. Foxall, Ekberg, and Griffith[15] found that wives of persons with chronic illness were more often dissatisfied with their present lives than husbands of spouses with chronic illness and more often wanted to leave home. Husbands more often than wives of individuals with chronic illness have difficulty sleeping and fatigue upon awakening.

Brooks[3] identified three types of family behaviors that sometimes emerge within family units of disabled clients. The *rejecting family* makes no place for the disabled person. The members are able to continue previous routines and activities without regard to the person's needs. This type of family seems to cope and hold the remaining members together by excluding and often ostracizing the incapacitated person. Sometimes divorce or institutional placements are the outcomes for the disabled person.

The second type of family response is the *sacrificing family* in which the individual becomes the center of all family routines. The family members overemphasize the disabled person's need for support. In doing so, they become overprotective, anxious, and foster dependent behaviors that may prevent total rehabilitation.[44] These actions can be seen in parents who are unable to relinquish the role of provider and counselor for the handicapped adolescent or young adult. They

may superimpose their fears and low expectations of performance and long-range capabilities on the disabled family member. Often families may force their opinions without regard for the client's interests or personal plans, resulting in client regression, depression, feelings of helplessness, and anxiety.[44] This type of sheltering by family members culminates in gradual decline in ability and loss of any rehabilitative gains.

The final type of family normalizes the experiences of the disabled person without sacrificing the needs of other family members. Traditional family roles are modified to keep the disabled individual in the family. Brooks[3] notes that flexibility and good communication skills are necessary to overcome the many physical, psychological, and social barriers asociated with disability. The estimated crucial time for the client and family members to form healthy adjustment behaviors toward the disability is during the first 3 or 4 weeks after the diagnosis.[44]

Rehabilitators believe in the value of family participation in the rehabilitation process and that family participation results in better ability to cope with disability. However, despite these beliefs and despite the philosophical stance in rehabilitation literature that the family be afforded every opportunity to participate in the rehabilitation process, Watson[47] found that 198 health professionals (72% of the sample consisted of nurses, occupational therapists, and physical therapists) from three rehabilitation hospitals believed in a directive model in which the family defers to the expectations of the rehabilitation team members.

NURSING ASSESSMENT

Illness and disability are subjective experiences, and the emotional impact of disability often varies from person to person. Different people also are able to cope better with illness than others The element of individuality is often the key to unlocking the gateway to a person's emotiona survival.[11] Therefore any effective nursing intervention begins with a compilation of baseline data that provides a framework from which appropriate nursing diagnoses are derived. The assessment is initiated during the first contact between a professional nurse and the client and is continued throughout the rehabilitation process. Subjective and objective data are obtained by asking the following questions:

Predisability life-style

1. What is your current occupation?
2. What was your occupation before the illness or injury?
3. What do you like to do in your spare time?
4. Do you spend most of your time inside or outside?
5. Do you live in a private home, apartment, duplex? Do you rent or own?

Past experience with disability

6. Do you know any other people who have a physical disability?
7. Do you know any other people who have a mental disability?
8. How did you describe disabled people before your illness/injury?

Coping styles

9. How are emotions handled in your family?
10. Have you had any losses in your life? If so, were you able to express your feelings at that time?
11. How do you handle stress in your life?
12. Has this way of handling stress had to change in any way since your illness/injury?
13. How would you describe your usual emotional state since your illness/injury?

Current knowledge of illness/injury

14. What have your doctors told you about your condition?
15. Are you satisfied with the amount of information you have received?
16. What else would you like to know?
17. What do you expect from this hospitalization?
18. What specific areas of expected improvement are most important to you?
19. How long do you expect to stay in the hospital?

Current stressors

20. What is your role (for example, breadwinner, homemaker, decision maker), within your family?
21. How many members are there in your family?
22. What are your major concerns outside the hospital (for example, spouse, children, money, job, housing)?
23. What emotional or physical supports do you expect from your family?

Available resources

24. What is your family's approximate yearly income?
25. Do you have any other source of income?
26. Are you a practicing member of any religious group?
27. What is your level of education?
28. Whom do you consider your closest friends? Do they live locally?
29. What people, animals, or things would you describe as helpful to you in your life at the present time?

Nurse interviewer's description of client's non-verbal behavior during the interview:

_____

_____

_____

_____

Subjective Data

Subjective assessment data pertinent to the psychological welfare of a client includes information related to eight areas: (1) life-style before the illness or injury, (2) antecedent personality, (3) experience with a disability, (4) usual style of coping, (5) current knowledge about the physical condition, (6) presence or absence of outside stressors, (7) type and amount of available resources, and (8) extent to which the disability has created disruptions in the client's and family's life.[4]

A person's predisability life-style must be taken into consideration or it becomes impossible for the nurse to understand where the disabled person's feelings come from and why he or she acts in a certain manner.[48] For example, the forest ranger accustomed to leading an active, outdoor existence may have a difficult time adjusting to a more confining, sedentary life-style after disablement. This individual might be expected to exhibit a lot of "acting out" and anger in a hospital environment. A young single girl whose life-style involved many social engagements, particularly in large mixed groups, may feel terribly isolated and depressed when relationships continue around her but gradually involve her less and less.

Personality patterns

Stewart and Rossier[41] noted that it is necessary to determine the client's antecedent personality structure when assessing disabled individuals. They suggested that awareness of the particular personality pattern could serve as a general guide to effective staff interaction. They identified several personality patterns.

Dependent, overdemanding clients usually make urgent requests for both physical and emotional attention from the nursing staff. When faced with a loss of function, these individuals become overwhelmed with a deep fear of abandonment and helplessness. They need frequent overt, verbal reassurances about their concerns and available support from the staff, especially after discharge.

Orderly controlled clients rely on the accumulation of knowledge and information to decrease anxiety after a disability. A number of disabilities create a frightening sense of lost control. Detailed descriptions of the condition and explanations of procedures seem to help these individuals.

Dramatic, emotional clients are perceived as being warm and expressive by staff and therefore well liked by all. For these individuals disability represents a personal weakness that tends to undermine interactions with and attractions to others. These clients need daily contact and verbal reassurance from health care professionals.

Conversely, *aloof* clients seem to require few emotional or physical contacts. Their interactions with others are often kept to a minimum in an attempt to protect themselves against painful reminders and disappointments. Hospitalization disrupts the life-style these clients have established, because it means forced close contacts with many people. For them, these interactions can be anxiety-producing experiences. They should be given privacy to promote adjustment to the disability.

Past experiences with disability

Another factor to include in a person's psychological assessment is the past experience one has had with other persons with disabilities. Someone with past exposure to a disabled person associated with a positive acceptance and outcome may be able to use this role model to help assimilate a new body image without serious effects on self-esteem. Another person may relate a disability to an acquaintance who had frequent problems with bowel and bladder control or a father who voiced disgust over any individual unable to be a "productive" member of society. The latter individual may certainly be expected to have more emotional hurdles to surpass before feeling "whole" again.

Coping style

One's coping style does not usually change with different types of stressors. A person develops a style of coping at an early age, along with development of a basic personality. There are several ways of coping with disabilities[45]:

1. Denial or minimization of the seriousness of the illness or injury
2. Isolation or disassociation of one's emotion from the distressing situation
3. Seeking verbal reassurance and emotional support
4. Requesting pertinent information about the physical condition in an attempt to restore one's sense of control
5. Active participation in specific illness-related procedures
6. Formulation of a personal philosophy or pattern of meaning related to the experience

Rehabilitation team members must be aware of individual coping styles in order to determine approaches consistent with each person's frame of reference. Persons who have handled stress alone for most of their lives may be reluctant to seek out or accept verbal help and support from a health care professional or family member. Actively respecting the need for privacy and providing support as requested is a way to approach this individual.

A study of 56 chronically ill adults sought to explain how disabled people cope. The most frequently used method of coping was determined to be an active searching for information about the physical condition and planned medical and nursing intervention. The second strategy used was to enhance one's spiritual life, and the third was to develop a method of self-distraction, such as watching television, doing needlecraft, or enlarging one's mental capacity by problem solving or meditating.[30] A nursing care plan that takes into account a person's coping style has a greater chance of success in assisting a person to achieve goals.

External stressors

The addition of one or more external stressors may place extra pressure on the individual during the course of rehabilitation. These stressors must be addressed and incorporated into an interdisciplinary rehabilitation plan if the client is going to adapt to the disability. Family expectations may be significantly higher for the client than he or she can be expected to achieve during the acute phase of illness or injury. The burden to perform beyond one's capabilities may only serve to remind the client of limitations rather than achievements. If this situation occurs regularly, it may result in a state of depression that is difficult to dissipate. Distractions from the rehabilitation process also may occur if the client is worried about financial problems or family responsibilities at home.

Available resources

A resource is viewed as something that fulfills a need, a "bank" that can be drawn upon in time of trouble or stress. For the disabled person, a resource is often multi-faceted and unique to the individual. It may be either concrete or obscure. Concrete resources such as monetary wealth, a person's educational background, social status, number of family members, and community agencies dealing specifically with the disabled usually can be identified. Examples of more obscure resources are a person's sense of humor, religious affiliation, chronological age, personal philosophy of life, value system, and the type of psychological and emotional support offered by family and friends. A critical element in learning to cope with disability is learning to use resources efficiently and effectively.[11] Some of the resources available to the family may be community support, including self-help clubs, cooperative attendant service for the disabled, and day care services for the disabled.[12]

Objective Data

Objective data pertinent to a person's ability to cope relates to direct observations made by rehabilitation team members. How do the client and family appear during the admission interview? Does the client have direct eye contact

during the discussion or look down or around the room a lot? Do the client and family members look well rested and neatly groomed? Or is there evidence of sleep deprivation and lack of interest in personal appearance? How do the family members relate to each other? Do they answer questions abruptly? Do they interrupt or contradict one another frequently? Does one family member answer most of the questions directed specifically to the client? Do they express feelings of anger, fear, shame, or depression? Are there signs of "hope" and determination in their responses? These observations are vital clues in determining how the client and family are or are not coping with the new situation.

Characteristic client and family behaviors that alert the rehabilitation nurse to difficulties in coping with the disability include the following:

1. Inability to concentrate
2. Verbalization of the inability to cope
3. Difficulty in meeting basic needs
4. Difficulty in making decisions
5. Difficulty in asking for assistance of others
6. Dependency on drugs or alcohol to solve problems
7. Crying frequently
8. Chronic fatigue
9. Withdrawal
10. Poor attention to personal appearance
11. Decreased appetite
12. Irritability or moodiness
13. Change in sleep pattern or eating habits
14. Denial of the loss
15. Reliving past experiences
16. Verbalization of discontent with physical or psychological self
17. Refusal to take care of or look at the altered body part
18. Verbalized fear of reaction or rejection from others
19. Decreased social interaction

NURSING DIAGNOSES

Accepted nursing diagnoses from the North American Nursing Diagnosis Association associated with coping and adaptation include the following:[19]

1. *Ineffective individual coping:* The lack of ability to psychologically deal with or adapt to a stressful event that leads to temporary or permanent changes in a client's behavior. Individuals may exhibit disorganization in thought processes

and productivity. They may refuse to actively participate in the rehabilitation plan by making negative remarks about the rehabilitation team's expectations or passively declining participation by avoiding staff interaction or scheduled appointments. Often this client will stay in bed, complaining of feeling too tired or too sick to do what is asked. Sometimes ineffective coping is identified when the individual needs frequent reinforcement of original teaching related to self-care, such as repeated instructions regarding self-catheterization, bowel and bladder elimination, putting on and caring for a prosthesis, or transfer techniques. The client who has difficulty coping may be trying to tell the nurse, "I can't deal with this situation; I still need your help and concern because I am afraid." Planning of nursing care is aimed at designing interventions that will arrest the ineffective coping pattern early enough so that the behaviors exhibited do not become permanent. Interventions should be directed at providing necessary emotional support to facilitate the client's adaptation to the disability and restoring the client to an optimum level of independence in decision making and self-care.

2. *Ineffective family coping:* The inability of the family to psychologically deal with or adapt to a stressful event. This event may lead to a breakdown in family organization, communication, relationships, and overall commitment to the disabled person. The family members may be unable to or do not desire to fully assume responsibilities once held by the client. Planning is directed at opening up avenues of communication between the individual family members and then between the client and family. Special attention should be given to the client's and family's adaptation to the community and to social interactions. Identifying and establishing a new or revised role within the family system that is mutually acceptable to the client and individual family members should be part of the planning.

3. *Dysfunctional grieving:* Feelings of sorrow stemming from the loss of a body part, function, or control over one's personal space and activity that remain at an intense level for an extended period of time and result in the failure or inability of the person to move through the stages of grief. This individual remains fixed at an early stage in the grief process, such as shock or denial, and is unable to completely resolve or work through the entire mourning process. Nursing goals and interventions are geared toward accepting the in-

dividual with a nonjudgmental attitude and allowing the person to express emotions and fears. Often various other rehabilitation team members, such as the psychologist or psychiatric clinical nurse specialist, must be incorporated into the plan for rehabilitation.

4. *Personal identity disturbance, self-esteem disturbance:* A lowered sense of personal worth and dignity originating either internally from the client or externally from the mirrored imagery of other's negative attitudes that are incorporated into the client's self-perception. Plans are directed at restoring the client's self-respect and self-esteem by encouraging verbalization of feelings, showing unconditional acceptance of the client, and providing a source of emotional support.

GOALS

The following are realistic goals mutually established with the client and family:
1. To maintain or restore self-esteem
2. To maintain or restore ability to perform activities of daily living
3. To maintain or restore role functions within the family network
4. To obtain emotional support during adjustment to the disability
5. To express grief
6. To openly communicate within the family network
7. To accomplish social adjustment goals
8. To use the expertise of rehabilitation team members as necessary

REHABILITATION NURSING INTERVENTIONS

Although grief is considered a normal reaction in people who have a severe change in their physical or mental status, this response is often overlooked by nurses and other health care professionals when caring for the disabled client. Often health care providers feel threatened by anyone who must adapt to other than a "normal" existence.[50]

Health care providers must understand that people have a *right* and a *need* to express their losses in different modes. It then becomes the nurse's responsibility to ensure that normal grief is not misinterpreted as a sign of weakness or dysfunction.[11] Health care professionals need to realize it is often their limitations and not those of the client that produce problems. The rehabilitation nurse should keep in mind that the newly disabled client is often a novice at dealing with the health care system. Aside from handling the physical assault to one's own body, the client is expected to adjust to various rehabilitation team members, other disabled clients, personal friends and relatives, and the general public after discharge. Since the nurse is often the first person a client deals with after a disability, the significance of the daily verbal and nonverbal communication between nurse and client must not be underestimated.[32]

General Considerations

While helping a client work through the stages of grief, the nurse would be wise to design interventions according to the level of expressed grief.[32] For example, during the stage of shock and disbelief, it would not be constructive to foster a client's independence, because this goal is not realistic during this stage. Emphasizing the nurse's dependability and consistency in executing basic nursing care procedures can help establish a sense of trust between the client and nurse. When the nurse carries out activities around the client's daily living and administers medications in a timely fashion and expert manner, the client begins to believe in the professional's capability.

A word of caution is advised when working with clients in a state of depression. It has been documented that nursing staff members caring for clients with spinal cord injuries had two typical reactions to depression.[44] Some of the staff members tended to deemphasize the client's sense of loss and expected the person to rapidly face and accept the disability. These staff nurses showed little tolerance for the client's expression of sadness, self-pity, or overall lack of enthusiasm. They expected the client to remain cheerful and grateful for any nursing interventions. This is of concern, because if clients pretend acceptance to win nursing approval, they are robbed of the chance to work through the feelings of anger and depression before leaving the rehabilitation setting. A total reversal in approach also was seen. Other nurses tended to rate the person with a spinal cord injury as being more depressed than they actually rated themselves. This view may cause nursing staff members to become overprotective and foster client dependence.

During the expression of anger, when the client acts out in an attempt to regain control, the nurse assists the client in understanding these symptoms and encouraging their expression in a constructive manner. To accomplish this, the nurse must be available to help the client identify and appreciate these feelings as normal and acceptable. Allowing the client to express feelings of anger within certain constraints also helps to establish trust. By accepting the behavior, the nurse demonstrates acceptance of the individual. Families also need guidance at this time to avoid personalizing any expressions of anger exhibited by the client. During this period, the client needs to experience some level of accomplishment. One way of achieving this is by setting short-term, obtainable goals. The nurse can foster higher levels of independence by encouraging the client to become involved in decision making and doing things his or her way rather than the professional's way.

Maintaining Hope

Hope is a powerful resource; it is anticipation of achievement or success. It also is feeling what is wanted will happen. Hope means becoming involved in a process. It implies that the individual refuses to give up or become a useless person in the face of diminishing health or disability.[49] Optimism, on the other hand, conveys a belief that good ultimately prevails over evil; it is a tendency of the person to take the most cheerful view.[48] Optimism denies the reality of the situation and does not permit real engagement of the nurse, client, and family with the true nature of the problem.[49]

Miller and Janosik[31] describe three levels of hope. The first is a hope for only superficial wishes in which there is little energy expended by the person. There also is distress noted when desires are not obtained. The second level of hope involves relationships, self-improvement, and self-accomplishment. The person's thoughts are goal directed and occupy considerable time and energy; if unobtained, they lead to feelings of anxiety. The highest level of hope involves seeking relief from constant suffering, personal ordeal, or entrapment. The person's energy is totally submersed in obtaining relief. Deep despair and a sense of "giving up" characterize the individual who loses the ability to hope.

Nurses must inspire hope, not the hope for cure, but the hope "to be": the hope to be alive, the hope to be of value, the hope to be productive, and the hope to be loved.[30] A sense of true hope enables a client to strive toward goals mutually established by the client and the nurse. Nurses who demonstrate faith and confidence in their clients' ability and help them maximize the smallest experience, such as watching a sunset, listening to a musical concerto, or playing with an animal, instill a feeling that they care for and about their clients.

In addition to true acceptance of the individual, nurses inspire hope by discussing the specific disability with the client and explaining the remaining options and abilities. Nurses who also take an active stand as advocate in initiating and supporting federal, state, and local legislation encourage clients to believe they are not obligated to accept things as they are. The client may become an active participant in determining the future of rehabilitative care.[1]

Inviting an occupationally and socially adjusted person with a disability to visit a newly disabled client in the hospital might offer a positive role model for the client to follow. This person also might share ideas and help the client to problem solve during hospitalization and even after discharge.

Restoring Self-Esteem

Brook's work[3] with multiple sclerosis clients demonstrated that people with disabling conditions can develop coping strategies to bolster their self-esteem, confront barriers, and exercise self-determination. The rehabilitation nurse can contribute to the development of a positive self-concept by teaching clients the skills that give one a sense of control over life.

By enhancing one's sense of personal worth or self-esteem, the nurse begins to assist the client in developing power. A high degree of self-esteem enables a person to become an active participant in care, develop confidence in interpersonal relationships, and enhance the success of role performance.[30]

Since the basic human need to be touched is the first form of communication a person experiences in life, the act of touching can be a powerful act of healing.[29] Touching a shoulder, holding a hand, and brushing a lock of hair are all acts that offer reassurance, a sense of comfort and encouragement to the client to open up and talk about feelings.

Rehabilitation nursing care of the chronically ill and disabled revolves around the concepts of caring, respect, empathy, and unconditional acceptance of the client. The following guidelines can be used to help restore the client's self-esteem:

1. Explore with the client the feelings and expectations of self for the purpose of developing the client's insight into the way in which the situation and future is viewed.

2. Develop the client's ability to care for self, because no matter how small the accomplishment, offering appropriate praise and recognition increases feelings of personal value.[30] Therefore enabling strategies or nursing interventions must be developed and used to facilitate self-care and effect greater client control.[34]

3. Alter any nursing care procedures to accommodate the client's wishes in order to increase the sense of control.

4. Determine with the client the time for scheduled appointments, the established routines for activities of daily living, and the type of prosthetic device or adaptive equipment that is to be ordered.

5. Show the client you are more interested in the person than the disease process by discussing general subjects of interest such as world events, hobbies, sports, and travel. Your expressed interest in the client's personality and life outside the hospital setting gives recognition to the client's worth and ability to establish relationships.

6. Pay specific attention to any facial expressions, quick gestures, or other nonverbal cues inadvertently conveyed to the client. A nurse's quiet manner or abrupt voice may be interpreted as a sign of rejection, aversion, or disgust at one's condition.

7. Encourage the client to become involved in social activities on the nursing unit. This gives the client the opportunity to practice interacting with other people in a controlled environment before actually facing the public upon discharge.

8. Encourage the client to develop undiscovered creative talents such as writing short stories or poems; doing needlework, ceramics, or painting; or tutoring young students in math or history. Any activity associated with a person's expenditure of energy af-

fords the nurse an opportunity to share in the client's sense of accomplishment and to give praise and respect for a task well done.

Nurses can assist clients in learning coping skills by helping them rehearse stressful events. A combination of progressive relaxation and coping self-statements are substituted for defeatist self-talk often used in stressful situations. First, an example of a stressful situation is enacted. Next clients are taught to use progressive relaxation techniques. Finally, they are taught to repeat coping skills statements until the situation can be rehearsed completely without feeling stressed. Davis, McKay, and Eshelman[10] state that progressive relaxation skills take approximately 1 to 2 weeks to master, and coping skills procedures can be mastered in about 1 week after that.

Coburn and Manderino[7] used coping skills training to assist a client with quadriplegia achieve the goal of improving coping strategies related to selected self-care tasks. Coping statements were used to assist the client during these stressful events. The coping statements were divided into statements used in preparation for, during, and after the stressful event. The following preparatory statements can be used before the event:

- What do I need to do to get ready for this?
- I can handle this.
- I will just stay with the facts and not exaggerate about what might happen.
- It is normal to take time to relearn how to make my body work.
- It is OK to not be 100% successful.

Statements used during the stressful event are:

- I will just concentrate on this task and stay with it.
- I am in control.
- I can take it step by step.
- I can do this just fine.
- I do not have to rush. I will just relax when I begin to feel nervous.
- I do not have to be perfect. It takes time for me and for other people to learn.

Statements made after the stressful event to reinforce success are:

- I did it! I kept to it and accomplished the task.
- I will get better every time I do this.
- I was able to keep this from becoming an overwhelming task.
- I was able to relax when I started to feel anxious.
- I was able to let myself make mistakes without being afraid.

Developing Power

Holistic nursing care of the person who is chronically ill and disabled promotes development of the individual's power resources or the ability to influence what happens to himself or herself. Nutrient power is that source of strength which assists the client in providing self-care, directing others regarding self-care needs, and becoming the ultimate decision maker regarding care.[30] According to Miller,[30] the three components that allow clients to maximize their power resources are (1) physical strength, (2) psychological stamina, and (3) a positive self-concept. The person's body build, height, and weight can be overt resources. Someone with maximum upper body strength will quickly learn transfer techniques, whereas another person will have to work hard at strengthening underdeveloped muscles before mastering the task of moving from the bed to the wheelchair with ease.

Psychological stamina is the unexplained phenomenon in which a person has the capacity to maintain a positive attitude despite overwhelming odds. This positive attitude provides the resilience needed to bounce back from adverse situations and prevents encounters with paralyzing anxiety.[31] No one knows why some individuals have this ability and others do not. Some innate quality enables some persons to fight or defend the essence of their inner being, whereas others passively accept situations thrust upon them from an outside source. A degree of psychological stamina seems to shield some persons from the feelings of powerlessness.

Maintenance of a positive self-concept is essential to maximizing power resources. The disabled client must integrate an accurate perception of the changed body part or of a changed functional level and recognize that the management of this new situation resides within the self. The nurse can assist the client in identifying activities that enhance self-esteem. Some of these activities are (1) emphasizing remaining personal strengths, (2) reviewing the person's accomplishments and intact roles, and (3) helping the client to see the positive aspects of any role change.[32]

Coping with the Reactions of Others

Clients who are disabled need the nurse to help them cope with the various attitudes displayed by family members and friends. Overprotection, hostility, disgust, rejection, condescension, fear, guilt, and pity may burden the client during the initial adjustment to the disability. Anticipatory identification of these reactions and early guidance by nurses and other rehabilitation professionals can offset the "hurt" and prepare disabled persons for comments and embarrassing situations that they may encounter.[49] Role playing and group discussion of problems help to bring these concerns into the open. Grief resolution is only delayed when open discussions about important feelings are avoided. Open discussions also may give the client a glance at some realistic situations that can occur in the world outside the rehabilitation unit.

Family Needs

Members of the rehabilitation team sometimes fail to realize the family system also is destabilized and going through a rehabilitation process. The family and health care system may take opposing positions, with the client in the middle, each vying for control of the client's care-taking needs.[44]

Throughout the grief response to loss of function, the nurse should remember the client and family need each other. Individuals belong to families; they do not usually resolve their problems independently, nor are they immune to the effects of the disability on other members of the family. When the stress is great and sufficiently prolonged, the buffer role of the family can be permanently incapacitated or even destroyed.

Most staff nurses acknowledge the concept of total client care, involving not only the client, but the family as well. They may even regard the family as the essential source of support to the disabled individual. All too often, however, the family is considered of secondary importance when the client is acutely ill or experiencing the grief process.

When the client experiences diagnostic tests, treatment, and evaluations, isolation from the family unit is almost inevitable. This isolation typically begins upon admission, when care is focused primarily on the client, and the family is placed in a secondary position.[2] Rehabilitation team members may choose to become the main source of support to the client, but it is also an important nursing responsibility to provide indirect rehabilitation through emotional support and instruction of the client's family and friends.

Involving the family in client care

Family members expect to share in control and decision making; they also expect nurses to appreciate the impact of disability and chronic illness on the family.[24] The family should be included in the rehabilitation process at the outset and should be an integral part of the process until both the client and family can cope by themselves or until other resources can provide the help they still need.[8] When the client is admitted to the rehabilitation setting, the family also is "admitted" and needs as much support and rehabilitation as the client.

I have often seen family members sitting at the client's bedside while nurses and other rehabilitation team members move in and out of the room with little acknowledgment that they are even there. Nurses can often be overheard describing clients' families as being "in the way," "asking too many questions," "interfering in the nursing management," "supportive" or "nonsupportive" of the client and staff.

Gardner and Stewart[16] state that family stresses may be alleviated by supportive care from rehabilitation team members. Appropriate staff interactions can help to decrease family anxiety, give reassurance, elicit cooperation, establish good rapport, foster understanding, and promote empathy and improved care. Conversely, when staff members interact inappropriately, family anxiety may increase, as well as fear, misunderstanding, mistrust, hostility, and even lawsuits. In this instance, the staff may not be able to obtain needed information about the client from the family.[16] Nurse interaction with family members benefits the family unit, clients, and the nurses themselves.

Nurses have an excellent opportunity to support the family because they are with the client and family at more regular intervals than any other rehabilitation team member. A therapeutic relationship requires an investment of time and energy. In a therapeutic relationship, some of the agony and suffering experienced by the client and family is shared by the nurse. Formation of a therapeutic trusting relationship *always* begins with the nurse.[13]

A critical step in establishing trust and rapport is getting to know the family members individually. The nurse must take responsibility for the therapeutic use of self to affect family care and establish an environment in which open communication with family members can take place. Therapeutic use of self refers to a personal trusting relationship between the nurse and family. The ability to gain this trust depends on the nurse's commitment to the client and the family and nonjudgmental acceptance of the family.

The client's physical environment, in addition to the emotional environment, also is important. Therefore any needs stemming from the client's physical, safety, and hygienic states must be met. Nurses should feel free to discuss the client's diagnosis, physical and emotional state, impending procedures, prognosis, and predictable physical and psychological reactions with the family.[16]

Respite care

As the number of chronically ill and disabled clients returning home increases, rehabilitation nurses need to be acutely aware of the family's capacity to deal with stress on a daily basis. They can make the family aware of the need for relief periods from caregiver responsibilities. Respite care was introduced to relieve family tensions and improve the long-range management of the client. It involves temporary care given to persons with disabilities for the purpose of a rest interval for the primary caregivers.

A 2-year study of 357 families, conducted in 1978, showed that respite care improved overall family functioning. Parents of disabled children reported an improved sense of satisfaction with life, an increased hopefulness about the future, and an improved attitude toward the disabled child. Therefore the nurse's role as client and family advocate might include the recommendation of respite care when indicated for the improvement of family "health."[8]

The nurse also can encourage family members to seek private, personal time of their own even though they may feel a little guilty doing this in the beginning. Such activities as learning and practicing relaxation techniques, participating in physical exercise, golfing, shopping, eating out with friends, and playing cards are some of the short-term methods that can be used to gain personal time. A lengthier "time out" can be obtained by taking a vacation when resources are available to take over caregiver responsibilities.[12]

One of the hardest tasks for family members is asking other relatives and friends for help. Often these other individuals may not be aware that help is needed or do not want to interfere. Learning to ask for help and appreciating this help can make others feel that they have a contribution to make in assuming some of the responsibilities involved when a person is disabled.

REHABILITATION TEAM INTERVENTIONS

Although the rehabilitation nurse has a vital role in assisting the client and family to cope with a disability, there are many instances in which the nurse's knowledge and expertise are not sufficient to meet the client's and family needs. A number of other rehabilitation team members assist the client and family in coping with a disability.

The psychologist and psychiatric clinical nurse specialist have expertise in the therapeutic use of self and various therapeutic communication techniques that facilitate the following:

1. Identification and ventilation of both the client's and family's feelings
2. Assessment of the client's mood swings and behavioral changes that may affect motivation
3. Counseling of the client and family regarding appropriate and realistic goals
4. Conducting family therapy sessions to improve communication and relationship problems within the family system
5. Consulting with all rehabilitation team members to foster the team effort and promote consistency in approaches to the client and family

The intervention of the team psychiatrist may be necessary if the use of medications such as mood elevators, antidepressants, and tranquilizers becomes necessary. These medications, however, should only be used on a short-term basis for situations of pathological grief and coping. The desired outcome is always expression rather than repression of feelings.

The social worker has an indispensable role in assisting the client and family to cope with actual and potential psychosocial problems. To recognize and anticipate these problems, the client's cultural, ethnic, and personal value systems are examined to identify their effects on adherence to the rehabilitation plan. The social worker assists the client and family in recognizing and obtaining financial, environmental, and community resources.

Physical, occupational, and recreational therapists all play an essential part in moving a client toward a positive self-image and in building self-esteem. Regularly scheduled therapy sessions encourage group participation and interaction between the client, other clients with disabilities, and therapists. These opportunities provide both mental and physical growth and function to maintain and restore the client's self-confidence.

The person who turns toward God during a personal crisis readily uses religious beliefs as a coping mechanism when faced with an uncontrollable event.[30] An atmosphere that encourages comfort in expressing those beliefs is essential to the holistic approach. The client's personal clergyman or the facility's chaplain may become a valuable rehabilitation team member. Scripture reading and regular visits from the clergy may inspire the growth of hope and be enough support to motivate the client to continue following the rehabilitation plan.

Any combination of these rehabilitation team members may organize and implement a supportive care group to encourage interaction, discussion, problem solving, and use of effective coping patterns by clients with disabilities and their families.

OUTCOME CRITERIA

The following outcome criteria are related to the client's and family's ability to cope:
1. The client:
   a. Sets realistic goals related to socialization, selection of an occupation, and performance of social roles
   b. Understands the emotional mood swings that occur during a normal grief response
   c. Describes own positive attributes
   d. Demonstrates a sense of self-esteem
   e. Displays pride in personal appearance
   f. Displays an attitude of self-confidence
   g. Is an active participant in decisions regarding care
   h. Performs self-care procedures within own optimum capabilities
   i. Seeks assistance from rehabilitation team members when experiencing difficulty in adapting to losses
2. The family:
   a. Speaks about the client in a positive manner
   b. Encourages the client to assume meaningful roles within the family system
   c. Encourages the client to perform self-care procedures within optimum capabilities
   d. Understands the emotional mood swings the client may experience during a normal grief response
   e. Reports any signs of beginning pathological grief after the client is discharged
   f. Asks for assistance of rehabilitation team members as needed

SUMMARY

The expression of grief and the emotional and psychological adjustments associated with chronic illness and disability are similar to responses to terminal illness. Since the disabled client often is a member of a larger family system, the various individual family members also are dramatically affected. Chronic illness and disability have the potential to fragment the family. Rehabilitation nurses have the potential of bringing the illness into focus and creating opportunities for the client and family to live a full life. Interventions of the rehabilitation team revolve around assisting the client to achieve a sense of independence, self-worth, and well being and in resuming former and new roles within the family.

TEST QUESTIONS

1. All of the following statements describe the family from a general systems approach *except:*
   a. A family contains inherent boundaries.
   b. Family members interact to achieve goals.
   c. External input has little effect on the family network.
   d. Family members are independent entities, yet each member is interrelated.
2. The stages of grief described by Engel include all of the following *except:*
   a. Restitution
   b. Acceptance
   c. Shock and disbelief
   d. Awareness

3. Loss of a client's physical function in any area may affect the client and family system by requiring that:
   a. Family roles and functions be reversed
   b. New sources of financial support be sought
   c. Community support systems be used
   d. All of the above
4. Subjective data related to coping elicited by the rehabilitation nurse during the interview are:
   a. Client and family's past experiences with physical disability
   b. Client and family's available resources
   c. Client and family's usual methods of coping
   d. All of the above
5. When assessing the disabled client and family, the rehabilitation nurse knows that the sacrificing family tends to relate to the disabled client by:
   a. Becoming overprotective
   b. Rejecting the client
   c. Placing the client in an institutional setting
   d. Modifying family roles to reestablish the client in the family network
6. Which of the following rehabilitation nursing interventions is appropriate to use when assisting a client in coping with a physical disability?
   a. Encourage the family to perform all the client's physical care.
   b. Work with the client to schedule occupational and physical therapy appointments.
   c. Let the client sleep as late as desired.
   d. Repeatedly discuss the client's limitations in order to force the client to face reality.
7. Which of the following rehabilitation nursing interventions is appropriate to use when assisting a family to cope with a client's physical disability?
   a. Encourage the client and family to communicate thoughts and feelings clearly and honestly.
   b. Encourage the client and family to keep thoughts and feelings to themselves to avoid hurting each other.
   c. Discourage family members from seeking respite because they will feel guilty leaving the client's care responsibilities to others.
   d. Discourage involvement of staff members with the client and family's long-term coping concerns.
8. When the rehabilitation team decides that medications such as mood elevators or antidepressants should be considered to treat a client experiencing a pathological grief reaction, the _____ is asked to evaluate the client.
   a. Social worker
   b. Psychiatrist
   c. Psychiatric clinical nurse specialist
   d. Physical therapist

Answers: 1. c, 2. b, 3. d, 4. d, 5. a, 6. b, 7. a, 8. b.

LEARNING ACTIVITIES

1. Assess your own feelings if faced with living with a disability. Identify how these feelings might impinge upon or enhance your ability to work with physically disabled clients and their family members.
2. Form a discussion group and share various ways that each member of the group is currently coping with stress or illness. Discuss whether these methods are effective or ineffective ways of coping.
3. Plan a coping skills training program for clients who are physically disabled. Incorporate relaxation skills and coping skills statements in your program. Determine with clients what situations should be used to simulate stressful events. Decide on how often these situations will be rehearsed and with whom.
4. Plan a family support group for families of clients you are seeing. Involve families in planning the support group. Determine how often the group will meet and who will facilitate the discussion. Elicit participation of other rehabilitation team members. Decide on goals, activities, and evaluation procedures. Determine if and when clients will join group.

REFERENCES

1. Berry J: The stage model revisited, Rehabil Lit 9:275, 1983.
2. Bond S: Communicating with families of cancer patients. II. The nurse, Nurs Times 78:1027, 1982.
3. Brooks N: From rehabilitation to independent living. In Ruskin A, editor: Current therapy in physiatry, Philadelphia, 1984, WB Saunders Co.
4. Carlson C: Methods of coping. In Martin N, Holt NB, and Hicks D, editors: Comprehensive rehabilitation nursing, New York, 1981, McGraw-Hill Book Co.
5. Charmaz K: The social reality of death, Menlo Park, Calif, 1980, Addison-Wesley Publishing Co, Inc.
6. Clark CC: Wellness nursing: concepts, theory, research, and practice, New York, 1986, Springer Publishing Co, Inc.

7. Coburn J and Manderino MA: Stress innoculation: an illustration of coping skills training, Rehabil Nurs 11:14 Jan/Feb 1986.

8. Cohen S: Supporting families through respite care, Rehabil Lit 43:7, Jan/Feb 1982.

9. Craven R and Sharp B: The effects of illness on family functions, Nurs Forum 11(2):186,1972.

10. Davis M, McKay M, and Eshelman E: The relaxation and stress reduction workbook, ed 2, Oakland, Calif, 1982, New Harbinger Publications.

11. Dell Orto A: Coping with the enormity of illness and disability, Rehabil Lit 45:22, Jan/Feb 1984.

12. Ekberg JY, Griffith N, and Foxall MJ: Spouse burnout syndrome, J Adv Nurs 11:161, 1986.

13. Engel G: Grief and grieving, Am J Nurs 74:93, 1964.

14. Eyres P: The role of the nurse in family-centered nursing care, Nurs Clin North Am 7:27, March 1972.

15. Foxall MJ, Ekberg JY, and Griffith N: Spousal adjustment to chronic illness, Rehabil Nurs 11:13, March/April 1986.

16. Gardner D and Stewart N: Staff involvement with families of patients in critical care units, Heart Lung 7:105, Jan/Feb 1978.

17. Goldberg I and Goldberg H: Family therapy: an overview, Monterey, Calif, 1980, Brooks/Cole Publishing Co.

18. Goldiamond B: Resocialization. In Martin N, Holt NB, Hicks D, editors: Comprehensive rehabilitation nursing, New York, 1981, McGraw-Hill Book Co.

19. Gordon M: Nursing diagnosis: process and application, ed 2, New York, 1987, McGraw-Hill Book Co.

20. Hafen B and Frandsen K: Faces of death: grief, dying, euthanasia, suicide, Englewood, Colo, 1983, Morton Publishing Co.

21. Hall AD and Fagen RE: Definition of a system. In Buckley W, editor: Modern systems research for the behavioral scientist, Hawthorne, NY, 1968, Aldine de Gruyter.

22. Kandzari J and Howard J: The well family: a developmental approach to assessment, Boston, 1981, Little, Brown & Co.

23. Klesper MJ: Grief: how long does grief go on, Am J Nurs 78:420, 1978.

24. Kodadek S: Family-centered care of the chronically ill child, AORN J 30:635, 1979.

25. Kubler-Ross E: On death and dying, New York, 1969, Macmillan Publishing Co.

26. Leavitt M: Families at risk: primary prevention in nursing practice, Boston, 1982, Little, Brown & Co.

27. Lewis K: Grief in chronic illness and disability, J Rehabil 49:8, July/Aug/Sept 1983.

28. Lindemann E: Symptomatology and management of acute grief, Am J Psychiatry 101:141, Sept 1944.

29. McAuliffe K and McAuliffe D: I care, Nursing '84 14:58, April 1984.

30. Miller JF: Coping with chronic illness, overcoming powerlessness, Philadelphia, 1983, FA Davis Co.

31. Miller JF and Janosik E: Family-focused care, New York, 1980, McGraw-Hill Book Co.

32. Mumma C, editor: Rehabilitation nursing: concepts and practice, a core curriculum, ed 2, Evanston, Ill, 1987, Rehabilitation Nursing Foundation.

33. Pereira B: Loss and grief in chronic illness, Rehabil Nurs 9:20, March/April 1984.

34. Pfister-Minogue K: Enabling strategies. In Miller JF, editor: Coping with chronic illness, overcoming powerlessness, Philadelphia, 1983, FA Davis Co.

35. Putt A: General systems theory applied to nursing, Boston, 1978, Little, Brown & Co.

36. Russell R: Concepts of adjustment of disability: an overview, Rehabil Lit 42:330, 1981.

37. Ryder C and Ross D: Terminal care: issues and alternatives, Pub Health Rep 2:20 Jan/Feb 1977.

38. Schilling J: Ethical issues related to chronic disease. In Anderson SV and Bauwens EE, editors: Chronic health problems: concepts, and applications, St Louis, 1981, The CV Mosby Co.

39. Servoss A: Depression and suicide in the disabled. In Krueger D, editor: Rehabilitation psychology, Rockville, Md, 1984, Aspen Systems Corp.

40. Sheehy G: Passages: predictable crises of adult life, New York, 1974, EP Dutton.

41. Stewart TM and Rossier A: Psychological considerations in the adjustment to spinal cord injury, Rehabil Lit 39:75, March 1978.

42. Strain J: Psychological reactions to chronic medical illness, Psychiatr Q 51:173, 1979.

43. Thompson L: Chronic grief. In Anderson SV and Bauwens EE, editors: Chronic health problems: concepts and applications, St Louis, 1981, The CV Mosby Co.

44. Tucker SJ: The psychology of spinal cord injury: patient-staff interaction, Rehabil Lit 41:114, May/June 1980.

45. Van Dyke C: Family-centered health care recognizes needs of patients, families, employees, Hosp Prog 61:54, Aug 1980.

46. Versluys H: Physical rehabilitation and family dynamics, Rehabil Lit 41:58, March/April 1980.

47. Watson PG: Family participation in the rehabilitation process: the rehabilitator's perspective, Rehabil Nurs 12:70, March/April 1987.

48. Webster's New World Dictionary: Compact school and office edition, Cleveland, 1975, William Collins & World Publishing Co., Inc.

49. Werner-Beland J, editor: Grief responses to long term illness and disability, Reston, Va, 1980, Res on Publishing Co, Inc.

50. Whall AL: Congruence between existing theories of family functioning and nursing theories, Adv Nurs Sci 3:60 Oct 1980.

51. Wilson HS and Kneisl CR: Psychiatric nursing, Menlo Park, Calif, 1979, Addison-Wesley Publishing Co, Inc.

ADDITIONAL READINGS

Baldree KS, Murphy SP, and Powers MF: Stress identification and coping patterns in patients on hemodialysis, Nurs Res 31:107, March/April 1982.

Bargagliotti LA and Trygstad LN: Differences in stress and coping findings: a reflection of social realities or methodologies? Nurs Res 36:170, May/June 1987.

Ben-Sira Z: Disability, stress and readjustment: the function of the professional's latest goals and affective behavior in rehabilitation, Soc Sci Med 23(1):43, 1986.

Brillhart B: Predictors of self-acceptance, Rehabil Nurs 11:8, March/April 1986.

Cohen CB: Patient autonomy in chronic illness, Fam Community Health 10(1):24, 1987.

Corbin JM and Strauss AL: Collaboration: couples working together to manage chronic illness, Image 26:109, Fall 1984.

Dembo T: Sensitivity of one person to another, Rehabil Lit 54:90, March/April 1984.

Fagin CM: Stress: implications for nursing research, Image 19:38, Spring 1987.

Jalowiec A, Murphy SP, and Powers MJ: Psychometric assessment of the Jalowiec Coping Scale, Nurs Res 33:157, May/June 1984.

Lowery BJ: Stress research: some theoretical and methodological issues, Image 19:42, Spring 1987.

McNett SC: Social support, threat, and coping responses and effectiveness in the functionally disabled, Nurs Res 36:98, March/April 1987.

Pollock SE: Human responses to chronic illness: physiologic and psychosocial adaptation, Nurs Res 35:90, March/April 1986.

Roche H: Experiencing loss. In Martin N, Holt NB and Hicks D, editors: Comprehensive rehabilitation nursing, New York, 1981, McGraw-Hill Book Co.

Shontz F: Psychological adjustment to physical disability: trends in theories, Arch Phys Med Rehabil 59:251, 1978.

PART IV

Evaluation of Rehabilitation Nursing

Functional Evaluation

Margaret M. Hens

OBJECTIVES

After completing Chapter 23, the reader will be able to:

1. Define functional assessment and functional evaluation.

2. Identify the purposes of functional evaluation at the client, team, and program levels.

3. List the basic elements of functional assessment instruments.

4. Describe six assessment instruments used to evaluate the functional status of clients during the rehabilitation process.

5. Discuss functional evaluation methodology as used in rehabilitation nursing.

6. Describe the development and refinement of client outcome criteria to evaluate functional status.

The process of rehabilitation directs attention to a client's functional performance. The maintenance and restoration of optimum function are goals of any rehabilitation effort, goals that mobilize many resources. The client's functional performance serves as the common denominator for the efforts of the interdisciplinary rehabilitation team. Assessment and evaluation of a client's functional performance are part of the rehabilitation nurse's responsibilities.

The conceptualization and analysis of functional performance are issues central to the nature and direction of planning, delivering, and evaluating rehabilitation care. The rehabilitation process and rehabilitation nursing are subject to evaluation by consumers and other professionals. Since the demand for cost-effective, high-quality care is of prime concern in health care delivery today, it is necessary to address questions about the characteristics of populations served by rehabilitation providers, the meaning of rehabilitation terminology, the methodologies used to assess and determine client needs, and the justification and evaluation of rehabilitation interventions. Answers to these questions provide the rationale for continuing and increasing the commitment of human and financial resources to rehabilitation. Since rehabilitation encompasses the client, family, and interdisciplinary team, each professional discipline faces the challenge of factoring out its own contributions, while viewing the composite outcomes of the collaborative effort.

Determination of client needs, justification and evaluation of interventions, administrative planning, and identification of information necessary for documenting cost-effectiveness and quality care specific to rehabilitation nursing and the rehabilitation process are included in the process of functional evaluation. This chapter addresses functional evaluation primarily from a nursing standpoint. Terminology, purposes of functional evaluation, and basic elements of functional assessment instruments are presented. A general review of the state of the art of functional evaluation is given. In addition, several instruments currently available for assessing and evaluating a client's functional performance are described, and the relevance and implications of functional evaluation data in the practice of rehabilitation nursing are discussed. This chapter concludes with a description of the development and refinement of client outcome criteria to evaluate functional status.

TERMINOLOGY

Functional evaluation incorporates three interrelated processes: (1) assessment of functional status, (2) classification based on functional abilities, and (3) evaluation of functional progress in relation to time, therapeutic interventions, and other factors that affect functional ability. Assessment, the first step of the nursing process, involves the systematic collection and subsequent organization of information about the client. Nurses working in any setting gather information about the client across a number of parameters using the techniques of interviewing, observation, inspection, auscultation, and percussion. Throughout the assessment, the nurse gathers and records data about the client's personal background; physical, functional, and psychosocial status; and responses to interventions. Nurses, by virtue of their professional orientation to the client's health and their close contact with the client, also are in a position to detect covert behavioral cues, which, when recognized, provide insight into actual and potential problems. The aforementioned areas have in common the concept of function.

The term *function*, when used in a rehabilitation context, is synonymous with performance. A client's ability to perform tasks deemed necessary for survival and participation in life has always received attention in rehabilitation. However, nurses have traditionally approached the assessment of a client's functional status qualitatively and subjectively. More recently, rehabili-

tation nurses have begun to formally assess the functional status of their clients using quantifiable data. Subsequent identification of problems, determination of goals and plans, implementation of plans, and evaluation of rehabilitation nursing therapies are contingent upon baseline and intermediate assessment data about the client's performance abilities. The rehabilitation nurse uses other assessment data as an adjunct in planning care and in helping to identify a client's strengths and limitations.

One of the earliest definitions of functional assessment was given by Lawton[19] in reference to a geriatric population. He defined functional assessment as "any systematic attempt to measure objectively the level at which a person is functioning in any of a variety of areas such as physical health, quality of self-maintenance, quality of role activity, intellectual status, social activity, attitude toward the world and toward self, and emotional status." More recently, Granger[14] defined functional assessment within the context of rehabilitation medicine as "a method for describing abilities and activities in order to measure an individual's use of the variety of skills included in performing the tasks necessary to daily living, vocational pursuits, social interactions, leisure activities, and other required behaviors." A salient similarity between these two definitions is the emphasis on making quantitative measurements across multidimensional functional areas. The very nature of the holistic philosophy of the rehabilitation process mandates this approach.

The concept of functional assessment is not new to nursing. Nurses have always assessed what clients can and cannot do in terms of meeting personal needs. They also have traditionally assimilated information about clients from a multidimensional perspective in order to develop nursing care plans that address physical, psychosocial, economic, vocational, and spiritual needs. Nurses have the advantage of observing the client in action. The astute nurse recognizes factors that enhance or restrain action and capitalizes on client strengths and available resources. Nursing assessment that incorporates functional assessment is most useful when it is validated with objective measures rather than with qualitative and subjective information.

Classification theory defines sets of phenomena so that categories are mutually exclusive. It provides a foundation for quantifiable and objective measurement of functional performance. Classification guides the selection of specific items used to describe and measure abilities and limitations within general areas of function. Classification methodology also imposes restrictions on the properties of a given category and clearly distinguishes between categories of function. It facilitates the definition of groups of individuals based on a common factor, which, in this instance, is functional status. If all clients within a given setting are judged according to the same parameters, then client profiles emerge that indicate groupings of similar and dissimilar abilities and limitations in function. These facilitate management and evaluation, not only on a case-by-case basis, but also on a programmatic basis. Classification of function focuses on two aspects: domains of measurement and quantified descriptor items.

Activities of daily living of either a personal care or instrumental nature are examples of domains of measurement. Personal care activities of daily living include the following tasks: bathing, feeding, bladder and bowel continence, grooming, and dressing. Instrumental activities of daily living include the tasks of shopping, preparing food, doing laundry, telephoning, managing money, performing housekeeping chores, getting around in the community, and managing a medication regimen.[19] Quantified descriptor items are the mutually exclusive explanations assigned a numerical value to identify the client's ability or inability to perform the task (domain of measurement). The numerical values are used to score domains of function.

Evaluation may be defined as an intellectual dynamic process whereby the nurse judges the effectiveness of care, draws conclusions, and gains additional insight into the assessment, planning, and implementation phases of the nursing process. Ideally, evaluation allows the nurse to measure progress toward goal achievement quantitatively. Functional evaluation may be defined as a dynamic, deliberate process involving initial and periodic quantifiable and objective collection of functional data to ascertain change in the client's performance of tasks in response to time, therapeutic interventions, and other variables that could influence performance abilities. This type of functional assessment is the only reliable basis for evaluating the influences on a client's and team's efforts to maintain and restore maximum functional independence. Evaluation makes it possible to target problem areas that need to be addressed.

PURPOSES OF FUNCTIONAL EVALUATION

Functional evaluation serves a number of purposes within each of the following three levels: client, rehabilitation team, and program. Functional evaluations at the client level help determine problems in the performance of activities and tasks and facilitate goals and plans for intervention. A comprehensive functional evaluation fosters a complete view of the client's function and ensures that all problems and potential problems are addressed and monitored.

Functional evaluation at the team level enhances communication and provides objective evidence about the effects of interventions. Functional evaluation data also help determine resources needed and serve as a basis for analyzing cost-effectiveness.

Functional evaluation at the program level provides a basis for quality assurance, nursing care audits, research, and overall program evaluation. There are several reasons for nursing-specific functional evaluations, and these are discussed in greater detail later in this chapter.

FUNCTIONAL ASSESSMENT INSTRUMENTS

Functional assessment instruments are used to guide functional evaluation. It behooves the rehabilitation nurse to have a working knowledge of the characteristics and properties of functional assessment instruments so that inaccurate conclusions are not drawn. Published functional assessment instruments may be categorized into three major groupings: (1) global scales, (2) activity of daily living scales, and (3) single categorical scales. Global scales incorporate multidimensional domains of measurement, including those categories of performance noted in the earlier definitions of functional assessment. Activity of daily living scales concentrate on activities of daily living as domains of measurement. Single categorical scales limit measurement to a single condition such as hand function, mental status, or mobility status.

Functional assessment instruments can apply to a very broad population, or they may be tailored to measure the functional status of a narrowly defined group. The Quadriplegia Index of

Function, discussed later in this chapter, was designed exclusively for functional assessment of persons with quadriplegia.[17]

There is consensus that the domains of activities of daily living and mobility require measurement in terms of functional level. The key factors in choosing other areas of function to be measured depend upon the needs of the client, team, and overall program. Once the major categories of function are chosen, descriptor items must exclusively target distinctions in level of performance of these functions.

Considerations when choosing a functional assessment instrument include the scoring mechanism, internal and external validity, and reliability. Scoring mechanisms quantify the client's ability to perform one or more tasks. Scores are considered to be ordinal or interval. Ordinal level scoring mechanisms attach a poverty of meaning to function and give an approximate value to the ability to perform. Interval level measurement, on the other hand, describes an actual amount of function. Statistically valid scaling construction dictates that each descriptor item be assigned a numerical value so that changes in functional ability can be shown within a specific domain of function. Scoring mechanisms must be derived empirically if the total score (sum of all scores on each domain of function) is to truly reflect functional performance. Foley and Schneider[11] note that many assessment methodologies used to determine placement decisions among the nursing home population are based on algorithms yet have been hastily adapted without scientific verification.

Any scoring system raises the issue of how best to weight one domain of function as opposed to another. For instance, along a continuum of measures, the question of how much the domain of mobility versus the domain of personal care should be represented, so that a total score truly reflects the degree of independent function, arises. The scoring mechanism must account for the client who is functionally adept in personal care activities of daily living, instrumental activities of daily living, and transfers but who is unable to ambulate. It also must account for the individual who can ambulate but who is limited or requires help with personal care and instrumental activities of daily living.

Descriptor items should be clearly defined to minimize bias resulting from inconsistent interpretations. For example, terms such as "independent," "dependent," "limited," "with help," and "with supervision" are not useful because they allow for varying interpretations. Rather, these items should be quantified in terms of levels of performance, for example, "dependent—client requires complete human or mechanical assistance to transfer from bed to chair."

A valid instrument should capture the domains of function to yield a composite picture of performance ability and allow extrapolation of data from a number of functional evaluations to predict needs of populations of people sharing a common medical diagnosis. In addition, a valid instrument should help predict functional status of these populations at intervals after discharge from the rehabilitation setting.

Reliable instruments should provide consistent results for functional status on the same client when used by different raters at the same time. The issues of scoring, validity, and reliability are major considerations in determining the usefulness of results obtained when using functional assessment instruments. Reliability and validity should be established and known to the users of these instruments.

STATE OF THE ART REVIEW

Although a number of measurement scales by which to assess functional status have been developed, a consensus on the domains and specific descriptor items that accurately describe task performance has not been reached. Keith[18] cites several major impediments to this apparent lack of a unified approach to the analysis of function: (1) a lack of standardized descriptor terminology, (2) basic methodological flaws, (3) proliferation of functional measurement scales with doubtful scientific merit, (4) failure to consider or inconsistency in accounting for the interplay of performance ability, physical-environmental setting, and the client's ability to learn and relearn necessary information, and (5) a lack of clearly conceptualized and stated outcome criteria based on valid analysis of functional status.

The literature on functional measurement scales in rehabilitation shows a trend toward increased research activity concerned with the refinement and adaptation of existing published instruments. Several published instruments have been used in rehabilitation settings. In addition to the elements of a functional assessment instrument previously discussed, selection of an appropriate instrument should be based on three other factors: (1) ease of administration, (2) practicality, and (3) client population. Ease of administration includes the time involved in gathering and scoring data, as well as the level of expertise required on the part of the rater. Directions for administration must include precise, easily followed guidelines. The instrument selected should provide the greatest amount of information required within the realistic constraints of the nurse's and client's time and the client's physical capabilities.

Practicality addresses the general and specific usefulness of the data collected via the instrument. The data must reflect concepts of function as a whole but target specific items. The instrument must blend with the daily routines of the rehabilitation setting. It should facilitate data collection by promoting time and energy conservation.

The nature of the client population also influences the selection of the functional assessment instrument. Some client populations, such as persons with quadriplegia, require a functional assessment instrument that is sensitive to small increments of change in function. Other client populations, such as individuals with lower limb amputation, do not require assessment with such highly sensitive and precise instruments.

DESCRIPTION OF SELECTED FUNCTIONAL ASSESSMENT INSTRUMENTS

A variety of instruments are used to measure functional status. The PULSES Profile, Barthel Index, Kenny Self-Care Scale, Quadriplegia Index of Function, Long Range Evaluation System, and Uniform Data System for Medical Rehabilitation are described.

PULSES Profile

The PULSES Profile, developed by Moskowitz and McCann,[22] is a global functional assessment instrument that yields a broad view of a client's well-being. (See box on p. 491.) Each letter in the acronym PULSES represents a domain of measurement. The "P" represents general physical condition; "U," use of the upper extremities; "L," use of the lower extremities; first "S," sensory status in the realms of vision, hearing, and speech;

"E," excretory status; and second "S," mental and emotional status. Each domain of measurement has four descriptor items that are weighted and scored. A number "1" descriptor item assigned to a domain represents no abnormality or restriction of function, and "2," "3," and "4" descriptor items, respectively, indicate increasing levels of dysfunction from minor to severe. The cumulative domain scores provide the PULSES Profile of the individual and give a very broad picture of function.

The original PULSES Profile, as well as a later adapted version by Granger and Greer,[15] has been used to assess, study, and monitor the functional status of clients involved in rehabilitation. The original authors have shown that the PULSES Profile is useful in classifying clients according to level of function over time and in predicting level of function in relation to medical diagnosis.

Barthel Index

Mahoney and Barthel[20] have shown that the Barthel Index is of value in obtaining baseline functional data and in monitoring improvement in mobility and self-care over time. The Barthel Index, shown in Table 23-1, measures performance ability in personal care activities of daily living and mobility. The client's ability to perform independently or with help is appraised and scored according to performance in 10 categories of function. The authors of this instrument devised a weighted scoring system that ranges from 0 to 100. A total score of 100 indicates complete independence, independent performance in all 10 domains. To be considered "independent" the client must not require assistance at any time, either before, during, or after the performance of the task.

Kenny Self-Care Scale

The Kenny Self-Care Scale measures six categories of function: (1) bed activities (including position changes), (2) transfers, (3) locomotion, (4) dressing, (5) personal hygiene, and (6) feeding. Performance is measured on a scale from 0 to 4, with 0 representing complete dependence and 4 representing complete independence. Each performance category is weighted equally.

Several investigators have examined the utility of the Kenny Self-Care Scale. Schoening and

PULSES Profile

P. Physical condition, including diseases of the viscera (cardiovascular, pulmonary, gastrointestinal, urological, and endocrine) and cerebral disorders that are not enumerated in the lettered categories below
   1. No gross abnormalities considering age of individual
   2. Minor abnormalities not requiring frequent medical or nursing supervision
   3. Moderately severe abnormalities requiring frequent medical or nursing supervision yet still permitting ambulation
   4. Severe abnormalities requiring constant medical or nursing supervision or confining individual to bed or wheelchair

U. Upper extremities, including shoulder girdle, cervical, and upper dorsal spine
   1. No gross abnormalities considering age of individual
   2. Minor abnormalities with fairly good range of motion and function
   3. Moderately severe abnormalities but permitting performance of daily needs to a limited extent
   4. Severe abnormalities requiring constant nursing care

L. Lower extremities, including pelvis, lower dorsal, and lumbosacral spine
   1. No gross abnormalities considering age of individual
   2. Minor abnormalities with fairly good range of motion and function
   3. Moderately severe abnormalities permitting limited ambulation
   4. Severe abnormalities confining individual to bed or wheelchair

S. Sensory components relating to speech, vision, and hearing
   1. No gross abnormalities considering age of individual
   2. Minor deviations insufficient to cause any appreciable functional impairment
   3. Moderate deviations sufficient to cause appreciable functional impairment
   4. Severe deviations causing complete loss of hearing, vision, or speech

E. Excretory function, that is, bowel and bladder control
   1. Complete control
   2. Occasional stress incontinence or nocturia
   3. Periodic bowel and bladder incontinence or retention alternating with control
   4. Total incontinence, either bowel or bladder

S. Mental and emotional status
   1. No deviations considering age of individual
   2. Minor deviations in mood, temperament, and personality not impairing environmental adjustment
   3. Moderately severe variations requiring some supervision
   4. Severe variations requiring complete supervision

Profile

P	U	L	S	E	S

From Moskowitz E and McCann CB: J Chronic Dis 5:343, 1957.

TABLE 23-1

Barthel Index

	With help	Independent
1. Feeding*	5	10
2. Moving from wheelchair to bed and return (includes sitting up in bed)	5-10	15
3. Personal toilet (wash face, comb hair, shave, clean teeth)	0	5
4. Getting on and off toilet (handling clothes, wipe, flush)	5	10
5. Bathing self	0	5
6. Walking on level surface	10	15
If unable to walk, propelling wheelchair (score only if unable to walk)	0	5
7. Ascending and descending stairs	5	10
8. Dressing (includes tying shoes, fastening fasteners)	5	10
9. Controlling bowels	5	10
10. Controlling bladder	5	10

From Mahoney FI and Barthel DW: Md State Med J 14:62, 1965.

*If food needs to be in cup, score as "with help."

associates[23] have shown that the Kenny scale is sensitive to changes in performance of self-care tasks and mobility. This scale also has been used to correlate the client's level of function with nurse staffing patterns.

Quadriplegia Index of Function

The Quadriplegia Index of Function, sections of which are shown in Figure 23-1, was developed by an interdisciplinary team for the sole purpose of measuring the functional status of persons with quadriplegia.[17] The index measures degree of performance ability in transfers, grooming, bathing, feeding, dressing, wheelchair mobility, and bed activities. It also measures degree of performance ability in management of bladder and bowel programs. Scoring criteria are meticulously outlined, thereby reducing observer bias.

Long Range Evaluation System

The Long Range Evaluation System (LRES), developed by Granger and McNamara,[16] is a diverse multidimensional functional assessment instrument. The LRES has several components: (1) an adapted PULSES Profile, (2) an adapted Barthel Index, (3) an ESCROW Profile (explained below), (4) limb functioning, (5) sensory abilities (communicative senses, including vision, hearing, speech), (6) use of health resources, and (7) feel-

ings and mood. The LRES also has components such as intellectual functioning and degree of unmet needs.

This instrument allows qualification and quantification of descriptor items of each domain contained in the PULSES Profile. Each descriptor item is tailored to show increasing degrees of required assistance. The 1 to 4 scoring mechanism was incorporated to reflect function in more quantifiable and broader terms. The adapted version of the PULSES Profile has been shown statistically to be valid, reliable, and predictive of function.

The modified version of the Barthel Index of Function incorporated in the LRES has a more detailed delineation of descriptor items and some additional activities of daily living and mobility tasks that more clearly capture and communicate the degree of assistance required for activities of daily living and mobility. The scoring system of the Barthel Index was concurrently modified to align the degree of assistance needed with a numerical value other than that assigned to the categories "independent" or "with help" in the original version.

The ESCROW Profile measures social support. Each letter of the acronym ESCROW represents an area of social function: *E*nvironment, *S*ocial interactions, *C*luster of family members, *R*esources, *O*utlook, and *W*ork, school, and vocational status. The LRES has four formats de-

Domain of measurement for bladder program (28 points)

Score inapplicable routine as *9.*

	4	3	2	1	0	9
A. 1. Voluntary voiding: toilet		3				
2. Voluntary voiding: commode						9
B. Intermittent catheterization program						9
C. Automatic bladder program						9
D. Indwelling catheter						9
E. Ileal diversion						9
F. Credé maneuver						9

Descriptor items for bladder program: scoring criteria

A. Voluntary voiding
1. Toilet
4 = Patient is completely independent, that is, needs no help in transfers, managing clothes, and cleaning self afterward.
3 = Patient is independent in transfers but may require assistance in *only* one of the following: managing clothes or cleaning self afterward.
2 = Patient is independent in transfers but requires assistance in managing clothes and in cleaning self
afterward.
1 = Patient needs help in transfers *and* in *one* of the following: managing clothes or cleaning self
afterward.
0 = Patient cannot do *any* of the above. Completely dependent.
2. Commode
3 = Patient is independent, that is, can get commode, requires no assistance in managing clothes or
cleaning self afterward.
2 = Patient can prepare commode but requires assistance in either managing clothes or cleaning afterward but not both.
1 = Patient can prepare commode but requires assistance in managing clothes *and* in cleaning afterward.
0 = Patient cannot do any of the above.
B. Intermittent catheterization program
3 = Patient needs *no* assistance in preparing, positioning, and disposing of equipment, manages
clothes; and cleans self afterward.
2 = Patient can manage clothes but needs assistance in *only* one of the following: preparing, positioning, and disposing of equipment and in cleaning self afterward.
1 = Patient needs help in all of the above but is able to instruct others in the necessary procedure.
0 = There is no bladder program, or patient does not possess sufficient knowledge to instruct others in
the necessary procedure.

Figure 23-1
Quadriplegia Index of Function. Domains of measurement and descriptor items. Client who
voids voluntarily on toilet. *(From Gresham GE and others: Arch Phys Med Rehabil 61:493,
1980.)*

Continued.

Descriptor items for bladder program: scoring criteria—cont'd

C. Automatic bladder program
>   3 = Patient is completely independent, that is, manages clothes, prepares, applies, and removes external device, *and* cleans self afterward without help.
>   2 = Patient manages clothes but needs help in one of the following: preparing, applying, and removing external device and cleaning self afterward.
>   1 = Patient cannot do any of the above but can instruct someone in the necessary procedure.
>   0 = Patient cannot do any of the above.

D. Indwelling catheter
>   3 = Patient needs no help in managing clothes, changing bags and catheters, positioning, and cleaning self afterward.
>   2 = Patient needs help in no more than two of the following: managing clothes, preparing catheters, changing bags, positioning, and cleaning self.
>   1 = Patient needs help in three or more of the above areas *but* can instruct someone in the necessary procedure.
>   0 = Patient is completely dependent and cannot instruct someone in the necessary procedure.

E. Ileal diversion
>   3 = Patient needs no help in managing clothes, changing bags, and cleaning self afterward.
>   2 = Patient needs help in one of the above.
>   1 = Patient needs help in two or more of the above *but* can also instruct someone in the necessary procedure.
>   0 = Patient cannot instruct someone in the necessary procedure.

F. Credé maneuver
>   3 = Patient needs no help in managing clothes, preparing supplies, doing Credé maneuver, and cleaning afterward.
>   2 = Patient needs help in only *one* of the above.
>   1 = Patient needs help in two or more of the above but can also instruct someone in necessary procedure.
>   0 = Patient cannot instruct someone in the necessary procedure.

Figure 23-1, cont'd
Quadriplegic Index of Function.

signed specifically for use on admission, discharge, and in outpatient and inpatient long-term care facilities.[16]

Uniform Data System for Medical Rehabilitation

Functional evaluation has been identified as the basis for developing a common language and documentation process for disability and rehabilitation outcomes. In 1983 the US Department of Education, National Institute of Handicapped Research, provided funding for the development of a uniform data system for medical rehabilitation. The American Congress of Rehabilitation Medicine and American Academy of Physical Medicine and Rehabilitation sponsored a task force for this purpose. The task force was charged with establishing a minimum data set of key functional characteristics in a format that could be easily administered, was statistically reliable and valid for measuring severity of disability and treatment outcomes, and was suitable for use by any discipline.[24] This project is headquartered at the State University of New York at Buffalo.

After review of existing functional assessment instruments, the task force developed the Uniform National Data Set format that includes an instrument known as the Functional Independence Measure (FIM) and then spent several years testing it at various facilities throughout the United States. The field testing included analyses of the FIM's statistical properties and resulted in instrument revision with repeated pilot tests.

The FIM measures disability in the following performance areas: feeding, grooming, bathing, dressing the upper body, dressing the lower body, toileting, bladder management, bowel management, bed/chair/wheelchair transfers, toilet transfer, tub/shower transfer, locomotion (walking or wheelchair), going up and down stairs, comprehension, expression, social interaction, problem solving, and memory. Each of these areas of function is measured on a seven-level scale that delineates strict differences in independent and dependent performance ability (actual percentage of helper effort required). Clients are rated on what they actually *do*, and no item is considered "not applicable." A FIM score ranges from a maximum total of 126 points, representing complete independence in all performance areas, to a minimum total of 18 points, representing total assistance in all performance areas.

The Uniform National Data Set format is also designed to collect additional data about the client, including demographic information, primary and secondary diagnostic codes, impairment group, duration of hospital stay, charges, program interruptions, and discharge destination (living arrangements).

An important part of the administration of the FIM is adherence to the guide that accompanies it and facilitates proper use. The guide offers explicit directions and definitions for the rating scale and variables to be measured. The Uniform National Data Set for Medical Rehabilitation permits, for the first time, an objective view of disability and the costs and benefits of rehabilitation. Data can be collected at admission, discharge, and follow-up. Acceptance of a consistent system for documenting disability permits facilities to judge their own clients and programs and to compare the outcomes of clients with the same diagnoses at different geographical points.

FUNCTIONAL EVALUATION IN REHABILITATION NURSING

The movement in the nursing profession toward developing methodologies for client need assessment, planning nursing care, allocating nursing human and financial resources, and evaluating nursing-specific client outcomes has paralleled the efforts in the rehabilitation field directed at assessing, planning, and evaluating rehabilitation interventions in general. To address the issues from a nursing perspective, the nursing profession has advocated three interrelated activities: (1) research and development of client-centered assessment-classification systems, (2) develop-

ment and use of a taxonomy of nursing diagnoses, and (3) integration of the nursing process to ensure a systematic approach to the delivery of client care. A fourth area that requires nursing attention is the development of outcome criteria to serve as a valid basis for evaluating the practice of nursing. The logical means for evaluating rehabilitation nursing is to develop outcome criteria that examine the effect of nursing interventions on the client's ability to perform self-care tasks and function in social roles.

The purposes of quantifiable functional evaluation in rehabilitation nursing are numerous. Dittmar[10] cites these purposes as (1) systematic identification of functional limitations requiring preventive, maintenance, and restorative actions; (2) recognition of client learning needs; (3) documentation of feedback about progression toward goal achievement; (4) allocation of nursing time, dollars, and staff; (5) coordination of care; (6) systematic nursing research and objective evaluation of care; (7) facilitation of placement decisions; (8) provision of objective data upon which to analyze costs, benefits, and quality of care; and (9) assistance for accreditation bodies, program evaluation, and third-party payers.

The development of client-centered assessment-classification systems has been associated with the determination of nurse staffing patterns. Formal client-centered assessment-classification systems were originally developed in acute care settings as part of an effort to allocate and assign nursing staff and resources based on the intensity of an individual's illness. An early study that had a major impact on subsequent classification attempts was conducted by the National League for Nursing (NLN) in 1937.[13] The major goal of the NLN study was to define the nursing care needs of hospitalized persons. Among the conclusions, the NLN recommended that 3.4 to 3.5 nursing hours per patient day be used as a care time guideline and that this guideline be further investigated to define the hours of nursing care required by different groupings of patients on a unit. Many hospital directors reviewed and adapted the NLN recommendation as a standard but for the most part ignored the qualification to the recommendation.[13]

During the 1940s and 1950s, nursing research indicated that some clients had similar nursing care requirements and could be classified accordingly. Another finding indicated that the intensity of a client's illness alone did not reflect the amount of nursing care needed. Often nurses found that clients who were moderately or mildly ill required more time for teaching and rehabilitation than did acutely ill clients who required treatments.[13] The studies conducted during these years included six descriptors: (1) degree of illness, (2) extent of activity, (3) number and complexity of treatments and procedures, (4) nature of adjustment, (5) teaching, and (6) rehabilitation.

With the advent of progressive patient care in the 1960s, classification of acute care patients went through three phases.[13] First, researchers concentrated on finding suitable professional versus nonprofessional nursing staff ratios. Second, they focused on the appropriate allocation of all health care resources. Third, they analyzed the 1937 NLN recommendations for nursing care time and concluded that the guidelines were no longer suitable as a basis for patient classification. This research encouraged analysis of length of stays and resulted in patient categorization based on "anticipated requirements for nursing care."[13]

The development of long-term health care (LTHC) client-centered assessment-classification systems has received attention only during the last 20 years. During the 1960s, several researchers recognized the shortcomings of applying acute care–based classification systems to the long-term care setting and sought alternatives that would address the needs of elderly, chronically ill, and disabled persons.

Burack[6] devised a four-category Interdisciplinary Classification for the Aged that described clients according to medical category, functional capacity, projected goals, and therapeutic category. McKnight[21] studied the nursing care requirements of a selected nursing home population. All of these research efforts provided insight for the future development of LTHC client-centered assessment-classification systems.[13]

In 1968 four multidisciplinary research groups from Case Western Reserve, Harvard, Johns Hopkins, and Syracuse Universities designed an assessment-classification instrument known as the Patient Classification for Long Term Care. This collaborative effort was a cornerstone in the development of subsequent LTHC assessment-classification systems. Five elements characterize the instrument: (1) it is client oriented rather than service or setting oriented; (2) it includes multidimensional assessment of 60 personal variables representing sociodemographic status, medical risk status, physical function, impairments, and

select medical conditions; (3) it employs objective terminology and guidelines; (4) it uses classification criteria deduced from empirical correlations between descriptor variables and outcomes; and (5) it incorporates flexibility so that it can be employed in a variety of settings to provide a varied amount of detail.[13] This instrument has been used to monitor the quality of care and assist LTHC policy planners. It has been used in education, training, and research.

A study that investigated the descriptor items assessed by the Patient Classification for Long Term Care was conducted by Cavaiola and Young.[8] They used the Patient Classification for Long Term Care as a basis for the development of An Integrated System for Patient Assessment and Classification and Nurse Staff Allocation for Long Term Care Facilities and identified 12 variables that yielded high appropriate prediction rates for skilled nursing and two distinctions of health-related levels of care. The following predictor variables were assigned weights through factor analysis: mobility level, walking, stair climbing, bathing, dressing, eating/feeding, toileting, behavior pattern, cigarette smoking, anemia, mental illness, and chronic respiratory care. The authors integrated the 12-variable assessment-classification system with data from nursing care time studies and constructed a model that associated client needs with the allocation of nursing staff.[8]

A noteworthy effort toward the development of valid and reliable LTHC client-centered assessment-classification systems has been made by Canadian researchers. Bay and her colleagues[1-3] proposed a sequential framework. These researchers designed a conceptual model based on four factors: demographic characteristics, physical status, psychosocial status, and self-care practices. Demographic characteristics included client descriptors similar to the Patient Classification for Long Term Care. Physical status included descriptors on extent of impairment and extent of diagnosed health problems. Psychosocial status included descriptors of level of mental functioning, personal adaptability, social adaptability, and quality of life-style. Self-care practices included descriptors of activities of daily living and therapeutics. Therapeutics was operationalized as the "patients' skill and judgment in carrying out prescribed treatments, management of medications, ability to contact health professional for assistance, and the need for supervision in managing treatments."[2] The assessment instrument also included information on the client's social and personal environment. When this instrument was tested, one of the most outstanding findings was a high interrater reliability on some of the psychosocial items.

The application of a client classification system in a rehabilitation setting to facilitate nurse staffing requires an instrument that identifies concrete domains of function to describe and predict client nursing care needs. Burgher and Hanson[7] developed a client classification system for nursing on a rehabilitation unit in response to the realization that clients involved in the rehabilitation process required different amounts of nursing care time than clients who were admitted to medical-surgical units. Reliability, validity, and ease of administration were methodological considerations in instrument development. The authors' first step was to delineate the total care indicators capable of predicting amount of nursing care required. They selected six domains of need: activities of daily living skills, bladder and bowel care, teaching/learning needs, presence or absence of aphasia, complex treatments, and behavioral problems. In selecting activities of daily living skills as a domain of care, the authors discovered a great discrepancy among nurses and other rehabilitation team members in their application of terminology to describe the client's amount of functional ability. Categories could not easily be differentiated according to the descriptor terms "standby," "independent," and "minimum, moderate, and maximum assistance." The authors increased reliability by defining dependency levels so that each category was mutually exclusive.

Clients were rated in the six domains of need and on two classification scales indicating total care needs. One scale listed four defined levels of care, and the other allowed ratings of clients according to a 10-point continuum that facilitated the comparison of a particular client to all other clients on the unit. The authors then correlated nursing care time requirements and identified three classification levels. The end product was a classification system capable of facilitating the prediction of the amount of nursing care time.

The use of nursing diagnoses is integral to the development and application of these classification systems in nursing. In addition to identifying nursing-specific client problems and potential problems, Warren[25] suggested that nursing diagnoses also (1) document nursing practice; (2) document nursing accountability; (3) facilitate communication between nurses and other health professionals by standardization of nursing terminology; (4) enhance the identification of client groups for purposes of research and long-range planning; (5) provide the foundation for quality assurance programs; (6) facilitate the research, development, and refinement of client outcome criteria, and (7) enhance the development of a computerized nursing data base, which in turn would facilitate clarification, research, theory analysis and synthesis, and evaluation of nursing practice. One cannot help but notice the similarities between the purposes of the nursing diagnosis and the overall purposes of functional evaluation in rehabilitation.

The nursing process is naturally linked to client-centered assessment-classification systems and nursing diagnoses. The nursing process is cyclical and dynamic; it organizes a myriad of information. The nurse arrives at a nursing diagnosis after a comprehensive assessment of the client that includes functional assessment. The subsequent steps of planning and implementation of interventions flow from nursing theories and the identified nursing diagnosis. The steps of evaluation necessitate scientific analysis of the client's response to the nursing interventions; consideration of intervening variables such as a complication or change in the client's physical, social, or environmental surroundings; and appraisal of the nursing resources, that is, nursing time, expertise, and dollars, that are part of the process of effecting change at the client level. Assessment, planning, implementation, and evaluation of nursing practice are major components of evaluation of the total program or process of care. An integral part of the nursing process is goal setting. Bower[5] outlines four steps in determining written goals:

1. Determine the desired outcomes.
2. Specify the nature, quality, and characteristics of the outcomes.
3. Check the outcomes to determine if they accomplish the task of meeting the need or of solving the problem.
4. Write the goal statement so that the action needed to attain the goal is included.

Stated goals address the behavioral areas: affective, psychomotor, and cognitive. Affective goals are concerned with the client's emotions, attitudes, beliefs, and feelings. Goals in the psychomotor realm are concerned with performance abilities. Cognitive goals focus on intellectual performance and the client's abilities to understand, hear, reason, analyze, and synthesize information.[5] Individuals function within all three contexts and affect and are affected by environmental situations.

The assessment of an individual's performance abilities and limitations has a direct influence on every nursing diagnosis, nursing intervention, and nursing-specific outcome criterion designed for or with the client. The client's functional status in the physical, cognitive-psychological-mental, and social spheres of life naturally impacts on the goal setting, design of interventions, and evaluation of interventions aimed at the following areas: eating and swallowing, bladder elimination, bowel elimination, sleep and rest, maintenance of skin integrity, personal hygiene and grooming, speech and language, vision and hearing, sensation and perception, movement, sexuality and sexual function, work and recreation, accessing the home and community, and coping.

Whether or not a formalized functional assessment instrument is used, the rehabilitation nurse assesses the functional status of the client and makes nursing judgments based on the information collected. Basic elements of function that influence gross and fine motor performance are endurance, stamina, strength, pain, age, physical build, sex, weight, cardiorespiratory status, coordination, and sensory status, that is, vision, hearing, vibratory sense, position, temperature, and touch. Another important influence on the ability to carry out or demonstrate motor performance is the cognitive ability to process the command and intention.

An area of necessary information in defining client needs is the determination of the degree of independence or the nature of assistance needed. The concept of independence conveys the idea that no physical assistance or supervisory assistance (the latter in the form of cueing, providing reassurance, or offering instructions) is needed. Physical assistance may take the form of help of another person or assistive equipment. The time required to perform a task also should be considered. What is gained if it takes someone 2 hours to dress just to sit in a wheelchair completely exhausted for the rest of the day if, with assistance, the same individual could be dressed in a fraction of the time but then be able to pursue a work or leisure activity?

The assessment of movement generally includes observations of the client's ability to move around in bed, transfer from one surface to another, manipulate a wheelchair, if appropriate, and ambulate. Specific items addressed in the assessment of bed mobility include the ability to roll from side to side and change position from supine to prone and vice versa. The client's ability to sit up, sitting balance, and ability to position the body in proper alignment also are assessed. In assessing transfer abilities, the nurse observes the client transferring from bed to chair or wheelchair and vice versa, into and out of a tub or shower, and on and off the toilet.

Assessment of wheelchair mobility requires observation of the client's ability to safely propel the chair, manipulate armrests and footrests, lock and unlock brakes, change position and posture, and care for the chair. Assessment of ambulation includes observation of the ability to walk and increase the distance of the walk and to ascend and descend stairs; gait pattern (foot placement); use of assistive devices; differences in performance on different floor surfaces; types of footwear; and condition of the feet.

Assessment of personal care activities of daily living includes observation of abilities in eating and swallowing, bladder and bowel elimination, grooming, bathing, and dressing. Eating and swallowing are basic to survival. Functional considerations for eating include ability to manipulate silverware, take food to the mouth, chew, open containers and packages of food, prepare meals, position self for eating, manage cups and glasses, pour liquids, and sip through a straw. The ability to eat and swallow also influences socialization because of social mores and personal feelings about eating in public in a socially acceptable manner.

Bladder continence has vital physical, social, emotional, and vocational components. Physical activity has a direct influence on bladder elimination. The natural anatomical positons for urination are a primary interest. Is the male client able to stand? Does the female client have adequate trunk stability to sit? Is the client able to drink sufficient daily fluids, or must another person govern intake? Does the client have adequate hand function and finger dexterity to perform facilitation techniques or to perform intermittent catheterization? Does the client require a wrist-hand orthosis or an assistive intermittent catheter device to improve hand and finger function? Is the client able to record intake and output? Is the client able to proceed to a toilet for urination in sufficient time to prevent incontinence?

Assessment of function when observing the client's ability to carry out the bowel program closely parallels the observation for ability in bladder elimination. Can the client assume the sitting position? Does the client have adequate hand function for cleansing and wiping after each bowel movement and for inserting a suppository? Can the client take laxatives by mouth? Is the client able to learn how to perform anal sphincter stretch when appropriate?

Functional assessment is directly linked to skin integrity. Development of pressure sores can prolong the rehabilitation process. Is the client able to inspect all skin surfaces for signs of redness and pressure? Does the client sense temperature, pressure, and pain? Does the client require special equipment such as an inspection mirror to view the back and buttocks? Is a special mattress or wheelchair cushion required?

Evaluation of the client's appearance directs attention to ability to dress and undress. Specific tasks observed include the ability to put on and take off a brassiere, blouse, polo shirt, undershirt, underpants, stockings or socks, dress, shirt, pants, shoes, and belt. The abilities of buttoning and unbuttoning, pulling a zipper up and down, and fastening and unfastening hooks and snaps are noted.

Assessment of bathing and grooming includes observation of the client's abilities to hold soap and a washcloth, wash the parts of the body, and dry the body. In addition, abilities in applying makeup, shaving, washing hair, combing and brushing hair, brushing and flossing teeth, performing denture care, and applying deodorant are observed.

The nursing process should result in nursing-specific outcome criteria. Several nurse researchers have devoted attention to the development and refinement of outcome criteria.

OUTCOME CRITERIA

When quantifiable objective functional evaluation data are used to monitor a client's functional status and when the nursing process is documented, outcomes of the nursing process are evident and

retrievable.[12] In discussing standards and criteria upon which to base evaluation of nursing practice, Ganong and Ganong[12] state:

> A standard is an acknowledged measure of comparison for quantitative or qualitative value, criterion, or norm. A criterion is a standard rule or test on which a judgment or decision can be based. It is essential to establish clinical nursing criteria against which to measure patient outcomes and the nursing process.

The development and refinement of outcome criteria based upon functional evaluation data are in their infant stages. Outcomes are the end products of a process. Client-centered outcomes in the rehabilitation process are concerned with changes in functional status. Rehabilitation nursing interventions are aimed at preventing a decline in functional status, maintaining current functional abilities, and restoring and maximizing functional independence. Outcome statements are explanations of how the client should look, feel, or act as a result of specific nursing interventions.[5] Dittmar[10] notes several issues that should be acknowledged in determining outcome criteria: (1) the feelings, behavior, knowledge, and health state of the client are affected by many factors other than nursing care; (2) many outcome criteria are not nursing specific; and (3) nurses commonly address the learning and psychosocial needs of the client, which are sometimes more covert than overt.

Bloch[4] proposes a process-outcome framework for developing outcome criteria. Her orientation toward outcome analysis favors dual consideration of the process and the expected outcome. She proposes development of client care outcome criteria by the rehabilitation team and simultaneous development of nursing-specific process-outcome criteria.

A methodology for developing outcome criteria upon which to base evaluation of nursing care of neurological clients was attempted by Waterman Taylor.[26] Her research focused on the development of an assessment instrument that would provide data to define criteria that would measure nursing care outcomes. Her approach did not specifically link the process of care with the outcomes of care in the manner recommended by Bloch[4]; however, her approach outlined several noteworthy steps involved with the process of outcome development for groups of clients: (1) definition of the clientele for whom the criteria will be applied, (2) identification of a time frame that specifies exact periods when some degree of benefit from nursing services should be evident, (3) identification of common and frequently occurring nursing problems shared by the group of clients, (4) clear statements indicating the expected result (outcome criteria), (5) specification of the realistic amount of progress toward goal achievement, (6) specification and standardization of the source of information, and (7) research and validation of a data collection instrument that would accommodate classification of clients based upon nursing care need or a common denominator reflecting nursing care need and refinement of criteria.

As stated earlier in this chapter, clients encountered in a rehabilitation setting share the common denominator of altered function. Rehabilitation nurses are challenged to address the issue of identifying client needs in direct relation to functional ability. Functional integrity may be compromised quite differently among clients sharing a common medical diagnosis, but nursing diagnoses are self-limiting. Goals derived from nursing diagnoses lend themselves to the development of outcome criteria that capture the change in the client's ability to perform in response to the planned nursing interventions. Although many changes in the client's level of functioning are the result of a collaborative effort involving the interdisciplinary team, nurses are responsible for assisting the client in performing physical, intellectual, and social functions. After discharge from a rehabilitation setting, the results of nurses' health teaching, adaptation to modified or different life-styles, and the management of complications could be measured.[26]

The measurement of outcomes in a rehabilitation setting is not new and has been used most often in the vocational/employment aspects of rehabilitation efforts. Recently, attempts have been made to develop long-term outcomes linked to independent living. Such long-term outcomes have relevancy at the social policy level as shown by DeJong and Hughes.[9] Their work centered on two issues against which the success of rehabilitation is judged at the social policy level: (1) the client being rehabilitated so as to live in the least restrictive environment and (2) the client becoming a productive member of society insofar as employment and community or social roles.[9] Reha-

bilitation nurses, as well as members of the rehabilitation team, design interventions that lead to increasing levels of independence that facilitate these outcomes. The authors acknowledge that these outcomes are not appropriate to all clients receiving rehabilitation services; however, their investigation shows how outcome measures can be developed by statistical means and applied at the long-range planning level.

SUMMARY

The current state of the art in functional assessment methodology and the number of available instruments suggest that the 1980s bear fruitful research efforts aimed at standardizing the measurement of functional status. The advantages of employing quantifiable and objective functional evaluation systems in rehabilitation are evident.

Quantifying functional evaluation is an invaluable methodology for guiding and enhancing the present and future planning and delivery of rehabilitation nursing care. The evaluation of nursing care based upon qualitatively and statistically questionable assessment instruments perpetuates inaccuracy, waste, and inadequate recognition of nursing resources and their potential effects. The application of quantified methodologies based on functional evaluation is an aspect of nursing care whose time is long overdue.

REFERENCES

1. Bay KS, Leatt P, and Stinson SS: Cross-validation of a patient classification procedure: an application of the U Method, Med Care 21:31, 1983.
2. Bay KS, Leatt P, and Stinson SS: A patient-classification system for long term care, Med Care 20:468, 1982.
3. Bay KS, Leatt P, and Stinson SS: An instrument for assessing and classifying patients by type of care, Nurs Res 30:145, 1981.
4. Bloch D: Evaluation of nursing care in terms of process and outcome, Nurs Res 24:256, 1975.
5. Bower FL: The process of planning nursing care: nursing practice models, ed 3, St. Louis, 1982, The CV Mosby Co.
6. Burack B: Interdisciplinary classification for the aged, J Chronic Dis 18:1059, 1965.
7. Burgher D and Hanson RL: Patient classification for nurse staffing in rehabilitation, ARN J 5:16, June 1980.
8. Cavaiola L and Young JP: An integrated system for patient assessment and classification and nurse staff

allocation for long term care facilities, Health Services Res 15:281, 1981.

9. DeJong G and Hughes J: Independent living: methodology for measuring long-term outcomes, Arch Phys Med Rehabil 63:68, Feb 1982.

10. Dittmar SS: Functional assessment in nursing. In Granger CV and Gresham GE, editors: Functional assessment in rehabilitation medicine, Baltimore, 1984, The Williams & Wilkins Co.

11. Foley WJ and Schneider DP: A comparison of the level of care predictions of six long-term care patient assessment systems, Am J Pub Health 70:1152, 1982.

12. Ganong JM and Ganong WL: Nursing management, ed 2, Germantown, Md, 1980, Aspen Systems Corp.

13. Giovannetti PBJ: Patient classification systems in nursing: a description and analysis, Hyattsville, Md, 1978, Health Resources Administration.

14. Granger CV: A conceptual model for functional assessment. In Granger CV and Gresham GE, editors: Functional assessment in rehabilitation medicine, Baltimore, 1984, The Williams & Wilkins Co.

15. Granger CV and Greer DS: Functional status measurement and medical rehabilitation outcomes, Arch Phys Med Rehabil 57:103, March 1976.

16. Granger CV and McNamara MA: Functional assessment utilization: the Long-Range Evaluation System (LRES). In Granger CV and Gresham GE, editors: Functional assessment in rehabilitation medicine, Baltimore, 1984, The Williams & Wilkins Co.

17. Gresham GE and Labi MLC: Functional assessment instruments currently available for documenting outcomes in rehabilitation medicine. In Granger CV and Gresham GE, editors: Functional assessment in rehabilitation medicine, Baltimore, 1984, The Williams & Wilkins Co.

18. Keith RA: Functional assessment measures in medical rehabilitation: current status, Arch Phys Med Rehabil 65 74, Feb 1984.

19. Lawton MP: The functional assessment of elderly people, J Am Geriatr Soc 19:465, 1971.

20. Mahoney FI and Barthel DW: Functional evaluation: the Barthel Index, Md State Med J 14:61, Feb 1965.

21. McKnight EM: Nursing home research study: quantitative measurement of nursing services, Bethesda, Md, 1971, US DHEW, Public Health Service, National Institute of Health, Bureau of Health Manpower Education, Division of Nursing.

22. Moskowitz E and McCann CB: Classification of disability in the chronically ill and aging. J Chronic Dis 5:342, 1957.

23. Schoening H and others: Numerical scoring of self care status of patients, Arch Phys Med Rehabil 46:689, 1965.

24. Task Force for Development of a Uniform Data System for Medical Rehabilitation: Uniform data system for medical rehabilitation, Buffalo, NY, 1986, Project Office, Department of Rehabilitation Medicine, Buffalo General Hospital.

25. Warren JJ: Accountability and nursing diagnoses, J Nurs Admin 13:34, Oct 1983.

26. Waterman Taylor J: Measuring the outcomes of nursing care, Nurs Clin North Am 9:337, 1974.

ADDITIONAL READINGS

Abdellah FG and Levine E: Better patient care through nursing research, ed 2, New York, 1979, Macmillan Publishing Co, Inc.

Austin E: How your nursing notes can rob your patients of benefits, Am J Nurs 78:58, Sept 1978.

Clark GS: Functional assessment in the elderly. In Williams TF: Rehabilitation in the aging, New York, 1984, Raven Press.

Crewe NM and Athelstan GT: Functional assessment in vocational rehabilitation: a systematic approach to diagnosis and goal setting, Arch Phys Med Rehabil 62:299, 1981.

Harvey RF and Jellinek HM: Functional performance assessment: a program approach, Arch Phys Med Rehabil 62:456, 1981.

Jacelon CS: The Barthel Index and other indices of functional ability, Rehabil Nurs 11:9, July/Aug 1986.

Jette AM: Functional capacity evaluation: an empirical approach, Arch Phys Med Rehabil 61:85, Feb 1980.

Katz S and others: Chronic disease classification in evaluation of medical care programs, Med Care 7:149, March/April 1969.

Posavac EJ and Carey RG: A method of program evaluation in rehabilitation settings, ARN J 4:5, July/Aug 1979.

Rameizl P: A case for assessment technology in long term care: the nursing perspective, Rehabil Nurs 9:29, Nov/Dec 1984.

CHAPTER 24

Quality Assurance:
Is Your Practice Effective?

Barbara Wisnom

OBJECTIVES

After completing Chapter 24, the reader will be able to:

1. Explain the relationship of quality assurance to professional nursing practice.

2. Define quality assurance.

3. List the basic components of a quality assurance system.

4. Identify the steps in the quality assurance process.

5. Discuss the relevance of quality assurance to the daily practice of rehabilitation nursing.

6. Apply a quality assurance model to measure the effectiveness of rehabilitation nursing care.

Belief in the individuality of the client and the role of the client in the rehabilitation process is basic to the premise that rehabilitation is integral to all nursing. Application of these beliefs to actual practice requires more than the knowledge and skill needed to execute them. It requires a commitment to excellence in the practice of rehabilitation nursing. More broadly, it requires commitment to the profession of nursing. Acknowledgment of accountability to the public, the client, and the profession is a characteristic of the professional. Being a professional is not a right. It is an earned privilege and a public trust. As such, it demands accountability as a moral and ethical duty. "A profession's concern for the quality of its service constitutes the heart of its responsibility to the public."[1]

To fulfill this responsibility, assurances must be made that the best care possible is given to clients. A system designed to measure, evaluate, and improve care, which has gained wide acceptance among health care professionals, is known as quality assurance. Simply put, it means providing the best care possible within available resources. This chapter deals with quality assurance and its application to the practice of professional rehabilitation nursing.

WHAT IS QUALITY ASSURANCE AND WHY IS IT NEEDED?

Professional nursing has been evaluating the quality of care it delivers for a number of years. As early as 1939, attempts were made to assess not only the quantity but also the quality of nursing service.[3] It was not until the 1960s, however, that the issue of evaluating quality became more widely applied. The Medicare legislation of 1965 addressed the standards of the Joint Commission on Accreditation of Hospitals (JCAH)* as norms by which the quality of care provided should be assessed.[6] Additional impetus was provided in 1972 by the passage of Public Law 92-603, which mandated professional standards review organizations.[3,11] These organizations were primarily physician-dominated review processes designed to evaluate medical care. The American Academy of Nursing responded shortly thereafter by stating "nurses should be included in quality assurance review organizations. . . ."[11] In 1974 the American Nurses' Association was awarded a contract by the federal government to develop methodologies "to measure the quality and effectiveness of nursing care."[3] Since that time, a variety of systems have been designed to improve quality through an evaluation of care.

To determine whether quality care has been given, the element of quality must first be defined. Criteria must be developed by which care can be measured uniformly. The process for doing this began with peer review efforts on a limited scale. Problems were identified through review of the client's medical record. The process was known as the audit system and was adopted primarily because it was systematic and objective. It incorporated a multidisciplinary study approach to review and could be applied to practice settings with uniformity.

Although the audit concept was sound, its application was often cumbersome. Many audit systems were designed so that methods and requirements of performing audits became the focus, rather than the correction of problems and the improvement of care.[8] Trying to learn the system was difficult. Frequently, individuals selected to serve on audit committees were the only ones who understood and used the system. Seldom did grass roots staff see, much less apply, final audit study results. Despite the fact that the system had the potential to improve quality of care, it frequently fell short of its goal. Consequently, the impact on the actual delivery of care to the client was rarely felt. Through attempts to determine

why audits were not effective, it became apparent that the reason was in the focus of the review process. Audits looked at paper, not at people!

The Joint Commission introduced the quality assurance standard in the 1979 *Accreditation Manual For Hospitals*. The initial interpretation of the standard was the application of the audit concept. JCAHO has studied and evaluated the system since its inclusion in the standards, and has continued to make modifications in an attempt to improve it. A new level of maturity was reached with the introduction of the 1984 standard. It described the quality assurance program as one "designed to enhance patient care through an ongoing objective assessment of important aspects of patient care and the correction of identified problems."[5] Subsequent revisions, including those published for 1988, have further refined this process. Although the basic goal remains the same—improving the quality of care—the method through which it can be achieved has changed considerably. Rather than depending primarily on a set number of medical record studies, components of care provided to clients are now an integral part of an ongoing monitoring and evaluation process. The primary target for improvement is people and not paper.

It would seem, then, that the charge of the profession to be accountable to the public, the client, and itself can be accomplished through a system of quality assurance.

Definitions

Among the various definitions of quality, a common one is a "degree or grade of excellence"; and of assurance, "a pledge or a guarantee." Quality assurance, therefore, can be stated as a "pledge of excellence." This definition is compatible with the simple definition given earlier: providing the best possible care within available resources. Other definitions come from a variety of sources but have essentially the same message. The JCAHO refers to quality assurance as a "program designed to objectively and systematically monitor and evaluate the quality and appropriateness of patient care, pursue opportunities to improve patient care, and resolve identified problems."[5] Zimmer[11] defines quality assurance as the implementation of a "systematic evaluation to make sure that delivered care is at the optimum achievable degree of excellence . . . and to continuously

---

*The JCAH acronym was changed in 1987 to JCAHO, the Joint Commission on Accreditation of Health Care Organizations, to more accurately reflect the wider range and diversity of health care providers that the organization serves.

take action to secure improvements." Dixon, Hopkins, and Walczak[4] define it as "the institution of formalized mechanisms for ensuring the detection and correction of factors hindering the provision of optimal achievable health care. . . ."

Importance of Quality Assurance

The abstract concept of a commitment to excellence can be translated into action in a variety of ways. One way is through professional accountability, which in turn must also be translated into action. Assuring the delivery of the best possible care is a means of doing this. If quality assurance is defined as a pledge of excellence, then the commitment to excellence can be realized through the use of its concepts in the rehabilitation nursing setting. Before this can be done, the importance of quality assurance must be grasped. If it is to be an effective system for evaluating and improving the care delivered to clients, it must be pertinent, meaningful, and easily applied to daily practice. To that end, a discussion of the importance of quality assurance to the individual rehabilitation nurse, to the client, to the institution, and to the public follows.

Individual rehabilitation nurse

If nursing is to control its own destiny, efforts toward quality assurance must begin within the profession itself. Only then can nursing collaborate with other professionals and with clients in the development of quality assurance systems of a broader scope. The concept of team, so important to rehabilitation, cannot be realized until each of the disciplines addresses its own concerns. Rehabilitation nurses therefore must first set down their own standards before they, with other disciplines and the client, can all work together to ensure quality care.

A joint committee of the American Nurses' Association Division on Medical-Surgical Nursing Practice and the Association of Rehabilitation Nurses did in fact establish such standards in 1977.[2] These standards, revised in 1986, will be used to demonstrate the applicability of quality assurance to rehabilitation nursing.[1]

Quality assurance is a vehicle for professional accountability through which care is evaluated, problems are identified, and corrective actions are monitored for effectiveness. Its significance lies in the ability of the system to continuously let the

rehabilitation nurse know about the quality of care given and the capability for providing that care. It provides an opportunity for the nurse to demonstrate a level of excellence using an objective approach with measurable results.

According to the JCAHO standards, nursing not only is responsible for the process of quality assurance, but also is charged with agreeing "on objective criteria that reflect current knowledge and clinical experience."[5] This statement recognizes the responsibility of nursing to be accountable to itself and the public trust through the development of methods for self-evaluation. This accountability does not preclude the involvement of other health care professionals, nor is it inconsistent with the team concept. Rather, it places "the primary focus [of the provision of nursing service] on the appraisal of quality through nursing methods developed and applied by nurses."[7] The *Standards of Rehabilitation Nursing Practice* represent a step in the development of such methods.

Client

When beset with an illness or disability, the client's energies are directed toward coping with the effect of that illness on present and future lifestyle. The assumption is made that those to whom the client has entrusted body and soul have the same goal in mind: to make the client well. The client further assumes, if thinking about it at all, that those who will make him or her well are qualified to do so. The client no more asks to see the educational credentials of the staff than does an airplane passenger ask to see the pilot's license! Nor should the client have to. The client has a right to expect the care received is of the highest possible quality. Furthermore, in this age of individual rights, the client demands quality care. Is this then automatic? Does the assumption lead to the fact? Of course not. The burden of proof is on the professional. Through use of an objective and systematic process of continuous evaluation and improvement, assurance can be made to the client of the best possible care, delivered safely, efficiently, and cost effectively. This process can be accomplished with quality assurance.

Quality assurance has other implications for clients, not only in the delivery of care but also in other timely issues. Cost-effective health care is a prime example. An efficient, well-defined quality assurance system has the capability of demonstrating that cost-effectiveness and quality are not mutually exclusive terms. In fact, one of the primary goals of quality assurance is cost-effectiveness.

Institution

Many of the elements that make quality assurance important to both nurse and client also are significant to management and the institution. The goals of these bodies do not conflict with the goals of the individual practitioner or the client. All desire quality. Management and the institution are accountable to the client and the public, much the same as the nurse. The institution and those responsible for running it want to know the capability of the staff for providing quality care. They too want to be able to demonstrate a level of excellence. A management commitment to quality assurance is a means of ensuring a reliable system that will, on an ongoing basis, monitor, evaluate, and improve care. Insistence on such a program, as well as active involvement on the part of management, further ensures that an awareness of quality will become a part of everyday life.

Other areas in which management is concerned with the implementation of a quality assurance system are related to complying with the requirements of the JCAHO and other accrediting and licensing agencies and to recognizing and meeting legal issues of professional liability (malpractice). The wise manager will recognize quality assurance as a management tool that will facilitate the accomplishment of institutional objectives.

Public

Accountability to the public trust is achievable through quality assurance. Why should healthy members of society be concerned with quality care or the lack of it within the four walls of a building that provides health care? Several reasons come to mind. One of these says, "If I'm not sick today, I could be tomorrow," or "One of my relatives could become ill." In that sense everyone, whether healthy or not, is concerned about quality care. The general population, however, does not usually deal with things that may affect them in the future, even if the future is tomorrow. So why the concern? Why do "letters to the editor" from lay people ask probing questions and make thought-provoking statements about the health care delivery system? The reason is quite simple—money! A significant portion of our gross national product is spent for health care. As inflation nibbles away at the income of the wage earner, the question of how and where dollars are spent becomes a major concern of the public. The consumer is becoming more discriminating. Despite the trend toward controlling one's well-being by keeping fit, one still does not have total control over disease and disability. So while a person may opt for purchasing foreign-made cars because they are perceived to be of higher quality, that option is not realistic when one becomes ill. The public expects, as does the client, that when health care is sought it not only will be of the highest quality possible but also will be affordable. Quality and affordability do not have to occupy opposite ends of the spectrum. Remember that a goal of quality assurance is to provide cost-effective care. It is no less than a responsible answer to the public trust.

ELEMENTS OF A QUALITY ASSURANCE SYSTEM

Now that a framework has been established defining the need for and importance of quality assurance, the basic elements of the system are presented. Knowledge of these elements is required before it can be applied to the rehabilitation practice setting.

First, the system must be a planned, systematic and ongoing process, a part of everyday life. It is not intended to be self-limiting, random, or haphazard.

Second, it must identify important aspects of client care that will be monitored. That is, its impact should be felt primarily at the bedside and not in the medical record. Review of the medical record is nonetheless important to the evaluation process and is included in the discussion.

Third, it must objectively and systematically assess both the cause and the scope of identified problems. It is important to evaluate why problems are occurring and how far they reach before appropriate action can be taken to correct them.

Fourth, priorities reflective of an impact on care must be established for the investigation and resolution of problems. Since problems do not occur in isolation and since resources to resolve them are not limitless, resolution must be focused on those having the greatest impact on care.

Fifth, actions must be initiated that will, as much as possible, eliminate identified problems.

Although it is recognized that not all problems can be completely resolved, it is expected that conscientious efforts will be made to at least minimize the potential for adverse effects on client care, while at the same time pursuing opportunities to improve care.

Sixth, actions implemented shall be monitored and tracked to assure that the desired result has been achieved and is sustained.

Last, the system must represent evaluation of care provided by all disciplines. Data obtained through the quality assurance system may then serve as an objective basis for staff appraisal via evaluation of clinical competence and performance.[5]

A quality assurance system, then, is one of continuous monitoring and evaluation of the quality and appropriateness of care through which problems are identified, corrective action is taken to resolve them, and the solutions are monitored for effectiveness. Opportunities to improve care are pursued, even when specific problems are not identified. The system is by nature flexible and dynamic. It can be accomplished by the staff nurse during interactions with clients. It can be designed in such a way that it interferes hardly at all with daily practice and lends itself well to multidisciplinary involvement. It is to be designed to meet the needs of the individual institution and the client population it serves. The system itself is to be evaluated and modified so that it is continuously effective in improving client care and is conducted in a cost-effective manner.[5]

How is this accomplished? A sophisticated approach with a shift in focus emerged with the JCAHO's system of continuous monitoring introduced in the 1984 standards. Initially a six-step process, it evolved in 1987 to nine steps. Just as the nature of health care is dynamic, so too is the nature of the JCAHO's standards, which will no doubt continue to evolve and be modified. Such modifications must therefore be looked upon not as a change of rules designed to frustrate harried hospital and nursing administrators (whose frustration inevitably filters down to staff) but as responsive and responsible modifications intended to be state-of-the-art standards. Given the opportunity for objective thought, one would not want the standards to stay the same, since they would not be useful to the professional practitioner as a guide to governing day-to-day practice.

Regardless of the number of steps printed in current JCAHO literature, the concept in a broad sense is essentially the same. Professional nurses must first define what they do that sets them apart and identifies them as professionals. This is accomplished through the setting of professional standards by peer groups both external to and within organizations. Once external and internal standards have been defined, the professional nurse must measure actual clinical practice against those standards using agency-specific criteria. The measurement will determine whether the practice meets or does not meet accepted and recognized standards as defined by peers. If practice is not consistent with existing standards, the professional nurse has a duty to take definitive steps to ensure that practice is improved to meet standards. Practice must continue to be monitored and evaluated to ensure continuing compliance with standards. Furthermore, as standards change to meet the changing face of health care delivery, practice must change and must be monitored continuously to ensure that it is responsive to the changes in standards.

APPLICATION OF QUALITY ASSURANCE TO REHABILITATION NURSING

To demonstrate how the basic elements of a quality assurance system can be applied to the practice of rehabilitation nursing, the process described is discussed in further detail. Standards and criteria specific to a rehabilitation setting have been chosen to illustrate the process.

Standards and Criteria Development

Each discipline is responsible for determining in advance standards to be monitored that affect client care. Once the standards are established, criteria are identified that define how each standard is met. These criteria are the specific means by which the professional nurse applies a standard to actual practice. It is incumbent on the professional to define not only what is important relative to client care, but also the skills, competencies, and judgments required to provide that care.[9] Criteria must be set down before determinations can be made about the presence or absence of quality care. Criteria define the elements of quality.

The decision about what criteria to use does not necessarily have to be difficult. Before making the decision, however, some ground rules need to be established if the system is to be effective. Criteria should be realistic, readily retrievable, and mutually agreed upon by the staff members who will be using them. "Realistic" means that the criteria should be applicable to the practice setting where they will be used and understood by those who will be using them. "Easily retrievable" means a minimum amount of staff time will be needed to review for their presence or absence. As much as possible, the staff using the criteria should agree about them in advance. Diversity of opinion is to be expected, of course, but unless there is at least general agreement, the staff will not use and apply the criteria consistently and uniformly. If there are strong differences of opinion about a particular criterion on the part of many of the staff members, it can be removed from the list for the time being. Agreement on criteria increases cooperation and is crucial to the effectiveness of the review process, particularly in the beginning of a program.

The next step in criteria development is the actual selection. Agency policies and procedures are a frequent source of criteria. These materials often have their roots in standards of practice established by experts in a particular field. Examples include the *Standards of Rehabilitation Nursing Practice* published in 1977 and revised in 1986 and the *Rehabilitation Nursing Standards* published by the JCAHO. Nurses working in a rehabilitation setting may decide to use these as a guide for writing policies and procedures and expand upon them to address the needs of the client population served.

The molding of nationally recognized and accepted rehabilitation nursing standards in this way provides assurance that care delivered to clients is based upon accepted scientific principles and theories of rehabilitation nursing; that the practitioners providing the care are guided by these principles and theories; that the management of the institution acknowledges the standards as benchmarks of quality and as levels of excellence to be attained; and that the *Rehabilitation Nursing Standards* will be used as the basis for evaluation of the care delivered. The *Standards of Medical-Surgical Nursing Practice*, from which the *Rehabilitation Nursing Standards* evolved, "provide a basic model to guide the development of criteria for evaluation of the quality of nursing. . . ."[2] Standards tell the individual rehabilitation nurse what is generally expected,

whereas policies and procedures provide the mechanics for application of the standards.

Professional Practice Standard IV of the *Standards of Rehabilitation Nursing Practice* states, "The nurse intervenes as guided by the individual care plan to prevent complications and promote, maintain or restore the individual's physical and psychosocial function at a realistic, optimal level. Nursing actions are consistent with the total rehabilitation program to achieve patient goals."[1] The process criteria state that the "nurse acts to ensure that rehabilitation care and goals are met by using nursing skills, such as teaching self-care . . . [the nurse] reviews and modifies interventions based on patient progress . . . and documents interventions and their effects on the client."[1]

The JCAHO's Physical Rehabilitation Services Standard, specific to rehabilitation nursing services, also addresses the use of the nursing process with the express goal of preventing complications and restoring the client to optimum function. These standards specify that rehabilitation nursing services will include interventions for physical care, including transfers of clients from one surface to another.[5]

These two standards serve as a base for the development of agency-specific policies and procedures that will guide the rehabilitation nurse in practice. Using both of these standards as a guide, staff members of the rehabilitation unit write policies and procedures covering general principles for all transfer techniques; techniques specific to certain disabilities (paraplegia, hemiplegia), transfers to and from surfaces (beds, wheelchairs), and definitive types of transfers (standing or sitting while needing total, partial, or no assistance). When broken down into component parts, the steps of the procedure become amenable to inclusion in a procedure for transfers. Translation of such procedural elements into evaluation criteria can now be accomplished (Figure 24-1).

Monitoring and Evaluation

Monitoring and evaluation constitute the second step in the process. This step determines whether problems are occurring. Criteria must be displayed in such a way that an evaluator can readily retrieve data needed to make an evaluation. A standardized format for data collection should be

---

Step 1   Use of *Standards of Rehabilitation Nursing Practice* and the Joint Commission's *Rehabilitation Nursing Services Standards* as resources

Step 2   Selection of specific standards

       A. *Standards of Rehabilitation Nursing Practice*

           Standard IV
              "The nurse intervenes . . . to prevent complications and promote, maintain, or restore . . . physical function."
           Process criteria 1-3
              "The nurse acts to ensure that rehabilitation care and goals are met by using nursing skills such as teaching self-care . . ., reviews and modifies interventions based on patient progress, . . . and documents interventions."

       B. Joint Commission's *Rehabilitation Nursing Services Standards*

           Standard Rh. 2.7.1
              Nursing interventions are designed to prevent complications and restore optimal function.
           Standard Rh 2.7.1.2
              Nursing interventions will include physical care for transfers of patients from one surface to another.

Step 3   Development of policies and procedures based on standards covering general principles for all transfer techniques by a committee of staff nurses

Step 4   Use of elements of the procedures as evaluation criteria

---

Figure 24-1
Criteria development using professional standards of practice.

developed. A sample of such a form is offered in Figure 24-2. This form should be used by all staff nurses as they participate in the evaluation.

The nursing staff members are instructed in the use of the form and are told to observe another staff member when the actual transfer is taking place. Both nurse and client behaviors are observed according to the items on the form. Either presence or absence of behaviors (criteria) is indicated by a check mark placed in the appropriate column. Comments are made to clarify or expand a particular point. The evaluator follows up with a client interview and a chart review. Evaluators are cautioned to make as few judgments as possible. For example, a "yes" response should not be given because the evaluator knows the staff member well and knows that person would "probably have put the client's shoes on, but she forgot." The response should be "no" because observation reveals the client had no shoes on. What the staff member usually does or might have

done is not being evaluated. The *actual* performance is.

A review of the responses will show the areas of weakness and reveal specifically why and how the standard is not being met. Lack of good body mechanics or instructions to clients would be readily apparent. Deficiencies in documentation of the nursing process also will be noted. This type of monitoring provides a three-part review: actual practice, client perception, and documentation. The criteria used are realistic and easily retrievable. Mutual agreement upon them is assumed because they originated from a procedure developed by a committee of staff nurses who used the *Standards of Rehabilitation Nursing Practice* and the JCAHO's *Rehabilitation Nursing Services Standards* as guides. Notations of deficiencies will help identify problem areas.

The example cited is just one of many lists of criteria that can be developed and implemented by rehabilitation nursing staff members involved

TRANSFER TECHNIQUES

INSTRUCTIONS TO THE EVALUATOR: Sometime during your shift, please complete this three-part review.

Part I: As unobtrusively as possible, observe another staff member performing the procedure described below. Make a check mark under the "yes" column if the staff member or the client is performing according to the description listed; put a check mark under the "no" column if the staff member or client is not. Under "comments" enter the code number and category of the staff member performing the procedure (for example, RN no. 012, LPN no. 076), and any other explanatory comments that are indicated.

OBSERVABLE CRITERIA	YES	NO	COMMENTS
A *Preparation*			
1. Client dressed properly (shoes, brace, and so on)			
2. Has transfer belt on			
3. Wheelchair positioned properly			
4. Safety considered (brakes, footrests)			
B. *Beginning the transfer*			
1. Client reaches sitting position in proper manner			
2. Nurse observes client for safety and balance			
3. Nurse is correctly positioned to assist client			
C. *Effecting the transfer*			
1. Nurse instructs and assists client in proper movements before standing			
2. Nurse uses proper body mechanics			
3. Nurse assists client to standing position using proper safety methods			
4. Nurse gives client time to achieve balance			
5. Nurse assists client into chair using proper method			
6. Client appears comfortable			

Part II: Within a reasonable time after the procedure is completed and when the client is resting comfortably, ask the client the following questions. Put check marks in the column appropriate to the client's response. Add other comments if necessary.

INTERVIEW CRITERIA	YES	NO	COMMENTS
1. Did the nurse explain the procedure to you?			
2. Did you understand what was explained?			
3. Did the nurse give you a chance to ask questions?			
4. Did the nurse give you enough time to prepare for the transfer?			
5. Did you feel safe?			
6. What comments or suggestions do you have so this could be easier or better for you?			

Figure 24-2
Quality Assurance Data Collection Form.   *Continued.*

TRANSFER TECHNIQUES—cont'd

Part III: After observing the procedure and interviewing the client, review the client's chart. Mark "yes" if the criterion element is present and "no" if it is not. Add comments as necessary.

DOCUMENTATION REVIEW	YES	NO	COMMENTS
1. Assessment of client's ability to transfer including status of: a. Physical condition b. Mobility c. Strength d. Endurance e. Balance f. Comprehension g. Motivation 2. Nursing diagnosis reflective of results of assessment 3. Type of transfer to be used 4. Equipment used 5. Evidence of instruction and comprehension 6. Client response to transfer to include a. Physical status b. Degree of mobility, strength, endurance, and balance c. Statements of how client felt about transfer 7. Evidence of client's ability to effect this kind of transfer 8. Modification of transfer plan to meet client's needs (if indicated)			

Figure 24-2, cont'd
Quality Assurance Data Collection Form.

in an evaluation of their own nursing care. It is not difficult to project how this method can be adapted to other standards and pertinent policies and procedures to be used, as in the process of criteria development.

The individual rehabilitation unit staff members decide in advance what policies and procedures to review. When the criteria are realistic, easily retrievable, and mutually agreed upon, all can participate with relative ease and a degree of interest. They will know ahead of time what is expected of them, both from the evaluator's and the practitioner's perspective. In fact, this methodology frequently raises the consciousness of the

staff to the point where the evaluator may find only minor deficiencies. Woody says that "people tend to perform most consistently those activities that are measured most frequently."[10]

Before the remaining steps are presented, note how this system can be used to monitor a number of procedures or aspects of client care simultaneously. The involvement of the entire professional staff is maintained, since they have selected the procedures to be reviewed and participate in the monitoring process.

The Quality Assurance Evaluation Assignment Sheet displays a proposed schedule for monitoring several aspects of care on a rehabilitation unit

	Week during which review and evaluation are to be done											
Procedures to be evaluated	Week 1	Week 2	Week 3	Week 4	Week 5	Week 6	Week 7	Week 8	Week 9	Week 10	Week 11	Week 12
Transfer techniques	A	B	C	D	E	F	G	A	B	C	D	E
Bed positioning	B	C	D	E	F	G	A	B	C	D	E	F
Preventive skin care	C	D	E	F	G	A	B	C	D	E	F	G
Bladder training	D	E	F	G	A	B	C	D	E	F	G	A
Bowel training	E	F	G	A	B	C	D	E	F	G	A	B

Reviews to be conducted by:	Day-shift RNs	Evening-shift RNs	Night-shift RN
	A	E	G
	B	F	
	C		
	D		

Figure 24-3
Quality Assurance Evaluation Assignment Sheet.

(Figure 24-3). Assume that the unit is staffed by four registered nurses on the day shift (*A, B, C,* and *D*), two on the evening shift (*E* and *F*), and one on the night shift (*G*). There also are other staff members working these shifts (licensed practical nurses and nurse assistants), the number appropriate to an average client census of 35. The professional nursing staff members select and decide on procedures to review using the Quality Assurance Data Collection Form. During a 1-week period, each registered nurse reviews and evaluates one client-staff interaction per week involving the procedure assigned. The data collection forms are kept in a central location so they are readily accessible to all staff. At the end of 4 weeks, each registered nurse has completed a reasonable number of client-staff interaction reviews.

The review has included the direct care provided, the client's response to the care, and the documentation. Over a period of 12 weeks, each registered nurse has participated in approximately the same number of procedure reviews. In addition, each procedure has been reviewed a total of 12 times, allowing for sufficient data collection.

According to the chart (Figure 24-3), five procedures were chosen by the staff of the rehabilitation unit for review. All of the procedures have a basis in the standards cited previously. Seven registered nurses were included in the review process, and all three shifts were represented. Each nurse conducted only one review per week. At the beginning of the next 12-week period, a number of options are available for continued monitoring and evaluation of care:

1. The same five procedures can be maintained for further review.
2. Any of the five can be deleted, and new procedures can be added.
3. All five can be eliminated, and five new procedures can be added for review.

The decision should be based on the results of the evaluations conducted. This will be discussed under "Problem identification."

The advantages of this method include:

1. A number of rehabilitation procedures are continuously monitored and evaluated.
2. No one individual on the staff is overburdened with too many reviews at one time.
3. All professional nursing staff members are included in the review process, and not just supervisory or administrative personnel.
4. The number of client-staff interactions evaluated is sufficient to allow for adequate data collection over a given period of time.
5. Review occurs as a part of routine work.
6. Nursing staff members are being updated continually on policies and procedures.

With several areas of care monitored by all of the professional staff, deficiencies in care and variations in standards will be noted on a more timely basis. The notation of deficiencies and variations leads to the third step in the quality assurance process—problem identification.

Problem Identification

The results of the criteria reviews are evaluated as they are completed by the individual nurse, and later on, collectively. Problems are then identified in two ways: (1) those that occur only once and are corrected immediately, and (2) those that occur on an ongoing basis and are observed for patterns or trends. Woody cautions evaluators against making generalizations too quickly when performing reviews. She cites "inadequate and insufficient data collection, and . . . premature action on inadequate information"[10] resulting in inaccurate conclusions. This is sound advice when using results obtained during an evaluation of criteria.

The nurses performing the review should understand the functions of problem identification ahead of time. One is to provide an opportunity to follow up on specific individual problems as they occur. Follow-up is done especially when these problems or deficiencies may adversely af-

fect the client if not corrected immediately (safety considerations, for example). The second is that less serious deficiencies (charting, for instance) are tracked over a period of time to observe for trends. An example is lack of nurse documentation regarding the client's level of understanding. Is it a one-time occurrence, or do nurses frequently neglect to document this element? The answer remains uncertain until the element is evaluated each time the procedure review is done and then is tracked over a period of time.

Deficiencies are displayed in the aggregate and monitored for patterns or trends. After a period of time, sufficient data will be available to identify problem areas. Problems will appear either insidiously or suddenly.

Consider a specific example. If transfer techniques are being monitored, there may be only one or two deficiencies noted the first month the review is done, then two or three the second, five the third, and six or seven during the fourth month. This gradual rise might not be noticed until after four or five months of review. It might be attributed to the fact that not all clients using transfer techniques were being evaluated or to the fact that the staff tended to do well in the beginning because they knew they were being evaluated but reverted to old habits as they became more comfortable with the process. What is significant, however, is that the problem may never have been noticed if the evaluations had not been conducted. By observing an insidious rise, deficiencies can be corrected before a major problem occurs. Assume the deficiency is "wheelchair brakes are not locked." One or two occurrences might be considered aberrations and corrected at the time on an individual basis. However, a gradual rise in the neglect of this important safety activity could result in a serious injury to a client if not brought to the attention of the entire staff.

Problems also may be identified when there is a sudden rise in a particular deficiency. Using the previous example, there may have been one or two deficiencies noted in the first few months of review. Suddenly, during the fourth month, the number of deficiencies jumps to 12! Again, the staff nurses who routinely review the data collection sheets would see this sudden rise immediately and should investigate the cause: more float personnel on duty than usual; a new employee on the unit; or malfunctioning wheelchair brakes. Regardless of the cause, corrective action must be initiated to resolve the problem. Problems should be corrected at the lowest level possible. Resolution should be as timely as practical and directly involve the person who is deficient.

When a problem is identified through an insidious or sudden rise in the number of deficiencies, that trend must be investigated to determine the cause. The scope is already known in most cases, having been defined by the number of deficiencies. When an investigation begins, more information may become known about the scope of the problem. If the cause is not readily apparent or attributable to an obvious cause (a new employee not familiar with procedures, for example), then more information is needed.

Since the reasons for problems are many, a few words are indicated regarding the importance of investigating the cause before taking corrective action. Remember Woody's advice about not making hasty judgments based on too little information. It is applicable here.

Causes can be internal (involving the staff of the rehabilitation unit) or external (involving other departments or staff). Causes may or may not be easy to control. If they fall outside the usual scope of the rehabilitation unit (budget and staffing decisions, for example), they probably will be more difficult to control and therefore to resolve. If corrective action is to be appropriate to the cause of the problem (and it must be to achieve sustained resolution), then identifying the cause is just as important as identifying the problem.

Consider this. When monitoring transfer techniques, assume that the staff on the rehabilitation unit used the Quality Assurance Data Collection Form. Suppose there has been an insidious rise in deficiencies for criteria B, no. 2 (observing client for safety and balance), and C, no. 4 (giving the client time to achieve balance). In addition, suppose that in question 4 (Did the nurse give you enough time to prepare for the transfer?) and 5 (Did you feel safe?) of the interview criteria, more clients than not have indicated that they did not feel safe or that the nurse did not give them enough time to prepare for the transfer. Since monitoring and evaluating for criteria B, no. 2, and C, no. 4, involve a degree of subjective judgment on the part of the evaluator, the client interview is particularly important in interpreting the results. Regardless of how the nurse felt, if the client's perception was one of feeling unsafe

or not having enough time, then the procedure was not as effective as it could have been despite the skill of the nurse assisting with the transfer.

The client's perception will influence the outcome of a procedure. If the perception is poor, there could be several adverse effects. Nervous clients do not listen well to instructions, and the resulting lack of comprehension will result in poor performance. Comprehension is especially important when the goal is to have the client perform the procedure alone. More seriously, as a result of poor comprehension and therefore poor performance, a fall could occur and result in injury. Injury would cause a setback in the rehabilitation process for the client, resulting in personal hardship and additional cost. Falls result in a high percentage of insurance claims, which, when paid, cause the institution's liability insurance premium to escalate. Increased length of stay because of a fracture costs medical insurance companies money, and this cost is passed on to the consumer. A less tangible result, but nonetheless serious, is the pain and suffering experienced by the client. The resulting loss of confidence and motivation often means the client has to start over again with the rehabilitation process. It is therefore clear that a problem in this area must be investigated and resolved.

It is unlikely that the cause of falls will be obvious. More information is usually needed. A study to evaluate the transfer procedure may involve more intensive monitoring over a 2-week period. The practitioners involved will be interviewed as to perceptions of their performance during the procedure. Additional duties and functions for which they are responsible will be taken into consideration. The orientation and in-service programs about transfer techniques will be included to see if there is emphasis on allowing the client sufficient time. Clients will continue to be interviewed to elicit their perceptions. Once all of the data are collected, this information will be reviewed and evaluated. Suppose that the results are that all of the above are implicated as causes for the problem! The nurses and aides do not see giving time to the client as a significant part of the transfer procedure. They feel overworked and understaffed. The educational programs do not place sufficient emphasis on giving the client time.

Corrective action would then have to be initiated to address all of the identified causes. Making assumptions about the cause without a thorough investigation is dangerous. It very often will result in lack of problem resolution. Without taking the time to determine the cause, corrective action will very likely be misdirected.

Corrective Action

Once the cause of the problem is identified, corrective action is indicated. Actions must be appropriate to the cause and scope of the problem. Of the several methods available, no one is necessarily better than others. The simplest, most direct action is the first choice and should be directed at the root of the problem. Whether or not it is a correct choice will not be known, however, until the quality assurance cycle is complete.

Corrective actions include, but are not limited to, the following:

1. An informal one-to-one contact between the practitioner responsible and an immediate supervisor
2. An educational program for the entire staff
3. Modification of an existing procedure to reflect more accurately client needs and staff capabilities
4. Development of a new procedure if the current one is completely inappropriate or if deficiencies point to the fact that no procedure exists to address a particular problem
5. Changes in staffing or allocation of client assignments
6. Repair of defective equipment or the purchase of new equipment
7. Disciplinary action according to agency policy

Deciding on the appropriate corrective action often taxes the creative problem-solving skills of even the most inventive rehabilitation staff nurse!

Problem Resolution

Problem resolution is probably the most frustrating step in the quality assurance process. The first four steps require direct involvement and action on the part of the rehabilitation nursing staff. Interest is at a peak and there is impatience to see results. The desire for instant gratification is common. Problems, however, do not emerge overnight. Neither will they be resolved quickly.

Problem resolution generally requires a wait-

and-see approach. Corrective action takes time to implement and often involves a series of activities. Unfortunately, the nature of most problems defies a quick solution. Blatant deviations from standards and procedures are rare. When they do occur, they are almost always immediately solved on a one-to-one basis.

A quality assurance system that uses continuous monitoring of more than one aspect of care at a time will solve two problems. The first problem concerns staff members' morale as related to involvement in quality assurance. When a number of procedures are monitored simultaneously, interest can be maintained while waiting to see if one particular problem has been solved. Quality assurance is a dynamic and cyclical process, not a start-stop-start activity. If it were, staff members would surely become bored while waiting to see the fruits of their labor.

The second advantage of continuous monitoring directly impacts on resolution of identified problems. Because the process is ongoing, criteria continue to be assessed. Whether the problem has been resolved will become evident as the results of evaluations are reviewed. Thus the final step—follow-up and monitoring for effectiveness—is crucial to the process.

Follow-Up and Monitoring for Effectiveness

Follow-up and monitoring for effectiveness constitute the most significant step in the overall system. Without it, the other steps are futile. All of the time and effort expended in criteria development, problem identification, and corrective action for problem resolution will be wasted if this step is overlooked.

As care continues to be reviewed and assessed, those elements where deficiencies were noted also are reviewed. Once corrective action has been implemented, the anticipated result is a decrease in the number of deficiencies. Regular evaluation of the Quality Assurance Data Collection Forms will clearly display whether deficiencies have actually decreased. Monitoring should continue periodically to see that the problem does not recur. When or if it does, the cause should be reinvestigated and alternate corrective actions considered. The process of ongoing review ensures that problems are not buried or forgotten. Critical aspects of care or areas where problems occur frequently and are difficult to resolve should be monitored indefinitely. Less critical aspects of care that are easily resolved may be dropped from the system so that others may be added. The dynamics of the system allow for give-and-take in the selection and use of standards and criteria.

Was the problem solved? This is the most important question. Everyone involved has a vested interest in the answer. The nursing staff members want to know that their efforts were not in vain and to feel they have a direct impact on care. The management of the institution wants to know so it can prove that quality care is given. Most of all, the clients want to know, since they are the primary recipients of benefits when problems related to their care are resolved. The public, too, has an interest, since it is ultimately their money and they wish it to be spent wisely.

SUMMARY

Regardless of the setting, the principles of rehabilitation are applicable to all nurses. Clients realize the benefits, no matter what their disability. The benefits of quality assurance also are applicable to all nurses and clients, because its components are interwoven into every aspect of care. It is clear that self-evaluation is an essential function of the professional nurse. Improvement of the care provided through self-evaluation is vital not only to the client but also to the nursing profession. It is a way of discharging the duty owed to the client, the public, and the profession. Quality assurance offers an opportunity for nurses to take responsibility for themselves and to be accountable.

REFERENCES

1. American Nurses' Association Division on Medical-Surgical Nursing Practice and Association of Rehabilitation Nurses: Standards of rehabilitation nursing practice, Kansas City, 1986, American Nurses' Association.
2. American Nurses' Association Division on Medical-Surgical Nursing Practice and Association of Rehabilitation Nurses: Standards of rehabilitation nursing practice, Kansas City, 1977, American Nurses' Association.
3. Bloch D: Evaluation of nursing care in terms of process

4. Dixon N, Hopkins J, and Walczak R: BAS basic audit seminar workbook, Chicago, 1964, JCAH.
5. Joint Commission on Accreditation of Hospitals: Accreditation manual for hospitals, 1988, Chicago, 1987, The Commission.
6. Joint Commission on Accreditation of Hospitals: Accreditation manual for hospitals, 1981, Chicago, 1980, The Commission.
7. Phaneuf M: Quality appraisal in nursing, the nursing audit, ed 2, New York, 1976, Appleton-Century-Crofts.
8. Roberts J and Walczak R: Toward effective quality assurance: the evolution and current status of the JCAH QA standard, Qual Rev Bull 10(1):11, 1984.
9. Walczak R: JCAH's new standard calls for more deliberate QA activities, Hosp Peer Rev 8(12):155, 1983.
10. Woody M: An evaluator's perspective, Nurs Res 29(2):74, 1980.
11. Zimmer M: Quality assurance for outcomes of patient care, Nurs Clin North Am 9(2):305, 1974.

ADDITIONAL READINGS

Carey RG: Integrating program evaluation, quality assurance, and marketing for inpatient rehabilitation, Rehabil Nurs 13:66, March/April 1988.

Courts NF: A patient satisfaction survey for a rehabilitation unit, Rehabil Nurs 13:79, March/April 1988.

Decker C: Quality assurance: accent on monitoring, Nurs Management 16(11):20, 1985.

DeVet CL: Nurses must broaden scope of monitors to meet JCAH Standards, Hosp Peer Rev 10(8):95, 1985.

Hamilton S: Unit-level quality assurance: essential for success, Rehabil Nurs 13:76, March/April 1988.

Joint Commission on Accreditation of Hospitals: Monitoring and evaluation: nursing services, Chicago, 1987, The Commission.

Joint Commission on Accreditation of Hospitals: Accreditation manual for hospitals, 1986, Chicago, 1985, The Commission.

Maloof M: Preparing for agency accreditation, Rehabil Nurs 11:11, Nov/Dec 1986.

Sabin S: Perspective: rehabilitation nursing opportunities and threats, Rehabil Nurs 11:22, Nov/Dec 1986.

Stearns G and Joseph E: Passing JCAH muster or 6 essential ingredients for a successful quality assurance program, Trustee 38(6):15, 1985.

Thompson TC: A proactive approach to accrediting standards, Rehabil Nurs 11:8, Nov/Dec 1986.

Walczak R: What happened to the problem-focused approach? QRC Advisor 1(6):2, 1985.

and outcome: issues in research and quality assurance, Nurs Res 24(4):256, 1975.

Determining the Cost of Rehabilitation Nursing

Margie L. Scott

OBJECTIVES

After completing Chapter 25, the reader will be able to:

1. Distinguish between direct and indirect nursing costs.

2. Describe the purposes and uses of client classification systems.

3. Analyze one client classification system.

4. Explain the characteristics of the DRG reimbursement plan.

5. Identify the benefits of a cost determination system for rehabilitation nursing.

The cost of health care in this country continues to escalate. Consequently, the need to curb rising health care costs, justify nursing service expenditures, and provide cost-effective quality care places far greater demands upon nursing administrators and leaders today than ever before. These factors challenge nurses to engage in more creative, realistic planning and decision making. Cost consciousness is especially critical if nursing is to become a more equitable, income-generating service.

The cost of nursing care has historically been measured on a per diem basis, which has not provided an accurate measure for determining the actual cost of nursing care. This method attempts to quantify nursing care by categorizing clients according to the amount of nursing resources consumed. For example, if a particular department of nursing service has five levels of care, level 1 might be individuals who required the least

amount of nursing care, or those persons who were independent in activities of daily living. Level 5 might be clients who required the most nursing care, or who were totally dependent upon nursing for performing their activities of daily living.

The per diem method has proven repeatedly to be inadequate in measuring care administered by a cadre of nursing personnel to clients with multiple problems and conditions. The inadequacies of this particular cost determination method have led nursing service departments to explore more creative, systematic, and accurate methods for determining the cost of nursing care. Cost benefit methods have been applied to health care for well over 2 decades in attempts to optimize efforts, identify the most effective alternatives in nursing care, and ensure that resources are wisely used.

This chapter provides insight into the current

situation and explores methods used today that attempt to put a price tag on nursing care. However, it is not feasible to discuss specific methods by which cost determinations of nursing care are made before first distinguishing between direct and indirect nursing care activities. These activities are the common elements required for the management and delivery of nursing care.

DIRECT AND INDIRECT NURSING CARE

Direct nursing care includes nursing activities that are client and family centered and carried out in their presence.[2] Direct nursing activities are the primary components of nursing care and depend largely upon the acuity of the client's condition, related nursing tasks, and the time required to perform these tasks.

The most obvious direct nursing care is hands-on-care activities necessary to provide daily care at the unit level. Costs to provide this care include salaries for personnel and equipment and maintenance of the care unit. More specifically then, hands-on care is necessary for the implementation of care regimens; documentation of care; client and family education; and management of care by clinical coordinators, head nurses, and clinical specialists.[9]

Indirect nursing care is somewhat more difficult to define and measure, perhaps because the costs involved are not clearly identified or directly involved with the implementation of client care. Costs include administrative overhead and depreciation. The most obvious costs are nursing administration at the nursing service level and nursing education. Supervision, staffing, orientation, in-service workshops, relations with departments such as personnel, purchasing, accounting, and medical records, and relations with the community also are included.[9]

Historically, nursing has absorbed the greatest portion of most hospital budgets. However, once the distinction was made between direct and indirect nursing activities, nurse administrators were able to begin to separate the actual cost of nursing care from the plethora of nonnursing tasks and services that often were included with nursing as a component of the room rate. Clearly, the distinction between direct and indirect costs allows nurse administrators to move toward obtaining greater financial solvency for their departments.[9]

CLIENT CLASSIFICATION SYSTEMS

The basis for beginning to make effective cost determination decisions about nursing care lies in the selection and use of a viable client classification system. Such a system provides a rational framework from which to operate in developing a model for application when attempting to determine the cost of nursing care. This is of particular significance since the advent of the new federal diagnosis-related group (DRG) reimbursement plan that has become the nationally accepted reimbursement method for calculating the cost of hospital care received by Medicare clients. Although rehabilitation services are currently exempt from reimbursement according to DRGs, some method will no doubt be used in the future to determine reimbursement according to functional progress or resource use. Correlating functional status, as determined by using the Uniform National Data Set discussed in Chapter 23, with costs and benefits of rehabilitation is one method that could be used.

A client classification system is one method of compiling information about clients relative to their characteristic needs and diagnoses. Clients are observed on both an individual and a collective basis to determine the cost of care for those who have similar problems and needs. Despite the potential of classifying schemes to assist with placing a more realistic price tag on specific levels of nursing care throughout a particular hospital, their effective use requires careful record keeping and extensive analyses of the data collected. Although there has been progress toward development of valid classification systems for standardizing care, a gap still exists between what nurses do and what they actually document and attempt to measure.[7] Despite the voluminous client classification systems in use today, the basic premise underlying all such systems is their usefulness in defining nursing care activities in behavioral terms that can then be converted to time standards.[7]

Setting differential charges for direct nursing care to clients has always been a difficult task despite the use of classification systems. Nursing service departments have fallen short in their efforts to legitimize methods for predicting staffing needs and to provide a data base for validation of budget requirements. Once a health care facility has chosen the client classification system that best meets its particular needs, time standards can be further converted to dollar costs to accurately determine the overall cost of nursing services.[7]

The literature suggests, overall, that there are immediate benefits to using client classification systems because these systems allow measurement of client acuity levels for specific nursing units. The use of classification systems to maintain standards and quality while containing costs has several advantages. It allows nurses to:

1. Define for the first time the cost of nursing services, thus placing a market value on these services.
2. Determine staffing needs by measuring acuity levels and categorizing clients according to number of hours of care they require, thus enabling more objective decisions to be made about future budgetary needs.
3. Reduce the problem of cross subsidization of other ancillary departments by the nursing department.
4. Monitor and use trends in client care needs to make more realistic budgeting predictions.
5. Document the care required by specific types of clients so that nursing care and nursing education can be better planned and implemented.[6]

Client classification systems in rehabilitation settings also would allow for determination of care needs according to the client's level of independence and address staffing needs. Since rehabilitation care is a complex, expensive, and long-term process, the need for reliable and valid outcome indicators is apparent.[5]

Many client classification systems in use today suggest the feasibility of documenting nursing activities. One such system is that used by the Lutheran Medical Center in Denver.

The Lutheran system is a weighted scoring system that requires the nurse on each shift to check the particular nursing activities provided to each client (Figure 25-1). The data from the check sheets are entered into a computer, which calculates the total times (including indirect times) needed to care for each client. Nursing care requirements are then calculated for each nursing unit and broken down by shift and job classification. Shift-by-shift data are collected for each biweekly time period. The computer compares

required client care time to the time actually spent on each unit (using payroll records of time worked by unit). The required and actual times also are compared with budgeted nursing time per client. These comparisons complete a comprehensive management information system (Figure 25-2).[7]

Since this system has been relatively stable for 7 years and since it provides comprehensive information on client needs and nurse staffing, it has been possible to identify client care trends, improve the efficiency of staffing, and gather a variety of statistical information to justify budgetary changes by nursing units.

In addition to using the client classification data in nursing, Lutheran's model has incorporated the information into a computerized utilization review program. The utilization review coordinator has computer screen access to each client's admitting and working diagnosis, surgical procedures, physician consultation, client classification category, and a listing of all the daily nursing care activities. If this information cannot justify hospitalization, individual chart review is done.

When the management team began to determine actual costs for providing service under DRGs, it was natural to look to the client classification system for help. With assistance from the data processing department, the team designed reports showing daily client classification categories for all clients. This information becomes available as soon as the client is discharged and includes total length of stay information. By multiplying the time allocation for each category by the average nursing salary, a cost for each classification category is determined. The computer can then show the actual costs of providing nursing care to each client. Currently, the computer program at Lutheran allows organization of data to show nursing care costs for each client, costs of nursing care by unit, nursing care costs for Medicare and non-Medicare clients by diagnoses, as well as average and total costs of Medicare and non-Medicare clients (Figure 25-3).

In a 2-week period, analyses of Medicare and non-Medicare data showed that Medicare clients required 10% more nursing resources per day and 40% more nursing time for their entire hospitalization. For certain diagnoses, the cost differential was minimal (for example, hyperplasia of the prostate), whereas for other diagnoses (for example, diverticulitis of the colon), the cost differential was marked.[7]

This type of system can be adapted easily for use in a rehabilitation setting if special consideration is given to the more time-consuming direct care activities such as listening, counseling, and teaching, and assisting with hygiene, elimination, turning and positioning, transferring, bathing and showering, and feeding, since these tend to require the largest percentage of time in rehabilitation nursing.

Most client classification systems in use today have been developed for use on medical and surgical nursing units. However, with slight modifications, they can be used in most rehabilitation settings. These systems are badly needed in rehabilitation. In a survey conducted by the University of Wisconsin Hospital at Madison, several rehabilitation facilities were contacted to determine (1) the state of the art in quantification of rehabilitation nursing and (2) what approaches and tools other facilities were using for classifi-

---

Write in "none" if no assistance needed. For multiple helpers, write in "M."

Date:

Activities of daily living (Check one in each category.)
Bathing, eating, dressing
1. Minimal assistance
2. Moderate assistance (M)
3. Dependent (M)

Limited mobility (transfer, ambulation)
4. Assistance needed (M)
5. Dependent (M)

Toileting
6. Bedpan or toilet assistance (M)
7. Dependent (M)
8. Totally dependent or comatose (M)

Treatments (Check all that apply.)
9. Minimal care drainage tubes (M)
10. Complex drainage tubes (M)
11. Skin traction, braces, or splints
12. Skeletal traction
13. Simple dressing (M)
14. Complex dressing (M)
15. Irrigations (M)
16. Complete isolation
17. Special treatments (M)
18. Simple treatments (M)
19. Symptomatic needs; requires > 2 hr/shift

Figure 25-1
Nursing Activities Index. *(From Nyberg J and Wolf N: J Nurs Admin 14:17, April 1984.)*   *Continued.*

Write in "none" if no assistance needed. For multiple helpers, write in "M."

Date: | | | | | | | | | | | | |
---|---|---|---|---|---|---|---|---|---|---|---|---|---

Medication (Check all that apply.)
20. Oral medications
21. IM or SQ medications
22. Multiple medications (five or more doses/shift; includes oral, IM, SQ)
23. IV (simple fluid administration, includes dressing)
24. INT medications or IV with medications   (M)

Tests (Check all that apply.)
25. Tests with preps or done by nurse
26. Complex tests (includes follow-up monitoring)

Monitoring (Check one if applicable.)
27. Special observation
28. Establish dosage of potentially dangerous drugs
29. Potentially unstable condition
30. Unstable or dangerous condition
31. Patient must be checked $\bar{q}$ 10 min

Teaching and counseling (Check only if specific need.)
32. Intensive teaching ($>$ 1 hr)
33. Teaching ($<$ 20 min)
34. Patient requiring special emotional support
35. Intensive psychological needs
36. Requires constant attendance (1:1)

Coordination and planning (Check only if applicable.)
37. Patient transferred
38. Extensive charting ($>$ 1 hr) or conferences
39. Admission
40. Surgical patient with routine operative course
41. Patient (medical or surgical) with complications occurring during hospitalization
42. Utilization review needed

Figure 25-1, cont'd
Nursing Activities Index.

Category	1	2	3	4	5	6	7	8	Total		Hours per pt day Budget	Required	Actual	Req/bdgt	Act/bdgt	% of performance
Pt avg	25.7	63.7	59.7	58.7	31.7	23.0	4.7	.3	267.3	PAT	5.850	6.13	6.06	104.79	103.59	101.16
YTD avg	30.7	67.8	55.5	50.2	29.0	18.3	3.8	.2	255.5	YTD	5.850	6.04	6.06	103.25	103.59	99.67
Pt %	9.61	23.83	22.33	21.96	11.86	8.60	1.76	.11								
YTD %	12.02	26.54	21.72	19.65	11.35	7.16	1.49	.08								

Patient totals Required hours	Actual hours
1,639.61	1,619.60

Census total	Census total	YTD totals Required hours	Actual hours
802	1,533	3,084.56	3,096.50

	Current FTE Required	Actual	Diff	YTD FTE Required	Actual	Diff
Mgt	.90	1.00	.10	1.80	2.00	.20
RN	14.56	14.97	.41	27.34	28.31	.97
LPN	2.88	2.60	-.28	5.27	5.23	-.04
A/O	.00	.17	.17	.00	.24	.24
WS	2.15	1.50	-.65	4.15	2.93	-1.22
MS	.00	.00	.00	.00	.00	.00
	20.50	20.25	-.25	38.56	38.71	.15

Figure 25-2
Example of biweekly nursing service staffing summary report. *(From Nyberg J and Wolf N: J Nurs Admin 14:17, April 1984.)*

From 08-01-83 to 08-14-83

Nurse unit breakdown: selected units

Diagnosis breakdown: all DX's

Payor breakdown: Med and Non-Med

Diagnosis	M/N	Visit no.	LOS	1	2	3	4	5	6	7	8
Diverticulitis of colon	M		14	1 32.00	2 80.00	3 147.00 980.00	2 128.00	1 78.00	5 515.00	0 0.00	0 0.00
	M	Total	14	1 32.00	2 80.00 Total patient cost:	3 147.00 980.00	2 128.00 Average daily patient cost:	1 78.00	5 515.00	0 0.00 70.00	0 0.00
	M	Average	14.0	1.0 32.00	2.0 80.00 Total patient cost:	3.0 147.00 980.00	2.0 128.00 Average daily patient cost:	1.0 78.00	5.0 515.00	0.0 0.00 70.00	0.0 0.00
	N		10	0 0.00	2 80.00	4 196.00 532.00	4 256.00	0 0.00	0 0.00	0 0.00 53.20	0 0.00
	N	Total	10	0 0.00	2 80.00 Total patient cost:	4 196.00 532.00	4 256.00 Average daily patient cost:	0 0.00	0 0.00	0 0.00 53.20	0 0.00
	N	Average	10.0	0.0 0.00	2.0 80.00 Total patient cost:	4.0 196.00 532.00	4.0 256.00 Average daily patient cost:	0.0 0.00	0.0 0.00	0.0 0.00 53.20	0.0 0.00
		DX (total)	24	1 32.00	4 160.00 Total patient cost:	7 343.00 1512.00	6 384.00 Average daily patient cost:	1 78.00	5 515.00	0 0.00 63.00	0 0.00
		DX (avg)	12.0	0.5 16.00	2.0 80.00 Total patient cost:	3.5 171.50 756.00	3.0 192.00 Average daily patient cost:	0.5 39.00	2.5 257.50	0.0 0.00 63.00	0.0 0.00

Patient categories (freq./cost)

Figure 25-3

Nursing costs by patient category. (Costs are illustrative, not actual.) M, Medicare; N, non-Medicare. (*From Nyberg J and Wolf N: J Nurs Admin 14:17, 1984.*)

cation of clients. Although some facilities were attempting to develop their own systems and others were modifying existing methodologies, they found that the quantification for this specialty was largely in its infancy.[2] The modified HEW rehabilitation tool is an example of one attempt at developing such a system for rehabilitation. This tool was adapted from Cleveland's and William's instruments. Both instruments are closely correlated, since client care intensities are arranged in four categories ranging from class I (low intensity) to class IV (high intensity). Although neither is a rehabilitation tool, the Cleveland instrument has social/emotional and teaching scales and uses rehabilitation language that encourages adaptation and use in a rehabilitation nursing setting.[2]

Staffing on rehabilitation units must be determined well in advance. To use personnel resources effectively, health care facilities must engage in more systematic measurement of client needs and requirements and conduct careful quality control evaluations.

Lately much attention has been given to the cost of rehabilitation nursing and medical care. More often than not, nursing administrators see reimbursement systems as methods of justifying care costs, whereas third-party payers and regulators use "cost effectiveness" to mean "cost cutting."

A nationwide survey on rehabilitation of clients with strokes estimated $3.26 billion in direct care costs and approximately $2.9 to $4.8 billion in indirect costs, including lost earnings each year.[10] Redford, Brostrom, and Gough[8] report that costs of care for totally dependent persons in extended care facilities are four times the cost of care of individuals who are mobile. Johnson and Keith[4] indicate that there is great potential to reduce costs by rehabilitating individuals and decreasing their dependence. They describe several studies to demonstrate that clients with a variety of diagnoses have improved function and rates of employment after a rehabilitation program.

DIAGNOSIS-RELATED GROUPS

Diagnosis-related groups, or DRGs, as these are most commonly called, are a concept that originated from Yale University as a management and utilization review tool. It has actually become the cornerstone of a federal prospective reimbursement plan mandating a change from a per diem to a cost per discharge system of reimbursement. The DRG system divides the client population into 23 major diagnostic categories (MDCs), which are further subdivided into 356 diagnostic-related groups according to age and the presence or absence of complications. A dollar figure based on retrospective cost data for a hospital and region is derived by averaging the cost of the care given to clients with a specific diagnosis with an adjustment made to account for inflation (based on a marketbasket index) plus 1%. Consequently, the amount of money the government will pay for the care of Medicare clients who are in each DRG will be determined by dividing the cost of the care the client has actually received by the number of clients discharged who have been assigned to that DRG. The actual income each hospital will receive for each DRG, then, is determined by multiplying the average cost by the number of clients assigned to that DRG.[1]

Before the emergence of DRGs, the most significant effort toward accomplishing a reimbursement plan for nursing care was the Relative Intensity Measure (RIM), which originated in New Jersey. RIMs are a method whereby nursing resources are measured in terms of minutes of nursing care received by clients. This method assumes the greater the number of minutes nursing staff spend with a client, the larger the nursing resources a client consumes. Although this method proved helpful in showing relationships between clients' consumption of nursing resources and their medical conditions, its use has not become widespread.[6]

Since hospital care for Medicare clients is currently reimbursed in approximately 46 states by the DRG method, it is imperative that nursing service departments begin to analyze their particular potential to justify cost for nursing service in a manner that correlates with the client's DRG, thus enabling them to receive an equitable share of DRG payments. For example, a department of nursing could develop 23 major care categories for its rehabilitation service that best correlate with the 23 MDCs. These would then be divided into 356 general nursing care strategies to correlate with the 356 DRGs. The general nursing care strategies are essentially detailed nursing care plans that include direct and indirect care needs of each of the 23 client groups. The care plan should allow for variances in both the interdependent and independent functions of nurses related to the client's severity of illness within each DRG.[1] Nursing care plans should be as detailed, clear, and concrete as possible and directly tied to specific client outcomes, a concept highly familiar to professional nurses since most are quite adept in the nursing process approach to planning and problem solving.

The DRG method of reimbursement is not without problems. A few of these are:

1. Inaccurate assignment of DRGs
2. Inaccurate nursing assessments of client needs
3. Allowance for the difference, if any, between the care needed and the care clients actually receive[1]

Much of the opposition against the use of the DRG economic model as a method of reimbursement for in-hospital care of Medicare clients centers around the controversy about its insensitivity to the stage of a client's disease and the varying intensity of the client's needs.[3] Although two clients may be hospitalized with the same diagnosis, there may be legitimate reasons why one might require more intensive, aggressive care that cannot be justified under the category of complications. For example, you may be caring for two clients who are the same age, both of whom have a diagnosis of cerebrovascular accident with right-sided hemiplegia. One might transfer and perform activities of daily living almost independently, whereas the other cannot perform these activities without maximum assistance. Or perhaps one client requires more supportive care than the other, which will probably increase that client's consumption of nursing care on that particular admission, yet not necessarily on subsequent admissions. Although time spent caring for clients is an average, care of these two clients may be significantly different and more time consuming for one than the other. For the most accurate reflection of care consumption, the DRG must be used carefully and in close relationship with the hospital's classification system.

Lagona and Stritzel[6] found in their study of nursing care requirements as measured by DRG that the immediate benefit of the client classification system was the ability to measure client acuity levels for each nursing unit. These values were used for determining later staffing requirements and in making budgetary projections. Although they found the ability to measure the cost of nursing care consumed by clients in a specific DRG to be extremely valuable to the nursing administration as a management tool, it was not particularly helpful in ascertaining the cost of caring for clients in any given DRG. They found data difficult to measure unless tabulated by client versus unit. This becomes difficult when clients are transferred from one unit to another. They concluded that clients must be observed closely and individual tabulations made from time of admission to time of discharge, thus providing a cross section of nursing units.[6] This may entail compilation of data when the client enters the emergency suite and when transferred to the intensive care unit, a medical floor, and a rehabilitation unit. Also, more careful assessments must be made to make tabulations as comprehensible as possible. By using nursing cost per DRG, the administration would be able to submit a simple, objective budget that would reflect accurately the monetary requirements needed to provide nursing care, therefore providing a more equitable means of allocating funds for nursing services.[6]

The inability of hospitals to accurately identify and justify their variable billing practices gave impetus to the emergence of DRGs. Perhaps if hospitals had initially been more conscientious in identifying costs of providing care, public understanding and economic pressures would not have become the problem they are today in challenging nursing personnel across the country to more accurately describe and quantify their contribution to client care.

APPLICATION TO NURSING

Regardless of the process used to determine the cost of rehabilitation nursing, more careful assessments must be made of the overall effect of DRGs and classification of clients on the improvement of practice. To effectively apply these processes in nursing, many questions must be addressed: Are all therapies under the realm of nursing actually nursing activities? Are these treatments considered by nursing when determining client acuity and nursing cost? Can nursing actually provide effective services now offered by another department, such as respiratory and physical therapy, at a lesser cost? And is one department subsidizing another?

As nurses begin to take a more active role in

determining the cost of nursing care, they will benefit. For nurses, the anticipated benefits are considerable. Nursing departments in many hospitals have traditionally lagged behind in financial acumen.[7] Nurses are perceived as an economic drain rather than as a financial asset. Determining the cost of and charging for nursing care should establish and validate nurses as income producers. This should greatly improve nurses' abilities to influence important decisions concerning nursing resources and practice.[9] Additionally, by generating revenue, a department of nursing could more freely explore new modes of health care delivery. It could obtain financial reimbursement for more highly qualified nurses to care for clients within specific DRGs, especially since nurses will need to be better prepared in order to implement the necessary care regimens under new time constraints. Finally, nursing services could contract with nurse consultants and clinical specialists to focus on client problems that are specific to a DRG.

When nurses gain the power and status that goes with recognition of their economic worth and when their role is more clearly defined through establishment of care levels, they may very well feel more committed to and satisfied with nursing, which is the key to high productivity[9] and the provision of the best possible care for all clients.

SUMMARY

The differences between direct and indirect nursing cost and the purposes and uses of client classification systems have been described. The client classification system used at Lutheran Medical Center in Denver has been analyzed for its application to a rehabilitation setting. DRGs, the federal prospective payment system, were explained. A cost determination system for rehabilitation nursing can help improve the quality and quantity of rehabilitation nursing services delivered to disabled clients.

REFERENCES

1. Curtain L: Determining cost of nursing services per DRG, Nurs Management 14:16, April 1983.
2. Davis AL: Classifying rehabilitation patients, Nurs Management 14:49, Feb 1983.
3. Grimaldi PL and Micheletti JA: Diagnosis related groups: a practitioner's guide, Chicago, 1985, Pluribus.
4. Johnston MV and Keith RA: Cost-benefits of medical rehabilitation: review and critique, Arch Phys Med Rehabil 64:147, April 1983.
5. Kutner B: Rehabilitation: whose goals? whose priorities? Arch Phys Med Rehabil 52:284, 1971.
6. Lagona TG and Stritzel MM: Nursing care requirements as measured by D.R.G., J Nurs Admin 14:15, May 1984.
7. Nyberg J and Wolff N: The D.R.G. panic, J Nurs Admin 14:17, April 1984.
8. Redford JB, Brostrom MA, and Gough KM: Reactivation programs and nursing care costs, Dimens Health Serv 51:14, Nov 1974.
9. Walker DD: The cost of NNurs Admin 13:14, March 1983.
10. Weinfeld FD, editor: National survey of stroke, Stroke 12(suppl 1):I-1, March/April 1981.

ADDITIONAL READINGS

Alward RR: Patient classification systems: the ideal vs. reality, J Nurs Admin 13:13, March 1983.
Fagin CM: Opening the door on nursing's cost advantage, Nurs Health Care 7:352, 1986.
Mason EJ and Daugherty JK: Nursing standards should determine nursing's price, Nurs Management 15:34, Sept 1984.
Mitty E: Prospective payment and long-term care: linking payments to resource use, Nurs Health Care 8:14, 1987.
Roddy PC, Korbin L, and Meiners MR: Resource requirements of nursing home patients based on time and motion studies. Long-Term Care Studies Program Research Report, DHHS pub no (PHS) 87-3408, US Department of Health and Human Services, Rockville, Md, April 1987, National Center for Health Services Research and Health Care Technology Assessment.
Shaffer F: Nursing power in the DRG world, Nurs Management 15:28, June 1984.
Staley M and Luciano K: Eight steps to costing nursing services, Nurs Management 14:35, Oct 1984.
Vanderzee H and Glusko G: DRG's, variable pricing and budgeting for nursing service, J Nurs Admin 14:11, May 1984.

Further Dimensions
in Rehabilitation Nursing

CHAPTER 26

Rehabilitation: Unlocking the Gates to Change

Judith A. Laughlin

OBJECTIVES

After completing Chapter 26, the reader will be able to:

1. Define change.
2. Identify the competencies required to be a successful change agent.
3. Outline the change process.
4. Identify approaches for overcoming obstacles that impede change.
5. Discuss two techniques that can assist the nurse in creating change.

Can the nurse have an impact in changing the behavior of a disabled client? The answers are obvious: yes, no, and sometimes. If the incentives and motivations are acceptable, the methods proposed for changing behavior are well planned and implemented, and these methods are seen as appropriate by those who are to be affected, planned change is most likely to occur.

Quality of life for the person who is disabled or who has a chronic disease is tied to the change process. The word "rehabilitation" implies change by its definition: "A creative process that begins with immediate preventive care in the first stage of accident or illness. It is continued through the restorative phase of care and involves adaptation of the whole being to a new life."[14] For adaptation to occur, change must take place.

Change means to make something different, to modify, vary, or alter it. People in general fear what is unknown to them, and change requires introducing the unknown. However, what is necessary to cope successfully with change is to act with anticipation; in other words, to use a method called planned change.

Planned change is a systematic process directed toward producing improvement in function, output, or solving a problem. The process is anticipatory and helps to make the unforeseen manageable. It is a process that nurses should be able to become comfortable with because it uses the same steps as those in the nursing process—assessment, planning, implementation, and evaluation.

The "change agent" was defined originally by social scientists who were the first to deal with planned change as a field of study. Two elements were identified as extremely important in facilitating planned change: (1) the personal characteristics of the individual who acts as the change agent and (2) the process used to accomplish the change.

THE CHANGE AGENT

When helping clients to change behavior, nurses must assume a number of roles that they judge to be appropriate for the client, the situation, and the nurse's own style. Bennis[2] identifies three roles for a change agent: consultant, fact finder, and educator. A fourth role, that of linker, was added by Menzel[10] and Havelock.[6]

The consultant role focuses primarily on developing action proposals for the client to consider. The fact finder dimension includes the ability to diagnose and develop techniques for identifying client problems and analyzing causes. As educator, the nurse must be able to teach concepts and skills to the client and others. The linker role requires the nurse to identify and match relevant resources to the needs of the client.

The nurse must develop or possess a multifaceted group of competencies to become a change agent in the rehabilitation process. In a 1976 study by Lippitt and Lippitt,[9] one of the respondents suggested that change agents have personal characteristics and skills that do not necessarily come from formal education. These include the abilities to be flexible, innovative, and creative; adapt to unfamiliar situations; be self-directed; demonstrate sensitivity toward others; be honest and ethical; deal successfully with ambiguity; genuinely desire to help others; respect self; be optimistic, self-confident, and sincere; and possess charisma. These qualities assist the change agent in developing credibility with the client and increase chances of success during the rehabilitation process.

The nurse in the change agent role will need to develop competencies in three major areas: knowledge, skill, and attitudes. The means of acquiring these needed competencies is through both formal and informal education.

Formal education can be accomplished by means of five methods. The first method includes review of the literature in the fields of behavioral science and rehabilitation. Literature review provides a foundation for the nurse in knowledge of change theory, conceptual models or frameworks, specific rehabilitation methods or techniques, and research tools. In addition, skills or abilities could

be improved upon by using knowledge gained about scientific methodology, teaching, communicating, and coping with realities.

A second method is to be tutored by experienced practitioners. This type of formal education would be invaluable to the nurse in a change agent role. Knowledge about change theory could be reinforced and enhanced. Specific rehabilitation techniques and research methods and techniques also could be demonstrated and tried. Skills in dealing with people and situations could be improved, because taking action would be a required part of the tutorial. Also the learner would be forced to suspect and diagnose problems, a skill that is needed by a change agent. The opportunity for the learner to work on specific teaching and communication skills would be available, as would immediate feedback by the experienced practitioner.

Training laboratories are a third method of formal education. These can be conducted by professionals who are actively involved with clients in various rehabilitation settings. These professionals have not only the appropriate academic preparation, but also the practical experience necessary to assist the nurse in focusing on skills through practice sessions. Some of the problems that may be included in training sessions are how to (1) stimulate a need for help, (2) develop a contract for collaboration, (3) be supportive of working through resistance, (4) stimulate change objectives or images of potentiality, (5) obtain feedback to guide the rehabilitation process, and (6) conceptualize criteria for making choices among alternative interventions.[9]

Training laboratories specifically assist the nurse in the development of skills for working with people, teaching and communicating, and diagnosing and detecting success or failure. In addition, knowledge of self will be gained, as well as improving attitudes related to trust, flexibility, desire to help, and honesty.

A fourth method of formal education is enrollment in university courses. Course work in the behavioral sciences, education, and rehabilitation will help the nurse gain skills in the use of scientific methodology, teaching, and rehabilitation techniques. Also, knowledge of change theory, learning theories, models or frameworks, research methods and techniques, and alternative methods will be enhanced.

The fifth approach to formal education is individual therapy and sensitivity training. This type of educational experience will force the nurse to become more knowledgeable about self. It allows for a one-on-one exploration of attitudes, especially those attitudes that have to do with openness, adaptability, honesty, desire to help, and learning. Skills and abilities needed to take action, deal with a variety of people and situations, teach, communicate, sense problems, and detect successes or failures will be upgraded. This type of educational experience gives depth, reality, and insight to one's role as a rehabilitation nurse.

Informal learning experiences also will aid the nurse in acquiring needed characteristics. Experience, of course, is the best teacher of the thinking practitioner in that knowledge of conceptual models and planning, as well as environmental and systems factors, will be tested. Also the nurse frequently will be faced with situations that require a flexible attitude. Discussion with peers, another informal learning experience, will help the nurse to grow in knowledge of self and increase trust and openness. Finally, experimentation will lead the nurse to become a better judge of personal effectiveness with use of skills, knowledge, and attitudes in scientific methodology, coping with people and situations, and interacting with the environment.

THE CHANGE PROCESS

Research in the area of change suggests the existence of identifiable ways of effecting change. Although no theories can predict the difficulties that arise in real-life situations, theories can be useful in providing direction.

Changed behavior of a disabled client during the rehabilitation process is the ultimate goal of a change strategy. Kurt Lewin,[8] the classic theorist of the change process, developed his model for change during the 1940s. Lewin's model considers behavior as a function of personality and environment. The interaction between the human aspects of personality and the environment (circumstances of the overall situation) is the dynamic component of any observed change in behavior. The personality element, however, is recognized as the most difficult aspect to control.

Lewin's theory comprises three phases: unfreezing, movement, and refreezing or stabilizing.[2] The unfreezing phase is the point at which there is an awareness of the need for change and a change relationship is established. The status quo is questioned, stimuli for change are created, and some discomfort or dissatisfaction with the present situation is induced. This phase may be the most difficult in the change process, since most people are creatures of habit. A client who is disabled because of an accident or chronic illness may be displeased with particular circumstances, but it is often less stressful to be dependent or continue certain behaviors than to face the real or imagined inconveniences that change may bring.

Movement, phase two, is the implementation of a new idea or plan designed to fit the need for change. During this phase, assessment and diagnosis of problems occur, options and alternatives are identified, goals are established, and action is actually taken, with evaluation the culmination of all of these events. The latter step is the time in which the client is the most vulnerable, because of taking the risk of moving from point A to point B. In addition, evaluation of the effectiveness of the change provides input for making additional changes before a change is viewed as permanent.

The crystallization of a new plan signals the start of the refreezing or stabilization phase. Refreezing is the end state. It is the functioning of a client after coming to a new desired level. In a sense, closure or termination occurs. This does not mean that a change is good or bad, but merely that it is complete. Refreezing is a phase in which the client functions at a level undisturbed by the mechanisms of change.

Another set of concepts that should be considered when examining change comes from general systems theory. These concepts assist in the description and analysis of activities that occur when change is attempted. A situation where a client is being helped through the rehabilitation process by a nurse would be described in terms of the open system concept. The open system is one that can receive and respond to information or stimuli from the environment. The closed system is one that lacks the quality of interchange with the environment.

Another concept of systems theory may be useful when considering change, that is, a change in any element of an open system will produce changes in other elements of that system. There is a tendency for a system to seek equilibrium or balance among the forces of its elements. This concept is analogous to the stabilization phase of Lewin's theory. Changing one element or function in a system creates an imbalance or disequilibrium in the system. The other elements then act to compensate or return the system's balance.

An open system does not imply an equal exchange of energy with the environment. When these concepts of systems are applied to the analysis of a nurse-client relationship during the rehabilitation process, the picture created is of a dynamic situation with numerous interdependent elements and one or more functions that will respond to a stimulus for change.

The relationship between change and the changer is another area around which change theories have evolved. Notably, Bennis[3] looked at change models from the perspective of collaborative and noncollaborative relationships. Collaborative means of stimulating change are most appropriate to rehabilitation environments, since collaboration implies mutual goal setting. Many nursing theorists view the nurse-client relationship from the perspective of the nurse who works with or assists the client in attaining an optimum level of functioning. This perspective is based on the idea that the client has ultimate responsibility for health. Ferguson[5] nicely summarized this viewpoint when she stated, "No one can persuade another to change. Each of us guards a gate of change that can only be unlocked from the inside."

OVERCOMING OBSTACLES THAT IMPEDE CHANGE

Many Americans believe that they have a right to health but not an obligation to improve it or maintain it. The nurse working with clients who are disabled therefore must be aware of current cultural attitudes toward health in general and the individual's perceived responsibility for personal health that may impact on the rehabilitation process.

The following five basic premises identified by Knowles[7] form the basis for these attitudes:
1. There exists a demand for instant gratification, living day to day, and a denial of death and disease.
2. Death and disease can be conquered by personal will or through scientific and technological advances.
3. Some people view old age as a set of

dispiriting conditions and decide that they would just as soon die early.
4. Individuals are chronically depressed to the point where they consciously or unconsciously wish for death and do not take care of themselves.
5. The physician, to whom Americans ascribe the ultimate wisdom about health, is not truly interested in the health of the American public.

These premises affect attitudes and values, which then impact on behavior. To successfully foster an environment of individual responsibility and positive health practices the nurse must be aware of a client's value system.

Current trends indicate that many people (particularly those under 40 years of age) are developing a new approach to health care. A sense of consumerism has pervaded the health care system. This is evidenced by improved dietary habits, regular exercise programs, awareness of environmental hazards, and a proliferation of self-help books. Such a philosophy is essential not only to instituting preventive measures, but also in circumstances where acute and long-term treatments become necessary.

The health belief model[12] can be used to explain behaviors that either enhance health or determine whether an individual will adhere to a treatment program during illness. This model was influenced by Lewin's ideas and therefore contains a strong component of motivation theory.

Essentially the model has three cognitive elements: (1) belief in a perceived personal susceptibility to an injury or disease threat, (2) belief that the disease or injury, if it occurred, would affect to some degree of severity part of an individual's life, and (3) belief that certain activities will either decrease its severity or do not entail barriers to action (that is, the activities can be accomplished).

Perceived susceptibility, the first element, refers to subjective risks of developing a condition. Individuals' beliefs about susceptibility range from one extreme to another. The client who had already been practicing risk-reduction behaviors and then became disabled would probably be more likely to comprehend the seriousness or severity of possible complications from lack of action (the second element). The third element, engaging in certain activities to decrease susceptibility or severity, will most likely occur if an action is seen as having a positive impact on the condition. Although a client may believe an action effective, that action may be impeded by certain barriers, such as cost, pain, inconvenience, or embarrassment. Whether the client takes action or succumbs to the barriers depends upon the degree of readiness to act and the perceived severity of the barriers.

At any point in the change process, resistance can arise. Resistance to change is considered a natural human behavior. The majority of human beings are reactive rather than proactive—they wait until a situation occurs before they act. Knowing that a change is not isolated in its application and effects provides the change agent with information needed to anticipate and avoid barriers to change.

The nurse needs to be able to identify barriers and aid clients in overcoming them. If the present situation or status quo is viewed as a barrier to change, then forces that will push a client to a new or changed position must be identified. The principle inherent in Lewin's force field analysis model is that to produce change, either restraining forces must be weakened or driving forces must be added or strengthened. The balance between restraining and driving forces must be altered if change is to occur.

Acceptance of change is affected by a number of important factors. First, if the client feels that the change is his or her own idea and is supported fully by significant others, resistance will be less. Second, resistance will decrease if the client sees the change as reducing present burdens, if the change is in accordance with one's values and ideals, and if autonomy and security will be increased as a result of the change. Third, the change experience will be met with less resistance if the client is part of assessing and diagnosing steps in the change process and agrees on the basic problem and solution alternatives.[16] The nurse/change agent must be able to empathize with the client and significant others, recognize valid objections, and take steps to relieve unnecessary fears. Finally, it is the decision making of the client that is critical to participation in health behavior changes. According to Roberts[11]:

> Personal decisions are affected by much within the individual—the cognitive, affective, and connotative elements—and by the situation in the sense of the psychological field, including,

among other forces, significant persons, the message, the channel of communication, and the agent of education. Any decisional movement itself is embedded in a complex process and is difficult to isolate, for there are predecisional forces and events. For us in health work, the postdecisional forces are important, for we have concern not only with the decision, but also with the maintenance of action resulting from the decision.

The nurse/change agent must listen to clients to learn attitudes, fears, values, needs, desires, priorities, and sources of information and their influence. Sometimes this means going ahead with clients on what they think they need first and that may be something other than the goals that the change agent has in mind.

TECHNIQUES FOR CREATING CHANGE

The techniques for creating change with clients must be carefully selected by the nurse. How directive or nondirective the change agent's role will be depends upon the client, the situation, and the change agent. The more directive role requires the nurse to assume leadership and direct the activity. If a more nondirective mode is the role selected, the nurse would then provide data and concepts or learning aids to the client as guides. The client then becomes the one responsible for self-initiation, implementation, and evaluation of the change process. Neither of these roles, however, is mutually exclusive. In fact, their manifestation may be seen in many ways and at any stage in a particular client situation.

One technique that can be used by the nurse to help clients achieve change is to teach the client skills of behavior modification. Farquhar[4] prefers the phrase "achieving self-directed change" that was suggested by the behavioral psychologist Albert Bandura because the client makes the changes while the nurse supplies the concepts to be learned and practiced. This technique is nondirective and probably would work best with clients who are not severely incapacitated.

Before embarking on a program of self-directed change, the nurse needs to make sure that the client has adopted the attitude that a change would be worthwhile. Without this positive attitude, the chances of successfully completing the six-stage program are highly improbable.

The self-directed program is made up of the

TABLE 26-1
Self-directed change

Stages	Steps
Stage I	
Identifying the problem	Become aware and collect data
	Set priorities
	Self-contract for change
	Analyze potential barriers
Stage II	
Building confidence and commitment to change	Make small changes first
	Deal with negative self-monologues
	Record positive self-statements
Stage III	
Increasing awareness of behavior through self-observation	Analyze behavior patterns in more detail
	Go back to problem identification and barrier analysis
	Self-record method
Stage IV	
Developing and implementing an action plan	Set long-range goals
	Identify steps and short-term goals
	Write self-contract
	Attempt change
	Achieve social support/helper
	Provide self-rewards
Stage V	
Evaluating the plan	Evaluate daily
	Evaluate at end of each self-contract
	List unexpected dividends
Stage VI	
Maintaining the changes	Return to methods used to achieve goals every so often
	Use monthly checklist as reminder to renew goal

following stages: (1) identifying the problem, (2) building confidence and commitment to change, (3) increasing awareness of behavior patterns by self-observation, (4) developing and implementing an action plan, (5) evaluating the plan, and (6) maintaining the changes.[15] Within each stage, Farquhar[4] recommends a number of stages and steps, outlined in Table 26-1.

If the self-directed change techniques are used, the nurse will be responsible for helping the client gain knowledge and skills through formal or informal training sessions and providing the learning tools such as books or audiovisual aids. In addition, the nurse can provide support, encouragement, and positive reinforcement when needed. The actual implementation of the change process, however, is the responsibility of the client.

Another technique that can help clients achieve change is to contract with them. "A contract is a mutual agreement between client and nurse concerning their expectations of each other. . . . Contracting is based on the premise that nurse and client are equal partners, each with different but equal responsibilities toward common goals. A contract makes expectations, goals and responsibilities explicit."[17]

Contracting is a more directive technique than the technique of self-directive change, but it is designed to help clients define what they need and want so as to increase the client's motivation to accomplish goals. Responsibility for carrying out the change process belongs to both the nurse and the client. A sense of equality must be established and requires that nurses verbalize their specific skills and limitations. Equality must exist between nurses and clients so that a sense of "we will work together on this" rather than "I have all the answers" is conveyed.

Four stages are involved in contracting with the client: (1) assessing the client, (2) planning the contract, (3) implementing the contract, and (4) evaluating outcomes. Assessment involves collection of data from client, environment, and significant others. Planning is accomplished with the client and includes establishing mutual goals, treatment methods, time frames, and responsibilities of the nurse and client or others. Implementing the contract involves translating expectations into actions that affect behavior. Evaluating outcomes determines how well goals were met and the degree of adherence and compliance to behavior changes.[13] Table 26-2 summarizes the stages and steps involved in contracting with the client.

The techniques of both self-directed change and contracting with the client provide valuable tools for rehabilitation nurses. Both techniques place ultimate responsibility for health status on the client. The nurse, however, must be effective in communications and interpersonal relations and be able to integrate these techniques into the

TABLE 26-2
Contracting with client

Stages	Steps
Stage I Assessing the client	Client's view of needed changes Client's environment Client's significant others
Stage II Planning the contract	Specific activities Duration of activity Methods to be used to evaluate activity Mutual responsibilities of client and provider
Stage III Implementing the contract	Translating expectations into behaviors Checkpoints for progress Teaching more about health (problem) Client's internal motivation Correction/reinforcement
Stage IV Evaluating outcomes	How well goals and objectives were met Improved adherence and compliance

nursing process to create a climate that opens the gateway to change.

SUMMARY

The nurse as a change agent should have a stable personality, conceptual sophistication, good interpersonal skills, and a good sense of timing. The change agent entering a client system needs a strong tolerance for ambiguity. The nurse's first encounter with a client may be marked by a certain amount of confusion that only time will resolve. Along with the change agent's tolerance for ambiguity must be patience and a high frustration level. Helping a client set goals and solve problems is likely to be a long and challenging experience. Quick results, full cooperation, and com-

plete success are unlikely. Resistance or dependency, resentment or overenthusiasm, and obstructionism or rationalization are just some examples of how clients may respond to attempts by the nurse to change behavior patterns or relationships. Therefore maturity and realism on behalf of the nurse are necessary to avoid reacting with the defeatism or withdrawal that commonly accompanies the frustration of a person's sincere efforts to help others. In addition, maturity is required if the change agent concludes that he or she cannot help the client, and referral to another professional is required. Finally, the best articulated plan for change can be destroyed if introduced at the wrong time. Knowledge of the client, the situation, and the nurse's own degree of patience is linked to timing. As one experienced change agent said: "Help is never really help unless it is perceived as 'helpful' by the person on the receiving end—regardless of the intention of the helper or consultant."[1]

REFERENCES

1. Beckard R: The leader looks at the consultive process, Washington, DC, 1971, Leadership Resources, Inc.
2. Bennis WG: Theory and method in applying behavioral science to planned organizational change. In Bartlett A and Kayser T, editors: Changing organizational behavior, Englewood Cliffs, NJ, 1973, Prentice-Hall, Inc.
3. Bennis WG: Changing organizations, New York, 1966, McGraw-Hill Book Co.
4. Farquhar JW: The American way of life need not be hazardous to your health, New York, 1978, WW Norton & Co, Inc.
5. Ferguson M: The Aquarian conspiracy, Los Angeles, 1980, JP Tarcher, Inc.
6. Havelock RG: The change agents' guide to innovation in education, Englewood Cliffs, NJ, 1973, Educational Technology Publications.
7. Knowles JH: The responsibility of the individual, Daedalus 106:57, Winter, 1977.
8. Lewin K: Frontiers in group dynamics: concept methods and reality in social science, Hum Relations 1:5, 1947.
9. Lippitt G and Lippitt R: The consulting process in action, San Diego, Calif, 1978, University Associates, Inc.
10. Menzel RK: A taxonomy of change-agent skills, J European Training 4(5):287, 1975.
11. Roberts BJ: Decision-making: an illustration of theory building, Health Educ Monographs 9:20, Nov 9, 1960.

12. Rosenstock IM: Historical origins of the health belief model, Health Educ Monographs 2(4):328, 1974.
13. Steckel SB: Contracting with patient selected reinforcers, Am J Nurs 80:1596, 1980.
14. Stryker R: Rehabilitative aspects of acute and chronic nursing care, ed 2, Philadelphia, 1977, WB Saunders Co.
15. Thorensen C and Mahoney M: Behavioral self-control, New York, 1974, Holt, Rinehart & Winston.
16. Watson G: Resistance to change, Am Behav Scientists 14:745, 1971.
17. Zangari ME and Duffy P: Contracting with patients in day to day practice, Am J Nurs 80:451, 1980.

ADDITIONAL READINGS

Bennis W, Benne K, and Chin R, editors: The planning of change, ed 2, New York, 1969, Holt, Rinehart & Winston.
Mauksch IG and Miller MH: Implementing change in nursing, St Louis, 1981, The CV Mosby Co.
McGovern WN and Rodgers JA: Change theory, Am J Nurs 86:566, 1986.
Olsen EM: Strategies and techniques for a change agent, Nurs Clin North Am 14:323, 1979.
Vanetzian E: Force field analysis: a person-centered approach to behavioral change, Rehabil Nurs 13:23, Jan/Feb 1988.
Welch LB: Planned change in nursing: the theory, Nurs Clin North Am 14:307, 1979.

Consultation in Rehabilitation Nursing

Jill A. Scott

OBJECTIVES

After completing Chapter 27, the reader should be able to:

1. Describe the services offered by a consultant.
2. Determine when to seek nurse consultation.
3. Identify ways in which to choose the appropriate nurse consultant.
4. Explain necessary considerations when negotiating with a nurse consultant.
5. Describe desirable characteristics of a contract.
6. State when and how the evaluation process should be used.

Consultation, the practice of seeking help or advice from colleagues, has been a long-established practice in the medical profession. The division of medical education and practice into various specialties and subspecialties has produced physicians who are experts in their areas of concentration. But in this age of specialization, there also is a renewed emphasis on the holistic approach to client care, an approach that has emphasized the necessity of treating the client as an integrated whole. The specialist, to truly respond to the total needs of clients, must seek the counsel of those who have expertise in areas other than one's own. This trend in medicine has had an impact on the education and practice of nurses as well.

The nurse of today, unlike counterparts in the era before 1960, is not and cannot be expected to be "all things to all people." Hospitals and clinics are divided into various specialties, and very early in the educational process and in clinical practice, the nurse is either placed in or chooses an area that begins to limit and intensify the scope of the selected area of practice.

In addition to this "bedside expert" in client care, there also has been a large increase in the numbers of nurses who seek to become clinical specialists by obtaining master's and doctoral degrees. It is not unusual to find, even in smaller, nonurban health care centers, nurses who act as consultants to their colleagues in the areas of obstetrics, cardiology, rehabilitation, neurology, and other specialized areas. "Consultation is an economical means to increase the technical competence of an organization."[3] The use of consultants to provide advice and guidance with patient care and with nursing management problems has been gradually increasing.

SERVICES OFFERED BY A CONSULTANT

The services offered by a consultant vary greatly, depending on a variety of factors. Some of the factors influencing the nature and result of a consultation include the expertise and background of the consultant, the setting in which the consultation takes place, the expectations of both the consultant and consultee, the problems and goals of both parties, and the methods chosen by the consultant.

Ferguson[2] believes that a consultant should assist the client (consultee) in identifying and clarifying alternative solutions to a given problem. "Generally, consultation is an advisement process in which the consultant provides suggestions and solutions ostensibly adapted to the special needs, problems, and situational constraints of the hiring agency, director, managerial group, or staff."[4] The consultant's experience and theoretical knowledge are used to help another person or group make better decisions or cope more effectively with problems. The nurse consultant in rehabilitation may function in any one or more of these ways:

1. As a knowledge resource and "expert" in clinical, client-centered matters
2. In identifying the need for change, planning for change, and helping the consultee implement change
3. As a teacher in staff development and inservice education
4. As a support person or sounding board in assisting clients to identify problems and possible solutions
5. As a liaison, bringing consultees together with other community agencies and resource persons

WHEN TO SEEK NURSE CONSULTATION

Rehabilitation can be treated either as a specialty or a vital part of every client's care. The services of a rehabilitation nurse consultant may be retained on a one-time basis to deal with a specific client, problem, or situation. Or, as in the case of an agency that houses large numbers of clients

with long-term or chronic illnesses, a contract may be made with the nurse consultant for ongoing, periodic visits to assure the continuity of rehabilitation nursing services within that institution.

Reasons for consulting a nurse specialist in rehabilitation might include:

1. To seek advice in adapting rehabilitation nursing services to a specific individual's situation, diagnosis, and personality
2. To coordinate the various rehabilitation disciplines to assure that the total needs of the client are being met
3. To evaluate, initiate, or upgrade policies and procedures
4. To develop, improve, and evaluate rehabilitation nursing skills and staff education
5. To organize an overall rehabilitation nursing program for a specific group of clients (for example, clients with spinal cord injury or stroke)

The services of a rehabilitation nurse consultant should be sought whenever those individuals usually concerned with overall care and rehabilitation lack the knowledge, skills, and expertise to offer a client the most comprehensive rehabilitation opportunities possible.

CHOOSING A CONSULTANT

In choosing a consultant, the client must consider the nature of the problem and the consultant's educational preparation, past experience, and credentials and references. The choice of who to approach should first be dictated by the nature of the problem. The client whose problem is organizing a spinal cord center within a general hospital obviously wants to seek the advice of a nurse with a strong background in theory and practice with spinal cord–injured clients. The consultee also would probably want someone with administrative and managerial skills, as well as an individual who is knowledgeable with regard to interpersonal communication and the hospital hierarchy. This consultant would probably have a master's degree in rehabilitation nursing along with several years of clinical and administrative experience in the area of spinal cord injury. In contrast, the nurse on a general medical unit seeking consultation regarding a specific client's pressure sore wants the consultant to be a nurse with extensive clinical experience and success in preventing and treating decubiti. The nature of the problem therefore is definitely the client's first consideration in choosing a nurse consultant.

Education

As already alluded to, the consultant's credentials are always evaluated with regard to the nature of the problem. Generally, however, the rehabilitation nurse consultant is a master's-prepared individual with a great deal of clinical experience in one or more subspecialties within rehabilitation nursing. The nurse consultant's master's degree in rehabilitation nursing lets the client know that the consultant has had theoretical preparation in the area of general rehabilitation, as well as clinical concentration and experience in one or more subspecialties within the field.

Past Experience

Past experience is often very important in choosing the appropriate consultant. This is especially true when the client requires assistance with matters that are essentially clinical. The nurse with graduate education and several years of experience in applying theory to actual clinical situations usually will offer clients the most relevant information and assistance.

Past experience in teaching also may be helpful. This experience indicates a certain expertise in communicating ideas to others, an important quality in many consultation situations. Similarly, administrative experience might also be a desirable quality of a good consultant.

Credentials and References

Before making the final decision as to the appropriateness of a particular consultant, the client should check the consultant's credentials. Where was the consultant educated? Is it a reputable school with current accreditation? Has the consultant written any articles or books in rehabilitation? A thorough review of the consultant's credentials is helpful in choosing the most appropriate person. Last, the consulting person or agency should check with others who have used the consultant's services. An extensive list of the consultant's credentials and experience along with persons who may be contacted as references is

obtained by requesting a copy of the consultant's curriculum vitae or resumé.

NEGOTIATING WITH THE CONSULTANT

Once the client has decided upon the most appropriate nurse consultant, an initial meeting is set up to establish the guidelines of the consultation. This initial meeting may involve only one or two key people from the agency and not all those who will eventually be involved in or affected by the consultation. Together with the consultant, they will agree on the structure of the consultation, discuss fees and time commitment, and share mutual expectations.

Fees

Generally the rehabilitation nurse consultant will fall into one of the following four categories where financial reimbursement is concerned: voluntary, salaried, flat fee-for-service, or hourly.

The conditions under which a consultant would donate services to an agency or organization are limited, but these do exist. A rehabilitation nurse might volunteer services to one or more community self-help groups with no formal ties to a health care agency or no financial backing. For example, groups of clients with multiple sclerosis or recovering stroke victims who have organized to provide mutual help and support might use the rehabilitation nurse as a knowledge resource and client advocate.

In institutions where there are large numbers of chronically ill and disabled clients, such as rehabilitation centers and nursing homes, the rehabilitation nurse may be a salaried member of the staff. As such, the nurse would provide rehabilitation nursing consultation to any staff member or client in that agency as a part of the consultation contract. This "inside consultant" has a distinct advantage over the consultant who comes from outside an agency when it comes to valuable knowledge about the agency's internal workings.

If it is not economically feasible to retain a rehabilitation nurse on salary, an agency or individual may contract a consultant's services as the need arises. If the consulting agency suspects from the outset that the nature of the problem or situation is one that will require an isolated consultation, the consultee may contract with the consultant for a flat fee covering a specified assignment. On the other hand, if the situation requires ongoing consultation, the consultant may set an hourly fee. This fee may include all hours the consultant spends on a specific project, whether in the agency or in outside preparation. More frequently, however, the fee covers hours spent in the agency or with the client and is set sufficiently high enough to cover preparation done elsewhere. Thus a fee of $100 per hour or above may sound inordinately high until one considers that for every hour spent at an agency, the nurse consultant has traveling expenses and preparation time averaging 2 or 3 hours. Where the consultation visit involves extensive travel and living expenses, these are usually negotiated separately from the standard consulting fee.

Time Frame

The nature of the problem or situation will dictate the time frame of the consultation and should be mutually agreed upon before the actual consultation process begins. In the ongoing consultative relationship, the two parties might agree on periodic visits by the consultant, for example, 2 or 3 hours monthly. In the self-limiting consultation, the consultant and client might agree upon an estimated time frame with target dates when specific parts of the project will be completed. In either case, both parties should agree on a time allotment that best suits their mutual needs.

The Client's Expectations

Once the matters of fee and time frame are decided, the client should share expectations about the consultative process with the consultant. Ideally consultation should be a collaborative effort. If this is to be true, the consultant must have a clear idea of what the client expects from the consultation to see if the client's expectations are reasonably compatible with the consultant's. A client who sees the nurse consultant as an expert with all the answers may be sadly disappointed when the consultant does not provide the solutions to the problems presented. Failure to explore the client's expectations may manifest itself in resistance to the consultation and eventual failure of the entire process and relationship.

The Consultant's Expectations

The expectations of the consultant also must be clearly outlined, understood by, and agreed upon by both parties in the consulting relationship. The nurse consultant is obligated to share with the client the way in which he or she operates, as well as perceptions of the situation at hand. The consultant's self-perception may be as an adviser, a resource person, a helper, or a catalyst.[1] The decision to function in one or all of these roles will depend upon the specific situation and the expectations the client and consultant have of one another.

Blumberg[1] sees the nurse consultant as responsible for several activities:

1. Meeting the expectations of the group, even when these are inconsistent with one's own ideas
2. Gaining the group's confidence by altering one's own thinking to coincide with the group's approach
3. Being supportive when the group becomes confused
4. Providing reassurance to the group regarding the worthwhile nature of their ideas
5. Maintaining an environment relatively free of criticism to encourage group participation
6. Assisting clients to define their own problems
7. Helping the group direct efforts and thinking toward the most critical aspects of the problem
8. Assisting clients to see where they fit with regard to the problem and its solution
9. Assisting the group with application of problem-solving methods to the particular situation

CONTRACTS

When the issues of salary, time, and mutual expectations are agreed upon by both parties, these should be formalized in a written contract. I favor a contract that can be renegotiated and terminated at any time by either party. This type of contract adds a flexibility to the consultation process that will, hopefully, have positive results, keeping the contract relevant to the consultation situation.

EVALUATION

Evaluation of the consultation, its process and relationship, should be conducted on an ongoing basis and upon termination of the consultation contract. Both parties should refer back to the contract for the guidelines for such an evaluation. The evaluation can be used as a learning tool in helping both parties with future consulting situations. Questions to be asked might include:

1. Was the problem correctly identified?
2. Were the client's expectations met? If not, why?
3. Were the consultant's expectations met? If not, why?
4. Were goals defined and met?
5. Are both parties satisfied with the outcomes?

Answers to these and other pertinent questions should be formalized in a written report with copies retained by the consultant and the original report submitted to the consultee.

SUMMARY

Nursing consultation is an efficient and economical method of sharing rehabilitation philosophy, theory, skills, and practice with colleagues. It also is a means of assuring coordinated, holistic care to chronically ill and severely disabled clients. The nurse who experiences a situation calling for rehabilitation knowledge and skills that he or she does not possess should explore nursing consultation as an effective avenue to gaining these skills and this information. Ultimately, the client-consumer of rehabilitation nursing services will be the beneficiary of this nurse's willingness to consult someone who can help obtain the knowledge and skills to deliver the best possible rehabilitation care to clients.

REFERENCES

1. Blumberg A: A nurse consultant's responsibility and problems, Am J Nurs 56:606, 1956.
2. Ferguson CK: Concerning the nature of human systems and the consultant's role. In Bennis W, Benne K, and Chin R, editors: The planning of change, ed 2, New York, 1969, Holt, Rinehart & Winston, Inc.
3. Lange FM: The multifaceted role of the nurse consultant, J Nurs Educ 18:30, Nov 1979.
4. Stevens BJ: The use of consultants in nursing service, J Nurs Admin 8:7, Aug 1978.

ADDITIONAL READINGS

Edlund BJ, Hodges LC, and Poteet GW: Consultation: doing it and doing it well, Clin Nurse Spec 1:46, Spring 1987.
Fitzsimons VM: Becoming a nurse consultant, Nurs Outlook 31:240, July/Aug 1983.
Gebbie KM: Consultation contracts: their development and evaluation, Am J Pub Health 60:1916, 1970.
Hough A: The nursing consultant role, Nurs Management 18(5):65, 1987.
Lippitt G and Lippitt R: The consulting process in action, San Diego, Calif, 1978, University Associates, Inc.
Miller LE: Resistance to the consultation process, Nurs Leadership 6:10, March 1983.
Mumma CM, editor: Rehabilitation nursing: concepts and practice, a core curriculum, ed 2, Evanston, Ill, 1987, Rehabilitation Nursing Foundation.
Noll ML: Internal consultation as a framework for clinical nurse specialist practice, Clin Nurse Spec 1:46, Spring 1987.
Norris CM: A few notes on consultation in nursing, Nurs Outlook 21:756, 1977.
Sedgwick R: The role of the process consultant, Nurs Outlook 25:756, 1977.
Walker ML: The clinical nurse specialist as a consultant, Nurs Management 17(5):61, 1986.

Research

Brenda P. Haughey

OBJECTIVES

After completing Chapter 28, the reader will be able to:

1. Explain why scientific research is important to the practice of rehabilitation nursing.
2. Describe the differences between the roles of consumer and producer of research.
3. Identify barriers to conducting, disseminating, and using rehabilitation nursing research.
4. Recognize the wide range of research problems and methods relevant to rehabilitation nursing research.
5. Identify future needs for rehabilitation nursing research.
6. Describe the major ethical issues surrounding research in rehabilitation nursing.

The history of nursing research spans many years, yet progress in this area of nursing has been slow and sporadic. Since the 1950s, however, commitment to scientific inquiry has grown immeasurably and research is now recognized as a responsibility of professional nurses. Nurses' involvement with research is vital to achieving the goals of the profession, and rehabilitation nurses, like those practicing in other clinical specialties, must accept responsibility for contributing to the research endeavor. "The provision of rehabilitation services that are grounded in systematic research is something owed the persons we serve and something required if our practice is to be viewed as credible by the informed public."[24]

The purpose of this chapter is to provide a broad perspective on nursing research overall and research in rehabilitation nursing in particular. The first section deals with the rationale for research in nursing. Roles in nursing research are then discussed. Following this, barriers to conducting, disseminating, and using nursing research are considered. To acquaint the reader with the diversity of research problems and approaches relevant to rehabilitation nursing, summaries of selected research reports are presented. Next an overview of future needs for research in rehabilitation nursing is given. The chapter concludes with a review of ethical considerations in conducting research. The research process is not dealt with directly in this chapter; however, references to basic nursing research texts are provided in the list of additional readings.

RATIONALE FOR RESEARCH

Nursing research can be defined as "a systematic inquiry into the problems encountered in nursing practice and into the modalities of patient care, such as support and comfort, prevention of trauma, promotion of recovery, health education, health appraisal, and coordination of health care."[28] Research is important to nursing for a number of reasons, but probably foremost is that it provides a scientific basis for nursing education, theory, and practice. As a practice profession, nursing must continuously expand, validate, and restructure the body of knowledge upon which the practice of its members is based. Gaps in knowledge need to be identified and nursing strategies need to be evaluated in terms of their effects on client outcomes. The contribution of research to meeting these needs can be significant, thus emphasizing the nurse's responsibility to actively engage in the research process and use research findings in clinical practice. Failure to accept this responsibility could have particularly unfavorable consequences for rehabilitation nurses who function as partners on the rehabilitation team. As Wahlquist points out: "For rehabilitation nurses to decide not to engage in research that is productive, scientifically rigorous, and credible will professionally cause us to wither and die. Other disciplines will continue to absorb us, conduct research, and then improve upon what we have been doing in the past."[64]

Many nursing research needs and problems are common to the entire profession; others are unique to individual specialty areas. Distinctions between specialties can be made on the basis of factors such as goals, methods, or intervention strategies, but a more fundamental differentiation can be made on the conceptual level.[46] The concepts of concern in rehabilitation research are disability and handicap, including the related human problems of adaptation.[27] Thus research emerging from specialty areas of practice has a dual purpose. The various ways in which nurses may articulate with the research process is the subject of the following section.

ROLES IN RESEARCH

Before considering the issue of role designation in research, it is useful to think about the broader context of research approaches, because these may ultimately have impact on the role the nurse assumes.

Three major models are used for conducting most nursing studies: academic or university based, agency based, and collaborative. Engstrom[22] suggests that the collaborative model has the most benefit for nursing in that it combines the advantages of the university- and agency-based models while decreasing their limitations. For example, university-based researchers have access to a wide range of resources that can facilitate their work. In addition, their efforts are encouraged and viewed as both legitimate and desirable. On the other hand, academic-based research may be somewhat "ivory tower" and not address questions that have relevance for clinical practice. Agency-based research, that is, research conducted in a health care facility by a nurse researcher or the members of a nursing research department, is more likely to be focused on practice problems and has the added benefit of being conducted in the "real-life" setting. However, these advantages may be realized at the sacrifice of generalizability of findings, investigator bias, and inattention to generating basic rather than practice-related knowledge.

The collaborative model is defined by Engstrom as a "research endeavor that pools the resources of any of a variety of researchers, agencies, scientists, clinicians, and representatives from different disciplines."[22] Interdisciplinary research is one example of a collaborative model, and it is one that has particular relevance for rehabilitation research. The team approach in the research setting is conducive to using this mode of inquiry, and the very complex nature of many rehabilitation nursing research questions often requires the input and expertise of other disciplines. This is not to suggest that alternative models are not viable or should be discouraged, but to heighten awareness that the interdisciplinary approach to research is one way to maximize the quality of outcomes, as is the team approach to client care. Further, interdisciplinary research efforts offer the possibility of combining resources and sharing burdensome tasks, providing new insights on the research problem, stimulating critical review and subsequent improvement of research design and methodology, and finally, of enhancing the likelihood of funding.[22]

Whatever the model used, the question remains as to the role of the nurse in research, with the major distinction being that between consumer and producer. Regardless of the clinical specialty, it is generally accepted that the appropriate role for nurses with baccalaureate education is that of consumer. Performance of this role requires an appreciation of its importance, knowledge and understanding of the process of scientific inquiry, and ability to evaluate research and determine its utility and applicability for clinical practice.[41] Because research is the responsibility of the profession overall, the significance of one's contribution is not determined by the particular role assumed. Consumers and producers have unique experiences and talents to offer the research effort. As suggested by Schlotfeldt,[55] the requirements for input are multiple and varied. Certain individuals may offer "conceptual ability sufficient to deal with abstractions and theoretical formulations, as well as with concrete evidence, . . . some will formulate research questions and suggest hypotheses worthy of testing, . . . some will explicate theories and take responsibility for formal research and for continuously restructuring nursing science and still others will function in the capacity of research assistants."[55] In brief, the consumer and producer roles are interdependent; practitioners may need the expertise of qualified researchers to help them test their hypotheses, but researchers are equally reliant on those in the practice setting to raise the relevant clinical questions.

To what extent are nurses in practice implementing the role of research consumer? The consensus in the literature seems to be that the research dimension of the professional role is not being performed adequately. This may be attributed, for example, to failure to internalize the importance of research, lack of experience with and knowledge about the research process, and insufficiently developed skills necessary for critical analysis of research findings.[22,41] Mallick[41] suggests that the problem may stem from a deficiency in the preparation of baccalaureate nursing students to fulfill the role of research consumer. In her words, the situation may relate to teaching strategies "that emphasize mastery of research terminology and concepts but that fail to instill students with an appreciation of the role of the research consumer or to teach them the skills to critically analyze reports for applicability to practice."[41] To study this problem, Mallick examined 15 introductory research texts to determine whether and to what extent the role of the research consumer was discussed. She found that of the 15 texts, only six made reference to the research consumer's role and the references made

were brief. Only two of the textbooks reviewed emphasized the role of the consumer throughout. Mallick also found that information concerning critiquing research findings was limited. Only eight of the books presented material on this topic, and its placement was mostly at the end of the text. The placement, she concludes, suggests that "critiquing is a second-rate activity that is undertaken only by those who cannot perform their own research."[41]

Jacox and Prescott[36] also have pointed out the importance to practicing nurses of knowing how to critique research and determine its relevancy for client care. Although they would agree that many nurses in practice may not be prepared to assess the technical aspects of research methods and statistical analyses, they give recognition to the practitioner's extensive clinical knowledge as an asset that can be brought to bear in evaluating the clinical significance of research findings.

The nurse working in a rehabilitation setting has valuable contributions to make as a research consumer. First, however, there must be a commitment to research as a professional goal as well as acceptance of responsibility for participation in the research endeavor. What we need to keep in mind is that "the key predictor of nursing's eventual fulfillment of its potential as a socially significant, scientific, humanistic, learned profession is commitment to research."[56] At most this text can only hope to encourage the practitioner to accept the many challenges to professional growth created by commitment to scientific inquiry.

As mentioned earlier, the consumer role also requires knowledge and understanding of the research process. This can be enhanced by a variety of activities, including, for example, obtaining formal education, reading research reports, discussing research findings with colleagues, attending research conferences and inservice education programs, serving on research committees, collaborating with nurse researchers, and participating as a member of a research team. The crucial point is the need to expose oneself to various aspects of the research process. By doing so, what initially seems unfamiliar and awesome may become increasingly clear and thus take on new meaning.

Another dimension of the consumer role, evaluating research findings and determining their relevance for practice, can be particularly difficult for new graduates and others functioning as practitioners. It is beyond the scope of this brief overview to describe the elements and steps of a research critique. However, it may be helpful to the reader to be aware that guidelines and approaches to evaluating research reports are available in the nursing literature. Several useful articles are included in the list of additional readings at the conclusion of this chapter.

From my perspective, one of the most salient contributions of the consumer in the rehabilitation process lies in the generation and clarification of research questions that need to be answered to elaborate a body of scientific knowledge upon which professional rehabilitation nursing practice can be based. As scientific findings accumulate, the development and testing of rehabilitation nursing theory, which is currently in its very early stages, is likely to be enhanced. Thus the depth of clinical knowledge and breadth of clinical expertise of the rehabilitation nurse have significant implications for the advancement of rehabilitation nursing science. The data base in rehabilitation research is growing, but much remains to be done to demonstrate the benefits of research.

What are the potential benefits of rehabilitation research? Although most health care providers in the field could probably respond to this question, there are relatively few research-based data that suggest answers. Fuhrer and others[25] addressed this question as part of a larger study to develop a cost-benefit model for evaluating rehabilitation research proposals. Their investigation was a multistage systematic survey of the opinions of experts working in rehabilitation-related roles. The potential advantages of research were dichotomized into those benefiting disabled individuals and those having impact on rehabilitation service systems or society (see box). The benefits are listed here in order of importance as judged by the study participants and include a fairly complete delineation of the legitimate uses of rehabilitation research.[25] For these outcomes to be realized, however, research must be conducted, disseminated, and used. It is important, then, to consider potential barriers to these processes and alternatives to overcoming them.

BARRIERS TO CONDUCTING, DISSEMINATING, AND USING RESEARCH

Rehabilitation nursing research has lagged behind research in nursing overall. This may be partly explained by the fact that rehabilitation nursing

---

Potential Benefits of Rehabilitation Research

Benefits to individuals
1. Enhancing quality and accessibility of services
2. Enhancing individual coping skills
3. Minimizing functional limitations and personal disability
4. Improving personal vocational status and material well-being
5. Encouraging individuals' social participation
6. Fostering consumer involvement
7. Improving physical environment
8. Containing personal costs and need for services
9. Containing institutionalization

Benefits to rehabilitation service systems or society
1. Enhancing effectiveness of service providers
2. Improving program development and evaluation
3. Expanding knowledge base
4. Improving program performance and performance measures
5. Facilitating societal change
6. Improving legislative impact and coordination of governmental entities
7. Developing and communicating policies, plans, and procedures
8. Facilitating administrative flexibility and improvement
9. Promoting generalizability of services

From Fuhrer MJ, Cardus D, and Rossi CD: Arch Phys Med Rehabil 60:239, 1979.

---

is a relatively new clinical specialty and the number of nurses practicing in this area is small. Other influences on conducting rehabilitation research are described.

Conducting Research

One of the major barriers to conducting rehabilitation nursing research is the lack of resources. For example, there is a shortage of nurses prepared to conduct research and serve as principal investigators. Availability of time for research is another important limitation. The constraint of time "prohibits the nurse with a 40-hour week work commitment to nursing service from undertaking these types of projects"[64]; other problems seem to have priority over clinical research. Another deterrent is the money required for research activities. Fewer dollars are being allocated to nursing research; thus competition for money is high and likely to increase as a greater number of nurses conduct and request financial support for this activity.[64] Although success in obtaining financial support may increase research productivity, many potential investigators may find the process of applying for funds too painful and may be discouraged by "environments that do not nurture research."[60]

Another potential problem is that scientific inquiry raises questions and threatens the status quo. Questioning tradition may be difficult but is necessary; "otherwise rehabilitation nursing will fall prey to intuitive, nonscientific nursing practices that might deter or impede quality care. Nurses will attempt to generalize from inadequate data bases, communicate with other health care providers in an unsound fashion, and probably arrive at inadequate conclusions."[7] Support to take on research activities is needed from organizations such as the Association of Rehabilitation Nurses. This organization awarded research grants for the first time in 1988 as a way of advancing research endeavors in rehabilitation nursing. Research productivity is proportional to the availability of resources[64]; thus the need to intensify efforts directed toward gaining financial, administrative, and organizational contributions to nursing research is obvious.

Barriers to conducting research also arise from the nature and complexity of research questions concerning the rehabilitation process and the related problems in research design and methodology. Also, there is no consensus about a theory of rehabilitation.[25,27] In the past, theories from other disciplines have been used. Although research guided by differing theoretical perspectives has added to our knowledge base, findings need to be synthesized into a framework of rehabilitation theory. The advantage of theories is that they "offer an opportunity for bringing together observed events and relationships, for explaining how and why phenomena are associated with one another, and for predicting the occurrence of future events and relationships."[49] The lack of a theoretical perspective in rehabilitation limits the generalizability or applicability of research findings and the ability to explain, predict,

and control the events of interest, namely, client outcomes. As noted by Goldberg, "rehabilitation research is concerned both with the consequences of disability for the disabled person and with the influence of the person himself upon the rehabilitation process."[27] These concepts are multidimensional and difficult to define and quantify. This may be a deterrent to undertaking a research project, especially for those having only beginning research skills. The reader is referred to the article by Suchman, listed in the additional references, for a more extensive review of models for research and evaluation in rehabilitation.

To reiterate, the issue of research design also may be an obstacle to conducting research. For example, studies that address client outcomes may require a prolonged time for completion and collection of data at several points within this time span. Collection of data is particularly likely to be necessary when determining various phases or levels of adaptation in the rehabilitation process is the objective of the research. The problem is not only the great investment of time but also financial requirements involved, factors that may have an effect upon the likelihood of obtaining funding. In addition, the investigator runs the risk of subjects dropping out of the study. Results may then be biased if the characteristics of those who continue in the study differ from those who do not. For example, individuals who have not successfully adapted or achieved a particular rehabilitation goal may be more inclined to withdraw from the research than those who have made more favorable progress. The difficulty in using the experimental approach to answer rehabilitation research questions also needs to be taken into account. Although the experimental design is the strongest in terms of making causal inferences, it is simply not a feasible method to study many rehabilitation research problems. One reason for this is the limited amount of scientific data available to justify the testing of experimental interventions. Another is the requirement of the true experimental design to include a control group of individuals not exposed to the experimental treatment who are comparable to the experimental group. Appropriate control groups are difficult to find for many of the questions addressed in rehabilitation research.[27] Finally, the experimental design calls for manipulation of the independent variable, the "presumed cause" of some outcome, the dependent variable. Given many of the outcomes of interest in rehabilitation research, manipulation may be both impossible and unethical.

Barriers to conducting research also stem from difficulty in obtaining a sample of subjects to study. Recruitment problems may arise from the small number of clients with the disease or disability of interest to the researcher and the reluctance of individuals to participate in a research project. Clients may be too ill or psychologically distraught to cooperate or may be discouraged from doing so by family members desiring to protect them. The investigator also may be faced with a dilemma in terms of data collection. Traditional methods may be inappropriate in light of the client's condition, thus creating the need to consider new approaches.

Sexton notes that studies "of chronically ill persons are difficult to design and manage, and the relative paucity of studies of persons with debilitating or progressive chronic illness (e.g., COPD [chronic obstructive pulmonary disease], multiple sclerosis, chronic renal disease) testifies to the difficulty."[57] She encourages nurses not to avoid doing research because of the difficulties involved. As noted, new designs and methods or adaptations of those more commonly used may be necessary to meet the needs unique to conducting research in rehabilitation nursing. For example, studies conducted at multiple health care agencies can increase the number of subjects available for study. This approach has the additional benefit of reducing the potential for bias associated with using a single facility. More extensive use of case studies also may be advantageous. Holm[34] suggests this method is underutilized in nursing research and ought to be given greater consideration.

As the foregoing indicates, there are numerous deterrents to conducting research on the rehabilitation process. Similarly there are barriers to disseminating research findings that have implications for their potential incorporation into practice.

Disseminating Research

The dissemination of research needs to be distinguished from its use. "Dissemination refers to the distribution process while utilization is concerned with the actual usage of the results by practitioners. Dissemination is a *necessary* prerequisite for utilization, but widespread availability of research reports does not *guarantee* that they will be read or used by the target audience."[14] Problems associated with dissemination of research findings span three key issues: researchers' inclinations to publish; the placement of research reports, that is, where they are published; and the manner in which the findings are communicated.

All researchers do not take seriously their responsibility to publish research results. As Fuhrer notes, "researchers are committed to the creation of reliable knowledge. Other goals, such as getting the knowledge utilized, are assigned less importance."[24] Thus in some cases the findings are lost to the rest of the professional community. It is probably true overall, however, that potential users of research suffer from the availability of too much information rather than too little.[24,53]

Researchers are more likely to transmit information if the intended recipients are research colleagues.[24] For this and other reasons, such as funding and prestige, scientific investigators tend to communicate findings in technical research publications.[24] In the research literature on rehabilitation, a unique problem stems from the fact that the specialty is multidisciplinary; thus reports are scattered in a wide range of publications. Important information may be missed by clinicians who tend to read in their practice areas even though journals of closely allied professions may include relevant research findings.[24]

To encourage the use of results, findings must be communicated in a manner that is appropriate for the needs of the potential consumers. Most reports, however, "are written for researchers and other academically-oriented persons and *not* for practitioners."[24] Practitioners and researchers have differing philosophies. Practitioners tend to protect the status quo, and researchers are oriented to raising questions that may foster change. The extent to which research findings threaten traditional clinical practices is related to their likelihood of being rejected. Thus inadequate or inappropriate dissemination of findings may create barriers to the use of research.

Using Research

Research use is directed toward "transferring specific research-based knowledge into actual practice."[29] However, studies by Stross and Harlan[61] and Ketefian[38] indicate that the use of research findings by physicians and nurses is limited. Several factors help account for this. For example, the large volume of research reports to which consumers are exposed "renders it impossible for either the researcher or practitioner to master and utilize relevant literature."[24] Practitioners may feel they have no time to read research reports, or the findings may be disseminated in such a fashion that they are simply ignored. In addition, potential consumers of research may have inadequate knowledge about scientific methodology and thus feel ill-prepared to evaluate research findings. Haller and others[29] suggest that we lack consistency in nursing in terms of the processes, criteria, and issues we take into account when determining a study's relevancy for practice. This conclusion is based on the results of their survey of nurse researchers who were asked to indicate those areas of clinical research they felt had been developed adequately enough to warrant incorporation into practice. In essence, responses ranged from none to all. Resistance to change also may contribute to the problem of using research findings in practice. The reader is referred to Chapter 26, in which the issue of resistance to change is explored in more detail.

Perhaps one of the most significant barriers to research utilization is the practitioner's assessment that the findings are irrelevant and inapplicable. Bolton points out that many studies do not have "input or participation from the practitioners who will ultimately constitute the vehicle for the application of research findings. When practitioners are not active participants in the design of studies, questions of major significance may be overlooked or inappropriately framed, and thus, the eventual results may be inapplicable."[14] This points to a gap between research and practice. Along this line, Abdellah and Levine[1] suggest that the gap between nursing faculty and those in clinical practice is widening and that this has a bearing on the problem of applying new knowledge to practice.

Haller and others[29] focus on differences in methodology between conducting and using research as a key determinant of the gap between research and practice. Research methods are systematic, rigorous, controlled, relatively inflexible, and designed to minimize the investigator's personal biases. The researcher uses logic and searches for commonalities in people or phenomena. Clinical measures, on the other hand, "may rely on precedent and call on clinical judgment.

The clinician takes an intuitive approach and views each case as unique."[29]

Insight into barriers to applying research to practice can facilitate attempts to overcome them, but resolution of the problems will no doubt require intense efforts, particularly on the part of nurse researchers, educators, and practitioners. The allocation of resources to the accomplishment of these efforts is justifiable, however, in light of the profession's goal to maximize the quality of care it provides. Some examples of contributions that have been made are included in the following overview.

OVERVIEW OF RESEARCH WITH IMPLICATIONS FOR REHABILITATION NURSING

Table 28-1 presents selected examples of research with potential implications for rehabilitation nurses. The studies included are not intended as an exhaustive review of the literature on each topic but highlight the broad scope of research questions pertinent to rehabilitation nursing and the variety of designs and methods investigators have used to study the problems at hand. For ease of presentation, the material is organized according to some of the major client problem areas requiring the attention of the rehabilitation nurse specialist. These include breathing, elimination, comfort, communication, mobilization/motor function, and coping. Except for those abstracts/summaries where the citation is preceded by an asterisk, all are reproduced with permission exactly as they appeared in the original publication.

As evidenced by the data in Table 28-1, there is much diversity in the research problems investigators have addressed. However, there are still many gaps in our knowledge that need to be filled.

FUTURE NEEDS FOR RESEARCH

The future needs for research in rehabilitation are numerous. One of the most important areas requiring further study is that of evaluating the nursing and team process in terms of client outcomes. We need to learn how nursing practices affect client care and to determine the factors that account for successes and failures.[1] Thus future research should focus on identifying client outcomes and developing precise instruments by

Text continued on p. 559.

TABLE 28-1 _____

Selected research with implications for rehabilitation nursing

Author/title/source	Abstract/summary
	Breathing
Fenton M and Gieske S: Relationship of the head-down position of postural drainage to lung parameters in chronic obstructive lung disease, Nurs Res 18(4):366, 1969.	Twenty hospitalized male subjects with chronic obstructive pulmonary disease were studied to determine some of the physiological effects of the head-down position of postural drainage. Pulmonary function measurements of tidal volume (TV), minute volume (MV), forced vital capacity (FVC), maximum expiratory flow rate (MEFR), and forced expiratory volume ($FEV_{1.0}$) were made. TV and MV were measured with a Tissot Spirometer using an open system with a two-way valve; FVC, MEFR and $FEV_{1.0}$ were measured on a Mc-Kesson Vitalor. Measurements were made in four positions ($15°$ prone, $15°$ lateral, $15°$ back, and $45°$ prone) and compared with the baseline performance of the patients. Findings indicated that in a majority of patients there was a decrease in lung function in the head-down position but there were no differences in functions with regard to the various head-down positions. Little or no change in subjective symptoms were noted and age of patient did not seem to affect the reaction to the head-down position.
Harris R and Hyman R: Clean vs. sterile tracheotomy care and level of pulmonary infection, Nurs Res 33(2):80, 1984. © The American Journal of Nursing Company.	As reported in the literature and observed in clinical practice, a variety of tracheotomy care procedures (tracheotomy suctioning and cleaning techniques) are currently used. The purpose of this research was to determine if clean tracheostomy care was more effective than sterile as measured by levels of postoperative pulmonary infection. Ten hospitals with large Head and Neck/ENT services were selected as data collection sites. At these centers a minimum of 15 tracheostomy patient charts were reviewed pre- and post-operatively for clinical and laboratory data related to infection. Patient level of infection was defined using the Weighted Level of Pulmonary Infection Tool, which was constructed for this study. Three categories of aseptic type emerged (clean, sterile, and mixed) because existing tracheotomy care procedures did not fall into one of the two hypothesized types. Data were analyzed using a maximum likelihood approach to mixed model analysis of variance or co-variance. The findings indicated significant differences among the three procedures with laboratory, but not clinical data. Laboratory data supported practicing clean procedures as those associated with the least post-operative infection.
Maloney FP: Pulmonary function in quadriplegia, effects of a corset, Arch Phys Med Rehabil 60:261, 1979	Fifteen quadriplegic patients underwent multiple pulmonary function studies performed in 2 positions, sitting and supine, and in both positions under 2 circumstances, wearing and not wearing a corset. Analysis of variance showed that 3 volumes were significantly improved ($p < 0.05$) supine, especially without the corset: vital capacity (VC), inspiratory capacity (IC) and tidal volume (Vt). Although most pulmonary function tests were improved when the patients were supine the trends when sitting were for improvement when wearing a corset. Most of these patients were studied at least 1 year postinjury and results are not substantially different from those 6 months postinjury. Corsets do not have an untoward effect on pulmonary function tests.

*Except for those abstracts/summaries where the citation is preceded by an asterisk, all are reproduced with permission exactly as they appeared in the original publication.

TABLE 28-1 _____

Selected research with implications for rehabilitation nursing—cont'd

Author/title/source	Abstract/summary
*Naigow D and Powaser M: The effect of different endotracheal suction procedures on arterial blood gases in a controlled experimental model, Heart Lung 6(8):808, 1977.	In an anesthetized hypoxemic animal model, 15 seconds of endotracheal suctioning, using a suction pressure of -170 mm Hg and endotracheal tube to suction catheter ratio of 1.87 to 1, produced a 13 mm Hg fall in arterial oxygen tension. Oxygen tension did not return to control level even at 5 minutes after suctioning. Giving 100% oxygen before suctioning prevented suction-induced hypoxemia during and immediately after suctioning, but at 5 minutes after suctioning, oxygen tension fell below control levels. Mechanical lung hyperinflation with room air after suctioning quickly raised arterial oxygen tension above control levels. When mechanical ventilation using 100% oxygen was maintained before, during, and after the suction procedure, arterial oxygen tension remained elevated at all times.
*Sitzman J, Kamiya J, Johnston J: Biofeedback training for reduced respiratory rate in chronic obstructive pulmonary disease: A preliminary study, Nurs Res 32(4):218, 1983. © The American Journal of Nursing Company.	The overall objective of this preliminary investigation was to determine whether breathing patterns of patients with chronic obstructive pulmonary disease could be altered by training patients to voluntarily change their breathing, using techniques of biofeedback training. Four ambulatory male patients were studied using a single-group repeated measures design. They participated in a biofeedback training program for a total of 19-22 trials over a two- to three-month period. Three to six 30-minute sessions per patient were used to establish pretraining baseline values of average resting respiratory rate, tidal volume, minute ventilation, and end-tidal CO_2, without feedback. Posttraining baseline values of these same measures occurred during the last three trials and at one-month follow-up. The authors concluded that some patients with chronic obstructive pulmonary disease can be trained with the aid of biofeedback training in the voluntary reduction of respiration rate and its associated increase in tidal volume. The effects of the training can carry over to baseline sessions conducted one month after training. However, the extent to which the voluntary reduction of respiratory rate is maintained beyond one month and is actually used in daily life is unknown. The course of improvement toward reduced respiration rates across the 12 training sessions indicated that the learning of reduced breathing rates that can be sustained over approximately 30 minutes requires several training sessions. Performance continues to improve over at least six sessions. This observation lends support to the idea that the sustained reductions of respiration rate and the associated increases in tidal volume are not easily explained as a result of the already available response repertory of these patients, but must be learned over the course of repeated training sessions. The data do not permit the conclusion that the training with respiration rate feedback was solely responsible for the learning, since subjects can be trained to some degree to slow their breathing by verbal instructions to relax, with or without actual feedback of their degree of muscular relaxation. The results of this study are clearly promising, although only further studies comparing the method of the present study with other methods can determine the relative utility of respiration-rate feedback.

Continued.

TABLE 28-1 _____

Selected research with implications for rehabilitation nursing—cont'd

Author/title/source	Abstract/summary
	Elimination
Champion V: Clean technique for intermittent self-catheterization, Nurs Res 25(1):13, 1976. © The American Journal of Nursing Company.	Seven patients with neurogenic bladder dysfunction who ranged in age from 16 to 54 years, and who had been on sterile intermittent self-catheterization, were changed to clean intermittent self-catheterization. Urine was monitored for one year after changing to clean technique. Urine specimens obtained while on clean technique were bacteriologically equivalent to urine specimens examined while patients were on sterile technique; the only exception to equivalent urine results were in patients who did not catheterize themselves at frequent intervals. Renal function tests on all patients were also normal. The clean, intermittent self-catheterization technique was effective, since infection did not seem to be caused by introducing bacteria into the bladder via the urethra.
Cornell S and others: Comparison of three bowel management programs during rehabilitation of spinal cord injured patients, Nurs Res 22(4):321, 1973. © The American Journal of Nursing Company.	To compare three approaches of providing bowel control for patients with recent spinal cord injuries 20 patients were assigned to each type of control: irritant-contact, stimulant, and mechanical. When effectiveness of the three approaches was measured for the time required for evacuation to occur after stimulation, the number of times evacuation did not occur from stimulation, and the number of accidental evacuations, the mechanical approach was found to offer the most effective bowel control during early rehabilitation programs.
Meshkinpour H, Nowroozi F, Glick M: Colonic compliance in patients with spinal cord injury, Arch Phys Med Rehabil 64:111, 1983.	While numerous communications have focused on urinary bladder dysfunction in the course of spinal cord injury, gastrointestinal disorders have received little attention. Abnormal bladder response to distension (automatic bladder) has been widely encountered among patients with complete thoracic spinal cord injury. To examine the similar concept in the colon intracolonic pressure changes were measured in response to variable volumes of water introduced into the organ. Eight patients with complete spinal cord injury at the thoracic region (T6-T10) and 10 healthy volunteers were studied. Water was infused into the colon and intracolonic pressure was recorded using a rectilinear dynograph. The procedure was continued until the pressure reached 40 mm Hg or 2500 ml of water had been administered. In spinal cord injury patients, the intracolonic pressure increased rapidly to a mean value of 35 mm Hg with as little as 300 ml of water, whereas in normal controls this pressure was achieved only after 2200 ml of water had been introduced into the colon. These findings indicate that the colon in patients with complete spinal cord injury of the thoracic region demonstrates an abnormal stretch response similar to that described in the bladder. This phenomenon could explain the frequent colonic symptoms experienced by these patients.
Reeves K, Furtado D, Redford J: Hydrogen peroxide: Potential for prophylaxis against bacteriuria, Arch Phys Med Rehabil 65:11, 1984.	The effect of dilute solutions of hydrogen peroxide, povidone iodine, and acetic acid on a chronic *Staphylococcus epidermidis* bacteriuria was studied to determine whether direct bladder instillation of the antimicrobial solutions would reduce or eliminate the bacterial count. In vivo instillation of volumes ranging from 50 to 400 ml and retained for 30 seconds to 40 hours was evaluated. The effect of the antimicrobial solution on bacterial survival in urine was also measured in vitro through quantitative analysis of the mixture at various times over 24 hours. Instillation of the antimicrobial solutions into

TABLE 28-1 ——
Selected research with implications for rehabilitation nursing—cont'd

Author/title/source	Abstract/summary
	the bladder had no measurable effect on the established bacteriuria. Symptoms of discomfort related to such a manipulation were least evident with hydrogen peroxide. In vitro, hydrogen peroxide had an antimicrobial effect as reflected by the reduction of the number of surviving organisms. Despite inefficacy in a case of already established bacteriuria, hydrogen peroxide appears worthy of study as a prophylactic agent against a variety of organisms because it exhibits in vitro efficacy and minimal in vivo symptoms.
Williamson M: Reducing post-catheterization bladder dysfunction by reconditioning, Nurs Res 31(1):28, 1982. © The American Journal of Nursing Company.	The purpose of this study was to determine the effect of reconditioning upon bladder dysfunction caused by prolonged catheterization. Eight women undergoing surgery with baseline residual urine volumes (RUVs) not greater than 25 ml and catheterization durations of 36 to 106 hours qualified as subjects. Immediately prior to catheter removal, the four treatment group subjects received reconditioning, a procedure in which their catheters were clamped for three hours followed by five minutes of urinary drainage. This cycle was repeated twice more, totaling nine hours ten minutes. The four control group subjects received no reconditioning. After catheter removal, reconditioned subjects resumed natural micturition significantly sooner than nonreconditioned subjects ($t = -2.82$, $df = 6$, $p < 0.05$). A t test showed no significant differences between the groups in post-indwelling catheterization RUVs following the first micturition, probably due to the small number of subjects, since the control group's mean post-catheterization RUV increased to a physiologically abnormal level (42.25 ml), while the reconditioned group's mean RUV stayed within normal limits. This study should be repeated to test for statistical significance in larger samples.
	Comfort
Barsevick A and Llewellyn J: A comparison of the anxiety-reducing potential of two techniques of bathing, Nurs Res 31(1):22, 1982. © The American Journal of Nursing Company.	This study compared the effects of the towel bath and the conventional bed bath on patient anxiety. The sample of 105 patients were divided into two groups—those who would be having invasive procedures and those with unrelieved pain. Anxiety was measured using the State-Trait Anxiety Inventory (STAI), the Palmar Sweat Index (PSI), and the Behavioral Cues Index (BCI). The scores from the STAI A-State subscale supported the hypothesis that the towel bath resulted in a significant decrease in anxiety for the sample as a whole and for the invasive procedure subsample. The hypothesis was rejected for the unrelieved pain subsample. Scores from the Palmar Sweat Index and the Behavioral Cues Index did not support any of the hypotheses. Based on the findings of this study, bathing is recommended for its anxiety-reducing effects.
Bohachick P: Progressive relaxation training in cardiac rehabilitation: Effect on psychologic variables, Nurs Res 33(5):283, 1984. © The American Journal of Nursing Company.	The purpose of this study was to investigate the effect of progressive relaxation training as a stress management technique for cardiac patients who were participants in a cardiac exercise program. After pretesting, 18 patients received 3 weeks of relaxation training in addition to their exercise therapy; a control group of 19 patients was not taught the technique. Pretesting used two instruments to measure stress levels—the Spielberger State-Anxiety Scale and selected dimensions of the Symptoms Checklist-90-Revised. At the completion of the relaxation training program, both groups of patients were retested on stress-level measures.

Continued.

TABLE 28-1

Selected research with implications for rehabilitation nursing—cont'd

Author/title/source	Abstract/summary
	Comfort—cont'd
	An analysis of covariance was used to test for the effects of the relaxation training program. The findings were: (1) posttreatment mean anxiety scores for the treatment group were significantly lower ($p < 0.05$) than that of the control group; and (2) the posttest scores for the treatment group were significantly lower for the dimensions of ($p < 0.01$) for somatization and interpersonal sensitivity and ($p < 0.05$) anxiety and depression than that of the control group. No systematic changes were induced in either the obsessive-compulsive or hostility dimension scores by the relaxation program.
Geden E: Effects of lifting techniques on energy expenditure: A preliminary investigation, Nurs Res 31(4):214, 1982. © The American Journal of Nursing Company.	A preliminary study of the effects of different lifting techniques (mechanical lift, rocking axillary, self-lift, shoulder assist, and straight-pull) was conducted. Fourteen female subjects participated. Measures of oxygen consumption, heart rate, respiratory rate, and blood pressure were recorded at six one-minute intervals during baseline and life phases. Analyses of variance (ANOVAs) were conducted on each measure for each phase using a two-factor repeated factor. In the baseline phase, no significant differences were obtained for the lift factor. The time factor yielded significant main effects for oxygen consumption, $p < 0.0001$, and heart rate, $p < 0.0001$.
	These effects were associated with one and two minutes following the subject's return to bed. In the lift phase, significant main effects were obtained for lift and time factors on oxygen consumption, $p < 0.0005$ and $p < 0.0001$. Significant main effects were obtained for the time factor on heart rate, $p < 0.0001$, respiratory rate, $p < 0.0006$, and systolic blood pressure, $p < 0.0045$. Finally, a significant main effect was noted for the lift factor on diastolic blood pressure, $p < 0.022$. These findings suggest that the mechanical lift is the most taxing on the person being lifted.
*Rettig F and Southby J: Using different body positions to reduce discomfort from dorsogluteal injection, Nurs Res 31(4):219, 1982. © The American Journal of Nursing Company.	The purpose of this experimental study was to ascertain whether discomfort from intramuscular injections in the dorsogluteal region could be reduced by the use of different body positions. Sixty subjects were randomly assigned to one of four treatment groups until 15 subjects were accrued in each group.
	Patients, in both the prone and side-lying positions, reported less discomfort more frequently when the femurs were internally rotated. The difference between the discomfort reported by patients in both positions with femurs internally rotated and with femurs externally rotated was significant at the 0.01 level. When the discomfort reported by patients in the prone position was compared to that reported by patients in the side-lying position there was no significant difference.
	It is concluded that patients may assume either the prone or side-lying position while receiving a dorsogluteal injection and that internal rotation of the femur is important to achieve muscle relaxation and decrease discomfort from the injection.

TABLE 28-1 _____

Selected research with implications for rehabilitation nursing—cont'd

Author/title/source	Abstract/summary
Rottkamp B: A behavior modification approach to nursing therapeutics in body positioning of spinal cord-injured patients, Nurs Res 25(3):181, 1976. © The American Journal of Nursing Company.	Ten spinal cord-injured patients at a rehabilitaton center were randomly assigned to two groups; one group received behavior modification training in body positioning, the other group received customary body positioning nursing care. Body positioning behaviors were modified through demonstration of body positions and shaping of body position moves with attention from the nurse as the positive reinforcer. Following treatment, the behavior modification group showed significant change in increased frequencies of daily changes of position and patient-initiated changes of position, in increased assistance needed for change of position, and in decreased frequencies of intervals of prolonged skin pressure. There was no significant change in frequency of face lying or participation in ward activities of daily living. Replications of the study are needed for confirmation of findings.
Steffel P, Schenk E, Walker S: Reducing devices for pressure sores with respect to nursing care procedures, Nurs Res 29:228, 1980. © The American Journal of Nursing Company.	In a study that focused on patient comfort and ease of performing nursing care activities 10 common pressure-reducing devices were evaluated for cost, stability, dimensions, positioning, temperature, bounce, noise, cleaning, leakage, weight, mechanical reliability, linen displacement, transfers, bathing, feeding, and dressing. Thirteen subjects—six quadriplegic patients, five paraplegic patients, and two patients with cerebrovascular accidents—and three nurses evaluated each device according to a prearranged schedule of daily patient care activity. Each subject tested five devices at least four times during two separate 24-hour periods. The devices were ranked and rated by subjects and nurses. When Kendall rank correlation coefficients were compared, the tau for ranking by subjects and nurses was 0.82; for rating, 0.42; and for ranking and rating combined, 0.73. Subjective comments by subjects and nurses were examined for relevant factors.
	Communication
Basso A, Capitani E, Vignolo L: Influence of rehabilitation on language skills in aphasic patients, Arch Neurol 36:190, 1979. © 1979, American Medical Association.	The influence of language rehabilitation on specific language skills (speaking, understanding, writing, and reading) was investigated in 281 aphasic patients (162 reeducated and 119 controls) who were subjected to a second examination no less than six months after the first. The relationship of the following factors to improvement was studied: (a) time between onset of aphasia and first examination; (b) type of aphasia; (c) overall severity of aphasia on first examination; (d) presence or absence of rehabilitation between first and subsequent examination. It was found that rehabilitation had a significant positive effect on improvement in all language skills. Time between onset and first examination and overall severity of aphasia were negatively related to improvement. The relationship of type of aphasia to improvement was not significant. Additional evidence of the efficacy of rehabilitation is provided by experience with patients who began language therapy several months or years after the onset of their language disorder.

Continued.

TABLE 28-1 _____

Selected research with implications for rehabilitation nursing—cont'd

Author/title/source	Abstract/summary
	Communication—cont'd
Beukelman D, Yorkston K, Waugh P: Communication in severe aphasia: Effectiveness of three instruction modalities, Arch Phys Med Rehabil 61:248, 1980.	In this study to determine which modality of instruction (verbal, pantomime, or combined verbal and pantomime) was the most effective in eliciting accurate and prompt responses from severely aphasic persons, subjects completed tasks involving body movements and object manipulation in response to each of the 3 modalities of instruction. Results showed that severely aphasic persons completed single-stage commands at least as accurately and depending on the task type, more accurately when given combined instructions than they did when given verbal or pantomimed instructions only. The combined instructions also resulted in a greater mean response promptness score (correct responses only) than either verbal or pantomimed instruction.
Heidt P: Effect of therapeutic touch on anxiety level of hospitalized patients, Nurs Res 30(1):32, 1981. © The American Journal of Nursing Company.	Effect of therapeutic touch on the anxiety of 90 volunteer male and female subjects between the ages of 21 and 65, hospitalized in a cardiovascular unit of a large medical center in New York City, was examined. The dependent variable, state anxiety, was defined as a transitory emotional state of the individual at a particular point and was measured by the Self-Evaluation Questionnaire x-1, developed by Spielberger, Gorsuch, and Lushene. Subjects were administered this tool pre- and postintervention. Three matched intervention groups were formed; each subject received an individual five-minute period of intervention by therapeutic touch, casual touch, or no touch. Subjects who received intervention by therapeutic touch experienced a highly significant ($p < 0.001$) reduction in state anxiety, according to a comparison of pre-posttest means on A-state anxiety using a correlated t ratio. Subjects who received intervention by therapeutic touch had a significantly ($p < 0.01$) greater reduction in posttest anxiety scores than subjects who received intervention by casual touch or no touch.
Kishi K: Communication patterns of health teaching and information recall, Nurs Res 32(4):230, 1983. © The American Journal of Nursing Company.	The purpose of the present study was to investigate verbal communication patterns between the health-care provider and the client in well-baby clinics, and then to investigate how these patterns relate to client recall of health information. The theoretical rationale derives from Flanders' (1960) idea of classroom interaction as a social structure in a social process. Communication patterns between health-care provider and client were analyzed by the Flanders Interaction Analysis System (FIAS, 1965). Four hypotheses were proposed: I. The higher the ratio of health-care provider indirect influence to health-care provider direct influence, the higher the client recall. II. The higher the frequency of health-care provider questions, the higher the client recall. III. The higher the frequency of client questions, the higher the client recall. IV. The higher the ratio of client talk to health-care provider talk, the higher the client recall. Hypotheses I, II, III, and IV were not supported. There was, however, a statistically significant inverse relationship between health-care provider questions and client recall.

TABLE 28-1 _____

Selected research with implications for rehabilitation nursing—cont'd

Author/title/source	Abstract/summary
Perry J: Effectiveness of teaching in the rehabilitation of patients with chronic bronchitis and emphysema, Nurs Res 30(4):219, 1981. © The American Journal of Nursing Company.	Twenty patients with diagnosed chronic bronchitis and emphysema, who participated in a rehabilitation program that incorporated principles of adult education reported on their ability to recognize and treat symptoms of their disease. Significant ($p < 0.05$) increases in knowledge and skills were found among study subjects.
Quinn J: Therapeutic touch as energy exchange: Testing the theory, Adv Nurs Sci 6(2):42, 1984. Reprinted with permission of Aspen Systems Corporation.	Previous investigators have suggested that the effects of therapeutic touch are the result of an energy exchange between the client and the nurse. In this investigation, the theory of energy exchange is viewed as part of the broader conceptual system proposed by Rogers. The theorem that the effects of therapeutic touch do not depend on actual physical contact is derived, tested, and supported via an experimental pretest-posttest design. Subjects treated with non-contact therapeutic touch demonstrated a significantly greater decrease in state anxiety than subjects treated with mimic control intervention. Implications for further theory development are presented.

Mobility

Baum H and Rothschild B: Multiple sclerosis and mobility restriction, Arch Phys Med Rehabil 64:591, 1983.	Examination of mobility restriction among multiple sclerosis (MS) patients and its relationship to selected disease and demographic characteristics was undertaken using data gathered in the National Multiple Sclerosis Survey. Whether and where an individual needed assistance and the types of assistance needed were the dependent variables. These data were crosstabulated with the following patient characteristics: sex, race, educational level, region of residence, age on prevalence day, marital status, awareness of diagnosis, diagnostic code, duration of disease and age at first diagnosis. More than half of the patients reported needing assistance both indoors and outdoors. Significant factors in increasing the percentage needing assistance were as follows: longer duration, older at the time of first diagnosis, admitted awareness of the diagnosis, currently unmarried, nonwhite, and a "probable" MS diagnostic code. Most patients relied on a wheelchair or a person's assistance for help while few relied on crutches or leg braces.
Hathaway D and Geden E: Energy expenditure during leg exercise programs, Nurs Res 32(3):147, 1983. © The American Journal of Nursing Company.	Comparisons of the effects of three exercise programs (active, passive, and isometric) and a rest program (control) on energy expenditure (oxygen consumption), heart rate, respiratory rate, and blood pressure were made. Thirty-six volunteers (18 men and 18 women) between the ages of 25 and 35 participated. Repeated measures ANOVAs (sex by program by time) were used to analyze the data. Significant program by time effects were obtained on oxygen consumption, heart rate, respiratory rate, and systolic blood pressure. In general, pair-wise comparisons indicate that for oxygen consumption and heart rate the isometric and active programs were comparable and significantly more demanding than either the passive or rest programs.

Continued.

TABLE 28-1

Selected research with implications for rehabilitation nursing—cont'd

Author/title/source	Abstract/summary
	Mobility—cont'd
Huang C and others: Prescriptive arm ergometry to optimize muscular endurance in acutely injured paraplegic patients, Arch Phys Med Rehabil 64:578, 1983.	This study compared the effect of (1) continuous, (2) intermittent, and (3) graded exercise on the cardiopulmonary responses of 12 acutely injured paraplegic individuals having neurologically complete spinal lesions, between T7 and T12, and seven able-bodied control subjects. Continuous exercise consisted of cranking an arm ergometer at a constant rate of 30 W. Intermittent exercise consisted of arm ergometry at 60 W for 30-second periods interspersed with 30-second rest periods. In graded exercise, subjects worked for consecutive two-minute periods at rates of 10, 20, 30, 40, and 50 W with no rest periods between work periods. Subjects exercised for 10 minutes or until they reached subjective fatigue. Heart rate (HR) and oxygen consumption (V_{O_2}) were measured during rest and work. Paraplegic subjects performed 4.93, 4.89, and 4.95 watt-hours of continuous, intermittent, and graded exercise, respectively. Comparable figures for control subjects were 4.98, 4.91, and 4.96 watt-hours. There was a high degree of correlation between HR and V_{O_2} in both paraplegic ($r = 0.80$) and normal ($r = 0.85$) subjects. Both V_{O_2} and HR were highly correlated with work load in each group.
	Paraplegic subjects had significantly higher HRs ($p < 0.001$), respiratory quotients ($p < 0.05$), and ventilatory volumes ($p < 0.05$) than control subjects. Graded exercise produced a significantly higher HR than continuous or intermittent exercise ($p < 0.001$) during the final data collection period. Oxygen consumption during graded exercise was higher than V_{O_2} for continuous or intermittent exercise ($p < 0.01$) during the final data collection period. There were no statistically significant differences between continuous and intermittent exercise in either V_{O_2} or HR. Serum lactate levels were significantly higher ($p < 0.05$) in paraplegic than among control subjects; however, the type of exercise had no significant effect on serum lactate levels.
Jamison S and Dayhoff N: A hard hand-positioning device to decrease wrist and finger hypertonicity: A sensorimotor approach for the patient with nonprogressive brain damage, Nurs Res 28(5):285, 1980. © The American Journal of Nursing Company.	To investigate whether a hand-positioning device placed in the palm of a patient with nonprogressive brain damage will decrease hypertonicity of the flexor muscles of the hand through proprioceptive sensory input to the alpha-gamma coactivation loop, a hard cone was placed in the affected hand of 11 subjects who had sustained cerebrovascular accidents and had flexor hypertonicity of the upper extremity. Measurements of hypertonicity and functionality were made weekly for four weeks. All subjects experienced a significant decrease in flexor hypertonicity. Only slight changes were observed in functionality.
Mitchell P, Ozuna J, Lipe H: Moving the patient in bed: Effects on intracranial pressure, Nurs Res 30(4):212, 1981. © The American Journal of Nursing Company.	Intracranial pressure (ICP) was measured in 20 patients before and after each of eight nursing care activities: turning the body to four positions, passive range of motion (arm extension and hip flexion), and rotation of the head to the right and to the left. Technically usable data was available for 18 patients. Mean ICP increased for at least five minutes in all patients after one of the four turns and in 88 percent after half the turns. Change in mean ICP with one pair of lateral or supine turns was strongly predictive of the direction of change (increase or decrease) of the other turn of the pair. Large increases in ICP occurred in the five patients for whom head rotation was done, while there was minimal change in ICP with both

TABLE 28-1 _____
Selected research with implications for rehabilitation nursing—cont'd

Author/title/source	Abstract/summary
	passive range of motion procedures. A cumulative increase in ICP occurred with activities spaced 15 minutes apart, regardless of the nature of the activity. No cumulative increase in ICP was found with procedures spaced at least one hour apart.

Coping

Author/title/source	Abstract/summary
Baldree K, Murphy S, Powers M: Stress identification and coping patterns in patients on hemodialysis, Nurs Res 31(2):107, 1982. © The American Journal of Nursing Company.	The types and severity of stressors and methods of coping with stress were assessed for 35 patients on hemodialysis. Coping was measured with a tested scale and stress was evaluated with a scale developed for the study. Test-retest reliability of the stressor scale was satisfactory ($r_s = 0.71$). Results indicated that stressors experienced by the hemodialysis patient can be measured with an objective tool; psychosocial stressors have an impact equal to that of physiological stressors. Fluid restriction was ranked as the highest psychosocial stressor, and the top physiological stressors were muscle cramps and fatigue. Patients on dialysis for one to three years indicated the greatest amount of stress. Patients used problem-oriented coping methods significantly more than affective-oriented methods ($t[34] = 7.06$), ($p < 0.001$). Optimism and controlling the situation were the two most common coping methods, and putting the problem out of one's mind and blaming someone else were the least important coping tools.
Chubon R and Moore CT: The cocoon syndrome: A coping mechanism of spinal cord injured persons, Rehabil Psych 27(2): 87, 1982.	Institutionalized spinal cord injured persons have been noted frequently to spend their bedrest and sleeptime with their heads covered with bed linens or pillows. A study was conducted to determine the prevalence of this head covering behavior among this disability group and to ascertain the etiology of the behavior. Comparison groups of spinal cord injured and non-spinal cord injured patients at two rehabilitation facilities were periodically observed during sleep and bedrest times for evidence of the behavior. Following the observation periods, the patients who manifested the behavior were interviewed to determine causal factors. The results clearly established a marked prevalence of the behavior in the spinal cord injured population compared to other physical disability types. Interview data suggest that the head covering behavior fulfills a variety of functions related to the coping process, but the reason for its prevalence in the spinal cord injured population remains uncertain.
Crewe N, Athelstan G, Krumberger J: Spinal cord injury: A comparison of preinjury and postinjury marriages, Arch Phys Med Rehabil 60:252, 1979.	A study of the preinjury and postinjury marriages of 55 spinal cord injured persons and their partners revealed several differences between the relationships. Although all patients had comparable levels of spinal cord injury, the disabled persons in preinjury marriages were judged to have less motivation for independence; a larger proportion of them received daily personal care assistance from their spouses. Furthermore, those in postinjury marriages were more likely to be employed and were judged to be better adjusted psychologically. Psychologists' assessment of marriages based on interviews with the spinal cord injured subjects and their spouses revealed that the postinjury marriages were happier than the preinjury marriages. Possible explanations for these findings are discussed, which include age and state of health, the impact of disability on the marital relationship and the personal assets of disabled persons who attract new partners.

Continued.

TABLE 28-1 _____

Selected research with implications for rehabilitation nursing—cont'd

Author/title/source	Abstract/summary
	Coping—cont'd
Dimond M: Social support and adaptation to chronic illness: The case of maintenance hemodialysis, Res Nurs Health 2:101, 1979.	The findings reported in the literature on the relationship between social support and adaptation to illness are ambiguous and, in some cases, contradictory. The present study sought to examine the relationship among support factors, medical status, and adaptation to chronic illness in 36 hemodialysis patients. Social support was measured on three dimensions: family environment (family cohesion and family expressiveness), level of spouse support, and presence of a confidant. Adaptation was assessed in terms of morale and changes in social functioning since the onset of dialysis. Data collection was done through unstructured interviews, mailed questionnaires, observation, and review of medical records. Correlation coefficients showed a positive association between the measures of social support and morale and a negative correlation among family cohesion, presence of a confidant, and changes in social functioning.
Dixon J: Group-self identification and physical handicap: Implication for patient support groups, Res Nurs Health 4:299, 1981.	Relationships between attitudes toward self and attitude toward handicapped persons based on semantic differentials and social distance measured for one nonhandicapped and five handicapped subsamples (n = 142) are presented. Among persons characterized by amputation, spinal cord injury, or stroke, over one third of the variation in evaluation of self was accounted for by elevation of persons with handicaps like one's own. Among persons characterized by arthritis or emotional disturbance and among the handicapped, evaluation of self was most closely related to evaluation of the average person. These results indicate strong group identification on the part of persons with more visible handicaps and a tendency toward dissociation on the part of those with less visible handicaps. The finding of high levels of identification within three of the five conditions studied suggests that group techniques may be beneficial in dealing with stigma and quality-of-life issues; the finding of dissociation among persons with other conditions suggests that such techniques should be employed with caution.
Lewis F: Experienced personal control and quality of life in late-stage cancer patients, Nurs Res 31(2):113, 1982. © The American Journal of Nursing Company.	This study examined the association of experienced personal control and quality of life for late-stage cancer patients within the context of Rotter's Social Learning Theory and Seligman's Theory of Learned Helplessness. It was hypothesized in late-stage cancer patients greater control would be associated with a higher quality of life as measured by self-esteem, anxiety, and perceived meaningfulness. The longer the history of the disease, the lower would be the individual's level of experienced personal control and quality of life. Fifty-seven late-stage cancer patients completed four standardized instruments: the Rosenberg Self-Esteem Scale, the Health Locus of Control Scale (HLC); the Lewis, Firsich, and Parsell Anxiety Scale; and the Crumbaugh Purpose-in-Life Test. As predicted, the measure of experienced personal control over life significantly correlated with scores on the self-esteem scale ($r = -0.33$; $p = 0.001$); the Purpose-In-Life Test ($r = 0.45$; $p = 0.001$), and the anxiety scale ($r = -0.30$; $p = 0.001$). Contrary to prediction, scores on the Health Locus of Control Scale were only significantly associated with scores on the Purpose-In-Life Test ($r = -0.18$; $p = 0.05$). Length of history of disease was significantly related to scores on the HLC

TABLE 28-1 _____

Selected research with implications for rehabilitation nursing—cont'd

Author/title/source	Abstract/summary
	Scale ($r = 0.27$; $p = 0.007$) and to scores on the anxiety scale ($r = 0.20$; $p = 0.03$) but was not significantly associated with scores on the self-esteem scale or the Purpose-In-Life Test.
Trainor M: Acceptance of ostomy and the visitor role in a self-help group for ostomy patients, Nurs Res 31(2):102, 1982. © The American Journal of Nursing Company.	The helper therapy principle, which underscores the benefits from helping another person, has been relatively unexplored in the self-help movement. This study examined whether persons enrolled in the United Ostomy Association, a self-help group for ostomates, who functioned in a helping role as visitors demonstrated a greater level of acceptance of their ostomy than those persons enrolled in the same group who have not served in the visitor role. Results indicated that visitors' acceptance of their own ostomies was significantly higher than nonvisitors'. The length of time since visitors and nonvisitors had their first ostomy surgery was not a significant factor in the person's acceptance of ostomy. There was a significant relationship between the person's level of acceptance of ostomy and the length of time the individual had served in the visitor role. Serving in the visitor role contributed significantly to predicting a higher level of acceptance of the ostomy. The length of time since surgery was a significant predictor to serving in the visitor role. Factors of age, sex, type of ostomy, and length of time since surgery did not contribute significantly to predicting a higher level of acceptance of the ostomy.

which these outcomes can be judged. Existing measures of quality of care are inadequate and require further refinement.[62] Also, more emphasis needs to be placed on assessments of functional status.[1] Most previous studies have not been concerned with client outcomes; to the contrary, the "trend has been to examine the process of nursing rather than the nursing process."[7] It is necessary to overcome this deficiency in future studies.

A related area requiring further study is the rehabilitation team concept. In response to a paper by Halstead,[30] Barnard concludes that "there is no real evidence that the costly rehabilitation team leads to the most favorable client outcomes."[7] In fact, she suggests that the team approach may even result in fragmentation of care. Specifically, then, the effectiveness of the team approach needs to be studied in various health care settings and among groups of clients who have differing characteristics, diagnoses, and health care needs. We need to determine, for example, whether and for whom primary nursing might be a more appropriate alternative.[7] According to Halstead, without more research "team care will remain as it is today, largely a matter of faith and the subject of many platitudes."[30]

One dimension of rehabilitation nursing and team outcomes, namely, their cost effectiveness, has not been adequately researched. Benefits of cost effectiveness have largely been viewed in terms of institutional rather than client needs.[62] "The number of procedures and treatments incorporated into rehabilitation without sufficient evaluation that are costly in time or resources is not known. It is clear, however, that without systematic, adequate evaluation, we cannot establish cost-effective, measurable rehabilitation nursing care that yields positive client outcomes."[7]

Many kinds of studies will be required to provide knowledge about the ways and degree to which the rehabilitation process influences client care. For example, Nagi[46] suggests that epidemiologic studies and research into the natural history of disability would be useful. Longitudinal studies that begin with the onset of disability also could generate important information. The process of rehabilitation is largely a reversal or prevention of the process of disability. An understanding of the course of the process of disability should provide a better basis for experimentation with the timing and techniques of intervention that would enhance the use of rehabilitation as a measure for the prevention rather than the remedy of disability.[46] Long-range successes of the rehabilitation process in terms of life adjustment need to be studied, as does the entire process of transition to and reintegration into the community after inservice care.[46] Results of prediction studies could be used as a basis for assigning clients to particular treatment regimens, thus having implications for improving rehabilitation services.[14]

More specific to rehabilitation nursing research is the need to make better use of and build upon data that already exist. Replication of previous research would be of benefit and must be done to allow generalizations to different groups. Descriptive studies also are needed in many areas. Results from such inquiries can help identify the independent variables that may influence rehabilitation outcomes and can suggest hypotheses that warrant further investigation.[7] As noted earlier, better use of case studies should be considered. Barnard points out that findings from intense studies of individuals can "identify variables that need to be measured, controlled, or manipulated in larger, more comprehensive studies."[7] Particular client problem areas that need the attention of nursing research include coping, self-care, mobility, sexuality, positioning, communication, maintenance of body functions, skin care, and sensation.[7]

Overall, we need to be concerned with increasing the commitment of rehabilitation nurses to research efforts and providing the necessary knowledge and skills to assure its implementation and use. Many needs for future studies have been delineated; however, one important aspect of nursing research, namely, ethical considerations, also should be addressed. This topic is the focus of the concluding segment of this chapter.

ETHICAL CONSIDERATIONS

Progress in science and technology has obvious advantages to society; however, some of the benefits simultaneously pose ethical concerns because they are accompanied by potential violations of human rights. One major issue that comes to mind is invasion of privacy. For example, think about the possible infringement of privacy created by the computerization of personal information, particularly when access to personal data is achieved easily. Within the health care sector, the newly developed capabilities for organ transplantation have raised questions about the definition of death and the appropriate criteria for selection of organ recipients. Similarly, the progress of nursing research and the increasing number of clinical studies involving experimentation with human subjects have brought to the attention of the profession the need to deal with ethical issues in the conduct of scientific inquiry. "By definition, the ethics of nursing research involve those aspects of research in nursing which relate to their moral and social impact on society . . . [and] the ethical limits within which clinical research may be undertaken because research on the human person presents unique hazards, risks, and responsibilities."[5] In this respect, concerns of rehabilitation nurses, whether consumers or producers of research, are consistent with those of the profession overall.

Conflicts Between Science and Society

As implied above, scientific progress and societal values may not be harmonious. Berthold notes that "the right of the individual in American society to dignity, self-respect and freedom for self-determination has conflicted with the rights and long-range interests of society on many occasions and on various issues."[11] Humanitarian, libertarian, and scientific values are integral aspects of the conflict. "Humanitarian values focus on respect for the sanctity of human life and the safeguards needed to protect the subject from physical or emotional harm. Libertarian values focus upon the individual's civil, political, and individual rights to dignity, self-respect, freedom of thought and action, and the safeguards needed to protect the individual from invasion of his privacy without his consent or knowledge. Scientific values focus upon the extension of knowledge for knowledge's sake and the safeguards needed to protect the right to know anything that may be known or discovered about any part of the universe."[11]

In summary, Berthold concludes that the "value conflict involves society's right to the extension of scientifically validated knowledge concerning the nature of man and his world, and human subjects' rights."[11] To put this in the context of nursing, "reverence for life and respect for human dignity have been distinctive attributes of true professional nurses."[5] However, because of this, ethical issues surrounding research endeavors can produce emotional conflict. It is important to be aware of the potential for such conflict, because it may affect attitudes toward and willingness to participate in and use research.

Issues in the Ethics of Research

Diener and Crandall[20] propose a series of ethical guidelines for research (see box on pp. 562-563). They categorize the ethical questions in research into three major areas: treatment of subjects, professional issues, and the relationship between science and society.

Treatment of subjects

Protection from harm. One of the basic concerns regarding the treatment of human subjects is that of harm that may be inflicted as a result of participating in the research. Harm is used in its broadest sense here and includes both physical and psychological injury or discomfort. One might ask if harm is ever acceptable, but there is probably no unequivocal answer to the question. A number of factors enter into determining whether a study can be ethically justified. One of these is the cost-benefit ratio, which takes into account evaluation of the potential risks entailed by the research in relation to the projected benefits of the investigation. A generally accepted guiding principle is that a study should create the least risk possible to test the study hypotheses.[20] Assessment of risk is not an easy task, however, especially in the domain of psychological harm. Another consideration pertains to the individual's knowledge of potential risks. Exposure to risks may be acceptable if the subjects understand them and voluntarily agree to exposure. Implicit here is the notion of informed consent.

Informed consent. Armiger[5] suggests that informed consent is the central issue in ethical research. In her view, informed consent means "that the person knowingly, voluntarily, and intelligently, and in a clear and manifest way, gives his consent to participation in the experimental procedures."[5] Facts that might affect the decision should be made known. These include, for example, resources such as time and energy, threats

to loss of dignity and autonomy, and the possibility of exposure to pain or injury.[11] The key factors involved in informed consent are summarized as follows:

1. Freedom to decide whether to participate without pressure or coercion.
2. Freedom to withdraw from the study at any time.
3. Knowledge about the potential benefits of the research.
4. Knowledge about the potential risks involved in participation.
5. Knowledge of alternative treatments, if applicable.
6. Information about what participation involves.
7. Assurance of confidentiality or anonymity.[5,20]

The decision about how much information to provide is sometimes difficult to make. It denpends in part on the characteristics of the subjects being studied and the nature and objectives of the research. May[43] has pointed out that there are potential problems with informed consent when the nurse is also the investigator because the client's perception of nurse versus researcher becomes an important variable. "In fact," she notes, "the subject's confusion about this dual role may increase the risk that he cannot give truly informed consent and consequently may fail to protect himself."[43] This and other issues pertinent to informed consent clearly warrant further study. However, the most important point of this discussion for the nurse to keep in mind is that the client has the right to make an informed decision about whether he or she wishes to be a research subject. Thus a key requirement for ethical research is informed consent of subjects.

Privacy. In essence, privacy refers to one's right to decide what and how much of himself or herself a person wishes to reveal. It is a right that is highly valued in our society. In the strictest sense, nearly all research on human subjects involves some degree of invasion of this right.[49] Of serious import, however, are invasions created by research conditions in which subjects are not clearly apprised of the nature of information to be obtained and the manner in which it will be used. According to Abdellah and Levine, "the test for undue intrusion is whether or not the intrusion is unreasonable or intolerable in terms of physical or psychic injury."[1]

Ethical Guidelines for Research

Sensitivity and responsibility

Ethical decisions are made by concerned and knowledgeable persons who realize the value implications of their choices. The ethical researcher is concerned about the well-being of research participants and about the future uses of the knowledge, and he or she accepts personal responsibility for decisions bearing on them. The basic ethical imperatives are that the scientist be concerned about the welfare of subjects, be knowledgeable about issues of ethics and values, take these into account when making research decisions, and accept responsibility for decisions and actions.

Precautions to safeguard participants

Research participants must be protected. In research exposing subjects to considerable risk, their safety must be ensured by stringent safeguards, including carefully selecting subjects and checking afterward for harmful effects. The scientist has a positive obligation to correct any harm that does befall a participant.

Informed consent

If the participants will be deprived of rights or exposed to serious risks, they should be informed and allowed to withdraw from the research. Subjects should usually be informed beforehand about aspects of the study that would affect their decision on whether to participate. They have the right to withdraw at any time, and strong pressure should not be used to gain cooperation. Even when no dangers are inherent in the research, subjects value informed consent, and it should be obtained whenever feasible.

The less powerful

Special care should be taken to protect the rights and interests of the less powerful participants in research, such as children, the poor, minorities, prisoners, and patients. Scientists should conduct more research on the concerns and needs of the less powerful and consider their viewpoints when formulating studies.

Privacy

Very private information about participants may be collected only with their consent. All research information on individuals should be strictly confidential and published only in summary form unless participants agree that they may be named in the report.

Deception

Research deceptions should never be practiced until an ethical analysis of the situation has been made. Are there other ways to obtain the knowledge? What will be the negative effects of the deception? Can safeguards such as forewarnings and debriefings be used? Deceptions vary from mild to blatant, and although many mild deceptions may be justifiable, large deceptions often are not. In addition to the ethical questions, deception research often suffers from methodological problems. Also, use of gross deceptions might seriously damage society's respect for the social sciences.

From Diener E and Crandall R: Ethics in social and behavioral research, Chicago, 1978, University of Chicago Press, pp 215-217.

The concept of privacy has several dimensions[20]:

1. The sensitivity of the information, for example, "how personal or potentially threatening it is."
2. The setting being observed. Settings range on a continuum from completely public to private. The home, for example, is private and "intrusions into people's homes without their consent are forbidden by statute."
3. Dissemination of information, for example, the number of people who "can connect personal information to the name of the person involved."

The more sensitive the information, the more private the setting, and the larger the number of people who may learn private information about individuals, the greater the concern must be about providing safeguards to protect subjects' privacy.[20] When possible, data should be elicited anonymously. When this is not possible, as is the case with many clinical nursing investigations, assurances of confidentiality become paramount, meaning that the information will not be divulged

Review by others

If the investigator is unsure about the ethics of the proposed research, he or she should seek the opinions of others. If subjects are to be exposed to risks or if the research raises serious value questions, it is wise to solicit the opinions of several reviewers. Disinterested persons may have a sounder ethical perspective than the scientist who is deeply involved with the research. It is often important to gain input from participants and from professional colleagues.

Experiments in change

When research is directed at changing individuals or a group, those who are the target of change should be consulted and their wishes and needs respected. Usually the target group can be involved in setting the goals of the change attempt. When various treatment groups are used in formal experiments, the scientist should carefully consider whether the various experimental manipulations are ethical. A group should not be placed at a serious disadvantage unless this possibility has been accepted by subjects or unless resources are insufficient to offer the most desirable treatment to all persons. Often the treatment that is found most effective can be offered to all participants after the study.

Objectivity and competence

Complete scientific objectivity is an ideal that cannot be realized in practice, but the scientist should strive to be as objective as possible in conducting research. Biases should never be deliberately introduced into the design or reporting of studies. Because poor research based on faulty method and design does not advance knowledge and wastes valuable resources, all social scientists have a responsibility to do the best research they are capable of. Results should be reported accurately and honestly, without omissions that would seriously affect their interpretation. Although values may influence the topic of research, the method should be designed to advance truth and not simply support a predetermined position.

Uses of research knowledge

Social scientists are responsible for how their discoveries are used. When a study is supported by a funding agency, the scientist must determine whether the research will be used for beneficial purposes. He or she should examine the possible applications of social scientific findings and endeavor to make these uses constructive. Before conducting a study the researcher must consider how the information will affect the people being studied. At a more general level, scientists have an obligation to speak out individually and collectively when they process expert knowledge that bears on important societal issues.

publicly. Protecting the subject's right to privacy, then, embraces the notion of protecting the individual against misuse of information.

Professional issues

Professional issues pertain largely to the personal attributes of investigators, which may have a bearing on the ethics of the research process. Characteristics of researchers are important because "convictions about individual dignity and autonomy help shape decisions about human subjects, control groups, and methodologic approaches.

Unquestionably, researchers reveal their belief about human dignity in the style, content, and interpretation of their reported findings."[5] Whether one is primarily a producer or consumer of research, awareness of potential breaches in ethics is essential.

Of particular importance is the need for scientists to have professional integrity and to be honest and accurate in their scientific endeavors. Although this may seem self-evident, it would be naive to assume that investigators are not confronted with many temptations to be dishonest.

Cases of data distortion and falsification can be found in the lay and scientific literature. The desire to make a significant contribution and the pressures of one's job to do research and publish are only two of many factors that may contribute to disregard of or inadequate attention to ethical standards.[20] Whether conscious or unconscious, investigator bias may be introduced into various phases and aspects of the research process, including design, data collection, analyses and interpretation of data, and reporting the findings of the research. Grant writing and crediting the contributions of others to the research project are other areas where the integrity of the investigator plays a major role.

In addition to integrity, the competence of the researcher is a significant consideration in assessing the ethical dimension of scientific inquiry. At the risk of sounding trite, it is nonetheless important to state explicitly the consensus that researchers need to be qualified to function as principal investigators. In fact, the earliest American Nurses' Association document to address ethics in nursing research stipulated that "research in nursing practice should be under the direction of a qualified nurse researcher."[4] Although the ultimate responsibility for carrying out ethical research no doubt lies with the individual investigator,[4] clinical agencies, funding agencies, and society also have responsibilities.[11]

Science and society

The relationship between the values of science and society was discussed earlier. An additional point that needs to be made, however, is that scientists have a responsibility to society because of the impact their efforts have on it.[20] Scientific data are used for many purposes, an important one being the substantiation of legislation and policy decisions. The contribution of nursing research to shaping the directions of health care has increased during recent years. As this growth continues in the future, societal accountability also will take on expanded dimensions.

Ethical Guidelines in Research

Although the history of ethical issues in nursing research is relatively short, ethical concerns are now a significant focus of attention within the profession. Ethics are addressed in two important papers published by the American Nurses' Association: *Code for Nurses With Interpretive Statements*[2] (Appendix B) and *"Human Rights Guidelines for Nurses in Clinical and Other Research."*[3]

Given the need for investigators to make multiple ethical decisions at each stage of the research process and in light of the responsibility of research consumers to assess the ethical components of research, the utility of ethical guidelines is apparent. "Ethical guidelines help insure that our research is directed toward worthwhile goals and that the welfare of research participants is protected."[20] Although primarily directed toward the area of social science research, the ethical guidelines proposed by Diener and Crandall[20] also have relevance for nursing. In addition, the substantive material included in the guidelines synthesizes and emphasizes some of the main points presented in this chapter.

SUMMARY

This chapter presents information concerning nursing research, with particular emphasis on research in rehabilitation nursing. Models for conducting research are presented and the roles of the research consumer and producer described. The aims and importance of scientific investigations are discussed, as are some of the major barriers to conducting, disseminating, and using research in nursing. Summaries of studies having relevance for rehabilitation nursing are included to provide the reader with a perspective on the wide range of pertinent rehabilitation research questions and the methodological approaches that have been used to try to answer them. Gaps in knowledge and needs for future research also are identified. Finally, ethical issues in conducting research are explored, and synthesis of this material is provided in the form of guidelines for action.

REFERENCES

1. Abdellah FG and Levine E: Better patient care through nursing research, New York, 1979, Macmillan Publishing Co, Inc.
2. American Nurses' Association: Code for nurses with interpretive statements, Pub No G56, 1985.
3. American Nurses' Association: Human rights guidelines for nurses in clinical and other research, Pub No D46, Kansas City, Mo, 1975, The Association
4. American Nurses' Association: The nurse in research: American Nurses' Association guidelines on ethical values, Nurs Res 17:104, 1968.

5. Armiger B: Ethics of nursing research: Profile, principles, perspective, Nurs Res 26(5):330, 1977.

6. Baldree K, Murphy JS, Powers M: Stress identification and coping patterns in patients on hemodialysis, Nurs Res 31(2):107, 1982.

7. Barnard RM: Research and rehabilitation nursing. In Murray R and Kijek JC, editors: Current perspectives in rehabilitation nursing, St. Louis, 1979, The CV Mosby Co.

8. Barsevick A and Llewellyn J: A comparison of the anxiety-reducing potential of two techniques of bathing, Nurs Res 31(1):22, 1982.

9. Basso A: Influence of rehabilitation on language skills in aphasic patients, Arch Neurol 36:190, 1979.

10. Baum H and Rothschild B: Multiple sclerosis and mobility restriction, Arch Phys Med Rehabil 64:591, 1983.

11. Berthold JS: Advancement of science and technology while maintaining human rights and values, Nurs Res 18(6):514, 1969.

12. Beukelman D, Yorkston K, Waugh P: Communication in severe aphasia: Effectiveness of three instruction modalities, Arch Phys Med Rehabil 61:248, 1980.

13. Bohachick P: Progressive relaxation training in cardiac rehabilitation: Effect on psychologic variables, Nurs Res 33(5):283, 1984.

14. Bolton B: Introduction to rehabilitation research, Springfield, Ill, 1974, Charles C Thomas, Publisher.

15. Champion V: Clean technique for intermittent self-catheterization, Nurs Res 24(1):13, 1976.

16. Chubon R and Moore CT: The cocoon syndrome: A coping mechanism of spinal cord injured person, Rehabil Psych 27(2):87, 1982.

17. Cornell S, Campion L, and Bacero S: Comparison of three bowel management programs during rehabilitation of spinal cord injured patients, Nurs Res 22(4):3321, 1973.

18. Crewe N, Athelstan G, Krumberger J: Spinal cord injury: A comparison of preinjury and postinjury marriages, Arch Phys Med Rehabil 60:252, 1979.

19. Diamond M: Social support and adaptation to chronic illness: The case of maintenance hemodialysis, Res Nurs Health 2:101, 1979.

20. Diener E and Crandall R: Ethics in social and behavioral research, Chicago, 1978, The University of Chicago Press.

21. Dixon J: Group-self identification for patient support groups, Res Nurs Health 4:299, 1981.

22. Engstrom JL: University, agency, and collaborative models for nursing research: An overview, Image 16(3):76, 1984.

23. Fenton M and Gieske S: Relationship of the head-down position of postural drainage to lung parameters in chronic obstructive lung disease, Nurs Res 18(4):366, 1969.

24. Fuhrer MJ: Communicating and utilizing research in medical rehabilitation, Arch Phys Med Rehabil 64:608, 1983.

25. Fuhrer MJ, Cardus D, Rossi CD: Judgments of the potential benefits of rehabilitation research, Arch Phys Med Rehabil 60:239, 1979.

26. Geden E: Effects of lifting techniques on energy expenditure: A preliminary investigation, Nurs Res 31(4):214, 1982.

27. Goldberg RT: Rehabilitation research as a specialization, Rehabil Lit 30(3):66, 1969.

28. Gortner SR: Research for a practice profession, Nurs Res 24(3):193, 1976.

29. Haller KB, Reynolds MA, Horsley JA: Developing research-based innovation protocols: Process, criteria, and issues, Res Nurs Health 2:45, 1979.

30. Halstead LS: Team care in chronic illness: A critical review of the literature of the past 25 years, Arch Phys Med Rehabil 57:507, 1976.

31. Harris R and Hyman R: Clean vs. sterile tracheotomy care and level of pulmonary infection, Nurs Res 33(2):80, 1984.

32. Hathaway D and Geden E: Energy expenditure during leg exercise programs, Nurs Res 32(3):147, 1983.

33. Heidt P: Effect of therapeutic touch on anxiety level of hospitalized patients, Nurs Res 30(1):32, 1981.

34. Holm K: Single subject research, Nurs Res 42(4):253, 1983.

35. Huang C, McEachron AB, and Kuhlenier KB: Prescriptive arm ergometry to optimize muscular endurance in acutely injured paraplegic patients, Arch Phys Med Rehabil 64:578, 1984.

36. Jacox A and Prescott P: Determining a study's relevance for clinical practice, Am J Nurs 78(11):1882, 1978.

37. Jamison S and Dayhoff N: A hard hand-positioning device to decrease wrist and finger hypertonicity: A sensorimotor approach for the patient with nonprogressive brain damage, Nurs Res 28(5):285, 1980.

38. Ketefian S: Application of selected research findings into nursing practice: A pilot study, Nurs Res 24(2):89, 1975.

39. Kishi K: Communication patterns of health teaching and information recall, Nurs Res 32(4):230, 1983.

40. Lewis F: Experienced personal control and quality of life in late-stage cancer patients, Nurs Res 31(2):113, 1982.

41. Mallick MJ: A constant comparative method for teaching research critiquing to baccalaureate nursing students, Image 15(4):120, 1983.

42. Maloney FP: Pulmonary function in quadriplegia: Effects of a corset, Arch Phys Med Rehabil 60:261, 1979.

43. May KA: The nurse as researcher: Impediment to informed consent? Nurs Outlook 27:36, 1979.

44. Meshkinpour H, Nowroozi F, Glick M: Colonic compliance in patients with spinal cord injury, Arch Phys Med Rehabil 64:111, 1983.

45. Mitchell P, Ozuna J, Lipe H: Moving the patient in bed: Effects on intracranial pressure, Nurs Res 30(4):212, 1981.

46. Nagi SZ: Some conceptual issues in disability and rehabilitation. In Sussman MB, editor: Sociology and rehabilitation, 1965, American Sociological Association.

47. Naigow D and Powaser M: The effect of different endotracheal suction procedures on arterial blood gases in a controlled experimental model, Heart Lung 6(8):808, 1977.

48. Perry J: Effectiveness of teaching in the rehabilitation of patients with chronic bronchitis and emphysema, Nurs Res 30(4):219, 1981.

49. Polit DF and Hungler BP: Nursing research principles and methods, Philadelphia, 1983, JB Lippincott Co.

50. Quinn J: Therapeutic touch as energy exchange: Testing the theory, Adv Nurs Sci 6(2):42, 1984.

51. Reeves K, Furtado D, Redford J: Hydrogen peroxide: Potential for prophylaxis against bacteriuria, Arch Phys Med Rehabil 65:11, 1984.

52. Retting F and Southby J: Using different body positions to reduce discomfort from dorsogluteal injection, Nurs Res 31(4):219, 1982.

53. Rogers EM: Research utilization in rehabilitation. In Neff WS, editor: Rehabilitation psychology, Washington, DC, 1971, American Psychological Association.

54. Rottkamp B: A behavior modification approach to nursing therapeutics in body positioning of spinal cord-injured patients, Nurs Res 25(3):181, 1976.

55. Schlotfeldt RM: Cooperative nursing investigations: A role for everyone, Nurs Res 23(6):451, 1974.

56. Schlotfeldt RM: Nursing research: Reflection of values, Nurs Res 26(1):4, 1977.

57. Sexton DL: Some methodologic issues in chronic illness research, Nurs Res 32(6):378, 1983.

58. Sitzman J, Kamiya J, Johnston J: Biofeedback training for reduced respiratory rate in chronic obstructive pulmonary disease: A preliminary study, Nurs Res 32(4):218, 1983.

59. Steffel P, Schenk E, Walker S: Reducing devices for pressure sores with respect to nursing care procedures, Nurs Res 29:228, 1980.

60. Stovlov WC: Rehabilitation research: Habit analysis and recommendations, Arch Phys Med Rehabil 64:1, 1983.

61. Stross JK and Harlan WR: The dissemination of medical information, JAMA 241(24):2622, 1979.

62. Thompson LF and Steffl BM: Research in gerontological nursing. In Steffl BM, editor: Handbook of gerontological nursing, New York, 1984, Van Nostrand Reinhold Co, Inc.

63. Trainor M: Acceptance of ostomy and the visitor role in a self-help group for ostomy patients, Nurs Res 31(2):102, 1982.

64. Wahlquist GI: Promoting research in rehabilitation nursing, Rehabil Nurs 7(1):19, 1982.

65. Williamson M: Reducing post-catheterization bladder dysfunction by reconditioning, Nurs Res 31(1):28, 1982.

ADDITIONAL READINGS

Abdellah FG: Approaches to protecting the rights of human subjects, Nurs Res 16(4):316, 1967.

Abdellah F and Levine E: Better patient care through nursing research, New York, 1978, Macmillan Publishing Co, Inc.

American Nurses' Association: Issues in research: Social, professional, and methodological, 1974, Publ No D44500.

Binger JL and Jensen LM: Lippincott's guide to nursing literature: A handbook for students, writers, and researchers, Philadelphia, 1980, JB Lippincott Co.

Burns N and Grove SK: The practice of nursing research: Conduct, critique and utilization, Philadelphia, 1987, WB Saunders Co.

Chinn PL and Jacobs MK: Theory and nursing, St. Louis, 1983, The CV Mosby Co.

Fawcett J: Utilization of nursing research findings, Image 14(2):57, 1982.

Gordon M: Determining study topics, Nurs Res 29(2):83, 1980.

Gorenberg B: The research tradition of nursing: An emerging issue, Nurs Res 32(6):347, 1983.

Gortner SR and Nahm H: An overview of nursing research in the United States, Nurs Res 26(1):10, 1977.

Haughey B: Considerations in applying research findings to practice, Dimens Crit Care Nurs 3(5):288, 1984.

Horsley J, Pelz DC, Guy JS: Using research to improve nursing practice, New York, 1983, Grune & Stratton, Inc.

Jacobsen BS and Meininger JC: The designs and methods of published nursing research: 1956-1983, Nurs Res 34(5), 1985.

Jacobson SF: Ethical issues in experimentation with human subjects, Nurs Forum 12(1):59, 1973.

Jacox A and Prescott P: Determining a study's relevance for clinical practice, Am J Nurs 78:1882, 1978.

Kerlinger F: Foundations of behavioral research, ed 2, New York, 1973, Holt, Rinehart, & Winston.

Kibrick AK: The emergence of research in nursing. In Wechler H and Kibrick A, editors: Explorations in nursing research, New York, 1979, Human Sciences Press.

LoBiondo-Wood G and Haber J: Nursing research: Critical appraisal and utilization, St. Louis, 1986, The CV Mosby Co.

Ozel AT and Kottke FJ: Research trends in physical medicine and rehabilitation, Arch Phys Med Rehabil 59:166, 1978.

See EM: The ANA and research in nursing, Nurs Res 26(3):165, 1977.

Snyder M, editor: A guide to neurological and neurosurgical nursing, New York, 1983, John Wiley & Sons, Inc.

Suchman EA: A model for research and evaluation on rehabilitation. In Sussman MB, editor: Sociology and rehabilitation, 1965, American Sociological Association.

Sweeney MA and Oliveri P: An introduction to nursing research, Philadelphia, 1981, JB Lippincott Co.

Werner EE and Weiner DL: Understanding the use of basic statistics in nursing research, Am J Nurs 83:770, 1983.

Wilson HK: Research in nursing, Reading, Mass, 1985, Addison-Wesley Publishing Co.

Wooldridge PJ, Leonard RC, Skipper JK: Methods of clinical experimentation to improve patient care, St. Louis, 1978, The CV Mosby Co.

Young C, Saelinger D, and Moore P: A conceptual framework for rehabilitation nursing, Rehabil Nurs 9:17, 1984.

Ethical Issues in Rehabilitation Nursing: A Case Study

Mila A. Aroskar

OBJECTIVES

After completing Chapter 29, the reader will be able to:

1. Identify ethical dimensions of nurse-client relationships in rehabilitation nursing.

2. Use ethical principles, concepts, and modes of thinking in making ethically sound choices in a client care situation.

CASE STUDY

Ann, a 21-year-old married college senior with a 6-month-old infant, was struck by a car 4 months ago while hurrying across the street to the agency where she was doing her public health nursing practicum. She is a paraplegic as a result of the accident and has recently arrived on your rehabilitation unit for further assessment and therapy after several surgical interventions. She is very discouraged and is described by some of the nurses as "depressed." She has told the nurses, her husband, and her parents that she is very concerned about the financial costs of her care, as well as the emotional and psychological costs to her husband and family. Her husband has recently taken two jobs in addition to his college studies to pay some of the hospital expenses because their health care coverage is minimal. Ann's mother has been caring for the baby since the accident. Ann told three of the nurses that she wants a weekend pass as soon as possible in order to go home and commit suicide. She sees this as a "rational way" to deal with the financial and emotional costs to those she loves. She does not want her family to know this and has asked the nurses to keep the information confidential. She also has been reluctant to participate in therapy for the past 2 days.

Clients with severe physical disabilities or chronic disease often confront nurses in rehabilitation settings with difficult and painful ethical circumstances or dilemmas. These questions and issues ought to be addressed *explicitly* in order for the client to receive care that takes the whole person into account in decision making and to preserve the nurse's personal and professional integrity.

ETHICAL DIMENSIONS OF THE NURSE-CLIENT RELATIONSHIP

The nurse-client relationship includes several important dimensions (Figure 29-1). The ethical dimension has always been an implicit part of the client care situation but has not always received explicit attention in decision making. Ethical dimensions of nursing and health care are receiving more specific attention as the availability of increasingly sophisticated and expensive technolo-

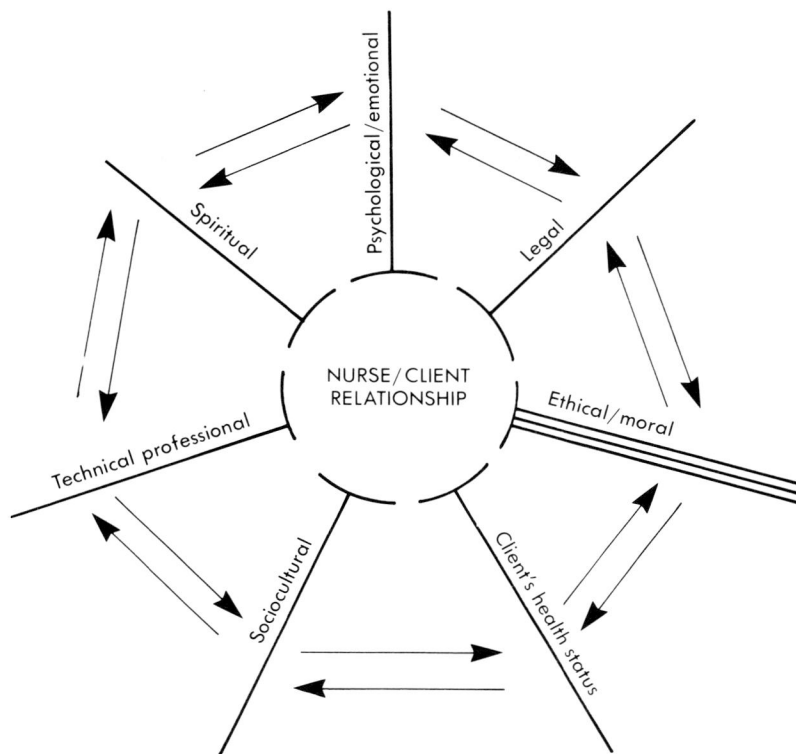

Figure 29-1
Interrelated dimensions of client care relationships.

gies make it possible to save lives that in the recent past would have been lost. At the same time, successful use of such technologies may allow survival of clients who, along with some health care professionals, may believe that an outcome such as living with a severe handicap is worse than dying. Such clients challenge the basic value structure of nurses and physicians who have learned to protect and support life in all circumstances. Nurses who find themselves struggling with such value conflicts will find no ready-made answers.

Rehabilitation nurses face ethical issues and dilemmas involving client rights, such as rights to refuse treatment and rights to confidentiality, as well as allocation and rationing of scarce nursing and other health care resources. Situations where the ethical dimensions predominate are identified by the following characteristics: (1) there is a conflict of needs, rights, or interests of the parties involved; (2) resolution requires reflective thinking using universal moral principles that can be justified; (3) decisions should be freely chosen and uncoerced; and (4) choices are affected by the feelings and values of the persons involved and the context of the situation. All of these conditions exist in the case study.

The nurses caring for Ann on the rehabilitation unit in a large general hospital are unclear about their obligations and what they ought to do with regard to the information Ann has given them. They decide to discuss their conflicts and questions in their biweekly interdisciplinary "ethics rounds." These rounds serve as one forum for reasoned discussion of the troubling ethical concerns in client care and help minimize the likelihood of ignoring them. Ideally, such discussion should occur as an integral part of all interdisciplinary and nursing client care conferences. In addition, ethical aspects of client care should be considered from a preventive perspective during the initial assessment period by each discipline and then brought to the interdisciplinary client care conference. This practice helps avoid crisis-oriented ethical decisions.

Initial ethical assessment would include assessing specific aspects of the client's situation that do or may raise ethical questions about the nurses' obligations in the present or future. The ethical principle of beneficence requires us to do good to and for all persons and to prevent or avoid doing harm to anyone.[11] This principle then requires that decision makers, such as nurses and physicians, are thoughtful and act with care. The following discussion includes but is not exhaustive of the ethical concerns of the nurses in their ethics rounds. It demonstrates a general process that nurses and others can use to make the most thoughtful decisions, taking ethical considerations into explicit account.

First, the nurses turn to the *Code for Nurses with Interpretive Statements*[1] (Appendix B) in hopes of finding solutions to their ethical concerns about their obligations in caring for Ann. The purpose of the code is to inform nurses and society of the profession's ethical values, obligations, and responsibilities. The 1976 and 1985 revisions of the code and the interpretive statements emphasize the accountability of nurses to clients. Earlier versions focused on the nurse's obligations to physicians and the employing institution. Items in the 1985 revision emphasize the provision of nursing service that respects the client's dignity and uniqueness. Human need is the major determinant in planning and implementing service, with respect for persons and their self-determination as a major value. Social or economic status, personal attributes, or the nature of the client's health problems do not determine nursing care according to the code.

The value and principle of respect for persons includes the moral right of each client to choose what will be done to his or her own person and to accept, refuse, or terminate treatment. The concept of respect for persons is complex and has been defined in various ways. It may be thought of as the principle that each person is seen as an individual, equal to every other individual and treated with consideration of his or her uniqueness. Morally compelling reasons are required to justify interference with a person's own purposes, privacy, and behavior.[10]

Such principles and values serve as general guides but do not help nurses to resolve specific ethical dilemmas like those in Ann's situation. There is a profound conflict of values for a nurse who values protecting and enhancing life and at the same time values client self-determination, which in this instance means that the client may make a choice with what the nurse and others would consider tragic consequences.

ETHICS ROUNDS DISCUSSION CONTENT

Failing to resolve the ethical issues and conflicts in Ann's situation through an appeal to the *Code for Nurses*, the nurses decide to engage in a process of systematic review of their ethical concerns similar to that of the nursing process. The nurses use the framework I developed for a discussion of their obligations to Ann and her family.[2]

Data Base

First the nurses consider the data base. Accurate information is a critical part of ethical inquiry and not always easy to accomplish when there is disagreement about the "facts" of the situation. They identify the people who are most closely involved in and affected by the decisions that Ann and others make with and for her. They include primarily Ann, her husband, parents, and infant son. Others secondarily involved and affected directly or indirectly are the rehabilitation team, which is responsible, with Ann, for her treatment plan; the institution; and the wider community. Further, the nurses obtain legal information from the hospital attorney as to relevant state law. One of the nurses also discusses the spiritual dimension, which includes a person's search for answers to ultimate questions about the meaning of life, death, and suffering.

Alternatives

The nurses think of several alternatives, including (1) respecting Ann's request for confidentiality and not telling her husband or parents, (2) telling Ann's husband and parents and asking them not to let Ann know that they have this information, (3) talking further with Ann in an attempt to assure that she makes any choices with adequate and accurate information and with hopes of influencing her decision toward life and ongoing therapy, in which she has been showing some progress in independence, and (4) discussing Ann's suicidal intentions and "depression" at the interdisciplinary ethics rounds, because it is only Ann's family from whom she explicitly wants her intentions withheld. The nurses are aware that choosing to make no decision as one option in this and similar instances is a decision with consequences. They also know that in the course of the ethics rounds discussion they may develop other options and may choose to consult a clinical specialist in psychiatric mental health nursing.

As the nurses consider the different choices they are concerned about jeopardizing the relationships of trust they are developing with Ann and wish to honor her request for confidentiality. They worry that if they do share this information with Ann's family and she discovers that they have, she will no longer trust anything they tell her. According to Childress,[7] trust is the expectation that others, such as caregivers, will respect certain moral limits. Accordingly, "trust includes the confidence that practitioners will provide personal care, respect us as persons, work for our life and health, and will not intentionally harm us."[7] The nurses are clearly seeking not to harm Ann and also want to work for her life and health.

Ethical Principles and Values

The principle of confidentiality claims that one has a duty to protect confidences against third parties under certain circumstances. Nurses might appeal to this principle in seeking to protect the information that Ann has given them. They feel bound to protect this knowledge even though given other circumstances they would feel bound to reveal this or similar information if the safety of others was in direct jeopardy. There are few who regard the principle of confidentiality as absolute, and most see those who seek to override the principle as having the burden of proving why they should do so. One of the nurses argues that, whereas the principle is not to be disregarded lightly, there are reasons to override it, for example, the consequences to Ann's family in terms of pain and suffering should she commit suicide. Ann's welfare is of primary importance yet the

welfare of others cannot be totally ignored. The nurses might then decide to talk explicitly with Ann about sharing her feelings with her husband and parents rather than keeping them to herself, with the additional burden of maintaining secrecy from those she cares about deeply. She may not have thought about taking the perspective of those who would be most directly affected by her actions and has only looked at her intentions from her own point of view. Bok, a philosopher, argues that although the premises supporting confidentiality are strong, they cannot support practices of secrecy by individual clients, professionals, or institutions "that undermine and contradict the very respect for persons and for human bonds that confidentiality was meant to protect."[5]

The nurses also are worried about negating the principle of autonomy or self-determination if they do not respect Ann's request. At the same time, they wish to protect and enhance their values for life and are very concerned about the consequences to Ann's family if she does carry out her intention to kill herself. Ann's family has continued to provide her with a strong caring support system from the time of the accident to the present. To their knowledge this has not changed.

Other consequences of the proposed choices are discussed, such as Ann's continuing conviction that suicide, with the intent or purpose of protecting her family from continuing emotional and financial burdens, is her best choice. Alternatively, Ann might change her mind and begin to participate actively in therapy again with the intent of attaining the highest level of independence possible in order to return home and care for her husband and baby.

Criteria

By taking any action, the nurses next consider what criteria other than Ann's medical status ought to be considered in making ethical decisions about their obligations. The criteria they consider further include social, psychological, and economic factors.

In thinking through the social and psychological aspects, the nurses recognize that Ann has not been declared "incompetent" to make her own decisions. She is still the primary decision maker, even though some would argue that a person thinking about suicide should not be making decisions alone. The nurses also are in a powerful decision-making position vis-à-vis the information that Ann has given them. They must make difficult choices in which they may decide to override the significant value of client self-determination and the principle of confidentiality with the argument that no one lives solely as an isolated autonomous individual. Ann is a spouse, mother, daughter, and member of the community. Before making a decision to override these values and principles, health care professionals must carefully assess Ann's decision-making capability. They decide to review the criteria developed by the President's Commission for the Study of Ethical Problems in Medicine and Biomedical and Behavioral Research.

Three general criteria for determining decision-making capacity suggested by the president's commission[12] are (1) the outcome of the decision, (2) the client's status or category, and (3) the client's functional ability as a decision maker. The first criterion of basing a determination of incapacity solely on the content of a client's decision because it is incongruent with the values of health care professionals and others was rejected. An ethical issue related to this criterion, which the nurses ought to consider, is paternalism. The concept of paternalism is discussed in many ways, and is generally considered to occur when others make decisions for a client based on what they consider to be in the client's best interests or when others interfere with the client's liberty in order to promote his or her welfare. One of the nurses argues, for example, that they should interfere with Ann's autonomy in decision making with the justification that the nurses know better than Ann how to promote her welfare at this time.

Brandt[6] argues that under certain circumstances a decision to commit suicide may be rational, but that a person who seeks to act rationally must also take into account various possible "errors" and make appropriate adjustments in his or her initial evaluation. He also discusses the danger of acting solely on the feelings and preferences one has today, suggesting that at any single moment many individuals might think it not worthwhile to go on living.[6]

There also are theological arguments (that is, arguments based on the study of God and his relationship to the world) against suicide that argue that we are stewards of our bodies and that as stewards we do not have the authority to end our lives simply because that is our choice. Arguments that go back to Aristotle are made that suicide does harm to other persons, which is the argument made by some of the other nurses who consider the potentially negative effects on Ann's family.

The second criterion of the president's commission would determine incapacity for decision making primarily on the client's membership in a particular category, such as age, mental retardation, or mental illness. This criterion is also rejected as a sole criterion and does not apply in Ann's case. It has been used to automatically deny young children and senile persons from participating in decisions about their own welfare in some instances.

The third criterion claims that decision-making incapacity is determined by an individual's lack of ability to make decisions that promote personal well-being as he or she sees it. This criterion requires health care professionals responsible for Ann's care to look beyond her choice for suicide simply because it conflicts with their own widely held values of enhancing and protecting life. If they decide to override Ann's autonomy the moral burden is on them to show that Ann is unable to make a decision that is congruent with her welfare as she sees it.

The nurses talk briefly about the economic criterion because Ann raised the issue of financial burdens to others. In the wider community, economic questions in health care are receiving much attention in an era of cost containment and competition. Although efforts at cost containment clearly raise questions of distributive justice or the fair distribution of benefits and costs of health care, it is difficult—if not impossible—to ethically justify decisions about individual client care decisions on dollar costs alone. Many say that financial costs should not be considered when individual client lives are at stake.

One of the nurses discusses an article he read recently on the economics and morality of caring for the terminally ill. Questions are raised as to whether a disproportionate, unreasonable, or unjust amount of money is being spent on care of the terminally ill in our society.[4] Ann is not terminally ill, but some of the same questions arise with regard to some forms of rehabilitation. An important and compelling point made in the article is that available data do not allow the conclusion that care of the terminally ill is unjust, unreasonable, or disproportionate. High costs alone do not justify such a conclusion. A further argument is made that simply belonging to a client category where the costs of care are high does not ethically justify thinking about denying or reducing care and treatment. The real problem is identified as the determination of when and how cost considerations are reasonable either in clinical or in administrative decision making. Acceptable criteria for making cost-conscious decisions might then be developed. The central dilemma is viewed as arising from the uncertainty regarding therapies that are only marginally useful in terms of benefits to the individual client, a dilemma that might be at issue in Ann's case. Although efforts to reduce financial costs of care are important, the authors conclude that great caution is required in making decisions for individuals based on financial considerations, because society has made no decisions and set no priorities for making client care decisions based on these considerations.

The issue of emotional and financial costs to Ann's family raises questions as to the community's obligation and responsibility to do as much as possible to modify this concern with regard to health care expenditures. Although there is some agreement in society about equity of access, there is no agreement that each person is entitled to whatever he or she wants or demands in terms of health care or that this is "owed" to all or any members of society.

Emotional and psychological costs to others may enter into consideration of alternative choices, but the client's welfare should always be of primary concern. In considering the emotional costs to others, there also may be some benefits that need to be assessed from the caregivers' perspectives in caring for a client. Ann's family may acknowledge that her situation is emotionally and financially costly but at the same time see Ann's continuing survival and progress as having far more benefits than costs. This is an example of the principle of proportionality. Proportionality requires weighing and balancing benefits and harms when they conflict in an attempt to produce a net benefit. If the choices are equally unattractive, we try to determine the best of the alternatives.[7]

Modes of Ethical Thinking

The nurses then look at their choices from the perspective of selected models of ethical reflec-

tion to see what this adds to thinking through the alternatives. The three models—consequentialist, deontologic, and pluralist—are discussed briefly here, as adapted from a discussion by Childress.[7]

The consequentialist model assesses the rightness or wrongness of actions based primarily on balancing benefits against risks. Choices are viewed in terms of consequences and results rather than duties and obligations. Decision makers try to determine the best set of consequences possible. A consequentialist generally avoids talking about rights of the individual because they cannot be quantified. Sometimes rights are translated into interests or needs so they can be balanced and trade-offs can be considered.

Utilitarianism is a commonly known type of consequentialism that is appealing to health care professionals because it considers harms and benefits to all and considers health as an independent "good." What is "good" is generally defined as happiness or pleasure, with "right" viewed as maximizing the greatest good and the least amount of harm for the greatest number of persons. This position assumes that one can weigh and measure harms and benefits and arrive at the greatest possible balance of good over evil for most people.

The nurses are aware that taking only consequences and results into account in making choices may be inadequate because some alternatives may seriously negate client autonomy, liberty, and rights. One of the nurses brings up the deontological model, which focuses on duties and obligations, for ethical reflection.

In the deontological model some acts, attitudes, and policies are inherently right (or wrong) apart from their efforts or consequences, as in the consequentialist approach.[7] Individual rights are emphasized rather than cost-benefit or harm-benefit analysis. One is required to universalize his or her actions and to never treat persons solely as means to ends but as ends in and of themselves. Fundamental values of this model include autonomy and self-determination grounded in respect for persons. The freedom and autonomy of the person, which has been a major point of discussion for the nurses, is critical in this model.

The pluralist model includes both consequentialist and deontological aspects. Although independent rights are emphasized, the importance of consequences and results also is recognized.

This is the model that is probably closer to the ways we think about situations in which there are conflicting values and obligations.[7] For example, in examining the choice of whether to talk with Ann's husband about her intention to commit suicide, the nurses may consider that the principle of autonomy and the duty of confidentiality may be overridden by the probable consequences that Ann's suicide would create for her husband and infant son. He cares deeply for Ann and her welfare, has not complained about his additional work since the accident, and provides much emotional support for Ann. He has often expressed hope to Ann and the nurses that she will soon be able to come home and that with some assistance they will once again be an intact family. He and Ann's parents have already made some modifications in their house so that Ann will have easier access with her wheelchair.

Rights

One of the nurses wants to review the American Hospital Association Statement on a Patient's Bill of Rights because she is concerned about Ann's rights as well as the rights of Ann's family. Claims to rights in the statement include rights to considerate and respectful care, to refuse treatment, and to have information about the medical consequences of refusal. Such claims do not deal adequately with the complexity of the situation confronting the nurses caring for Ann when claims of such rights conflict with other fundamental values. Simply stating rights as claims does not begin to resolve moral issues in client care.

Rights can be discussed in many ways, for example, as negative rights and positive rights. A negative right is the right not to be killed. A positive right is a claim of the right to die with dignity. Rights may be divided broadly into legal and moral rights, which may or may not have legal support. Moral or human rights are considered to be of fundamental importance and take priority over other rights; they are shared equally by all human beings.[3] Fundamental rights of persons include being treated as ends, never solely as a means to the ends of others, such as researchers or medical personnel. The notion of human rights is based on "basic protection for individuals to demand that states protect and provide basic goods, services, and liberties for people."[9] When moral rights are ignored or violated, there is a sense that grave injustice has occurred.

Churchill and Simán[8] make several important points about rights as claims and their relationship to broader ethical concerns. The nurses discuss these points in light of Ann's claim that she has a right to do whatever she wishes with her life. Often rights language takes on a sense of absolutism in which rights language is used simply to make claims against others. This makes wider exploration of ethical concerns involving rights almost impossible. Rights as claims are only one dimension of the moral significance of rights, and rights often conflict. A more meaningful discussion of rights must include other major dimensions of the moral life, such as responsibilities and the role of persons in the larger community and as interconnected members of society. Rights discussions should include considerations of both individual liberties and rights and a recognition of our social interdependence. This is an essential perspective for both clients and health care professionals recognized by Ann's nurses in their discussion.

The mere assertion of rights does not settle issues such as individual claims to a right to die or a right to refuse treatment. Treating rights as absolute possessions of individuals that they may exercise at their own discretion is to abuse them and to misunderstand the role of rights and their status in moral arguments in which one is also concerned about what individuals ought to do, as well as what it is possible to do socially and legally.

Often when an individual makes a rights claim it becomes adversarial against others and does not recognize the interdependence of individuals in families and communities. Also, making a rights claim, such as "I have a right to die," may point to a need for moral certainty about one's choice. That is, an individual such as Ann, in making her claim, has a need to guarantee the rightness of her choice in advance and without regard to the context of the choice.

The major argument made by Churchill and Simán[8] is that rights are social and relational, not simply private possessions of individuals. Personal rights and social interdependence are inseparable aspects of human existence. Rights do not make sense alone and require that attention is paid to the social side of rights as well as the individual side.

Making moral judgments, then, about ourselves and others is not simply a matter of examining isolated acts, such as Ann's claiming a right to die or to refuse therapy. Such claims demand explicit consideration of our interdependences, as well as our claims of rights to self-determination. The "right" of Ann's son to have his mother choose life rather than death may override claims of individual rights in this instance. It does matter whether individuals make decisions and take action out of selfishness alone, with no regard for others. Ethical reflection requires that one identify and be sensitive to the interests and values of others, not solely those of self.

In summary, following Churchill and Simán's[8] points, rights are public and social, not solely private or individual. They indicate relationships between and among persons. Rights are not merely personal possessions. Rights delineate mutual respect and moral equality in community. They do not guarantee the rightness of particular choices in advance or in general. Discussion of rights alone does not exhaust the possibilities for moral discussion or necessarily take priority over other elements in ethical reflection. Focusing on individual rights alone is too narrow and leads to the danger of reducing ethical decisions to a formula that is implied in many discussions of rights in which rights are simply claimed and considered to be the conclusion rather than the beginning of ethical inquiry. The nurses take into account Ann's claim to self-determination and freedom of choice and also examine consequences to others, an example of the pluralist model of ethical reflection.

DECISIONS AND ACTIONS

The nurses do not have unlimited time available for their ethics rounds, so they decide that they have at least discussed a broad range of moral considerations relevant to Ann's situation and considered their obligations. Although they do not have a "moral stamp of approval" for any one course of action, they will make their decisions based on careful thinking and reasoned discussion that enhances the moral principles of beneficence and autonomy. They acknowledge how deeply they care about Ann's welfare and the welfare of all their patients. At the same time that they care

about each person as a unique individual, they also care about them as members of families in the past, present, or future and as members of the human community. A sense of community responsibility for its members follows from these considerations and reminds the nurses that they wish to discuss the principle of justice more thoroughly in their next ethics rounds. The mention of the article on economics and morality increased their interest in pursuing the topic further in light of concerns about how social and health care resources should be allocated or rationed and by whom when they believe that health care should be based primarily on need. They also realize that others in society have different ideas for distributing burdens and benefits and that often these decisions are made in administrative or political arenas.

Decisions for action that grew out of the discussion in the nurses' ethics rounds include talking with Ann about the ethics rounds, the other alternatives suggested, and the moral and ethical questions and worries discussed. They also decide to hold an interdisciplinary rehabilitation team conference among those team members working with Ann and to recommend that, on the basis of their discussion, passes be withheld for a limited period, during which every effort will be made to include Ann in discussion of therapy and her future. The team had been conducting these conferences without Ann's participation because of a cutback in staff. The nurses are convinced through their discussion that this will enhance Ann's autonomy and sense of personal dignity. At the same time, the health care professionals' value of caring for and protecting life also will be enhanced.

We do not know the final outcome, but the nurses are convinced that open discussion of the ethical aspects of client care in a forum such as ethics rounds on their unit has enhanced decision making with and for clients and that communication between the nurses and other caregivers has become more respectful and caring.

REFERENCES

1. American Nurses' Association: Code for nurses with interpretive statements, Pub No G56, Kansas City, Mo, 1985, The Association.
2. Aroskar M: Anatomy of an ethical dilemma: The theory, Am J Nurs 80:658, 1980.

3. Bandman B: The human rights of patients, nurses, and other health professionals. In Bandman EL and Bandman B, editors: Bioethics and human rights, Boston, 1978, Little, Brown & Co.

4. Bayer R and others: The care of the terminally ill: Morality and economics, N Engl J Med 309:1490, 1983.

5. Bok S: The limits of confidentiality, Hastings Cent Rep 13:24, 1983.

6. Brandt RB: The morality and rationality of suicide. In Beauchamp TL and Perlin S, editors: Ethical issues in death and dying, Englewood Cliffs, NJ, 1978, Prentice-Hall, Inc.

7. Childress JF: Priorities in biomedical ethics, Philadelphia, 1981, Westminster Press.

8. Churchill LR and Simán JJ: Abortion and the rhetoric of individual rights, Hastings Cent Rep 12:9, 1982.

9. Jameton A: Nursing practice: The ethical issues, Englewood Cliffs, NJ, 1984, Prentice-Hall, Inc.

10. Jonsen AR and Butler LH: Public ethics and policy making, Hastings Cent Rep 5:25, 1975.

11. Muyskens JL: Moral problems in nursing: A philosophical investigation, Totowa, NJ, 1982, Rowman & Littlefield.

12. President's Commission for the Study of Ethical Problems in Medicine and Biomedical and Behavioral Research: Making health care decisions, vol 1. Washington, DC, 1982, US Government Printing Office.

ADDITIONAL READINGS

Abramson M: A model for organizing an ethical analysis of the discharge planning process . . . of the chronically impaired older person from an acute care hospital to the community or an institution, Soc Work Health Care 9(1):45, 1983.

Banja JD: Proxy consent to medical treatment: Implications for rehabilitation, Arch Phys Med Rehabil 67:790, 1986.

Bayer R: Ethics in home care and quality assurance, Caring 5(1):50, 1986.

Brown BA, Miles SH, Aroskar MA: The prevalence and design of ethics committees in nursing homes, J Am Geriatrics Soc 35:1028, 1987.

Cox B and Roy MM: Nursing ethics can improve quality long term care, Am Health Care Assoc J 11(6):48, 1985.

Huckabay LMD: Ethical moral issues in nursing practice and decision making, Nurs Admin Q 10(3):61, 1986.

Murphy CP: The changing role of nurses in making ethical decisions, Law Med Health Care 12(4):173, 1984.

Nadolsky JM: Ethical issues in the transition from public to private rehabilitation, J Rehabil 52(1):6, 1986.

Poletti RA: Ethics of death and dying, Int J Nurs Stud 22(4):329, 1985.

Smith SF: Withholding or withdrawing food and fluids: An ethical question, Calif Nurs 81(8):4, 1985.

Stewart-Amidei C: Editorial: Are we creating our own ethical dilemmas? J Neurosci Nurs 20:71, 1988.

Tammelleo AD: If you want to stop treating a patient . . . to dialyze a terminally ill double amputee, RN 49(6):59, 1986.

Vogel AC: Supportive care only: Guidelines for making a major ethical decision, Consultant 25(2):116, 1985.

Future Directions in Rehabilitation Nursing

Sharon S. Dittmar

OBJECTIVES

After completing Chapter 30, the reader will be able to:

1. Discuss the current emphasis on cost containment in health care delivery.
2. Describe the concern with quality of care within the current cost containment atmosphere.
3. Recognize the need for increasing knowledge in rehabilitation nursing.
4. Predict changes in rehabilitation nursing practice.
5. Discuss the importance of establishing a scientific base for rehabilitation nursing practice.

The decade ahead holds many challenges and opportunities for nurses. The past has brought rehabilitation nurses to the realization that a specialty group cannot act in isolation, but through collective action within the nursing profession can achieve one strong voice for the discipline of nursing. Trends in health care delivery facing the nursing profession require unity, negotiation, compromise, participation, and leadership in order that we as rehabilitation nurses can continue to provide the best possible nursing care to rehabilitation clients. Cost containment, quality rehabilitation care, and progressive professional development of the specialty area are some of the trends that rehabilitation nurses can influence.

COST CONTAINMENT

Cost containment in health care delivery will be the major sociopolitical issue of the next decade.

According to Colachis, "medical care costs have increased from a predicted 3% of the total national income in the early part of this century, to more than 10% today. When Medicare was established in 1965, the costs were $3 billion/year. In 1984, Medicare spent 40 billion dollars or 70% of its budget on hospital services. Medicare provides 40% of the income of the average hospital. Although the explosion in high technology and in costly procedures have prolonged life, we are faced with ever greater financial costs."[4]

The federal government is retreating from shouldering the burden of medical care expenses. One of the indicators of this shift is the establishment of prospective payment systems whereby Medicare reimburses hospitals according to Diagnostic Related Groups (DRGs) rather than reimbursing them, as previously, according to length of stay in the hospital. Many smaller hospitals have experienced financial difficulties with prospective reimbursement and have already closed their doors. Paralleling this development, an increasing number of multicorporate organizations, often with substructures including health maintenance organizations, ambulatory care centers, free-standing emergency centers, and home health care agencies now characterize the health care system. Because Medicare payment for inpatient operating costs is predetermined for each client according to average cost of the identified diagnostic group, clients are being discharged "quicker and sicker" from acute care facilities to other levels of care. Rehabilitation services were exempt from DRGs during the first 2 years of their implementation. Their impact, however, has had rippling effects, and demands are now being made to justify the costs of rehabilitation. Some adaptation of the DRG payment system will affect rehabilitation services in the very near future.

These new economic policies will have a major impact on the future of rehabilitation nursing. Consequently, nurses must become more astute in recognizing the impact of cost containment policies on client care and rehabilitation nurses. Some of the possible effects include the following: (1) Hospitals will curtail educational and service programs that do not result in adequate pay adjustments. (2) Tertiary hospitals may lose financially if there are not greater adjustments for clients who require longer stays for intensive rehabilitation. (3) Home care and noninstitutional settings will be used by hospitals more frequently as clients in need of continuing care are discharged. (4) Many nursing homes will not have adequate staff for the sicker clients being admitted. (5) Home health care agencies will not have the time to upgrade staff skills and technology to provide care to sicker clients. There also will be possible effects on rehabilitation nurses, including (1) hospital layoffs of nurses and team members, (2) possible shifts from quality of care to cost savings, (3) emphasis on discharge planning, with larger caseloads for discharge planners resulting in overwork, less training, and little client advocacy, (4) use of contracted services rather than obtaining the best services for the individual client, and (5) less time for counseling.[21] The wise nurse will watch the financial reports of his or her institution and those of other health care institutions in the community, because the financial status of the institution will affect the care provided and the economic status of the nurse.[8]

A number of strategies are available to rehabilitation nurses for maintaining and improving services to rehabilitation clients within the cost containment policies. Now is the time for nurses to seek and secure funding for community nursing centers to serve the growing market for community-based rehabilitative and preventive services for the elderly and the clients who are discharged sicker and quicker from acute care institutions. Nurses also must increase their knowledge about sources of health care delivery funds and effects of legislation on the economy. Furthermore, nurses must "cost out" nursing services if these services are to be viewed as something other than "hotel costs" lumped with all other institutional services. Nurses can provide cost-effective care delivery alternatives when there is more knowledge and sophistication about how the economy works.[8]

Cost-Effectiveness of Rehabilitation Nursing Practice

Rehabilitation nurses will have to develop a level of expertise in demonstrating the difference they make in terms of cost. Although studies focused on cost effectiveness of rehabilitation services and rehabilitation nursing are sparse, some studies have been conducted. Pozen and others,[15] over a 15-month period, studied 102 sequential clients who had experienced a myocardial infarction. Findings suggested that a critical care unit (CCU)–based nurse rehabilitator was effective in increasing return to work, teaching clients, and decreasing smoking.[15] Luginbuhl and others[9] report that prevention and rehabilitation have a far greater effect on cost-containment than dramatic technological interventions.

A study done by Kottke[7] lends support to the current trend to contain costs by increasing independence. In 1972 conservative estimates placed the costs of institutional maintenance of a totally dependent individual at approximately $8,300 annually. By improving this individual's function so that he or she could feed himself or herself, the costs were reduced to $6,000 annually. If the same individual could become partially independent by achieving limited self-care, the annual costs would be decreased to $4,600. With complete independence but need for room and board, the annual cost would be decreased still further to $2,400. If this individual had family or support services and could live at home when reaching partially or completely independent levels of function, the institutional costs would be totally eliminated. We need only multiply this client's situation by several thousand individuals and today's costs to demonstrate that the savings would be enormous.

Rehabilitation nurses must develop methods to reflect accurately the time consumed in client education, psychosocial support of clients and families, and development and implementation of care plans. Further, client outcomes related to nurse-specific strategies must be documented in terms of cost effectiveness. For example, assisting clients to increase independence in self-care skills is one area in which nursing should be able to demonstrate that initial expenditures result in long-term cost savings.

Quality of Care

Quality of care issues will be reexamined in the future in light of the emphasis on cost containment Application of extraordinary measures to save and prolong life will come under increasing scrutiny. Questions will arise about the use of advanced technology to save lives of severely physically and mentally handicapped persons. Decisions made by individuals, families, health care providers, and society in these situations will become much more complex and involve new ethical dilemmas. The rehabilitation nurse will be increasingly in need of professional networks in which to discuss these dilemmas with colleagues and arrive at conclusions that are personally and professionally comfortable.

Experts predict a number of possible advantages and disadvantages with application of the DRG prospective system. DRGs have inspired nursing to seek ways to document nursing care in a quantifiable form; high-risk clients may benefit from early identification and preadmission screening and testing with more appropriate care; better client follow-up in ambulatory clinics may prevent unnecessary readmissions; and client education programs may be upgraded. Conversely, DRGs may result in inappropriate admissions and readmissions of persons with multiple chronic conditions, underutilization of tests and procedures to save money in the short run, avoidance of expensive and complicated treatments, use of lower quality drugs and equipment, use of labor-

intensive rehabilitation services only when such services can demonstrate cost reduction, and decline in high-risk care because it may prove too expensive.[21]

Consumer involvement in quality issues

Disabled consumers have become activists, are more vocal in demanding access to better care, and are more likely than in the past to question the care they receive. These people continue to want integration into community life, accessible housing, employment, public buildings, transportation, and recreation. Rehabilitation nurses, along with other members of the rehabilitation team, will be required to be more creative than in the past in assuring that the disabled receive appropriate services and have the opportunity to assume their rights to participation in community life. According to Symington, it is up to health care professionals to "translate these desires into specific goals with a time frame for completion."[19]

The changed attitudes of consumers demonstrate increased involvement in rehabilitation, but services have not been able to meet expectations. One response of consumers has been to establish self-help groups, which have become very common as clients seek information, additional services, and social support not provided in the acute care setting. Consumers also have become more aware of their rights to litigate and have increasingly brought legal suits against health care providers and institutions for lack of care or negligent care. The activism of consumers has brought additional pressure on rehabilitation nurses and rehabilitation team members to provide more services with less monies while at the same time maintaining quality.

Responses of professional organizations to quality issues

The cost containment policy will continue to be a major issue in health care delivery and has potential for affecting quality of care both negatively and positively. Rehabilitation services have not been free from waste. For example, clients have sometimes waited needlessly for referral to rehabilitation programs, have not been evaluated for admission to rehabilitation programs at the earliest time, and have not always been taught as quickly as possible to perform self-care activities. Professional organizations have responded by taking steps to promote and maintain quality in rehabilitation nursing and rehabilitation services.

The Association of Rehabilitation Nurses (ARN) has developed certification procedures to ensure professional competence in the delivery of rehabilitation nursing services. This is a beginning step in monitoring the quality of rehabilitation nursing care. Further steps should include development of certification examinations geared to differing levels of nurse education. Revised standards of care for rehabilitation nursing were published in 1986. A core curriculum identifying knowledge necessary for rehabilitation nursing practice has been published, and a revision of this curriculum reflecting the current state of the art and science of rehabilitation nursing was published in 1987.

Concern for quality of services also dominates the home care scene. Recently the National Association of Home Care (NAHC) was formed to develop standards of care and guidelines for the administration of home care services. This organization also seeks to overcome gaps in service for home care clients.[11]

In 1979 The Commission on Accreditation of Rehabilitation Facilities (CARF) developed program evaluation standards.[16] Rehabilitation facilities apply for and are reviewed to meet these standards and receive accreditation from this organization. In the future, most rehabilitation facilities will seek CARF accreditation.

Other leaders in rehabilitation indicate that by the 1990s the concern for quality will shift from concern with credentials of employees and accreditation of facilities to concern with quality of service delivered. Nadolsky[13] predicts that the organization's ability to meet the needs of recipients of rehabilitation services will be more likely to determine quality than the external accomplishments of service providers (certification) and the programs (accreditation) they represent.

Federal and state funding of rehabilitation services and their continuation, however, will not rest solely on quality but on a combination of quality and outcome criteria. Attention to client outcomes as a measurement of nurse-specific and team-specific interventions will be required to document effectiveness of rehabilitation services and to substantiate the necessity of government funding for the improvement of rehabilitation services. Decisions for government allocation of resources to rehabilitation nursing and rehabilitation services will be based on quantitative "dollars and cents" data.[10] Norms can be established for improvement in function for specific conditions through the use of aggregate data. The quantitative determination of degree of client progress allows for evaluation of rehabilitation programs and of improvements in rehabilitative care.[14]

PROGRESSIVE DEVELOPMENT OF REHABILITATION NURSING AS A SPECIALTY

Progressive development of rehabilitation nursing as a specialty within a cost-conscious health care delivery system mandates increasing knowledge, changing practice, and establishment of a scientific base for practice. Rehabilitation nurses must propose, implement, and evaluate changes to keep pace with societal shifts and to positively affect the future of rehabilitation nursing.

Increasing Knowledge

Until recently, few basic nursing programs offered courses specifically developed to teach philosophy, concepts, principles, and practice of rehabilitation nursing. Despite advances in curricula at the undergraduate level, there continues to be a need for more emphasis on basic rehabilitation nursing content in baccalaureate degree programs, and this need should be communicated to faculty until such time when all students graduate with beginning competencies in rehabilitation nursing.[2] In addition to basic knowledge and skills in rehabilitation nursing, students must be prepared in managerial skills, including marketing and budgeting. Contemporary and future practice demands that nurses define and quantify their services, and to accomplish this task some educational preparation is required.

Entry into practice, an issue with which nurses have been struggling for many years remains controversial, but progress has been made in achieving consensus within nursing. The rapid changes in health care delivery and in the nursing profession have given momentum to problem resolution. The two major nursing organizations, the American Nurses' Association (ANA) and the National League for Nursing (NLN), maintain that there should be two levels of nursing education. In July 1985 the ANA House of Delegates recommended retention of the title "professional nurse" for the professional practitioner prepared at the baccalaureate degree level and establishment of the title "associate nurse" for the technical practitioner prepared at the associate degree level. NLN and ANA councils have been working together to define the scope and practice of nursing within these levels. Titling and licensing procedures will require close communication between these two groups and support from the nursing population as they strive to find the most agreeable solutions.[20] It behooves rehabilitation nurses to support the efforts of these two organizations as they attempt to resolve professional and public confusion over the multiplicity of entry levels to nursing. Leaders in rehabilitation nursing have been in the forefront of support for an academic base for rehabilitation nursing that is firmly established in institutions of higher learning.[2,23]

There continues to be a shortage of rehabilitation nurses academically prepared for leadership roles. In 1980 approximately 5% of all nurses (85,000 nurses) held masters and doctoral degrees.[22] The need remains for nursing leaders who can function as managers of rehabilitation nursing units, nursing homes, and home health care agencies; as researchers in clinical nursing; and as educators in schools of nursing. Only five graduate programs in the United States offer specialty preparation at the graduate level in rehabilitation nursing. Bryce predicts that "with society's burgeoning need in both nursing practice and education for well-prepared rehabilitation nurses, the number of graduate programs in rehabilitative nursing should be doubled, perhaps tripled during the '80s."[2] Thus far only two new programs have been developed and implemented.

Changing Practice

The rehabilitation nurse of the future will function in different practice roles and settings and be more active in the legislative process as an advocate of the disabled consumer. She or he will become knowledgeable and skillful in the application of high technology—technology used to improve the management of rehabilitation facilities, control client environments, assist with learning, improve client and family communication, and increase function for disabled persons. The shift to community care, participation in the legislative process, and use of advanced technology are some of the factors that will affect practice.

Shift from hospital settings to community settings of practice

The provision of rehabilitation services is shifting from acute rehabilitation centers to rehabilitation in ambulatory settings, long-term care facilities, and the home. Consistent with this shift, the home health care industry is booming and new companies are forming every day. In the past home health care was nonacute and nontechnological.[20] Procedures once performed only by professional nurses are now being performed by family members and ancillary health care providers. Intravenous therapy, renal dialysis, and home respiratory therapy have become common practice in the home. Home health care nurses are confronting new practice problems as they care for clients who are discharged quicker and sicker from acute care settings.

In the future, the demand for rehabilitation nursing care in the home, in long-term care facilities, and in ambulatory care settings will be greater than ever before. Numbers of persons cared for in nursing homes will quadruple by the turn of the century. These clients will require a high level of rehabilitative, psychosocial, and custodial nursing care.[18] The need for rehabilitation nurses to work in these agencies and assist nurses currently employed in community settings is apparent.

The NLN has been approached by an insurance company to explore the possibilities of a demonstration project of nurse-provided care for the chronically ill elderly.[20] Nurse-managed community centers are one alternative to expensive institutional care. Rehabilitation nurses have the knowledge and skill to develop and implement other cost-effective methods for providing care to the disabled and elderly. For example, Emick-Henning[5] discusses what nurses should know about the types of adult day care available, the funding for these centers, and the services offered. Developing and managing adult day care centers is another way rehabilitation nurses could contribute to cost containment and quality of rehabilitation services.[5]

Societal, institutional, and self-expectations of the professional rehabilitation nurse will include greater accountability and independence in nursing practice. Rehabilitation nurses have functioned more independently than most nurses in areas of nursing diagnosis, nursing therapy, and nursing evaluation of nurse-directed care in long-term care and rehabilitation facilities. New models of care will increase the opportunities for nurses to exercise independence and accountability in nursing practice.

Twenty-five states now have health insurance laws that legitimize reimbursement for nursing services.[20] As a result, more rehabilitation nurses will establish their own offices and work on a fee-for-service basis. This arrangement benefits the nurse who in this role can apply knowledge and skill as an accountable professional and the client who can have a choice of entry to the health care system. Rehabilitation facilities also benefit without the need for creating additional salaried positions. Examples of services that might be provided are discharge planning and education of clients and families; consultation to institutions and clients about rehabilitation equipment; direct rehabilitation services in the home; education of nursing personnel in institutions, nursing homes, and home health care agencies; and guidance on cost containment for rehabilitation services.

Rehabilitation nurses have traditionally worked for insurance companies in the private sector, providing disability management and assistance with cost control of rehabilitation services.[24] Self-employed nurses could offer these services to multicorporate organizations and to long-term care facilities within the health care industry.

Participation in the legislative process

A number of years ago, Rothberg pointed out that "rehabilitation represents a social phenomenon that has evolved over the centuries and brought us a sense of responsibility for others and a concern for human welfare."[17] Predictions for the future suggest that there will be a shift away from the traditional view of health care as a social good to an economic view subject to the influence of supply, demand, and price.[1]

A basic principle of rehabilitation is that there is an ongoing need for federal and state support of rehabilitation to meet the needs of those who are disabled and who do not have the financial resources to overcome the effects of their disability.[12] To ensure that rehabilitation services remain available to disabled individuals, rehabilitation service providers must be constantly vigilant socially and politically in advocating continued government support of these services. Re-

habilitation nurses, other team members, and disabled citizens will have to rally together to meet the onslaught of predicted cuts in government support to rehabilitation services and lobby to maintain current levels of service.

Rehabilitation nurses can participate in the legislative process in a number of ways. First, we can become more aware of proposed legislation by reading newspapers, legislative columns in professional journals, and reports from congressmen and by participating in professional and consumer organizations. Second, we can write to elected representatives expressing our opinions and rationale for these views. Third, we should all be registered voters and regularly cast informed votes in each election. Fourth, we can contribute money to campaigns of legislators whose platforms we support. We also can run for elected office and cast votes for programs supportive of the disabled population.

Use of advanced technology

Advanced technology presents both threats and opportunities. Some of the high tech procedures require more skilled nursing care; others decrease the amount of nursing care and time. Through the application of advanced technology, the medical profession has been able to decrease the number of invasive procedures used for diagnosis and treatment. At the same time, ethical questions related to cost arise when a large amount of time and money are used for procedures that benefit only a few individuals. The same use of resources could contribute to care and rehabilitation of large numbers of clients with chronic disease and disability.[18]

Rehabilitation nurses will learn to use and instruct clients in the use of high tech equipment designed to improve function. Some disabled clients are now using sophisticated equipment, including microputers, to perform a number of self-care activities. Research conducted at Wright State University makes use of computerized systems to substitute for neural circuits and enable individuals who are paralyzed to walk. Computer systems activated by voice recognition and touch are being used to assist immobilized individuals in performing self-care tasks; software communication packages are being used to assist disabled persons with speech impairments and severe motor involvement; and computer-aided braille trainers are used to teach braille to blind persons.

Unfortunately, high tech equipment is still too expensive to purchase for every disabled person who could benefit, but costs are decreasing each day.

Some nurses will become expert in developing computer programs to aid disabled clients. Nurses with a special interest in this area may develop computer-aided instruction programs for clients and families; construct data bases that supply information about what equipment can be purchased, where it can be purchased, and at what cost; and design innovative systems to help save time in routing clients to rehabilitation therapies, recording discharge plans for long-term care facilities and home health care agencies and referral agencies; and in documenting rehabilitation nursing care and client outcomes. Computerized systems can save time and money over the long run and assist nurse researchers in obtaining data bases for investigation of variables affecting the outcomes of rehabilitation nursing care.

Establishing a Scientific Base for Rehabilitation Nursing Practice

The future of rehabilitation nursing as a specialty area within nursing depends upon identifying and developing a scientific base for nursing practice. The need to develop a scientific base for practice has received increasing attention during the last 20 years. Prior to 1969, only one center for nursing research existed, at Teacher's College, Columbia University, in New York City. In the ensuing years several research centers in nursing have been established.[3]

The federal government has traditionally been a major proponent and source of funding for nursing research. The Institute of Medicine (IOM) report recommended that an organizational entity be established within the federal structure to place nursing in the mainstream of scientific inquiry and accountability.[6] Recent passage of legislation creating a National Center for Nursing Research within the National Institutes of Health indicates the strong commitment of the federal government and is likely to give a strong impetus to nursing research.

Some areas that require investigation by rehabilitation nurses are:

1. Strategies to prevent primary disability.
2. Promotion of health, well-being, and independence in activities of daily living and social roles among those who are disabled.
3. Prevention of secondary complications of disablement that have potential to reduce productivity and quality of life.
4. Identification of constructive and destructive coping mechanisms of individuals and families experiencing disablement.
5. Quantitative evaluation of functional improvement over time of disabled clients participating in rehabilitation programs.
6. Therapeutic environments for rehabilitation.
7. Effectiveness of high technology in improving function.
8. Rehabilitation in the home.
9. Development and evaluation of team-specific and nursing-specific client outcome criteria.
10. Effective resource utilization of personnel and equipment.
11. Cost effectiveness of rehabilitation nursing.
12. Rehabilitation program evaluation.

Rehabilitation nurses in practice settings and nurse researchers can combine talents to most effectively advance the science of nursing. Many of the areas listed also would lend themselves to rehabilitation team research. The viability of the specialty depends upon participation in and initiation of research to improve practice and demonstrate cost effectiveness.

SUMMARY

Rehabilitation nurses must remain flexible and be able to influence changes in health care delivery as well as adapt to them. The quantity and quality of rehabilitation nursing care based on client outcomes must be documented in a variety of rehabilitation settings. Roles of the rehabilitation nurse and settings in which rehabilitation nursing practice takes place will change. The rehabilitation nurse will be required to act more assertively as a client advocate as the government retreats from financing health care. The rehabilitation nurse also will become more knowledgeable about cost and technology. All rehabilitation nurses must become involved in establishing a scientific base for rehabilitation nursing practice. The future lies with each rehabilitation nurse. Rehabilitation nurses can help solve the problems in delivery of rehabilitation services, or they can contribute to these problems.

REFERENCES

1. The health care system in the mid-1990s: A study conducted for the Health Insurance Association of America, Arthur D Little, Inc, 1985.
2. Bryce RH: The challenge of rehabilitation nursing in the '80s, Rehabil Nurs 5:8, 1980.
3. Carnegie ME: Quo vadis? Nurs Res 27:277, 1978.
4. Colachis SC: New directions in health care, Arch Phys Med Rehabil 65:291, 1984.
5. Emick-Henning B: Adult day care: Support system for the disabled elderly and their caregivers, Rehabil Nurs 8:29, 1983.
6. Institute of Medicine, Health Care Services Division, Nursing and Nursing Education Committee: Nursing and nursing education: Public policies and private actions, Washington, DC, 1983, National Academy Press.
7. Kottke FJ: Historia obscura hemiplegiae, Arch Phys Med Rehabil 55:4, 1974.
8. Lauver EB: Where will the money go? Economic forecasting and nursing's future, Nurs Health Care 6:132, 1985.
9. Luginbuhl WH and others: Prevention and rehabilitation as a means of cost containment: The example of myocardial infarction, J Public Health Policy 2:103, 1981.
10. McFarlane FR and Frost DE: Rehabilitation directions: Feast, famine, or distinction in the 1980's, J Rehabil 47:20, 1981.
11. Morris EM and Fonesca JD: Home care today, Am J Nurs 84:341, 1984.
12. Nadolsky JM: The "1984" crisis in rehabilitation, J Rehabil 50:4, 1984.
13. Nadolsky JM: The evolution of rehabilitation in a service society, J Rehabil 51:7, 1985.
14. Posavac EJ and Carey RG: Using a level of function scale (LORS-II) to evaluate the success of inpatient rehabilitation programs, Rehabil Nurs 7:17, 1982.
15. Pozen NW and others: A nurse rehabilitator's impact on patients with myocardial infarction, Med Care 15:830, 1977.
16. Program evaluation in inpatient medical facilities, Chicago, 1979, Commission on Accreditation of Rehabilitation Facilities.
17. Rothberg JS: The challenges of rehabilitative nursing, Nurs Outlook 17:37, 1969.
18. Stevens BJ: Facing changes head on, Nurs Health Care 6:27, 1985.
19. Symington D: The goals of rehabilitation, Arch Phys Med Rehabil 65:427, 1984.
20. Ten trends to watch, Nurs Health Care 7:16, 1986.
21. The wonderful awful truth about DRGs, The Coordinator, p 18, June 1984.
22. US Health and Human Services Department: The registered nurse population, Washington, DC, 1983, US Government Printing Office.
23. Watson P: Components of rehabilitation nursing practice advancement, Rehabil Nurs 10:28, 1985.
24. Weiner SM: Rehabilitation nursing in the private sector, Rehabil Nurs 8:31, 1983.

ADDITIONAL READINGS

Aiken LH: Nursing priorities for the 1980's: Hospitals and nursing homes, Am J Nurs 81:324, 1981.
Aiken LH: Nursing's future: Public policies, private actions, Am J Nurs 83:1440, 1983.
Kelly LY: Nurses of the third wave, Nurs Outlook 28:330, 1980.
Levine E and Abdellah FG: DRGs: A recent refinement to an old method, Inquiry 21:105, 1984.
Naisbitt J: Megatrends, New York, 1984, Warner Books.
Rothberg JS: The rehabilitation team: Future direction, Arch Phys Med Rehabil 62:407, 1981.
Schaffer FA: Nursing power in the DRG world, Nurs Manage 15:28, 1984.
Steel JE: Designing the future, J Neurosci Nurs 19:321, 1987.

Appendixes

Standards of Rehabilitation Nursing Practice*

PROFESSIONAL PRACTICE STANDARDS
Standard I. Data Collection

The nurse continuously collects data that are systematic, comprehensive, and accurate. The nurse uses a data collection framework that facilitates an examination of the client's health status, incorporates information on the client's relationship to the environment, and provides data for nursing diagnosis.

Standard II. Nursing Diagnosis

The nurse analyzes the data derived from the assessment to determine the nursing diagnosis.

Standard III. Planning and Goal Setting

The nurse collaborates with the individual, family, significant others, and representatives of other disciplines to formulate a realistic plan that identifies goals, specific nursing actions, and resources to meet the individual's needs.

Standard IV. Intervention

The nurse intervenes as guided by the individual care plan to prevent complications and promote, maintain, or restore the individual's physical and psychosocial function at a realistic, optimal level. Nursing actions are consistent with the total rehabilitation program to achieve patient goals.

*From Standards of Rehabilitation Nursing Practice. Copyright American Nurses' Association, 1986. Published by the American Nurses' Association. Reprinted by permission.

Standard V. Evaluation

The nurse evaluates the individual's responses to nursing actions. If the goals have not been attained, the data base is examined, further data are collected as needed, and nursing diagnoses and care plans are revised.

PROFESSIONAL PERFORMANCE STANDARDS
Standard VI. Professional Development

The nurse assumes responsibility for continuing education and professional development and contributes to the professional growth of others.

Standard VII. Interdisciplinary Collaboration

The nurse collaborates with the interdisciplinary team in assessing, planning, implementing, and evaluating the individual's care, rehabilitation programs, and related rehabilitation activities.

Standard VIII. Quality Assurance

The nurse participates in peer review and interdisciplinary program evaluation to assure that high-quality nursing care is provided to individuals in a rehabilitation setting.

Standard IX. Research

The nurse contributes to the scientific base of nursing practice and the rehabilitation field through the review and application of research.

American Nurses' Association Code for Nurses*

1. The nurse provides services with respect for human dignity and the uniqueness of the client, unrestricted by considerations of social or economic status, personal attributes, or the nature of health problems.
2. The nurse safeguards the client's right to privacy by judiciously protecting information of a confidential nature.
3. The nurse acts to safeguard the client and the public when health care and safety are affected by the incompetent, unethical, or illegal practice of any person.
4. The nurse assumes responsibility and accountability for individual nursing judgments and actions.
5. The nurse maintains competence in nursing.
6. The nurse exercises informed judgment and uses individual competence and qualifications as criteria in seeking consultation, accepting responsibilities, and delegating nursing activities to others.
7. The nurse participates in activities that contribute to the ongoing development of the profession's body of knowledge.
8. The nurse participates in the profession's efforts to implement and improve standards of nursing.
9. The nurse participates in the profession's efforts to establish and maintain conditions of employment conducive to high-quality nursing care.
10. The nurse participates in the profession's effort to protect the public from misinformation and misrepresentation and to maintain the integrity of nursing.
11. The nurse collaborates with members of the health professions and other citizens in promoting community and national efforts to meet the health needs of the public.

*From Code for Nurses with interpretive statements. Copyright American Nurses' Association, 1985. Published by the American Nurses' Association. Reprinted by permission.

APPENDIX C

Audiovisual Aids

Audiovisual aids are listed chronologically from 1973 to 1987. Within each year aids are arranged in alphabetical order. Where available, the rental or purchase price of each item is listed. Members of Rehabilitation International, USA (RIUSA), subscribers to Rehabfilm Newsletter, and members of any organization in the RIUSA Council of Organizations receive a rental discount. Many of these audiovisual aids are available from rehabilitation centers. When rehabilitation centers are not the distributors and when addresses of the distributors are not listed, audiovisual aids can be requested from Rehabfilm, Suite 704, 1123 Broadway, New York, NY 10010. Rehabfilm materials are only available for rental to organizations in the United States, Canada, and Puerto Rico.

Like Other People
England, 16 mm, col, 37 min, 1973. Producer, Kestrel Films; sales distributor, Perennial Education. Rental $60.
Summary: Highly praised film depicts the lives of a young man and woman who have severe and moderate degrees of cerebral palsy, respectively. Covers their lives together as lovers and conveys the social prejudices they suffer, the social pleasures they share. Presents topics of sexuality, marriage, and individual dignity.

Access
Canada, 16 mm, col, 15 min, 1975. Producer and sales distributor, Social Planning and Review Council of British Columbia. Rental $60.
Summary: Shows that architectural barriers affect both able-bodied and disabled. Examples are given of problems of people who are confined to wheelchairs and people whose limi-

tations are the result of physical size, age, or burden. Also shows successful access design for old and new buildings and problem situations with solutions.

Balance and Gaiting Using the Scott-Craig Long Leg Brace
Videorecording. Craig Hospital, Physical Therapy Department, Englewood, Colo., Rocky Mountain Regional Spinal Injury Center, Inc., 1977. One videocassette (45 min), sd, b&w, ¾". Purchase $100.
Summary: Describes the use of the Scott-Craig long leg brace, which enables spinal cord injury patients to become ambulatory. Illustrates proper gaiting and balancing techniques.

Deaf Patients: Special Needs, Special Responses
Videorecording. Loraine DiPietro, Washington, DC, the National Academy of Gallaudet College, 1978. Videocassette (24 min), sd, col, ¾", plus booklet. Captioned for the hearing impaired.
Summary: Introduces nurses to deafness and deaf people and stresses the adjustments necessary to achieve effective communications with deaf patients in a medical situation. Identifies and demonstrates means of communicating with deaf patients and ways of increasing the deaf patient's ability to communicate.

Feeding Techniques for Adult Dysphagic Patients
Videorecording. Chicago, Rehabilitation Institute of Chicago, 1979. One videocassette (30 min), sd, col, ¾", plus guide. Credits: Sandra Lindaman.
Summary: Illustrates and discusses the mechanics and problems of feeding adult dysphagic patients.

Grooming, Bathing, and Skin Care for the Physically Disabled
Slide. Minneapolis, Sister Kenny Institute, 1979. 57 slides, col, and audiocassette (20 min), plus script.
Summary: Demonstrates care with a variety of infirmities. Adaptive equipment is shown. Emphasizes importance of providing patient with opportunity to practice new techniques and learn at own rate.

I Am Not What You See
16 mm, col, 28 min, 1979. Purchase $425; rental $45. Videocassette, purchase $375. Produced by Canadian Broadcasting Corporation; distributed by Filmakers Library, Inc.
Summary: Portrays the difficulties experienced by a woman severely crippled by cerebral palsy. This woman is currently a practicing psychologist and champion for the rights of the disabled.

I Had a Stroke
16 mm, col, 28 min, 1979. Purchase $425; rental $60. Videocassette, purchase $375. Discussion guide available. Produced by Grania Gurievitch and Dr. John Downey for the Department of Rehabilitation Medicine, Columbia University; distributed by Filmakers Library, Inc.
Summary: Portrays the experiences of a 36-year-old professional woman, an elderly man with severe speech difficulties, a woman who was unable to return to work, and a young man with a spastic arm. Emphasis is on the problems of transition from hospital to home and the adaptations necessary to resume everyday life.

What is Spinal Cord Injury?
Slide. Englewood, Colo., Craig Hospital, Rocky Mountain Regional Spinal Injury Center, 1979. One hundred thirty-four slides, col, plus audiocassette (18 min). Inaudible signal. Purchase $146. Credits: Donna D. Zingleman.
Summary: Describes the functioning of the body's nervous system. The relationships of the brain, spinal cord, spinal nerves, and peripheral nerves are discussed.

Learning About Disabled Workers, Parts 1-10
Slide. Austin, The Commission, Washington. Distributed by National Audiovisual Center, 1980. Eight hundred three slides, col, 2×2 inches, plus cassette (125 min).
Summary: Contents: 1, Learning about disabled workers; 2, Dealing with disabilities; 3, The mentally retarded worker; 4, The epileptic worker; 6, The mobility-impaired worker; 7, The blind/visually impaired worker; 9, Psychological-social disabilities; 10, The physically disabled worker.

Patterns of Pain
16 mm, col, 28 min, 1980. Purchase $425; rental $45. Videocassette, purchase $375. Produced by Canadian Broadcasting Corporation; distributed by Filmakers Library, Inc.
Summary: A professor of psychology, a zoologist, and a physician describe the perception of pain in the nervous system. Absence of pain, perception by the wounded during battle; pain control through hypnosis, acupuncture, and yoga; thresholds of pain; the body's ability to release its own analgesic; and new surgical techniques for implanting electrodes in the brain to block the perception of chronic pain are illustrated and discussed.

Sykes
16 mm, col, 13 min, 1980. Purchase $293; rental $30. A film by Deirdre Walsh; distributed by Filmakers Library, Inc.
Summary: Portrays a blind, elderly man who refuses to allow either age or infirmity to dampen his spirits.

Total Back Care, Phase II
Slide. Minneapolis, Sister Kenny Institute, Abbott-Northwestern Hospital, 1980. One hundred thirteen slides, col, plus cassette (40 min), plus script.
Summary: Provides a detailed description of the anatomy of the spinal column and function of the lower back. Illustrates proper standing, sitting, and lying postures, correct procedures for lifting. Describes effects of degeneration and injury to the spinal column.

Discussion with Dr. Frank Bowe

USA, U-matic, col, 30 min, 1981. Produced by American Telephone and Telegraph Corporate Television. Rental $50.

Summary: Discussion edited from a presentation made by Dr. Bowe at AT&T. Focus is attitude toward disabled people of private sector employers, and discussion covers what needs to be done to increase employment figures, job evaluation suggestions, reasonable accommodation, and possible areas of support by state rehabilitation agencies.

Intensive Caring: A Patient's Perspective

USA, ¾" videocassette, col, 80 min, 1981. Produced and distributed by Twentieth Century Fox, 23705 Industrial Park Dr., Farmington Hills, MI 48024.

Summary: In this two-part video presentation, Elaine Lowenthal discusses and answers questions about being afflicted with Guillain-Barré syndrome at an adult age.

Pins and Needles

16 mm, col, 37 min, 1981. Purchase $450; rental $70. Videocassette, purchase $400. Produced by Genni and Kim Batterham; distributed by Filmakers Library, Inc.

Summary: Film about a young woman's experiences after being diagnosed with multiple sclerosis. Expresses many major issues including sexuality, self-esteem, dependency, denial of reality by family, the appropriateness of occupational workshops, and the problems of access.

Rehabilitation: A Patient's Perspective

16 mm, col, 28 min, 1981. Purchase $425; rental $45. Videocassette, purchase $375. LC 73-702361. Produced by Grania Gurievitch and Dr. John Downey for the Department of Rehabilitation Medicine, Columbia University; distributed by Filmakers Library, Inc.

Summary: This is a film written to sensitize professional staff members to emotional needs of patients. A patient with Guillain-Barré syndrome is followed from her initial helplessness to her discharge from the hospital. The film emphasizes her inner feelings during the rehabilitation process and stresses the special relationship between patient and therapist in promoting progress.

Rehabilitation of the Elderly Patient

Videorecording. An essential aspect of geriatric medicine. The Jewish Institute for Geriatric Care, St. Louis, The CV Mosby Co., 1981. Videocassette (30 min), sd, col, ¾", plus booklet. Credits: Leslie S. Libow, MD.

Summary: Illustrates the rehabilitation program for and progress of patients recovering from strokes, hip fractures, and amputations of lower limbs.

The Economics of Disability

USA, U-matic, b&w, 30 min, 1981. Produced by AT&T; sales distributor MGS Services. Rental $50.

Summary: Edited from an appearance made by Dr. Frank Bowe for Bell operating company representatives. Topic is affirmative action and its relationship to the economies of any given company or of the United States. Includes federal spending trends and costs for a disabled person and federal support rolls versus rehabilitation costs. Captioned.

The Facts of Life: Cousin Geri Returns

USA, ¾" videocassette, col, 30 min, 1981. Produced by Jerry Mayer for NBC-TV; distributed by ATAT. Production Company, c/o Embassy Television, 100 Universal City Plaza, Universal City, CA 91608.

Summary: The Facts of Life is a spin-off from the popular NBC series Diff'rent Strokes. This particular episode features comedienne Geri Jewel, who has cerebral palsy. Geri's disability creates some concern for her friends at the Eastland School, who fear she might experience rejection from a young man she's been dating. Geri assures them of her capabilities despite her disability.

The People You Never See

16 mm, col, 28 min, 1981. Purchase $425; rental $45. Videocassette, purchase $375. Produced by Canadian Broadcasting Company Corporation; distributed by Filmakers Library, Inc.

Summary: Describes several young people with cerebral palsy. One young person is wheelchair bound and barely able to speak. Her efforts to learn to communicate with Bliss symbols and a typewriter are portrayed. Six other adults who live in the community as an extended family are seen. Their efforts to negotiate the environment are shown. Their struggles are a strong argument for accessibility for the disabled.

To Live On

16 mm, col, 26 min, 1981. Purchase $425; rental $45. A film by Daniel Hess. Available from Filmakers Library, Inc.

Summary: Describes the unique program of the Bulova School and the importance of vocational rehabilitation. Disabled people are seen not only repairing watches but achieving financial independence, pride, spirit in learning together, and living a full and active life.

Transfer Techniques

Videorecording. Harmarville Rehabilitation Center, Educational Resources Division, Pittsburgh. Harmarville Rehabilitation center, Educational Resources Division, 1981. Videocassette (46 min), sd, col, ¾". Contents: Part 1, An introduction to transfer methods; Part 2, Standing transfer; Part 3, Sitting transfer; Part 4, Dependent transfer; Part 5, Car transfer.

Access to Emergency Treatment: Deaf/Hearing Impaired

USA, ¾" videocassette, col, 27 min, 1982. Produced and distributed by Zelma & Grossman Productions, Inc. 174 Fifth Ave, New York, NY 10010.

Summary: Discusses and illustrates how to inform and alert personnel at institutions with emergency facilities as to how to recognize and diagnose deafness and, once recognized, how to communicate in an emergency situation.

Attitudes: The Second Handicap

England, ¾" videocassette, col, 50 min, 1982. Produced by Chris Davies in association with Don Coutts, British Broadcasting Corp.; distributed by The BBC Community Programs Unit, BBC Television Centre, Wood Lane, London W12 8QT, United Kingdom. Signed and captioned by BBC-TV program; produced by Chris Davies, who is sensitive to issues on awareness of disability. Mr. Davies himself has athetoid cerebral palsy.

Summary: Includes discussions of employ-

ment, accessibility, social awareness, political response, education. Twenty-member discussion panel composed of disabled people, employers, and members of Parliament.

Berta Bobath: Assessment and Treatment Planning, and Adult With Hemiplegia, Part 1

Videorecording. University of Maryland, School of Medicine, Department of Physical Therapy, Video Services, Baltimore, The University, 1982. Videocassette (54 min), sd, col, ¾", plus accompanying material *The Bobath Approach*). Credits: Berta Bobath.

Summary: Focuses on Berta Bobath's assessment and treatment planning for an adult with hemiplegia.

Chillysmith Farm

USA, 16 mm, col, 55 min, 1982. Produced by Mark and Dan Jury; distributed by Filmakers Library, 133 East 58th St., New York, NY 10022. Rental $75.

Summary: Chillysmith Farm was home to Gramp, whose last years were memorably documented in the photo-essay *Gramp*. Here we meet the whole family, four generations who live together and care for one another through birth, aging, illness, and death.

Choices: In Sexuality With Physical Disability

USA, 16 mm, col, 56 min, 1982. Produced by Mercury Productions; distributed by New York University, Institute of Rehabilitation Medicine, 400 East 34th St., New York, NY, 10016. Rental $75.

Summary: The disabled recount their own struggles with sexuality, considering such issues as seeing one's self as a sexual person, finding partners, fears of rejection, telling about one's disability, beginning relationships, and so on. In the second part of the film, specific problems in regard to sexual activity are dealt with, including incontinence, loss of sensation, and mobility and positioning.

Disabled Women's Theatre Project

USA, ¾" videocassette, col, 58 min, 1982. Produced and distributed by Patricia Regan and the Disabled Women's Theatre Project, 192b Lancaster St., Albany, NY 12210.

Summary: Original material performed by this acting company of women with a variety of physical disabilities. A blend of humorous and dramatic portrayals of the reality of disability progressing from a series of group living scenes through individual vignettes.

Dystonia
USA, 16 mm, col, 30 min, 1982. Produced by Barnett Addis, Ph.D.; distributed by the Behavioral Sciences Media Laboratory, University of California at Los Angeles, 760 Westwood Plaza, Los Angeles, CA 90024.
Summary: This film documents the experiences of six individuals afflicted with dystonia musculorum deformans, a rare and often misdiagnosed neurological condition that impairs muscular function. Also touches on the psychosocial effects on sufferers and family members.

Finding A Voice
USA, ¾″ videocassette, col, 60 min, 1982. Produced by Martin Freeth, WGBH-Boston; distributed by Time-Life Video, 100 Eisenhower Dr., Paramus, NJ 07652.
Summary: A WGBH-Boston/"Nova" program about the development of electronic aids for the communications-impaired population. Concentrates on the visit of an Englishman with cerebral palsy, Dick Boydell, to the Artificial Language Center in East Lansing, Michigan. Under the supervision of the Center's Director, John Eulenberg, appropriate technology for Mr. Boydell and others is devised.

Nursing Management in Neurogenic Bladder. Part I. Mechanism of Impairment in Spinal Cord Injury
Slide-tape. Rehabilitation Institute of Chicago, 1982. Cassette; 53 slides; b&w, col; study guide, 9 pages. Credits: Yeong Chi Wu, MD, Rosemarie King, MS, RN, and Winona Griggs, MSN, RN.

Nursing Management in Neurogenic Bladder. Part II. Urologic Nursing Care of Patients With Spinal Cord Lesions
Slide-tape. Rehabilitation Institute of Chicago, 1982. Cassette; 77 slides; b&w, col; study guide, 12 pages. Credits: Yeong Chi Wu, MD, Rosemarie King, MS, RN, and Winona Griggs, MSN, RN.

Nursing Management in Neurogenic Bladder. Part III. Assessment and Management After Stroke
Slide-tape. Rehabilitation Institute of Chicago, 1982. Cassette; 59 slides; b&w, col; study guide, 9 pages. Credits: Yeong Chi Wu MD, Rosemarie King, MS, RN, and Winona Griggs, MSN, RN.

Progressive Development of Movement Abilities in Children
Videorecording. Produced by Indiana University, Audio-visual Center, Bloomington Indiana, The University, 1982. Videocassette (13 min), sd, col, ¾″. Credits: David L. Gallahue.
Summary: Traces the phases of motor development from birth through childhood. The aim is to understand the progressive development of children's fundamental movement patterns.

Rehabilitation After Myocardial Infarction
Videorecording. Chicago, American Medical Association, 1982. Videocassette (50 min), sd, col, ¾″, plus guide (American Medical Association, Video Clinics). Credits: Deeb N. Salem, MD.
Summary: Provides clinical guidelines for the rehabilitation of patients with myocardial infarction. Identifies components of rehabilitation programs, including physical activity, functional evaluation, exercise training, patient and family education, counseling, and possible effects of certain medications on the patient's sexuality.

The Elephant Man: ABC Theatre of the Month
USA, ¾″ videocassette, col, 96 min, 1982. Produced by Richmond Crinkley for ABC-TV Theatre of the Month.
Summary: The Elephant Man is based on the real-life history of an Englishman named John Merrick, a deformed person of inner beauty, talent, and wit who in his time (late nineteenth century) was regarded as a curious freak of nature. The television show is adapted from the Tony Award–winning play, not the film.

The Silent Epidemic: Alzheimer's Disease
England, 16 mm, col, 25 min, 1982. Produced by Granada Television International; distributed by Filmakers Library, 133 East 58th St., New York, NY 10022.

Summary: Describes Alzheimer's disease and the problems raised by its increasing incidence. We meet two people married to persons with Alzheimer's disease and learn of their problems in coping. Also explored are the problems of providing proper treatment facilities for persons with Alzheimer's disease and the difficulties of integrating them into nursing homes.

The Wilson Crisis

USA, ¾″ videocassette, col, 56 min, 1982. Produced by Williams Whiteford and Susan Hadary Cohen; distributed by the Department of Physical Therapy, University of Maryland, 32 South Greene St, Baltimore, MD 21201.

Summary: This program documents the impact of a medical crisis on the lives of a 76-year-old, Glenn, and his son, Warren. After his stroke, Glenn is overwhelmed by the changes he experiences and becomes dependent upon his son. The tape follows Glenn's movement from dependency to rehabilitating himself physically and mentally.

We Won't Go Away

England, 16 mm, col, 52 min, 1982. Produced by Patricia Ingram for Central Independent Television; distributed by ACC House, 17 Great Cumberland Place, London W1, England.

Summary: A film about the struggle for their civil rights by the disabled people of America. The reporter, Rosalie Wilkins, herself in a wheelchair, interviews several disabled activists, including Ed Roberts and Judy Heumann.

Code Gray: Ethical Dilemmas in Nursing

Videorecording. Fanlight Productions, Boston, Fanlight Productions, 1983. Videocassette (26 min), sd, col, ¾″, plus guide. Credits: Ben Actenberg.

Summary: Examines the moral and ethical issues of health care delivery. Nurses confront ethical dilemmas in four actual work situations. Raises issues for discussion.

Easy Rolling

USA, U-matic, col, 18 min, 1983. Producer and sales distributor, Medical Center Rehabilitation Hospital. Rental $50.

Summary: Shows wheelchair maintenance and repair; tightening of spokes; wheel alignment; removal, packing, and installation of bearings; proper tightness of rear and front wheels; replacement of handrim clips. Also includes safety tips for falling forward or backward.

It's Not a Question of If . . .

USA, 16 mm and U-matic, col, 18 min, 1983. Producer and sales distributor, Sojourn Productions. Rental $60.

Summary: Presents current state of research on reversal and cure of paraplegia and quadraplegia resulting from spinal cord injury. Interviews conducted with prominent researchers including Petrofsky, Faden, Green, Hauseabout, Burnstein, Brucker, and Hoffer. Also covers the importance of immediate posttrauma care (4 to 24 hours after injury).

Parkinson's Information Exchange

Videorecording. Video Forum, Hoag Hospital, Parkinson's Educational Program, Newport Beach, Calif., 1983. Two videocassettes (120 min), sd, col, ¾″. Credits: William Cox. Contents: Part 1, Overview (30 min) and role of physical therapy (30 min); Part 2, Speech therapist (30 min) and occupational therapist (30 min).

Patient Teaching: A Nursing Process Approach

Slide. Author, Susan Toth; editor, Robin Wells. Philadelphia, JB Lippincott, 1983. Four hundred sixty-one slides, col, plus five audiocassettes (12, 13, 13, 14, 15 min each), plus instructor's guide. Contents: Part 1, Introduction to patient teaching; Part 2, Assessment of learning needs; Part 3, Planning of teaching and learning; Part 4, Implementation of teaching; Part 5, Evaluation of learning.

Summary: Presents principles of patient teaching, emphasizing their application in everyday nursing practice. Provides the basic knowledge and specific skills needed to become an effective teacher of patients.

Wilderness Access

USA, U-matic, col, 28 min, 1983. Producer and sales distributor, Octavio Molina. Rental $50.

Summary: Documentary about an organization

in Minnesota called Wilderness Inquiry II, which takes integrated groups of able-bodied and disabled people into the wilderness for rugged adventures in canoes. Participants are very enthusiastic about the program.

Assessment of Adult Hemiplegia.
Videorecording. University of Maryland, School of Medicine, Department of Physical Therapy, Video Services, Baltimore, Md., 1984. Videocassette (47 min), sd, col, ¾". Credits: Susan Ryerson.
Summary: Assesses an adult patient who has had a stroke. Four different positions for components of function and movement are shown. Also depicted is an evaluation of the patient's visual, sensory, and hearing ability.

Going to the Edge Working With Cancer Patients
Videorecording. University of Michigan, Medical Center Media Library, Ann Arbor, Michigan, The University, 1984. One videocassette (33 min), sd, col, ¾", plus one booklet. Credits: Claudia W. Kraus.
Summary: Physicians, social workers, and a nurse clinician discuss their personal responses to the emotional issues involved in working with cancer patients, and the patient/professional relationship, its satisfactions, and its power to sustain them in their work.

The Family Caring
Videocassette. 29 min, 1984, Crosspoint Communications, 105 Market St., Pittsburgh, PA 15222. Rental $55; purchase $225-$450.
Summary: Describes methods of caregivers in three families who are coping with a family member with a prolonged illness: Alzheimer's disease, multiple sclerosis, and cerebral palsy, respectively.

Intermittent Catheterization: Self-Care
Slide-tape module, 60 slides, 1 audiocassette, 12 min, Rehabilitation Institute of Chicago, 1984. Purchase $115.
Summary: Entertaining animation and clear presentation of difficult subject. Basic parts and functions of urinary system; advantages and steps of an intermittent catheterization program; significance of low residual urines; and problems resulting from overdistention and delayed bladder emptying.

Say Goodbye to Back Pain
Videorecording. ½", 96 min. Narrated by Alexander Melleby. West World Productions, Inc., 1985.
Summary: Provides a progressive, 6-week series of 16 easy exercises to eliminate or reduce back pain. Based on work of Hans Kraus.

Functional Assessment of the Elderly
Video. 28 min, study guide. Contents: Part 1, Cognitive and special senses; Part 2, Activities of daily living. Hospital Satellite Network, 1986. Rental: Part 1 $60, Part 2 $60. Purchase: Part 1 $275; Part 2 $275; Parts 1 and 2 $450.
Summary: Prepares nurses to evaluate the functional abilities of elderly clients. Describes physical skills and normal age-related changes. Common problems, developments that warrant referral, and possible nursing interventions are described. Can be used for undergraduate and graduate nursing programs and for hospital, nursing home, and home care nursing staffs.

Complications of Spinal Cord Impairment
Video. 28 min, study guide. Hospital Satellite Network, 1987. Rental $60, purchase $275.
Summary: Stresses importance of suspecting spinal cord injury in every accident victim. Illustrates techniques for immobilizing a patient's spine and provides information on how to distinguish between spinal and hypovolemic shock. Shows common injuries that may cause partial or complete spinal cord impairment and shows how these injuries affect systems of the body. Correlates level of injury and potential level of function in persons with spinal cord injury.

Nursing Management of Dermal Ulcers
Video. 28 min, study guide. Hospital Satellite Network, 1987. Rental $60, purchase $275.
Summary: Clear illustration of preventive measures for dermal ulcers. Skin risk factors, causes, steps in prevention, treatment methods, and various stages of dermal ulcers described.

Welcome to My World
Videorecording. 38 min. By Ann Shuel and Betsy Farkas. Available from Educational Communication Center, State University of New York at Buffalo, 1987.

Summary: Describes the situation of people coping with a disability or chronic illness and discusses how others can be more sensitive to their needs.

Multiple Sclerosis: Update and Management
Video. 28 min, study guide. Hospital Satellite Network, 1986. Rental $60, purchase $275.
Summary: Covers various types of multiple sclerosis: benign, relapsing/remitting, remitting/progressive, and progressive. Explores the diagnostic process and its difficulties while emphasizing the neurological examination, patient history, symptoms, drug treatments for specific symptoms, and nursing interventions.

The following tapes are available for rental or purchase from the National Head Injury Foundation, Inc., PO Box 567, Framingham, MA 01701. Rental $35 per tape plus $35 per tape refundable deposit for a 5-week period starting from the day of shipment. Videocassettes, purchase, $70 each.

A Fate Better than Death
18 min. Produced in Boston. Features four head-injured young adults. This emotionally charged film includes an interview with the co-founders of the National Head Injury Foundation. Focuses on support groups and the comments of families as they cope with the devastating effects of head injury. Available as ½″ VHS.

Head Trauma—The Silent Epidemic
8 min. Produced by the Bryn Mawr Rehabilitation Hospital of Pennsylvania. Introduces the lay person to current rehabilitation techniques and team approaches to head injury management. Would be helpful to insurance claims people, state agencies, vocational rehabilitation therapists, special education teachers, and mental health personnel. Available as ½″ VHS.

Coma
15 min. A five-part series done for Boston television station WNEV. Explores the issues and myths surrounding coma. Ms. Young interviews staff members inside the Greenery Nursing Home in Brighton, Mass., and films them in the rehabilitation setting. Included is a poignant and emotional meeting of a parents' support group. This tape is an excellent vehicle for introducing the complexities of coma and its effects on the family to both family members and health care professionals. Available as ½″ VHS.

APPENDIX D

Equipment Resources

Alimed Inc.
297 High St.
Dedham, MA 02026
(800)225-2610
(617)329-1560
1, 3, 4, 5, 6, 7

All Orthopedic Appliances
P.O. Box 488
Greenwood, SC 29648
(800)327-3288
(803)233-2564
1, 2, 4, 5, 7, 17

American Automobile Association
8111 Gatehouse Rd.
Falls Church, VA 22047
(703)222-6000
(Supplies free list of hand control manufacturers
The Handicapped Driver's Mobility Guide)

Key
1, ADL and homemaking aids
2, Ambulation and standing aids
3, Bathroom aids
4, Beds
5, Chairs, wheelchairs, and mobility and positioning devices
6, Clothing and dressing aids
7, Cushions, mattresses, and pressure pads
8, Diabetes supplies
9, Peritoneal dialysis supplies
10, Drug delivery, feeding systems, and nutritional supplies
11, ECG and heart rate monitors
12, Urinary and incontinence supplies
13, Heating pads, and heat and cold therapy
14, Lifts and lifting aids
15, Ostomy, skin, and wound care supplies
16, Respirator, suction, and inhalation supplies, including apnea monitors
17, Traction equipment
18, Communication aids
Source for key: Am J Nurs 84:350, 1984.
A comprehensive directory of products can be found in The Association of Rehabilitation Nurses *Membership Directory and Product Guide 1984-1985*.

American Stair-Glide Corp.
4001 E. 138th St.
Grandview, MO 64030
(816)763-3100
3, 5, 14, 16

Bruce Medical Supply
411 Waverly Oaks Rd.
P.O. Box 9166
Waltham, MA 92254
(800)225-8446
(800)342-8955 (in Mass.)
(617)894-6262
1, 2, 3, 5, 6, 8, 12, 15, 18

Cleo, Inc.
3957 Mayfield Rd.
Cleveland, OH 44121
(800)321-0595
(216)382-9700
1, 2, 4, 7

Dixie U.S.A., Inc.
P.O. Box 55549
Houston, TX 77255
(800)231-6230
(713)688-4993
1, 4, 5, 7, 8, 11, 12, 13, 15, 16

Everest & Jennings
3233 Mission Oaks Blvd.
Camarillo, CA 93010
(800)235-4661
(805)987-6911
1, 2, 3, 4, 5, 6, 14

Extensions for Independence
635-5 Twin Oaks Valley Rd.
San Marcos, CA 92069
(619)744-4083
(For Sit 'n Ski and other adapted ski equipment)

FashionAble for Better Living, Inc.
5 Crescent Ave.
Rocky Hill, NJ 08553
(609)921-2563
1, 2, 3, 4, 5, 6, 7, 12, 13, 14

Gaymar Industries, Inc.
Route 20 A, 10 Centre Dr.
Orchard Park, NY 14127
(716)662-2551
4, 7, 13

Graham-Field, Inc.
415 2nd Ave.
New Hyde Park, NY 11040
(800)645-8176
(516)328-0500
1, 2, 3, 4, 5, 6, 7, 10, 11, 12, 13, 15, 16, 17

Handicapped Driving Aids of Michigan, Inc.
4020 2nd Way
Wayne, MI 48184
(313)595-4400
3, 4, 5, 6, 14

Invacare Corp.
899 Cleveland St.
Elyria, OH 44036
(800)321-5715
(216)329-6000
2, 3, 4, 5, 6, 14, 16, 17

LIC Care Inc.
102 Kalmus Dr.
Costa Mesa, CA 92626
(800)854-6900
(714)957-1071
1, 2, 4, 17

Medline Industries, Inc.
1200 Town Line Rd.
Mundelein, IL 60060
(800)323-3743
(312)949-5500
1, 2, 3, 4, 5, 6, 13, 14, 16

J.T. Posey Company
5635 Peck
Arcada, CA 91006
(818)443-3143
1, 4, 5, 6, 12

St. Louis Ostomy & Medical Supply
10821 Manchester Rd.
St. Louis, MO 63122
(314)821-7355
1, 2, 3, 4, 5, 7, 8, 10, 11, 13, 14, 15, 16, 17

Sammons, Inc. (Fred)
P.O. Box 32
Brookfield, IL 60513
(800)323-5547
(312)325-1700
1, 2, 3, 4, 5, 6, 7, 12, 13, 18

Sherwood Medical Co.
Hospital Products Division
33 Benedict Pl.
Greenwich, CT 06830
(203)661-2000
10, 12, 15, 16

Suburban Ostomy Supply Co.
1 Watson Pl.
Framingham, MA 01701
(800)225-4792
(617)877-8140
1, 2, 3, 4, 5, 7, 8, 9B, 10, 12, 13, 15, 17

Truform Orthotics & Prosthetics
3960 Rosslyn Dr.
Cincinnati, OH 45209
(513)271-4594
2, 3, 4, 5, 7, 13, 17

Ventura Research & Rehabilitation for
Handicapped, Inc.
35 Lawton Ave.
Danville, IN 46122
(317)745-2989
2, 3, 4, 5, 6, 7

APPENDIX E

Organizations for the Disabled

Alexander Graham Bell Association for the Deaf
3417 Volta Pl. NW
Washington, DC 20007
(202)337-5220

American Association of Diabetes Educators
500 N. Michigan Ave., Suite 1400
Chicago, IL 60611
(312)661-1700

American Association of Retired Persons
1909 K St. NW
Washington, DC 20049
(202)872-4700

American Cancer Society
90 Park Ave.
New York, NY 10016
(212)599-3600

American Civil Liberties Union
132 W. 43rd St.
New York, NY 10036
(212)944-9800

American Council of the Blind
1010 Vermont Ave. NW, Suite 1100
Washington, DC 20005
(202)393-3666

American Deafness and Rehabilitation
Association
Box 55369
Little Rock, AR 55369
(501)663-4617

American Diabetes Association
505 8th Ave.
New York, NY 10018
(212)947-9707

American Foundation for the Blind, Inc.
15 W. 16th St.
New York, NY 10011
(212)620-2000

American Heart Association
7320 Greenville Ave.
Dallas, TX 75231
(214)373-6300

American Lung Association
1740 Broadway
New York, NY 10019
(212)315-8700

American Parkinson Disease Association
116 John St., Suite 417
New York, NY 10038
(212)732-9550

American Speech, Language, Hearing
Association
10801 Rockville Pike
Rockville, MD 20852
(301)897-5700

Amyotrophic Lateral Sclerosis Association
15300 Ventura Blvd., Suite 315
Sherman Oaks, CA 91403
(818)990-2151

Architectural and Transportation Barriers
Compliance Board
330 C St. SW, Room 1010
Washington, DC 20202
(202)245-1591

Arthritis Foundation
1314 Spring St. NW
Atlanta, GA 30309
(404)873-3389

AT&T Communications
Reston, VA
(800)222-4474
Responds to customers who use telecommunications devices for the deaf. A National Special Needs Center has also been formed to answer questions concerning the special equipment.
(800)833-3232 (TDD)
(800)233-1222 (voice only)

Better Hearing Institute
Box 1840
Washington, DC 20013
(703)642-0580

Clearinghouse on the Handicapped
Department of Education
330 C St. SW
Washington, DC 20202
(202)732-1723

Disability Rights Center
1616 P St. NW, Suite 435
Washington, DC 20036
(202)328-5198

Epilepsy Foundation of America
4351 Garden City Dr., Suite 406
Landover, MD 20785
(301)459-3700

Guide Dog Users, Inc.
12 Riverside St., Apt 1-2
Watertown, MA 02172
(617)926-9198

Guide Dogs for the Blind
P.O. Box 1200
San Rafael, CA 94915
(415)479-4000

Guiding Eyes for the Blind
Yorktown Heights, NY 10598
(914)245-4024

Help for Incontinent People
P.O. Box 544
Union, SC 29379
(803)585-8789

Independent Living for the Handicapped
Department of Housing and Urban Development
HUD Building
Washington, DC 20410
(202)755-5720

Information Center for Individuals with Disabilities
20 Park Plaza, Room 330
Boston, MA 02116
(617)727-5540

International Association for Enterostomal Therapy, Inc.
2081 Business Circle Dr., Suite 290
Irvine, CA 92715

Leukemia Society of America, Inc.
733 3rd Ave.
New York, NY 10017
(212)573-8484

The Library of Congress
Division of the Blind and Physically Handicapped
1291 Taylor St. NW
Washington, DC 20542
(202)287-5100

Mainstream, Inc.
1030 15th St. NW, Suite 1010
Washington, DC 20005
(202)898-1400

Mended Hearts, Inc.
7320 Greenville Ave.
Dallas, TX 75231
(214)706-1442

Muscular Dystrophy Association, Inc.
810 7th Ave.
New York, NY 10019
(212)586-0808

Myasthenia Gravis Foundation, Inc.
53 W. Jackson Blvd., Suite 909
Chicago, IL 60604
(312)427-6252

National Amputation Foundation
12-45 150th St.
Whitestone, NY 11357
(718)767-0596

National Association for Home Care
519 C St. NE
Washington, DC 20002
(202)547-7424

National Association for the Visually Handicapped
22 W. 21st St.
New York, NY 10010
(212)889-3141

National Committee on Treatment of Intractable Pain
P.O. Box 9553
Friendship Station
Washington, DC 20016-1553
(202)944-8140

National Congress of Organizations of the Physically Handicapped
16630 Beverly
Tinley Park, IL 60477

National Council on Aging
600 Maryland Ave. SW
West Wing 100
Washington, DC 20024
(202)479-1200

National Easter Seal Society
2023 W. Ogden Ave.
Chicago, IL 60612
(312)243-8400 (voice)
(312)243-8880 (TTY)

National Eye Institute
Information Officer
Building 31, Room 6A32
Bethesda, MD 20205

National Foundation for Ileitis and Colitis
444 Park Ave. S
New York, NY 10016
(212)685-3440

National Foundation March of Dimes
1275 Mamaroneck Ave.
White Plains, NY 10605
(914)428-7100

National Head Injury Foundation
333 Turnpike Rd.
Southborough, MA 01772
(617)485-9950

National Institute on Aging
National Institutes of Health
Building 31, Room 5C35
Bethesda, MD 20105
(301)496-1752

National Jewish Center for Immunology and Respiratory Medicine
1400 Jackson St.
Denver, CO 80206
(303)388-4461

National Multiple Sclerosis Society
205 E. 42nd St.
New York, NY 10017
(212)986-3240

National Rehabilitation Information Center
4407 8th St. NE
Catholic University of America
Washington, DC 20017
(202)635-5826
(202)635-5884 (TDD)

National Society to Prevent Blindness
500 E. Remington Rd.
Schaumburg, IL 60173
(312)843-2020

National Spinal Cord Injury Association
600 W. Cummings Pk., Suite 2000
Woburn, MA 01801
(617)935-2722

National Spinal Cord Injury Hotline
Patients with spinal cord injury (SCI) and their families can learn what programs and facilities are available to them in their own communities. The hotline has toll-free lines active 24 hours a day to offer information, referral, peer support, and hope for those who have SCI-related problems.
(800)526-3456
(800)638-1733 (in Md.)

Occupational Safety and Health Administration (OSHA)
Office of Public and Consumer Affairs
US Department of Labor, Room N3637
200 Constitution Ave. NW
Washington, DC 20210
(202)523-8148

Paralyzed Veterans of America
801 18th St. NW
Washington, DC 20006
(202)872-1300

Parkinson's Disease Foundation
William Black Medical Research Building
Columbia University Medical Center
640-650 W. 168th St.
New York, NY 10032
(212)923-4700

President's Committee on Employment of the
Handicapped
111 20th St. NW, Room 636
Washington, DC 20036
(202)653-5044

Recording for the Blind, Inc.
20 Roszel Rd.
Princeton, NJ 08540
(609)452-0606

Rehabilitation International
22 E. 21st St.
New York, NY 10010
(212)420-1500

Rehabilitation Services Administration
Office of Special Education and Rehabilitative
Services
Department of Education
330 C St. SW, Room 3431
Washington, DC 20202
(202)723-1282

SATH
26 Court St.
Brooklyn, NY 11242
(212)858-5483

Self-Help for Hard of Hearing People
7800 Wisconsin Ave.
Bethesda, MD 20814
(301)657-2248
(301)657-2249 (TTY)

Self Help Center
1600 Dodge Ave.
Evanston, IL 60201
(312)328-0470

Sex Information and Education Council
of the U.S.
32 Washington Pl.
New York, NY 10003
(212)673-3850

Society for the Rehabilitation of the Facially
Disfigured
550 First Ave.
New York, NY 10016
(212)340-5400

Stroke Club International
805 12th St.
Galveston, TX 77550
(409)762-1022

Telecommunications for the Deaf
814 Thayer Ave.
Silver Spring, MD 20785
(301)589-3006

United Cerebral Palsy Association, Inc.
66 E. 34th St.
New York, NY 10016
(212)481-6300

United Ostomy Association, Inc.
2001 W. Beverly Blvd.
Los Angeles, CA 90057
(213)413-5510

Publications for the Disabled

About Stroke
(Sister Kenny Institute Staff, 1978)
Sister Kenny Institute
Abbott Northwestern Hospital, Inc.
800 E. 28th St. at Chicago Ave.
Minneapolis, MN 55407
$7.50

Accent On Living
Cheever Publishing
P.O. Box 700
Gillum Road and High Dr.
Bloomington, IL 61701
Quarterly, $6.00/yr

Access: The Guide to a Better Life for Disabled Americans
(Bruck L, 1978)
Random House
201 E. 50th St.
New York, NY 10022
$5.95

Adaptations and Techniques for the Disabled Homemaker
(Strebel MB, 1978)
Sister Kenny Institute
Abbott Northwestern Hospital, Inc.
800 E. 28th St. at Chicago Ave.
Minneapolis, MN 55407
$8.75

Adult Aphasia Program
(Bullock K and McLoughlin J)
Word Making Productions
70 W. Louise Ave.
Salt Lake City, UT 84115
$13 plus $1.50 handling
Covers 14 language-deficiency areas (e.g., auditory recognition, comprehension, naming, functional writing), with step-by-step lessons in each.

An Adult Has Aphasia
Interstate Printers and Publishers Inc.
Danville, IL 61832
Written to help families better understand the nature of the aphasic's problems and to make suggestions for assisting in his or her progress.

Be Good to Your Back
(Burton C, Nida G, 1980)
Sister Kenny Institute
Abbott Northwestern Hospital, Inc.
800 E. 28th St. at Chicago Ave.
Minneapolis, MN 55407
$6.00

Clothing for the Handicapped: Fashion Adaptations for Adults and Children
(Strebel MB, 1978)
Sister Kenny Institute
Abbott Northwestern Hospital, Inc.
800 E. 28th St. at Chicago Ave.
Minneapolis, MN 55407
$6.00

Prices, when listed, are subject to change related to increases in printing costs, advertising, and marketing. Purchasers are advised to contact the publishing company or agency for current price listings.

Coping with Chronic Pain: A Patient's Guide to Wellness
   (Florence D, Hegedus F, Reedstrom D, 1982)
   Sister Kenny Institute
   Abbott Northwestern Hospital, Inc.
   800 E. 28th St. at Chicago Ave.
   Minneapolis, MN 55407
   $5.25

Disability and Rehabilitation Handbook
   (Goldenson RM, editor in chief, 1978)
   McGraw-Hill, Inc.
   1221 Avenue of the Americas
   New York, NY 10020

Disabled USA
   President's Committee on Employment of the Handicapped
   Washington, DC 20210
   (202)653-5044
   Quarterly, single issue $4.50, four issues $9.50

Getting There: A Guide to Accessibility for Your Facility
   (Lifchez R et al.)
   College of Environment Design
   University of California
   Berkeley, CA

Home Health Care Resources
   Sears Special Catalog
   Sears, Roebuck and Co.
   Sears Tower
   Chicago, IL 60684
   Free

Home Safety Round-Up
   National Easter Seal Society
   2023 W. Ogden Ave.
   Chicago, IL 60612
   6 pages, 100 copies $4.00
   (send stamped self-addressed envelope with request)

ILRU Sourcebook: A Technical Assistance Manual on Independent Living
   (Frieden L, Richards L, Cole J, Bailey D, 1979)
   The Institute of Rehabilitation and Research
   1333 Moursund
   Houston, TX 77030
   $19.95

International Rehabilitation Review
   Rehabilitation International
   25 E. 21st St.
   New York, NY 10010
   (212)420-1500
   Irregular, $20.00/yr

Living with Chronic Neurologic Disease: A Handbook for Patient and Family
   (Cooper IS, 1976)
   W.W. Norton & Co., Inc.
   500 Fifth Ave.
   New York, NY 10110

Low Back Care Manual: A Patient Guide
   (Beehler K, Gullickson S, Loeper J, Loux E, 1983)
   Sister Kenny Institute
   Abbott Northwestern Hospital, Inc.
   800 E. 28th St. at Chicago Ave.
   Minneapolis, MN 55407
   $4.50

Mainstream
   Magazine of the Able-Disabled
   2973 Beech St.
   San Diego, CA 92102
   10 issues, $14.97/yr

Ostomy Quarterly
   United Ostomy Association, Inc.
   2001 W. Beverly Blvd.
   Los Angeles, CA 90057

Paraplegia News
   Paralyzed Veterans of America, Inc.
   5201 N. 19th Ave., Suite 1L
   Phoenix, AZ 85015
   (602)246-9426
   Monthly, $12.00/yr

Rehabilitation Gazette
   4502 Maryland Ave.
   St. Louis, MO 63108
   Biennial, individuals $15.00, institutions $20.00

Rehabilitation World
   Rehabilitation International USA
   1123 Broadway
   New York, NY 10018
   (212)741-5160
   Quarterly, $25.00

Sex and the Male Ostomate
United Ostomy Association, Inc.
2001 W. Beverly Blvd.
Los Angeles, CA 90057

Sex, Courtship, and the Single Ostomate
United Ostomy Association, Inc.
2001 W. Beverly Blvd.
Los Angeles, CA 90057

Sex, Pregnancy, and the Female Ostomate
United Ostomy Association, Inc.
2001 W. Beverly Blvd.
Los Angeles, CA 90057

Sexuality and the Spinal Cord Injured Woman
(Bregman S, 1975)
Sister Kenny Institute
Abbott Northwestern Hospital, Inc.
800 E. 28th St. at Chicago Ave.
Minneapolis, MN 55407
$6.00

The Sourcebook for the Disabled. An Illustrated Guide to Easier, More Independent Living for Physically Disabled People, Their Families and Friends
(Hale G, ed, 1979)
Paddington Press Ltd.
Grosset & Dunlap (distributor)
51 Madison Ave.
New York, NY 10010

Speech and Language Rehabilitation: Workbook for the Neurologically Impaired
(Keith R)
Interstate Printers and Publishers Inc.
Danville, IL 61832
$5.95
Designed for the client who is not able to receive continuous therapy by a speech pathologist. Meant to improve family and client involvement.

Sports 'N Spokes
PVA, Inc.
5201 N. 19th Ave., Suite 111
Phoenix, AZ 85015
(602)246-9426
Bimonthly, $5.50/yr

Table Manners: A Guide to the Pelvic Examination for Disabled Women and Health Care Providers
Sex Education for Disabled People
477 15th St.
Oakland, CA 94612

Toward Intimacy: Family Planning and Sexuality Concerns of Physically Disabled Women, ed 2
(Task Force on the Concerns of Physically Disabled Women, 1978)
Human Sciences Press
72 Fifth Ave.
New York, NY 10011

What You Should Know About On-the-Job Hearing Conservation, 1983 ed
Channing L. Bete Co., Inc.
South Deerfield, MA 03173
A scriptographic booklet.

When You Meet a Person in a Wheelchair
(Ellefson MA, Ellefson D, 1983)
Sister Kenny Institute
Abbott Northwestern Hospital, Inc.
800 E. 28th St. at Chicago Ave.
Minneapolis, MN 55407
$0.35

Workbook for Aphasia
Wayne State University Press
5959 Woodword Ave.
Detroit, MI 48202
$9.95 plus $1.00 handling
Contains exercises for the redevelopment of higher-level language functioning.

APPENDIX G

Organizations for Rehabilitation Nurses

American Association of Neuroscience Nurses
218 N. Jefferson St.
Chicago, IL 60606
(312)993-0043

American Burn Association
c/o Shriners Burn Institute
202 Goodman St.
Cincinnati, OH 45219

American Congress of Rehabilitation Medicine
130 S. Michigan Ave., Suite 1310
Chicago, IL 60603
(312)922-9368

American Medical Association
535 N. Dearborn St.
Chicago, IL 60610
(312)645-5000

American Nephrology Nurses' Association (ANNA)
Box 56, N. Woodbury Rd.
Pitman, NJ 08071
(609)589-2187

American Nurses' Association
2420 Pershing Rd.
Kansas City, MO 64108
(816)474-5720

American Society of Ophthalmic Registered Nurses (ASORN)
P.O. Box 3030
San Francisco, CA 94119
(415)561-8513

Association of Rehabilitation Nurses
2506 Gross Point Rd.
Evanston, IL 60201
(312)475-7300

Commission on Accreditation of Rehabilitation Facilities (CARF)
101 N. Wilmot Rd., Suite 500
Tucson, AZ 85711
(602)748-1212

Joint Commission of Accreditation of Health Care Organizations
875 N. Michigan Ave.
Chicago, IL 60611
(312)642-6061

National Association of Orthopaedic Nurses
Box 56, N. Woodbury Rd.
Pitman, NJ 08071
(609)582-0111

National League for Nursing
Ten Columbus Circle
New York, NY 10019-1350
(212)582-1022

Otorhinolaryngology and Head/Neck Nurses
c/o Warren Otologic Group
3893 E. Market St.
Warren, OH 44484
(216)856-4000

National Institute of Neurological and Communicative Disorders and Stroke
9000 Rockville Pike
Bethesda, MD 20892
(301)496-9746

APPENDIX H

Information Sources for Rehabilitation Nurses

JOURNALS

Journals of particular interest to rehabilitation nurses are listed in alphabetical order. Addresses for subscription requests are given, as are frequency of publication and subscription rates for individuals for 1 year within the United States (rates for institutions and individuals in other countries are higher). Subscriptions are often included in membership dues to professional organizations. Subscription rates may increase each year related to increases in printing costs, advertising, and marketing. Purchasers are advised to write to the publishers for current prices.

Advances in Nursing Science
Aspen Systems Corporation
16792 Oakmont Ave.
Gaithersburg, MD 20877
Quarterly, $46.50

American Journal of Nursing
(official journal of the American Nurses' Association)
American Journal of Nursing Co.
555 W. 57th St.
New York, NY 10019-2961
Monthly, $24.00

American Journal of Occupational Therapy
(official journal of the American Occupational Therapy Association)
1383 Piccard Dr., P.O. Box 1725
Rockville, MD 20850-4357
Monthly, $25.00

Archives of Physical Medicine and Rehabilitation
American Congress of Rehabilitation Medicine and The American Academy of Physical Medicine and Rehabilitation
78 East Adams St.
Chicago, IL 60603
Monthly, $50.00 (reduced rates for students)

Computers in Nursing
J. B. Lippincott Co.
Downsville Pike
Route 3, Box 20-B
Hagerstown, MD 21740
Bimonthly, $30.00

Geriatric Nursing
American Journal of Nursing Co.
555 W. 57th St.
New York, NY 10019
Bimonthly, $20.00

International Journal of Rehabilitation Research
HVA-Edition Schindele
Hugo-Stotz-Str.
D-6900 Heidelberg 1
Federal Republic of Germany
Quarterly, $28.00

Journal of Gerontological Nursing
Slack, Inc.
6900 Grove Rd.
Thorofare, NJ 08086
Monthly, $28.00

Journal of Neuroscience Nursing
(official journal of the American Association of
Neuroscience Nurses)
American Association of Neuroscience Nurses
National Office
218 N. Jefferson St.
Chicago, IL 60606
Bimonthly, $30.00

Journal of Nursing Administration
J. B. Lippincott Co.
Downsville Pike
Route 3, Box 20-B
Hagerstown, MD 21740
11 issues/yr, $37.00

Journal of Rehabilitation
(official journal of National Rehabilitation Association)
633 S. Washington St.
Alexandria, VA 22314
Quarterly, $35.00

*Journal of Rehabilitation Research and Devel-
opment*
Superintendent of Documents
US Government Printing Office (GPO)
Washington, DC 20402
Stock Number 051-000-00175-3
Quarterly

Nursing Administration Quarterly
Aspen Publishers, Inc.
7201 McKinney Circle
Frederick, MD 21701
Quarterly, $59.59

Nursing Economics
Anthony J. Jannette, Inc.
North Woodsbury Rd., Box 56
Pitman, NJ 08071
Bimonthly, $28.00

Nursing and Health Care
10 Columbus Circle
New York, NY 10019-1350
Monthly except July and August, $20.00

Nursing Outlook
American Journal of Nursing Co.
555 W. 57th St.
New York, NY 10019-2961
Bimonthly, $25.00

Nursing Research
American Journal of Nursing Co.
555 W. 57th St.
New York. NY 10019-2961
Bimonthly, $23.00

The Occupational Therapy Journal of Research
The American Occupational Therapy Foun-
dation, Inc.
1383 Piccard Dr.
Rockville, MD 20850
Bimonthly, member $35.00, nonmember
$45.00

Orthopaedic Nursing
(official journal of the National Association of
Orthopaedic Nurses)
North Woodbury Rd., Box 56
Pitman, NJ 08071
Bimonthly, $21.00

Physical and Occupational Therapy in Geriatrics
The Haworth Press, Inc.
75 Griswald St.
Binghamton, NY 13904
Quarterly, $32.00/vol

Physical Therapy
(official journal of the American Physical Therapy Association)
American Physical Therapy Association
1111 N. Fairfax St.
Alexandria, VA 22314
Monthly, member $11.00, nonmember $50.00

Rehabilitation Nursing
(official journal of the Association of Rehabilitation Nurses)
2506 Gross Point Rd.
Evanston, IL 60201
Bimonthly, $30.00

Rehabilitation Psychology
  (official journal of Division 22 of the American
  Psychological Association)
  Springer Publishing Co.
  536 Broadway
  New York, NY 10012
  Quarterly, $28.00

Topics in Acute Care and Trauma Rehabilitation
  Aspen Publishers, Inc.
  16792 Oakmont Ave.
  Gaithersburg, MD 20877
  Quarterly, $48.00

Topics in Geriatric Rehabilitation
  Aspen Publishers, Inc.
  16792 Oakmont Ave.
  Gaithersburg, MD 20877
  Quarterly, $44.00

OTHER SELECTED SOURCES OF INFORMATION FOR REHABILITATION NURSES

The Clearinghouse on the Handicapped
Department of Education
330 C St. SW
Washington, DC 20202
(202)723-1723
  Serves as an information center on federal
  funding, legislation, and programs and on
  sources of information for professionals in the
  handicapped field and consumers.

Sister Kenny Institute
Abbott Northwestern Hospital, Inc.
800 E. 28th St. at Chicago Ave.
Minneapolis, MN 55407
(612)863-4457

Materials Development Center (MDC)
Stout Vocational Rehabilitation Institute
School of Educational Rehabilitation Institute
School of Education and Human Services
University of Wisconsin-Stout
Menomonie, WI 54751
(715)232-1342
  National Center for the collection, develop-
  ment and dissemination of materials in the
  areas of vocational work evaluation, work ad-
  justments, and sheltered workshop manage-
  ment.

National Clearinghouse of Rehabilitation
Training Materials (NCHRTM)
Jean Hudder
Oklahoma State University
115 Old USDA Building
Stillwater, OK 74074
(405)624-7650
  Distributes publications and audiovisuals use-
  ful in the development of rehabilitation profes-
  sionals.

National League for Nursing
Resource and Studies Service
10 Columbus Circle
New York, NY 10019
  Programmed instruction and rehabilitation as-
  pects of nursing.

National Rehabilitation Information Center
(NARIC)
4407 Eighth St. NE
The Catholic University of America
Washington, DC 20017
(800)34-NARIC
(202)635-5826
(202)635-5884 (TDD)
(202)635-6090 (ABLEDATA)
  Offers two databases:
  REHABDATA contains more than 9,000 rehabil-
    itation research reports and other docu-
    ments in the field.
  ABLEDATA is a file of more than 8,000 citations
    on commercially available aids and devices
    for disabled persons.

Index

Page numbers in *italics* indicate illustrations; page numbers
followed by *t* indicate tables.

Neurogenic bladder
autonomous, 154-156, *156*
classification of, 154
complications associated with, 160-165
intermittent catheterization of client with, 177-178
reflex, 154, *155*
research on, with rehabilitation nursing implications, 553t
uninhibited, 156-158, *157*
voiding maneuvers for client with, 176-177
Neurogenic bowel, 204-205
autonomous, 205-206
nursing intervention for, 221
etiology, incontinence pattern, and bowel program, 222t
reflex, 205
nursing intervention for, 220
uninhibited, 205
nursing intervention for, 218, 220
Neurological conduction disorders, respiratory muscle fatigue and, 88
Neuromuscular disease, dysarthrias and, 292
Neurons, motor; *see* Motor neurons
Nightmares, 231
Nipride; *see* Nitroprusside
Nitrogen balance, negative, immobility and, 373
Nitroprusside (Nipride), 160
Nits, infestations of, 268
treatment of, 273-274
Nociceptors, 315
Nocturia with uninhibited neurogenic bladder, 157
Nocturnal myoclonus, 231
Noise, hearing damage from, 355
North American Nursing Diagnosis Association (NANDA), diagnostic categories of, 53-54
Nurse, rehabilitation; *see* Rehabilitation nurse
Nurse-client relationship
ethical dimensions of, 576-578
King's nursing theory and, 25
Nursing, rehabilitation; *see* Rehabilitation nursing
Nursing Activities Index, 519, *520*
Nursing care; *see also* Health care
classification of, 496-497
cost of, by patient category, *523*
determining cost of, 517
direct and indirect, 518
rehabilitation; *see* Rehabilitation nursing
Nursing diagnoses
for altered body temperature, 129-130
for communication deficits, 324-325
for coping, 473-474

Nursing diagnoses—cont'd
definitions and uses of, 53
for eating and swallowing difficulties, 143-144
for environmental access, 449
for grooming deficits, 272
for hearing impairment, 354
for hygiene deficit, 272
for impaired bladder function, 173-174
for impaired breathing, 100-101
for impaired skin integrity, 249
for impaired vision, 343
for impaired work or recreational ability, 434-435
for mobility deficit, 371-372
NANDA-approved, 54
purposes of, 498
for sexuality, 416-417
Nursing education, 587-588
Nursing intervention
defined, 55
Orem's nursing theory and, 24-25
Nursing process, 45-62
components of, 46-56
documentation of, 56-61
goal-setting component of, 498-499
Nursing research; *see* Research
Nursing standards, 508
Nursing theory, 16-17
Nutrition
alteration in, nursing diagnosis of, 100-101
brain and, 138
and changes in nails, 268
maintenance of, with respiratory impairment, 112
pressure sores and, 246, 252
Nutritional deficiency, respiratory muscle fatigue and, 88
Nutritional status
assessment of, 47
with impaired sense of taste, 325
Nutritionist, role of
on rehabilitation team, 37
with respiratory impairment, 113
Nystagmus, optokinetic, hygiene and, 270

O

Objectives, 67, 68
Occupational therapist, role of
with communication deficit, 305-306
with grieving client, 480
with hygiene and grooming deficits, 283
with perception or sensation impairment, 329
on rehabilitation team, 36
with respiratory impairment, 113

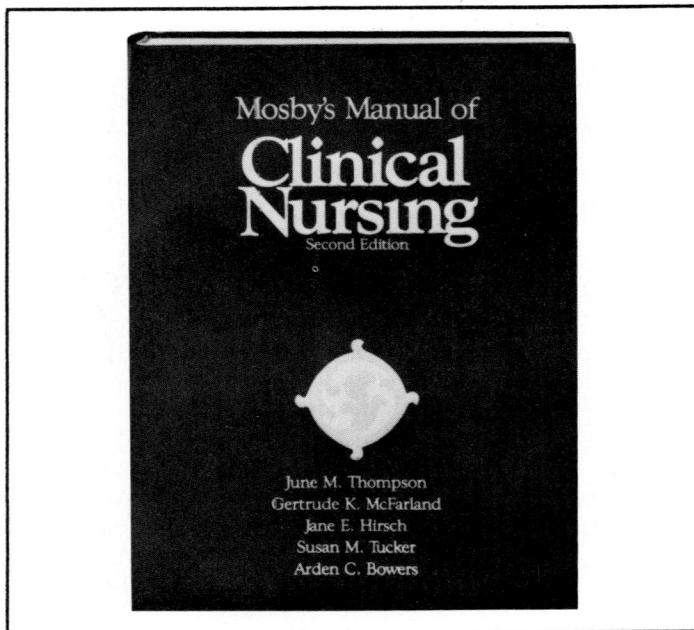